ompany, LLC

m

Joseph Morita
r Premedia Services Private Ltd

-4054 8
-0-8261-4089-0

4-4028

2 1

l the publisher of this Work have made every effort to use sources believed to be reliable to pro-
on that is accurate and compatible with the standards generally accepted at the time of publica-
medical science is continually advancing, our knowledge base continues to expand. Therefore, as
ion becomes available, changes in procedures become necessary. We recommend that the reader
t current research and specific institutional policies before performing any clinical procedure. The
ublisher shall not be liable for any special, consequential, or exemplary damages resulting, in whole
om the readers' use of, or reliance on, the information contained in this book. The publisher has
bility for the persistence or accuracy of URLs for external or third-party Internet websites referred
ublication and does not guarantee that any content on such websites is, or will remain, accurate or

iscounts on bulk quantities of our books are available to corporations, professional associations, phar-
al companies, health care organizations, and other qualifying groups. If you are interested in a custom
cluding chapters from more than one of our titles, we can provide that service as well.

ails, please contact:
Sales Department, Springer Publishing Company, LLC
st 42nd Street, 15th Floor, New York, NY 10036-8002
: 877-687-7476 or 212-431-4370; Fax: 212-941-7842
l: sales@springerpub.com

d in the United States of America by Gasch Printing.

ANNUAL REVIEW OF NURSING RESEARCH

VOLUME 34, 2016

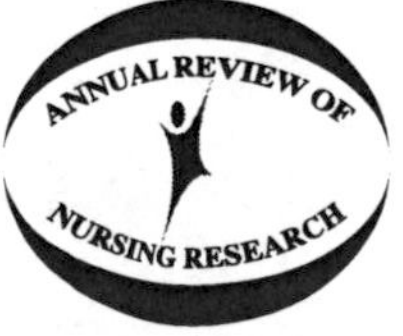

SERIES EDITOR

Christine E. Kasper, PhD, RN, FAAN, FACSM
Department of Veterans Affairs
Office of Nursing Services, Washington, DC
and
Professor, Daniel K. Inouye School of Nursing
Uniformed Services University of the Health Sciences,
Bethesda, MD

VOLUME EDITORS

Susanne W. Gibbons, PhD, C-ANP, C-GNP
Asssistant Professor, Daniel K. Inouye Graduate School of Nursing
Uniformed Services University of the Health Sciences

Michaela R. Shafer, PhD, RN, CLNC
US Air Force (retired)

Ann
Nur

Nursing Ethics:
Changin

VOL

Series E

CHRISTINE E. KASPER, P

Volume Edi

SUSANNE W. GIBBONS, Ph
MICHAELA R. SHAFER, P

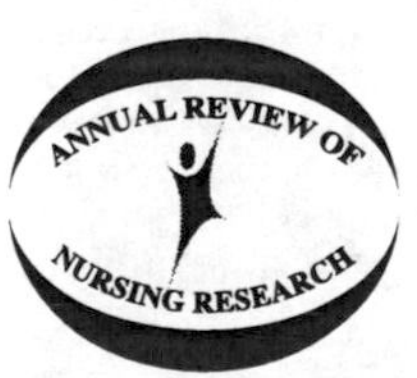

SPRINGER PUBLISHING COMPAN
NEW YORK

Contents

Systems of Care

Research

About the Volume Editors

Susanne W. Gibbons, PhD, C-ANP, C-GNP, is an assistant professor in the Daniel K. Inouye Graduate School of Nursing at the Uniformed Services University of the Health Sciences (USUHS) who teaches across Doctor of Nursing Practice and Doctor of Philosophy programs. Dr. Gibbons has a Bachelor of Science from the Johns Hopkins University School of Nursing, a Master of Science from the University of Maryland, School of Nursing, and she received her PhD in Nursing Science from the Catholic University of America. Although her primary position is with the University, she also maintains a part-time primary care practice in the community. Dr. Gibbons has been recognized for her teaching and contributions to USUHS with multiple teaching awards and a University Medal for Outstanding Service. She is a member of several professional organizations that include the American Nurses Association, Sigma Theta Tau International, and the Southern Research Association where she serves in a variety of capacities. She is an accomplished author and has made significant contributions to the literature related to self-neglect in older adults, and military health-care provider stress and coping during deployment. Her current research involves the social experience of cancer family caregiving dyads. Dr. Gibbons' career has focused on vulnerable groups and their nursing needs.

Colonel Michaela R. Shafer, PhD, RN, CLNC, recently retired after serving over 30 years in the U.S. Air Force. She has a baccalaureate degree in nursing from the University of North Carolina, a master's in critical care nursing, and a PhD in biomedical research and nursing, both from the University of Texas. She has been a critical care and flight nurse for 40 years and has served in a variety of leadership positions that include commander of a Level I trauma center, director of nursing, chief of hyperbaric nursing for the Department of Defense, and, most recently, assistant professor at the Uniformed Services University of the Health Sciences in Bethesda, Maryland. Her most recent focus has been on leadership and ethics in the military and studying the care and outcomes of trauma in war. She has several funded studies and recent publications primarily articulating the moral grief experienced by health-care providers caring for those in harm's way. She continues to consult on Veterans' issues for several universities including the

University of South Florida, University of Texas, Baylor, and Rice. She is a member of the board of directors for the Center for Medicine after the Holocaust and participated on the research subcommittee developing the new American Nurses Association *Code of Ethics for Nurses with Interpretive Statements*. Her ethics consulting service advises local hospitals and central institutional review boards on ethical issues related to human subjects' research.

Contributors

Janice Agazio, LTC (Ret) USA, PhD, CRNP, FAANP, FAAN
Assistant Dean for Doctoral Programs
School of Nursing
The Catholic University of America
Washington, DC

Suzanne Bakken, PhD, RN, FAAN, FACMI
Alumni Professor of Nursing and Professor of Biomedical Informatics
School of Nursing
Department of Biomedical Informatics, and Irving Institute for Clinical & Translational Research
Columbia University
New York, NY

Patrick Barrett, PhD
Chair
School of Social Sciences
University of Waikato
Hamilton, New Zealand

Mary Butler, NZROT, PhD
School of Occupational Therapy
Otago Polytechnic
Dunedin, New Zealand

Jane Chung, PhD, RN
College of Nursing
University of New Mexico
Albuquerque, NM

Rita D'Aoust, PhD, MS, BSN
Associate Dean for Academic Affairs, Director of Interprofessional Initiatives
College of Nursing
University of South Florida
Tampa, FL

Mary Rose Day, DN, MSSA, BSc, RPHN, Dip. Mang. (RCSI), RM, RGN
College Lecturer
Catherine McAuley
School of Nursing & Midwifery
Brookfield Health Science Complex
College of Medicine & Health
University College Cork
Ireland

George Demiris, PhD, FACMI
Department of Biobehavioral Nursing and Health Systems
School of Nursing
University of Washington
Seattle, WA

Petra Goodman, COL (Ret) USA, PhD, WHNP-BC
Assistant Dean for Research and Faculty Development
School of Nursing
The Catholic University of America
Washington, DC

Susanne W. Gibbons, PhD, C-ANP/GNP
Assistant Professor
Daniel K. Inouye Graduate School of Nursing
Uniformed Services University of the Health Sciences
Bethesda, MD

Pamela J. Grace, RN, PhD, FAAN
Associate Professor of Nursing and Ethics
William F. Connell School of Nursing
Boston College
Chestnut Hill, MA

Beatrice Hale, PhD
Independent Researcher
Dunedin, New Zealand

Elizabeth (Betsy) S. Hopkins, BS, MLS
Nursing and Communication Disorders Librarian
Brigham Young University, Provo, UT

Edmund (Randy) Howe, MD, JD
Professor of Psychiatry, Associate Professor of Medicine
Director, Programs in Ethics
Senior Scientist, Center for the Study of Traumatic Stress
Uniformed Services University of the Health Sciences
Bethesda, MD

McKenna Hughes
Research Assistant
Brigham Young University
Provo, UT

E. Ann Jeschke, PhD, MTS
Graduate Research Assistant
Gnaegi Center for Health Care Ethics
St. Louis University
St. Louis, MO

Patricia Leahy-Warren, PhD, MSc (Research), BSc, Hdip PHN, Dip. Mang., RPHN, RM, RGN
Senior Lecturer
Catherine McAuley
School of Nursing & Midwifery
Brookfield Health Science Complex
University College Cork
Ireland

Ann Maradiegue, PhD, FNP-BC, FAANP
Nurse Practitioner Consultant
James Madison University
Falls Church, VA

Geraldine McCarthy, PhD, MSN, Med, Dip. Nursing, RNT, RGN
Emeritus Professor
University College Cork
Ireland

Patricia McMullen, PhD, JD, RN, CNS, WHNP-BC, FAANP
Dean
School of Nursing
The Catholic University of America
Washington, DC

Marìa Elisa Moreno-Fergusson, DNS, BSN
Titular Professor
Faculty of Nursing and Rehabilitation
Universidad de La Sabana, Colombia

Oluwakemi Opanubi, MSN, RN
PhD Student
School of Nursing
The Catholic University of America
Washington, DC

Nancy Reame, PhD, RN, FAAN
Mary Dickey Lindsay Professor of Disease Prevention and Health Promotion in the Faculty of Nursing
School of Nursing and Irving Institute for Clinical & Translational Research
Columbia University
New York, NY

Alicia Gill Rossiter, DNP, MS, BSN
Military Liaison, Instructor, Sequence Director, Veteran to BSN Program
College of Nursing
University of South Florida
Tampa, FL

Michaela R. Shafer, PhD, RN
Colonel, USAF (Ret)

Jamie L. Shirley, PhD, RN
Lecturer
Nursing and Health Studies
University of Washington, Bothell Campus
Seattle, WA

Hilaire J. Thompson, ACNP-BC, CNRN, FAAN
Department of Biobehavioral Nursing and Health Systems
School of Nursing
University of Washington
Seattle, WA

Laura Bentley Webster, MA, RN
Ethics Consultant
UWMC & HMC and Staff ICU/ED RN
University of Washington Medical Center (UWMC) and Harborview Medical Center (HMC)
Seattle, WA

Karen J. Whitt, PhD, FNP-BC, AGN-BC
Assistant Professor
College of Nursing
Brigham Young University
Provo, UT
Professorial Lecturer
School of Nursing
The George Washington University
Washington, DC

Foreword

> Most people, under most circumstances, generally will do what is right, if they know what is right, and if the temptation to err is not too great.
>
> —Luther Christman (1976; cited in Pittman [2005])

Ethics is a branch of Western philosophic thought dealing with moral behavior of individuals or specific conduct. Socrates, regarded as the father of ethics, taught, "There is only one good, knowledge, and one evil, ignorance." In other words, people will do what is correct if they know what is right. Wrong action is the result of ignorance. Traditionally, there are three branches of ethical study. The first derives from the work of Aristotle (384–322 BCE) and states that virtues provide individuals guidance on how to act so that both the person and society benefit. The second branch of ethics was defined by Kant (1724–1804 CE), which sees the concept of duty as central to morality. For example, humans have a duty as rational beings to respect other rational beings. Finally, the utilitarian school of thought asserts that conduct should be the cause of the greatest number of people. In essence, ethics studies, catalogs, and recommends concepts of right and wrong conduct in response to questions of behavior such as "What do I do . . .?"

As with changes in the social order over millennia, behaviors and beliefs once ethical in the time of ancient Greece have morphed into new common understandings, at least in modern Western societies. Universal values are regarded as the essential equality of men and women, human or natural rights, importance of education, the centrality of justice in human endeavors, and the fundamental oneness of humanity.

To be able to engage in right action and thought, one must be acutely aware of self, that is, how we think and what has contributed to our personal beliefs, assuming a lack of psychiatrically defined personality disorder, which makes discernment of truth somewhat challenging. Thus the famous admonition "Know thyself" on the wall at the entrance to the temple of the Oracle of Delphi in ancient Greece. Being intimately aware how and why we behave the way that we do is fundamental to being able to ethically operate in the world as an individual and as a health-care professional. More importantly, culture, religious beliefs, family values, extent of educational achievement, and political beliefs color and influence the way that we operationalize our ethics in the world. To ignore that these factors operate in other health-care professionals as well as our patients and their families is narcissistic at best and potentially harmful to our mission as nurses to alleviate suffering. The world is not created in our own image. Perhaps, that is why Socrates famously stated, "the unexamined life is not worth living" (Plato, 1989).

Luckily, as nurses we have the *Code of Ethics for Nurses with Interpretive Statements* (American Nurses Association [ANA], 2015). Historically, Florence Nightingale taught that a nurse's ethical duty was first to the care of the patient. This principle underpins all forms of ethical discussion and research in the profession of nursing. The ANA adopted the first formal code of ethics in 1950 and the International Council of Nurses established their code of ethics in 1953. As health-care delivery and systems have exponentially increased in complexity since that time, updates to the Code have periodically been made, with the newest this year.

The ANA states that the Code serves the purposes of: (a) it is a succinct statement of the ethical values, obligations, duties, and professional ideals of nurses individually and collectively; (b) it is the profession's non-negotiable ethical standard; and (c) it is an expression of nursing's own understanding of its commitment to society (ANA, 2015). Nursing research has been active and abundantly productive in examining and forwarding the field of modern ethics in nursing, which is the topic of the present volume. Each chapter presents a new and intriguing review of a unique aspect of research in nursing ethics. We are grateful to the volume editors Drs. Gibbons and Shafer for their work in compiling the various subject matter experts, and indebted to those authors for the time and effort required to synthesize their individual chapters.

Christine E. Kasper, PhD, RN, FAAN, FACSM
Series Editor

REFERENCES

American Nurses Association. (2015). *Code of ethics for nurses with interpretive statements*. Washington, DC: Author.

Pittman, E. (2005). *Luther Christman: A maverick nurse, a nursing legend*. Victoria, BC, Canada: Trafford.

Plato. (1989). *Symposium* (A. Nehamas & P. Woodruff, Trans.). Indianapolis, IN: Hackett Publishing Company.

ANNUAL REVIEW OF NURSING RESEARCH

VOLUME 34, 2016

CHAPTER 1

Nursing Ethics

A Lifelong Commitment

Susanne W. Gibbons and E. Ann Jeschke

ABSTRACT

Over the past 30 years, the health-care context as well as the roles and responsibilities of nurses have drastically changed. Leaders in nursing around the world recognize that the health-care system is stressed and the well-being of the nursing workforce plagued by the pressures and challenges it faces in everyday practice. We do not intend to make a strong normative argument for why nursing ethics education should be done in a certain way, but instead show from where we have come and to where we can go, so that educators are positioned to address some of the current shortcomings in ethics education. Our goal is to provide an illustration of ethics education as an interwoven, ongoing, and essential aspect of nursing education and professional development. By developing professional identity as character, we hope that professional nurses are given the skills to stand in the face of adversity and to act in a way that upholds the core competencies of nursing. Ultimately, health-care organizations will thrive because of the support they provide nurses and other health-care professionals.

http://dx.doi.org/10.1891/0739-6686.34.1

INTRODUCTION

The evolution of ethics teaching in nursing education has gone from a period of little or no curricular emphasis to a resurgent effort aimed at producing a competent professional nurse. Although the professional nurse aims at achieving an overarching social good by fostering health and wellness, nursing has traditionally achieved this broader goal by forging bonds of loyalty with the particular patient being served (Allmark, 1995; Woods, 2005). Over the past 30 years, the health-care context as well as the roles and responsibilities of nurses have drastically changed. In many health-care settings, nurses have little patient contact since medical technicians and nursing aides perform many of the duties previously assigned to nurses. Examples of such health-care tasks include checking blood pressures, giving bed baths, and setting up meals. These responsibilities allowed the nurse to remain in constant contact with the patient. Now, hospital nurses spend a lot of their time administering medications and documenting patient clinical status as opposed to ministering to the patient's bedside needs. Advanced practice nurses who provide services like primary care, anesthesia care, and psychiatric counseling still maintain a high level of contact with their patient. For example, in the United States, many nurse practitioners perform simple office procedures, like suturing, and have the authority to write prescriptions to treat a variety of acute and chronic health conditions. This medicalization of nursing and the other changes described are slowly eroding the nurse's traditional caring role as patient advocate who metaphorically (and in many cases literally) holds the patient's hand by providing support and reassurance.

As hospital nurses take on more administrative and procedural functions while advance practice nurses take on more roles and responsibilities of the physicians, the professional nurse is challenged to balance competing demands while keeping the central focus on the patient. These are only a few examples of the types of changes in health care that have resulted in uncertainties for educators when deliberating what to teach and how to teach it, when it comes to health-care ethics. Nurses realize they are not alone and that all health professionals must work together to safeguard professional values and create environments where ethical practice is possible. The former concern is the focus of this chapter namely, how to create professional nurses who are able to negotiate, adapt, and provide excellent care to patients within the complexities of a dynamic and evolving health-care setting.

By "professional nurses," we mean those who are constantly striving to develop character through the ongoing practice and refinement of requisite skills attendant to the profession of nursing. By skills, we mean clinical skills as well as ethical decision-making skills that provide the structure for a nurse to faithfully deliver patient care to the best of his or her ability. This occurs within the particular context in which the nurse operates, while utilizing available resources. The previous two definitions operate on the assumption that the provision of excellent patient care requires the professional nurse to balance many competing interests both inside a highly integrated health-care team and outside from various sectors of the broader health-care industry. Finally, these definitions allow us to subsume nursing policy and regulations under a more ancient Aristotelian account of ethics wherein excellence of character is typified by a disposition to act in the right way within a specific context. This disposition is not solely formed by sharpening analytic skills in order to deliberate which course of action is the most ethical. These skills are an aspect of developing an ethical disposition, but they fundamentally rely on the development and constant refinement of particular habits within the practice of nursing. These habits become the foundation of a fine-tuned ethical sensitivity that gives rise to a propensity to act in a certain way and allows the professional nurse to navigate and negotiate competing demands without losing the center of balance, which should always be focused on patient care.

This chapter is primarily descriptive and exploratory in nature. We do not intend to make a strong normative argument for why nursing ethics education should be done in a certain way, but instead show from where we have come and to where we could go so that educators can address some of the current shortcomings in ethics education. Our goal is to provide an illustration of ethics education as an interwoven, ongoing, and essential aspect of nursing education and professional development. To achieve our goals, we start by describing the current health-care context in which professional nurses operate as well as trends in nursing ethics education. Within this section, we identify elements of nursing ethics education that are meant to assist with ethical decision making and describe some of the ways in which this current model is insufficient in helping nurses remain focused on the patient. Thereafter, we discuss the importance of forming a nurse's character by developing a broad set of competencies that become the foundation of a professional nurse's identity. Shifting to a focus on character formation allows us to identify a broad set of skills without making a hard-and-fast distinction between practical skills and ethical decision making. Ultimately, we wish to promote character formation by integrating theory and practice in an effort to establish classroom ethics education as the first step in a lifelong, dynamic process that extends beyond formal education far into the nurse's professional career.

THE CURRENT SITUATION

Leaders in nursing around the world recognize that the health-care system is stressed and the well-being of the nursing workforce plagued by the pressures and challenges it faces in everyday practice. Professional nurses are compelled to provide excellent patient-centered care while being harried by an economically driven health-care system that values productivity and outcomes often defined in monetary terms (Sellman, 2011). One of the competing demands that can easily decenter the nurse is resource restriction imposed by insurance companies. Clearly, insurance companies authorize the payment of equipment, medicine, and treatment methods. In many instances, the nurse is not able to provide the patient with the most appropriate care due to restrictions for payment. Another challenge is the ever-increasing pace at which services are expected to be rendered to the patient. It is not the quality of time spent with each patient that counts in terms of productive output but the number of tasks that can be performed in a shorter period of time. These time restrictions devalue reflection and critical thinking, both essential aspects of professional nursing care that allow the nurse to bond with the patient. Within the context of a high-technology health-care system, the nurse's focus can inadvertently be shifted from the well-being of patients to the proper functioning of machines or computers. Finally, the nurse, as a member of a highly integrated, interdisciplinary health-care team, constantly faces being pulled away from the patient's needs when attempting to integrate the expectations of team members, authority figures, as well as family members. Even the patient's expectations can come into conflict with the nurse's ability to achieve such expectations due to limited resources or a clash in what is perceived to be the most beneficial mode of providing care.

National and international concerns about the quality of care provided by professional nurses have led to ensuring ethical standards are upheld by outlining core competencies for nurses. The guidelines of the World Health Organization (WHO) and the International Council of Nurses (ICN) for professional behavior are intended to help nurses—as well as other health-care providers—navigate everyday choices by providing them with a list of actions and skills that must be performed in order to uphold the standards of excellent nursing care. They also detail the rights of a professional nurse (International Council of Nurses, 2012; World Health Organization, 2015). While such professional codes specify what actions a professional nurse is ethically required to achieve or forbidden to do, they provide only a skeleton of ethical competency. Checklists of rules of conduct, responsibilities for the profession, and rights of the nurse provide a start for ethical professional nursing practice. However, they do not thoroughly explore how the professional nurse should develop the core competencies that will enable him or her to remain centered on the patient in environments defined by constantly competing demands. Furthermore, these rules and regulations do not explore how the professional nurse becomes recentered on the patient's care once the nurse's professional balance is lost.

Graduating student nurses and practicing nurses report an inability to resolve ethical dilemmas faced in their practice, and, as a result, frequently endure moral distress which can, and often does, lead to burnout and attrition (Pauly, Varcoe, Storch, & Newton, 2009; Ulrich, Hamric, & Grady, 2010; Whitehead, Hebertson, Hamric, Epstein, & Fisher, 2015). Moral distress occurs when an individual's moral integrity is seriously compromised either because he or she feels unable to act in accordance with core values and obligations or because the attempted actions fail to achieve the desired result (Jameton, 1984). Besides an increase in moral distress among professional nurses, in recent years, there has been a decline in public trust toward the health professions in general (Crigger & Godfrey, 2014). In terms of nurses, this professional distrust may exist because nurses often look toward managers and other leaders within the organizational structure for guidance. They also tend to adhere to the majority view of their staff, often putting their own opinions aside and changing decisions based on input from other providers—issues that potentially interfere with providing competent care and with fostering an ethical work environment. Many believe that the professional nurse's tendency to be a rule follower may, in fact, be a breakdown in ethics when considering the broader health-care context in which patient care must be performed.

In the United States, the landmark 2010 *Future of Nursing Report: Leading Change, Advancing Health* by the Institute on Medicine was a disappointment to many nurse leaders because the report failed to address the everyday ethical issues confronted by nurses who work in diverse roles and settings as well as the challenge of a prevalent conformist attitude in nursing (Hylton-Rushton & Broome, 2015). The American Nurses Association (ANA) responded with a summit meeting composed of 50 nurse leaders who met to address nursing ethics for the 21st century. They developed a blueprint identifying initial steps in an effort to lay the groundwork upon which to begin developing a more robust understanding of the ways in which nurses can be created to not only balance competing demands but also revitalize and foster health-care settings that support ethical nursing practice (American Nurse Today, 2015). Their premise is that professional nurses need to be supported in a more comprehensive way in order for them to develop their core professional competencies that will enable them to do the right thing for the right reasons. Both can be combated with a more robust and comprehensive ethics curriculum.

As nursing educators and practitioners, we agree with the ANA's assessment and realize that creating a competent professional nurse requires a lot more than simply acquainting students and nurses with rules, regulations, and policies. It seems that more needs to be done in order to integrate ethics into all levels of the nursing curriculum from the moment a nursing student enters into the classroom until he or she decides to exit the profession. Simply providing information about what a professional nurse should or should not do does not assist in translating the rule into the nurse's ethical behavior while going about the business of day-to-day patient care in a context that challenges his or her ability to achieve excellence. While the formation of clinical skills is masterfully performed in nursing schools nationwide, incorporating ethics into the standard curriculum in such a way that students can translate their ethics knowledge into the practice setting still seems to stymie nurse educators (Hamric, 2001). Nursing competency occurs through not only the acquisition of clinical skills, but ethical ones as well. A professional nurse's ability to assess and diagnose a patient's problem is no less important than the ability to advocate for proper resources for a patient who has a terminal diagnosis. Next, we turn to the importance of character development as professional identity as a broader foundation for understanding ethical action within the practice of nursing.

DEVELOPING PROFESSIONAL CHARACTER

It has been said that professional nursing is an intrinsically moral practice because it is concerned with care of the most vulnerable and sometimes marginalized persons in our society (Gastmans, Schotsmans, & Dierckx de Casterle, 1998). Put differently, every aspect of professional nursing dwells in the realm of ethics. As such, professional competencies cannot easily be divided into ethical and clinical skills, since nursing is, in fact, always bound up in an "ethical way of being" as the professional nurse provides patients with the most excellent care possible. Those who enter nursing school and graduate to become professional nurses as well as nurse educators bring their own set of values that guide and inform their practice of nursing and achievement of core competencies. Upon entering nursing school, a professional identity develops, as a student's values are shaped by a theoretical and practical understanding of the profession, which is constantly aimed at learning how to care for the patient's well-being. As such, ethical development goes hand in hand with identity formation as students begin to see how their own personal values resonate with what they are learning in the classroom.

Initially, students are socialized into the nursing profession by teaching them to strive to follow the rules, standards, and codes of discipline that define and orient the nursing profession around the goal of achieving excellent patient care. However, as the educational process continues, students start to emulate those teachers and clinicians who express values that are consistent with their own understanding of excellent patient care as well as those concepts and skills they have learned in their coursework. One of the most important aspects of developing a professional identity is the emulation of teachers and clinicians who are able to display both theoretical and practical knowledge how to embody, in their action, values consistent with the profession of nursing (Benner, Sutphen, Leonard, & Day, 2010). The expression of excellent care occurs when the professional nurse is able to transfer expert knowledge and skills to the care of the patient (Vanlaere & Gastmans, 2007). In other words, in addition to rules and regulations, student nurses need role models who can help guide them to develop nursing character through theoretical learning and clinical enculturation in both the classroom and clinical setting.

Eventually, upon entering the field of nursing, professional nurses are able to demonstrate their character by competently tending to the patient's healthcare needs with courage, humility, integrity, and compassion (Crigger & Godfrey, 2011; Lachman, 2007; McCammon & Brody, 2012; Vanlaere & Gastmans, 2007). Thus, we see the professional nurse's character development as a compass guided by ethics education. This compass makes nurses more able to embody their professional core competencies in the everyday practice of professional nursing. Having briefly discussed how we see character formation and ethical action as intimately intertwined with professional identity and the achievement of excellent patient care, respectively, we turn next to what ethics education might look like.

ESSENTIAL ELEMENTS FOR ETHICS EDUCATION

Throughout the first half of this chapter, we have been referring to professional nursing's core competencies that should enable a nurse to more adroitly provide excellent care for the patient. Our goal is not to identify a new, different, or broader set of competencies than already exists in the various professional codes of ethics. It is simply to suggest how nurse educators could provide a more comprehensive mode of ethics education. As has already been noted, it is important that student nurses follow rules and regulations. Therefore, ethics education must start in the classroom where students will learn the various roles and responsibilities they are expected to assume. In addition, all nursing students benefit from exposure to ethical theories and principles as tools for ethical analysis.

The general consensus is that ethics education is best addressed first through specific courses on ethics as opposed to lectures integrated throughout into the curriculum. This is supported by research suggesting that students who have been provided specific ethics courses experience an increase in moral sensitivity and moral reasoning (Grady et al., 2008; Park, Kjervcik, Crandell, & Oermann, 2012; Woods, 2005). However, in order to truly achieve ethics in practice as a disposition of character, which enables the professional nurse to act in dynamic real-time scenarios, ethics should be taught throughout the curriculum, woven into theoretical as well as clinical coursework. Ethics education should be integrated, whenever it is possible, to reinforce theories, to enable the process of having to analyze situations in confusing and complicated settings, and to assist nurses with balancing competing demands. Content can be tailored to particular academic learning needs and clinical experiences within the setting in which the student nurse is operating (Kalb & O'Connor-Von, 2007).

Nursing ethics education is not about presenting definitive choices, or right answers, but more about being ready to confront whatever situation presents before the professional nurse in an optimal way, while choosing among multiple options in circumstances that range from simple to complex. Nurses also need to know when to refer to a wider, more representative group of decision makers like an ethics committee or other consulting group. Through the ability to think about problems critically, and by providing role models in clinical practice settings, nursing ethics education will better prepare professional nurses to manage stressful situations as well as boost their confidence and their ability to achieve excellence. Achieving professional competence is therefore more than understanding ethical theories. It is a process of ongoing development that includes gaining the requisite information concerning professional identity as well as core competencies; learning about ethical theories; and training in clinical settings that promote constant reflection, analysis, and reasoning of how ethics is integrated into all aspects of patient care. In such a way, ethical reflection and behavior will come to permeate all of the student nurse's skills that have been cultivated throughout the education, and the professional nurse will be able to apply these into the practice setting (Cannaerts, Gastmans, & Dierckx de Casterle, 2014).

The Importance of Good Teachers

One aim of ethics education is to break open the student's and practitioner's worldview so that they can attempt to see the value in other ways of approaching ethical situations that may not have previously been considered. In the beginning, this approach can cause student uncertainty and vulnerability because students are asked to question their own values. For this situation to result in ethically sensitive professional nurses, nurse educators must support their students during this difficult "insecure" stage. Therefore, ethics teachers should strive to create a positive learning atmosphere that not only allows for free exchange of ideas but also increases student comfort and acceptance (Cannaerts et al., 2014). Teachers are the ones who create the pedagogical context for learning by providing a caring attitude and cultivating the competencies associated with the profession. Educators who are knowledgeable as well as supportive are more likely to stimulate, challenge, and encourage students, allowing them to flourish in a safe and comfortable learning environment (Hsu, 2011; Kyle, 2008; Numminen, van der Arend, & Leino-Kilpi, 2009).

As previously discussed, ethics role models, both formal and informal, as well as experiential encounters in clinical learning settings broaden a student's perspective on ethics by illustrating how ethics is infused in all the activities. Ethics educators include the classroom teacher as well as other mentors in clinical settings, where these teachers are seasoned clinicians who not only impart knowledge, but also establish initial impressions as competent professional nurses with a fine-tuned ethical sensitivity to the way they provide patient care (Cannaerts et al., 2014; Woods, 2005). Students' ability to think and act with ethical sensitivity will be more likely to increase with the guidance of strong role models, professional practice, and professional maturity. Their development in a positive direction is enhanced by ongoing reinforcement of ethics frameworks by revisiting foundational philosophy, theory, and professional codes to analyze problems as well as by constant refinement of their understanding as they gain more experience. Monteverde (2014) proposes that practice-based learning should enable students to consider ethical theories as tools that help them "name" and "frame" practice issues. Similarly, their daily life should be a playground on which students can test out how these theories work in the real world. We hope that such an orientation to nursing ethics education will develop more mature nurses whose behavior becomes habitual as they strive to perfect their professional character.

Moral Reasoning and Group Interactions

Although there are many options for ethics content delivery, students prefer real-life experience case studies that are contextually relevant to their practice, and they prefer group discussions to traditional lectures (Kyle, 2008; Nasrabadi et al., 2009; Numminen et al., 2009). It is up to the ethics teacher to bridge the theory practice gap so that nursing ethics education is grounded in day-to-day clinical practice; however, peers and other instructors can also be instrumental in this regard. To develop ethical competence, students need to question their own values and convictions as they reflect on their practice and other professional behaviors. A variety of learning strategies are useful for exposure, illustration, and practice with ethical concepts (Kalb & O'Connor-Von, 2007). Group discussion forums allow students to exchange ideas in relation to a real-life problem, give them the opportunity to express a variety of positions, and, depending on the composition of the group, offer them the opportunity for intradisciplinary (e.g., a variety of nursing specialties with different levels of education and experience) and possibly interdisciplinary (e.g., medicine, social work, psychology) interaction that exposes them to the views of other health professions (Cannaerts et al., 2014).

Problem-based learning may be a structured, student-driven form of group learning that features a problem that is real, encourages thinking in terms of the problem, and requires knowledge acquisition from other sources as needed for problem-solving (Lin, Lu, Chung, & Yang, 2010; Monteverde, 2014). Innovative adjunct approaches to ethics education such as diaries or journals (Durgahee, 1997), simulated scenarios (Vanlaere & Gastmans, 2007), and blended learning that integrates traditional classroom teaching with web-based learning or similar electronic modalities (Cho & Shin, 2014; Hsu, 2011; Hsu & Hsieh, 2011) enhance learning while offering students options for reflection and expression that can be private with the added benefit of being anonymous. However, developing moral sensitivity and learning how to reason morally is best achieved through emphasis on actual experiences, making connections to the real world, and by addressing issues that meet the needs of the student audience (McLeod-Sordjan, 2014; Park et al., 2012).

The more exposure students and nurses have, the more likely they develop the ability to recognize moral conflicts when they exist, assess the situation, use strategies for considering alternative solutions, and check their decisions (Grace, 2014; Pinch & Haddad, 2008). However, as practicing nurses know, in the real world, this is often an interdependent, as opposed to an independent, activity. Interactions with others to analyze and address ethical issues should begin early in the nursing education and continue throughout the professional career. Especially since moral distress and ethical climate are correlated, guiding nurses and other health-care providers to work together as a team has many advantages (Corley, Minick, Elswick, & Jacobs, 2005; Pauly et al., 2009).

Interprofessional Opportunities for Growth

Health-care professionals and students who adopt a worldview of their profession often see the world through that professional eye without the ability to frame the problem from the perspective of the other professions. Therefore, providing interprofessional experiences from which student nurses can develop an understanding of how other professions approach common situations will help the students to function more collaboratively in the current health-care context without losing sight of their goal of providing patient-centered care. Health-care providers often do not recognize the ethical elements of everyday clinical encounters they share with patients. By developing approaches to patients that address a variety of issues in an interdisciplinary group, student nurses can learn to recognize the ethical elements in everyday issues as they unfold and will be more able to address them. As participants of interprofessional discussions dissect their own style of communications with patients, individuals in the group have the opportunity to uncover their own biases, emotions, values, perceptions, and professional goals that influence what they say and how they act (Truog et al., 2015). Interdisciplinary forums for ethical discussions, therefore, increase health-care providers' self-awareness, making them better providers and better members of the health-care team.

Professional Competence: A Lifelong Quest

For nurses to become professionally competent, they need to have the ability and the opportunity to perceive, reflect, and remove obstacles that prevent them from focusing on excellent patient care. Individual education and practice in ethical decision making is a long-term individual commitment that requires practice in a safe, supportive environment. Our hope for professional nurses who have moved beyond the classroom setting is that they continue to develop their character as a way of increasing their professional competence. For professional competence to become a lifelong quest, not only the individual nurses, but also the health-care organizations for whom they work have to support professional nurses' efforts to do the right thing for their patients. At the organizational level, a supportive environment for ethical decision making, collaboration, and communication with peers and other professionals are major factors affecting the work environment (Poikkeus, Numminen, Suhonen, & Leino-Kilpi, 2014). Leadership has a key role in providing opportunities for character development and growth in the understanding of core competencies by professional nurses. Similarly, without the necessary infrastructure that empowers and supports the professional nurse's ability to act in the best interests of the patient, it becomes impossible for the professional nurse to attain the goal of professional excellence.

Suhonen et al. (2011) found considerable room for health-care managers to create positive ethical environments, accomplished by flattening out the decision-making hierarchy so that more members of the health-care team are able to voice their ethical assessment of the patient's situation (McDaneil, 1998). In many instances, such a change also facilitates a decrease in moral distress among the health-care team members and increases collaboration (Kalvemark Sporrong, Arentz, Hansson, Westerholm, & Hoglund, 2007; Tang, Johansson, Wadensten, Wenneberg, & Ahlstrom, 2007). Ethics consultation is a way to enhance clinical work while simultaneously working to ensure a high level of organizational ethics (McGee, Caplan, Spanogle, & Asch, 2001). An increase in ethical climate has not only been associated with an increase in employee morale, but has also been found to be associated with organizational commitment, fostering an engaged and retained workforce (Shirey, 2005). In summary, the combination of professional competence and fostering a positive ethical climate not only contributes to the quality of patient care but also increases the overall success of the organization.

CONCLUSION

Since the 1980s, the control of health-care systems has shifted from professionals to health-care managers known as managed care organizations. The resulting concern voiced by nursing leaders is that individual patient needs are secondary to the demands of the organization and the financial bottom line. While educators have the responsibility to lay the foundation for professional identity, ethical decision making, and interprofessional practice, it is up to practicing nurses to be advocates for patients, families, and health-care teams. Nurses continue to face challenging issues in their everyday clinical practice that will only increase with an aging and chronically ill society. None of these issues has gone unnoticed since national and international nurse ethics experts recognize the urgent need to develop strategies that more effectively address practice concerns in an effort to retain a qualified workforce (Goethals, Gastmans, & Dierckx de Casterle, 2010; Suhonen, R., Stolt, Virtanen, & Leino-Kilpi, 2011; Ulrich et al., 2010).

Ethical work environments are those that allow individual ethical values to guide behavior, which includes setting priorities for the ethical treatment of patients (McDaniel, 1998). We would like to encourage nurses to have the courage to assess the situations in which they work and act in the patient's best interest even when it is difficult to do so (Lachman, 2007). By developing professional identity as character, we believe that professional nurses will have the skills to stand in the face of adversity and act in ways that uphold the core competencies of nursing. Ultimately, health-care organizations will thrive because of the support they provide nurses and other health-care professionals. Nurses must have the fortitude to push forward—change can only occur if nurses have the integrity, courage, and character to ride the waves of change.

REFERENCES

Allmark, P. (1995). Uncertainties in the teaching of ethics to students of nursing. *Journal of Advanced Nursing, 22*, 374–378.

American Nurse Today. (2015, February). *Nursing ethics for the 21st century*. Retrieved from http://www.americannursetoday.com/nursing-ethics-21st-century/

Benner, P., Sutphen, M., Leonard, V., & Day, L. (2010). *Educating nurses: A call for radical transformation*. San Francisco, CA: Jossey-Bass.

Cannaerts, N., Gastmans, C., & Dierckx de Casterle, B. (2014). Contribution of ethics education to the ethical competence of nursing students: Educators' and students' perceptions. *Nursing Ethics, 21*(8), 861–878.

Cho, K. C., & Shin, G. (2014). Operational effectiveness of blended e-learning program for nursing research. *Nursing Ethics, 21*(4), 484–495.

Corley, M. C., Minick, P., Elswick, R. K., & Jacobs, M. (2005). Nurse moral distress and ethical work environment. *Nursing Ethics, 12*(4), 381–390.

Crigger, N., & Godfrey, N. (2011). *The making of nurse professionals: A transformational, ethical approach*. Sudbury, MA: JB Learning.

Crigger, N. & Godfrey, N. (2014). From the inside out: A new approach to teaching professional identity formation and professional ethics. *Journal of Professional Nursing, 30*(5), 376–382.

Durgahee, T. (1997). Reflective practice: Nursing ethics through story telling. *Nursing Ethics, 4*(2), 135–146.

Gastmans, C., Schotsmans, P., & Dierckx de Casterle, B. (1998). Nursing considered as moral practice: A philosophical-ethical interpretation of nursing. *Kennedy Institute on Ethics Journal, 8*(1), 43–69.

Goethals S., Gastmans C., & Dierckx de Casterle B. (2010). Nurses' ethical reasoning and behaviour: A literature review. *International Journal of Nursing Studies, 47*(5), 635–650.

Grace, P. J. (2014). *Nursing ethics and professional responsibility in advanced practice* (2nd ed.). Burlington, MA: Jones & Bartlett Learning.

Grady, C., Danis, M., Soeken, K. L., O'Donnell, P., Taylor, C., Farran, A., et al. (2008). Does ethics education influence the moral action of practicing nurses and social workers? *American Journal of Bioethics, 8*(4), 4–11.

Hamric, A. (2001). Ethics development for clinical faculty. *Nursing Outlook, 49*, 115–117.

Hsu, L. L. (2011). Blended learning in ethics education: A survey of nursing students. *Nursing Ethics, 18*(3), 418–430.

Hsu, L. L., & Hsieh, S. I. (2011). Effects of a blended learning module on self-reported learning performances in baccalaureate nursing students. *Journal of Advanced Nursing, 67*(11), 2435–2441.

Institute of Medicine. (2010). *The future of nursing: Leading change, advancing health*. Washington, DC: National Academies Press.

International Council of Nurses (ICN). (2012). *The ICN code of ethics for nurses*. Retrieved June 14, 2015 from http://www.icn.ch/images/stories/documents/about/icncode_english.pdf

Jameton, A. (1984). *Nursing practice: The ethical issues*. Englewood Cliffs, NJ: Prentice.

Kalb, K. A., & O'Connor-Von, S. (2007). Ethics education in advanced practice nursing: Respect for human dignity. *Nursing Education Perspectives, 28*(4), 196–202.

Kalvemark Sporrong, S., Arentz, B., Hansson, M. G., Westerholm, P., & Hoglund, A. T. (2007). Developing ethical competence in health care organizations. *Nursing Ethics, 14*(6), 825–837.

Kyle, G. (2008). Using anonymized reflection to teach ethics: A pilot study. *Nursing Ethics, 15*(1), 6–16.

Lachman, V. D. (2007). Moral courage: A virtue in need of development? *MedSurg Nursing Journal, 16*(2), 131–133.

Lin, C. F., Lu, M. S., Chung, C. C., & Yang, C. M. (2010). A comparison of problem-based learning and conventional teaching in nursing ethics education. *Nursing Ethics, 17*(3), 373–382.

McCammon, S. D., & Brody, H. (2012). How virtue ethics informs medical professionalism. *HEC Forum*, *24*, 257–272.

McDaniel, C. (1998). Enhancing nurses' ethical practice: Development of a clinical ethics program. *Nursing Clinics of North America*, *33*(2), 299–311.

McGee, G., Caplan, A. L., Spanolge, J. P., & Asch, D. A. (2001). A national study of ethics committees. *American Journal of Bioethics*, *1*(4), 60–64.

McLeod-Sordjan, R. (2014). Evaluating moral reasoning in nursing education. *Nursing Ethics*, *21*(4), 473–483.

Monteverde, S. (2014). Undergraduate healthcare ethics education, moral resilience, and the role of ethical theories. *Nursing Ethics*, *21*(4), 385–401.

Nasrabadi, A. N., Joolaee, S., Parsa-Yekta, Z., Bahrani, N., Noghani, F., & Vydelingum, V. (2009). A new approach for teaching nursing ethics in Iran. *Indian Journal of Medical Ethics*, *6*(2), 85–89.

Numminen, O., van der Arend, A., & Leino-Kilpi, H. (2009). Nurse educators' and nursing students' perspectives on teaching codes of ethics. *Nursing Ethics*, *16*(1), 69–82.

Park, M., Kjervcik, D., Crandell, J., & Oermann, M. H. (2012). The relationship of ethics education to moral sensitivity and moral reasoning skills of nursing students. *Nursing Ethics*, *19*(4), 568–580.

Pauly, B., Varcoe, C., Storch, J., & Newton, L. (2009). Registered nurses'perceptions of oral distress and ethical climate. *Nursing Ethics*, *16*(5), 561–573.

Pinch, W. J., & Haddad, A. M. (2008). *Nursing and health care ethics: A legacy and a vision*. Silver Spring, MD: Nursebooks.org, The publishing program of American Nurses Association.

Poikkeus, T., Numminen, O., Suhonen, R., & Leino-Kilpi, H. (2014). A mixed methods systematic review: Support for ethical competence of nurses. *Journal of Advanced Nursing*, *70*(2), 256–271.

Rushton, C. H., & Broome, M. (2015). Safeguarding the public's health: Ethical nursing. *Hastings Center Report*, *45*(1). http://dx.doi.org/10.1002/hast.410

Sellman, D. (2011). Professional values and nursing. *Medical Health Care and Philosophy*, *14*, 203–208.

Shirey, M. R. (2005). Ethical climate in nursing practice: The leader's role. *Journal of Nursing Administration: JONAS Healthcare Law, Ethics, Regulations*, 7(2), 59–67.

Suhonen, R., Stolt, M., Virtanen, H., & Leino-Kilpi, H. (2011). Organizational ethics: A literature review. *Nursing Ethics*, *18*(3), 285–303.

Tang, P. F., Johansson, C., Wadensten, B., Wenneberg, S., & Ahlstrom, G. (2007). Chinese nurses' ethical concern in a neurological ward. *Nursing Ethics*, *14*(6), 810–824.

Truog, R. D., Brown, S. D., Browning, D., Hundert, E. M., Rider, E. A., Bell, S. K., et al. (2015). Microethics: The ethics of everyday clinical practice. *Hastings Center Report*, *45*(1), 11–17.

Ulrich, C. M., Hamric, A. B., & Grady, C. (2010). Moral distress: A growing problem in the health professions? *Hastings Center Report, 40*(1), 20–22.

Ulrich, C. M., Taylor, C., Soeken, K., O'Donnell, P., Farrar, A., Danis, M., & Grady, C. (2010). Everyday ethics: Ethical issues and stress in nursing practice. *Journal of Advanced Nursing*, *66*(11), 2510–2519.

Vanlaere, L., & Gastmans, C. (2007). Ethics in nursing education: Learning to reflect on care practices. *Nursing Ethics*, *14*(6), 758–766.

Whitehead, P. B., Herbertson, R. K., Hamric, A. B., Epstein, E. G., & Fisher, J. M. (2015). Moral distress among healthcare professionals: Report of an institution-wide survey. *Journal of Nursing Scholarship*, *47*(2), 117–125.

Woods, M. (2005). Nursing ethics education: Are we really delivering the goods? *Nursing Ethics*, *12*(1), 5–18.

World Health Organization (WHO). (2015). *The WHO Global Competency Model*. Retrieved June 14, 2015 from http://www.who.int/employment/WHO_compentencies_EN.pdf

CHAPTER 2

Shattered, Suffering, and Silenced

Sharon's Story

Michaela R. Shafer

ABSTRACT

This chapter presents a case study of a 30-year-old female news reporter in Albuquerque, New Mexico, named Sharon Fullilove. The case is presented as a personal narrative by her mother, who is a critical care nurse, former chief nurse, Level I trauma unit commander, and colonel in the U.S. Air Force. The narrative is followed by excerpts from Sharon's chart that confirm a series of decisions made by both the hospital and the providers. The subsequent narrative is meant to give the reader an opportunity to reflect on the variety of clinical ethics questions that emerge when a patient enters into a contract with a physician and hospital for care. The goal is not to perform a thorough ethical analysis of the case but to let the reader experience what it is like when best practice standards, attention to patient care, and compassionate concern for family members are set aside. The case concludes with a set of broad questions that can be used for further discussion. Hopefully, this case will bring to the forefront the centrality of ethics in professional decision-making within the context of medical care.

http://dx.doi.org/10.1891/0739-6686.34.15

BACKGROUND

Despite an increased focus on patient safety and programs to prevent errors, a report published in the *Journal of Patient Safety* (James, 2013) reveals new statistics showing that between 210,000 and 440,000 patients die from preventable harm while seeking care. Hospital errors and medical mistakes are now considered the third leading cause of death after only cancer and heart disease (James, 2013). Many argue about the statistics, but Dr. Lucian Leape, a Harvard pediatrician, who is often referred to as the "father of patient safety" has expressed great confidence in the estimates put forth by James (Allen, 2013). Additionally, Dr. Mayer, vice president of quality and safety at MedStar Health, states that people may argue about the statistics but "all the estimates, even on the low side, expose a crisis" (Allen, 2013). For someone who preached patient safety throughout her career, it was devastating to see my daughter die at age 30 in a hospital that provided less-than-adequate care. The following case presents Sharon's story, which is not a pathography, "where the author's experience of her illness and her encounters with the health system supply plot, narrative drive and reflection" (Berlinger, 2005, p. 7), because Sharon is no longer able to orate her own tale. Instead, it is my own story, which I present as an account of a nurse and mother who was done harm when her daughter's life was cut short during a procedure that had a low probability of being life-threatening.

PERSONAL NARRATIVE

Since this is my personal narrative, the meanings herein are mine; however, as is always the case with narratives, I am opening myself up for various new interpretations of meaning as the reader picks up my story. It is my wish that in sharing this gut-wrenching experience, Sharon's story will provide a piece of pedagogical literature that provokes rigorous ethical discussion and debate concerning what went wrong and right in terms of the care she received as she was (or was not) escorted to her death. Losing my daughter due to medical errors has impacted not only me but my entire family in ways that I could not have comprehended during my 40 years as both a civilian and military nurse. It is important to note that my experience is colored by my practice as a critical care nurse, surgical supervisor, chief nurse and commander of a Level I trauma center; particularly, as a military officer where I have seen extraordinary acts of heroic medicine take place on a daily basis when we went about the business of saving our wounded with devastating injuries. Having sat on numerous risk-management and patient-safety committees, my extensive background in health care cements the foundation upon which I stood as I watched the events of my daughter's death unfold. As I entrusted the care of my oldest daughter, Sharon, to the cardiologists at the largest hospital in New Mexico, I was involved not only as an expert nurse, but more importantly as a mother of a beloved child. These two roles are inextricably interwoven in the story you are about to experience.

As a 30-year-old news reporter at a local station in Albuquerque, New Mexico, Sharon was somewhat of a local celebrity (Figure 2.1). Overall, she was a healthy young woman who would do nearly anything to get to the bottom of a story. While covering the local state fair, she injured her shoulder. After going to a doctor, she was told she needed a magnetic resonance image (MRI) to diagnose her injury. Unfortunately, Sharon had a pacemaker and could not have the test. Her pacemaker was placed at approximately age 25 due to an "overactive vagus nerve" as she described it. At times, she would become very dizzy and faint and during a tilt table test, we discovered she would go into third degree heart block during these times. To prevent her from completely passing out, it was decided to place a pacemaker to maintain her heart rate and blood pressure, which for the most part was extremely successful. It certainly never stopped her from attempting anything, be it dangerous or not. So to facilitate diagnosis of her shoulder injury, she asked about having an MRI-compatible pacemaker placed.

A local cardiologist in Albuquerque stated that he could do the procedure. In helping Sharon understand the risks associated with such a procedure, both she and I asked a myriad of questions. During our consultation with the physician he assured us that if there were any problems, the operating room would be on standby and they would be able to have her chest opened in five minutes as

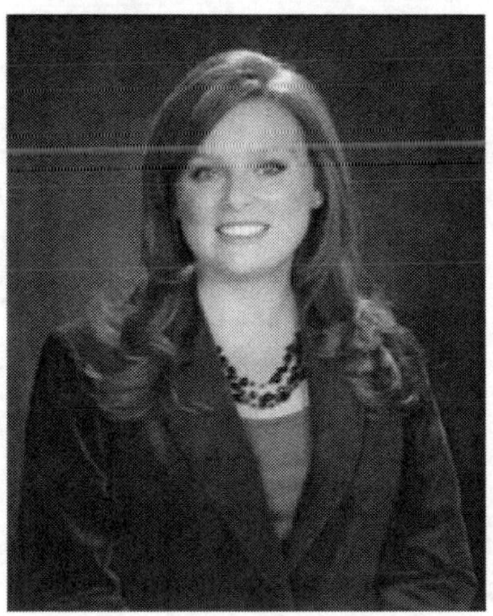

FIGURE 2.1 Sharon Fullilove.

the standards required. He described the procedure using a laser extractor with visualization via a trans-esophageal echocardiogram. Blood would be on standby as would the thoracic surgeon. He stated that this was an outpatient procedure and Sharon should expect to be home that same evening. As is normal, the physician provided us with the usual list of everything that could go wrong. As a nurse who had listed all of those complications a million times on consent forms (including death), I did not believe that with the proper procedures in place and a skilled physician doing the procedure Sharon would be at high risk for dying, especially since she was only 30 years old and otherwise healthy.

I personally had never been involved with the procedure Sharon was about to undergo, so I pulled the document, *Transvenous Lead Extraction: Heart Rhythm Society Expert Consensus on Facilities, Training, Indications, and Patient Management* published by the Heart Rhythm Society in conjunction with the Cleveland Clinic (Wilkoff et al., 2009). It was really the only document that outlined the requirements for performing the transvenous lead extraction. I was concerned about the death rate that was reported since it was 0.8%, but my daughter said, "Mom, I was in the office and I don't think anybody was under the age of 80 in there. Surely, I am not the one that will have that complication. I am young and healthy." I remember thinking to myself, "I really hope so, Honey! I really hope that is true." Like most young active adults, she was impatient to find a way to fix her shoulder which bothered her much more than her heart.

During her preoperative visit, she put me on speaker phone as she asked her questions. I followed with questions more in line with the guidance I had from the Heart Rhythm Society. In response, we were assured that Sharon's cardiologist had experience doing the procedure. It was reinforced that the operating room would be on standby if there were any complications. I asked about potential complications and the cardiologist explained about perforation and bleeding, but again assured me that they could see if there was any bleeding with the trans-esophageal echocardiogram that would be placed. If any complications occurred, Sharon would be rushed to surgery where a thoracic surgeon was on standby. After all of our questions were answered, I said for the first of two times to the cardiologist, "Please, this is an elective procedure, so do not do anything that would put her in danger. Just stop and she will have to live with the old pacemaker since it works just fine." He stated that he understood and that all possible precautions would be taken.

Sharon postponed the surgery for a couple of weeks so she could join our entire family for her uncle's wedding. We all had a wonderful time together as a family. Certainly, none of us suspected that this would be the last time many would see her alive. It is strange that my brother feels guilty for having the wedding. Somehow he feels that he delayed her surgery and maybe she wouldn't have died if he had not been married. I, on the other hand, am thankful that we all had time together before we lost her.

A few days later I traveled to Albuquerque to be with Sharon for the procedure. Before I left home, I remember being nervous and even said to a coworker "I sure hope this goes well." I look back and now realize that I had a gut feeling from the beginning that she should not do this, but passed it off as a mother worrying too much. The day before the procedure, we went to the hospital to fill out forms and were told to report to the hospital at 10 a.m. the next morning. We went to dinner and then talked late into the night before deciding we had better get some sleep.

We were awakened by the phone at 6:30 a.m. with a frantic voice asking where we were. Confused, we were told to get to the hospital immediately. Sharon quickly took a shower and we headed to the hospital. I remember feeling very uneasy as soon as we got there. It was very frenetic. There must have been eight people in the room, starting intravenous lines (IV), getting an electrocardiogram, talking to her about anesthesia, hanging antibiotics, and so forth. I distinctly remember being annoyed with the anesthesiologist as he was in such a hurry and turned up her antibiotic drip way too fast. I went over and slowed it down and told Sharon that it was not okay to turn up the antibiotic just because they were in a hurry. She just said "Mom, stop it! It will be fine." I was wondering what the big hurry was. I finally said to the nurse, "Everyone seems a little crazy. Can we please just slow down and get this all done right?" She sort of laughed and told me she would make sure that everybody took a deep breath and Sharon would be fine. All of a sudden, the team came in and off Sharon went yelling at me to take a picture of her with her famous thumbs up as she left the room. I did and it was the last conversation we ever had.

I knew the procedure might be lengthy as they removed one set of leads and placed another so I was not concerned as time passed. However, about an hour into the procedure, the cardiac catheterization lab nurse came out and said, "Could you please sign this new consent form? Unfortunately, Sharon signed the wrong one." I looked at her and told her I was not the next of kin. Her husband was in the military, and therefore not there, so I had no authority to sign the document. I asked her what form Sharon signed and the nurse explained that several things were left off the first document. I remember not being surprised since everything was so hectic when we arrived. However, I did not suspect anything was wrong. Another couple of hours passed and I saw a man dressed in scrubs run through the lobby past me and out the door. He was panicked and did not stop to talk to anyone. An hour or so later, I saw the same man run back into the facility and he stopped abruptly in front of me and said, "Where have you been?" I told him I had never moved from that waiting room, and asked why he was looking for me.

He said, "We had a lot of trouble getting the lead out but everything is okay now." He ran off before I had a chance to ask him why he had run out of the building. I breathed a sigh of relief as I knew that getting the old lead out was the most dangerous part of the procedure and I assumed that was already done based on his comments, which I later found out were not true. In fact, he had gone to another hospital to pick up a laser extractor since the team was having difficulty removing the pacemaker with the equipment on hand at the hospital.

The afternoon continued without any further communication and then I heard a chilling voice over the loud speaker saying, "Code Blue, elevator 3. Code Blue, elevator 3." As a critical care nurse, I shuddered remembering the days of transporting a coding patient in an elevator. Seldom did that scenario result in a good outcome. I immediately felt sympathy for the patient, family, and health care professionals involved. I had a momentary thought, "Oh no, please don't let it be Sharon." However, I quickly remembered the conversation with the gentleman in the scrubs implying the worst was over so I relaxed and began to casually talk on the phone while I waited. After another couple of hours, I got concerned having heard nothing since the man in scrubs frantically passed. I went to the phone in the waiting room and called the cath lab. A nurse answered and said that the doctor was going to be out in just a minute. I sat right by the door so he would not miss me.

The door opened and the cardiologist walked out with his head hanging down. I took one look at him and knew something horrible had happened. He shook his head and I began to scream, "NO, NO!!!" I am not sure if I collapsed to the floor or just stood there screaming. The next thing I remember was being whisked (even though it all seemed to happen in slow motion) from the waiting room and was put in the room where Sharon had been prepped for the procedure. The cath lab nurse and the cardiologist sat down next to me and asked if I wanted to call someone and did I want a chaplain? All I remember hearing was that "Sharon died in the cath lab during the procedure and they have taken her to the operating room where they are trying to save her." The cardiologist then said the strangest thing to me: "I prayed every minute I was in there. Honestly, I think it was just Sharon's time." I looked at him in disbelief, but could not scream the things I was thinking, "It was not her time! What happened in there that she is now dying?" I was alone. Honestly, I do not remember ever being so alone in my life. I knew I had to call her husband, my husband, and my other two kids in order to get them all to Albuquerque as soon as possible. I was shaking so violently that I could not dial any number without help. I do not remember talking to anyone—I have no idea what I said as I was in complete shock, but my other daughter can tell you the exact place and time I called and gave her the news. I spent the next several hours feeling completely alone.

The chaplain stayed with me as I tried to reach family and friends. The cardiologist came back and forth with news every half hour or so. Each time he appeared more gray and dejected. Finally, around 5:30 p.m., I was told they had repaired Sharon's heart and that she was in the ICU, but nobody knew how long she was without oxygen and no one had any idea if she would survive or not. Again, the cardiologist said, "If she has left this earth, it was just her time to go and God would welcome her home." Now I must interject here that I am a Christian and believe in God and heaven, but I was appalled that the blame for this mishap was being attributed to God! It was the one statement that I could not get past and was infuriated every time he mentioned the prospect of her being "called home." I was taken to the ICU waiting room with the chaplain, who was wonderful and did not take the same view as the cardiologist about what had happened. She was thoughtful, compassionate, and I was thankful she was there to physically and emotionally hold me up.

We waited for what seemed like an eternity. I literally felt like I could not breathe and knew that I would not be better until I saw Sharon. Finally, I was escorted to her room. You must remember that I am a long-time trauma and critical care nurse. For the most part, I knew what I was walking into that night. But the sight of my daughter (Figure 2.2), swollen three times her normal size from fluid resuscitation, head packed in ice, attached to 18 IV delivery machines, hearing the cyclic whoosh of the ventilator, the strange thumping noise of the balloon pump and the totally normal sounding rhythm of her heart on the monitor was

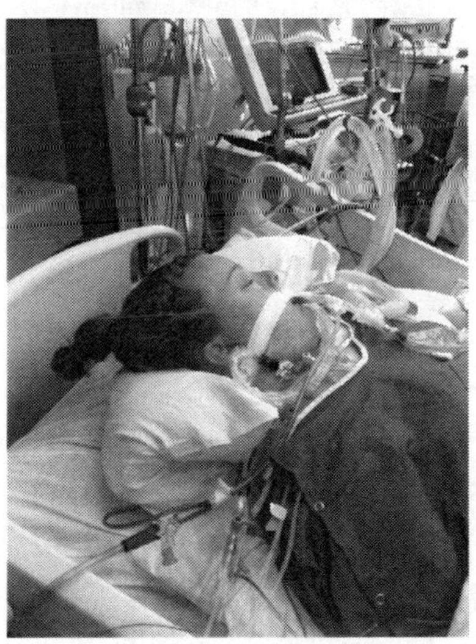

FIGURE 2.2 Sharon in the intensive care unit.

at once terrifying, heartbreaking, confusing, overwhelming, and nauseating. I halted at the door to register the shock and slowly walked over to Sharon and whispered to her that I was with her.

Then the begging began. I told her she was tough and if anybody could survive this, it was her. She had already endured so much in her short life and yet, always seemed to find the joy in life when others tried to extinguish it from her. I wondered what had she ever done to deserve all of this. I felt extreme guilt for not protecting her and was sure this was my fault. I should never have let her do this! Why did I let her do this? And then I apologized to her for not protecting her again. Upon my advice once before, she had gone to the Air Force Academy and been raped by an upper classman. She valiantly fought the system to no avail, but lost her innocence in those years after that event as the Air Force, the Academy and others tried to crucify her for telling the truth about the cover up of women being raped at these institutions. It was horrible for us both and I felt guilty then that I had not done my homework and allowed her to enter a place that was not safe for women at the time. Again, I felt as if I had not done my due diligence in finding out about this hospital, this doctor, or this procedure. I was not yet angry; I was simply grief-stricken and guilt-ridden.

The ICU nurse started to describe all the medications hanging and I told him that in this moment I could *not* be an ICU nurse and did not want the details of what was happening. I was just her mom and I really could not deal with trying to take care of her physically, as I needed to care for her emotionally as well as our whole family. I spent that night alone sitting by her bed, stroking her face and holding her hand. At 4 a.m., I felt a chill come over me and then mysteriously something whooshed past me. No one was there and I looked at Sharon and knew that she had left this earth in that moment. Her spirit had moved past me. I was sure that the rest was just a waiting game until all of the family got there and the surgeon felt he could finally give up trying to save her.

The next morning, my husband and daughter arrived. I sat and watched as each new person walked in and saw her lying there. Every expression on each visitor's face is indelibly imprinted in my brain. Friends came. Some rushed to hug her, some ran into an invisible wall at the door and could not make themselves enter, some cried and would not get near her, and some brought gifts. Maggie, a coworker, brought in a bear (Sharon's nickname was Share Bear) and a blanket that she loved to snuggle in when Sharon visited her home. Maggie carefully placed the bright orange blanket over the sterile white sheets and quietly sat and read her *People* magazine every time she visited. Others brought cards and put pictures of Sharon and her friends all over the walls. I found these expressions of love so comforting in this place that seemed cold and aloof. This was a strange feeling because I had always found comfort in the hospital as being a nurse was my profession. When my son finally arrived a couple of days later, my heart broke as he walked over and told his sister he loved her and then came and held me.

As each member of my family arrived, I watched as they grieved in their own way. My other daughter became the cheerleader, giving pep talks to Sharon about how and when to wake up. My son comforted both sisters and honestly looked helplessly on not knowing how to help. My husband held me and tried to coordinate the parade of people who began to show up to talk to us and particularly to me.

I quickly became more aware of my surroundings and remember a hospital official coming to say that they needed to disguise Sharon as she was a local celebrity and we did not want people from the community just dropping in to see her. Her television name was different than her given name so I assured them that no one would know her real name and that was not a concern. I did not want our friends to be blocked from visiting or calling. I came to realize later that this was the beginning of what I felt to be the cover up by the hospital.

The thoracic surgeon became the primary provider for Sharon in the ICU. He kept assuring me that he had gotten to her quickly and that she had never been without cardiopulmonary resuscitation. He believed he had saved her. He used those words—"I saved her." I thought, "typical surgeon," but was relieved that someone still thought she had a chance for survival. The cardiologist continued to come by and invariably wanted to pray with me and was always negative about her chances for survival. In retrospect, he was the one who really knew what had happened in the cath lab. I should have realized then that he knew she had been without oxygen too long to survive. I quickly grew tired of his attempts to pray and telling me about how he prayed during the procedure. I do not remember if at this point, he implied or actually said that if God had wanted her to live, he would have helped him in the lab. In either case, he continually blamed the outcome on God. I now suspect that he was overcome with guilt and needed me to forgive him, but that was never explicitly communicated. Instead his gestures literally felt like he was stalking me. I would see him down the hall and run to avoid him. My husband repeatedly asked him to leave me alone as I did not appreciate his tone or innuendos. Once I was hiding in an empty room in another hallway, and yet, he searched me out and began his religious rituals with me despite my obvious discomfort. His affect was so strange, particularly when countered with the optimism of the surgeon and the guarded discussions with the nurses.

Often there were as many as 10 visitors in Sharon's room at any one time. No one dared to ask any of us to leave. My husband told me later that many people came in and each one made a beeline for me. They ignored everyone else in the room. You see, they all were aware of my status as a critical care nurse, a colonel in the Air Force, and a commander of a hospital. The head of the heart team came to tell me that he was sorry and that they would surely find out what happened so that it never happened again. He gave me his card. The nurses told me stories. They focused particularly on a 17-year-old girl down the hall that had collapsed in cardiac arrest on the street and was able to be resuscitated. She was doing well. I remember trying to be happy for her, but all I could do was ponder how someone could survive collapsing on a street or survive horrific injuries in a war and my daughter lay dying while cared for in a major medical center. I wish I could tell you that I had much hope at this point for a miracle, but I had seen this scenario too many times. It was heart-wrenching watching everyone else expecting her to wake up and be her normal jubilant self.

One evening, the thoracic surgeon came in and began to fiddle with the IV drips. The ICU nurse was quite agitated that he was even touching them and tried to ask him to please just describe what he wanted and the nurse would adjust the drips. The surgeon didn't listen. He just kept fiddling. As soon as he left, the nurse went over and changed all the drips back to the original settings and said he would be right back after checking the chart. He informed me that they were new pumps and he wished that the doctors who were never trained on them would leave them alone. As foggy as I initially was, my perception shifted to crystal clarity at some point so that every detail of every day became distinctly clear. I watched how people reacted particularly when I asked questions. Once, I asked about an intensivist and why the surgeon was caring for my daughter. They said he likes taking care of his own patients. Then I asked about brain resuscitation and the nurse said, "We are doing the best we can with cooling her down. We are trying to get in touch with a neurologist to come in and see her." This was at least 24 hours after being admitted to the ICU. The neurologist finally showed up and announced that he was not happy that he had to be there as he was retired. He callously said to do an electroencephalogram (EEG) and start to rewarm her, then repeat the EEG in 48 hours to confirm she was brain-dead. Then he walked out. He never said he was sorry, never explained what he was doing and he had the most horrible attitude and bedside manner. The ICU nurse told me that they had to call him in from his retirement since they did not have any active practicing neurologists available to help. The nurse then told us that he was a motorcycle rider and that he hoped he never got in an accident in New Mexico because there was no one to do any brain resuscitation. It was a death sentence. Any hope we had was slowly drifting away.

Sometime in the next day or so, the surgeon stated that we needed to try to rewarm Sharon to see if we could elicit any neurologic response. The ice bags were removed from her head and she was slowly rewarmed. Her body temperature did not return to normal as quickly as the surgeon would have liked so he ordered warm blankets be placed over her to try to accelerate the process. That continued for several hours. By this point I was completely exhausted, so my family insisted I return to the hotel to get at least one night's sleep knowing that the next day would be very emotional one way or the other. I am not sure how the following scenario actually occurred so I will simply describe the encounter. I was lying in the bed and all of a sudden Sharon appeared at the foot and said, "Mom, it is time to let me go, I am absolutely fine. It is okay." I was sure she was standing right in front of me and was acutely aware that the next day was going to be the end of this ordeal. I knew she was really gone.

On the fourth day after surgery, I got dressed and went back to the hospital. Shortly after I arrived I was called to the nurses' station directly outside of Sharon's room. I was told there was a phone call for me there. When I answered, the man on the phone identified himself as the anesthesiologist for Sharon's procedure. He seemed distraught and said, "I have never been part of anything so horrible in my life. She was such a wonderful girl. We had such fun together joking around before the procedure. I just wanted you to know that it was a mess in there and I am so, so sorry." He hung up and I stood there stunned. He had just confirmed for me that something had gone horribly wrong during the procedure. In all of my years in nursing, I have never seen a physician admit to such a thing and I was sure he had called to make sure that I knew that this was way outside of normal. I suspected that his conscience was overcome with remorse and he needed to get it off his chest.

By the time I reentered the room, Sharon's body temperature had returned to normal and so it was decided to perform another electroencephalogram. We were all taken to the waiting room just outside the ICU. Before we left her room, I distinctly remember my other daughter telling Sharon to wake up and surprise everybody because if anybody could beat this mess, it was her big sister Sharon. We spread out to wait and I paced up and down the hallway. I was unaware of everyone else except my husband who kept going down to peek in Sharon's room to see what was going on. Finally, he came back with tears in his eyes and held me in the hallway and said, "There is nothing there, just nothing." I knew this was going to be the end and I braced myself for the discussion that was coming. My family walked in and most sat down as the surgeon waited to tell us the news. He started by saying he was sorry, but he had never seen someone with absolutely no brainwaves at all. She was brain-dead and he had pronounced her before we came back in the room. Everyone was sobbing and I walked over to hold my baby in my arms. I told her I was sorry for all of this and I felt as though I would faint from the realization that I would never see my beautiful baby sing, dance, and be her silly self ever again.

Without missing a beat, Laura, the organ donor representative, came into the room. She and the surgeon discussed organ donation with us. If Sharon had indicated that she was an organ donor, they really needed to know it now. I knew Sharon had specifically written down that she wanted to be an organ donor since she had heard so much about how this helped people from her nurse parents. Fortunately, she had not only consented to organ donation, but had actually listed every single body part on this form and so the decision was easy or so I thought. Her father became quite upset and said "Please, I do not want her cut up and sent to different people. I really cannot stand anyone taking her eyes." I tried to explain that she had wanted this and we needed to honor her wishes. This began what most in our family would say was the worst 48 hours of the entire ordeal.

Not only was our beautiful baby dead, but we had to endure another two days of waiting until the organ recovery teams came to harvest her organs. During the signing of paperwork, it became apparent that the hospital had chosen not to do an autopsy. I was shocked, as I had assumed it would be done for anyone who came in healthy and became an unexpected death. I inquired as to why and was told that there was a note in the chart by the charge nurse that stated that they were not doing an autopsy due to hospital policy. I asked the staff to reconsider but they declined. I was told in no uncertain terms that the hospital would not pay for an autopsy. I got on the phone on a Saturday morning and called the Medical Examiner (ME) myself. They were shocked that a mother was calling, but I begged them to do an autopsy. Between tears, I explained the circumstances of Sharon's death and they told me that if the hospital had chosen not to do the autopsy, I would have to pay for it myself. I agreed and went back to be with my family in Sharon's room. Shortly thereafter, I received a call from the ME's office and they said that they had talked about it and under the circumstances, the hospital should have ordered the autopsy and that it would be charged to the facility. By now my guard was up and I felt that there was a real attempt on the part of the hospital and staff to cover up much of what had gone on in surgery. Once I was assured that the autopsy would be done, our attention was moved to preparing ourselves for the agonizing process of waiting.

A time for the team to arrive was established and a countdown began. Every four hours, someone would come in and give us a time hack. Each and every time, we were pulled to Sharon's bedside to say goodbye. It happened over and over until I nearly collapsed. The staff changed focus to saving organs, not my daughter. As the hours passed by, the odor of dying flesh began to fill the room. Her friends had now left as there was nothing else to do there leaving only our immediate family and closest friends there to wait out this drama. The transplant coordinator kept us busy making posters of Sharon and writing goodbye notes on each of them so that the transplant team could see and read about Sharon and how much she meant to each of us. Each was a love note to a daughter, sister, wife, and friend. We were encouraged to go get some sleep as the next day would be extremely difficult. Family and friends took turns staying with her so she was never left alone.

The next morning when I arrived, I experienced one of the only moments during this entire ordeal where I felt as if someone recognized my daughter's humanity. The night nurse in the ICU had asked to work that final night with Sharon even though it was her day off. She had bonded with all of us and during this final night she had washed Sharon from head to foot, including her beautiful reddish blonde hair. She had braided her hair across the front to keep the hair from her face. Crisp white sheets were placed over her with her favorite blanket still atop the sheet. Even though she was still attached to so many machines and tubes, she looked like a human being for the first time in this ICU. All around the room were pictures of flowers painted on typing paper and folded to make cards (Figures 2.3 and 2.4). At first, I did not understand the meaning of the flowers. The nurse told us that before bathing Sharon, she had taken each toe and each finger and dipped them in paint to make these flowers. She had also made a plaster mold of her hand and that was sitting on the bedside table with a bright red rose lying across her palm. I had been an ICU and trauma nurse for over 40 years and I had never in all that time seen anything so genuinely kind and thoughtful. I completely broke down, thanked her profusely for understanding that Sharon was a person who loved us and we loved her. For a moment, our baby was treated with the respect that she deserved. I will forever be grateful for that nurse—she helped me live through a horrific day.

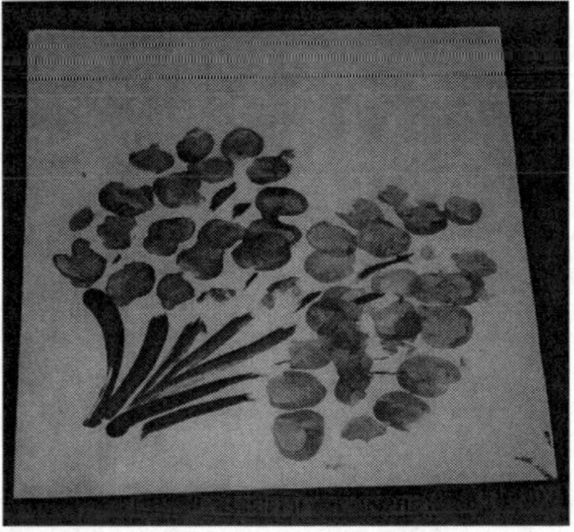

FIGURE 2.3 Sharon's finger and toe print flowers.

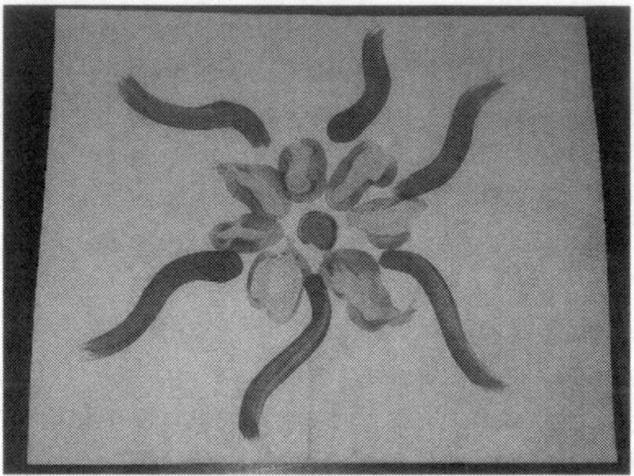

FIGURE 2.4 Flower from Sharon's fingerprints.

The day droned on with the inevitable four-hour time hacks continuing, despite our need to stop them, because each four hours that passed meant we were closer to never seeing her again. The chaplain came in to pray with us when we heard the transplant teams had arrived and my son and other daughter had to hold me up to keep me on my feet. I was overcome with agony, pain, and loss all in that moment. We were pushed to the side of the room so the team could prepare the equipment for transfer to the operating room. They seemed uncomfortable that we were there and even more so when we accompanied them all to the door of the operating room. There we kissed our beautiful girl goodbye and somehow walked out of the hospital. I don't remember anything until we exited when I saw the helicopter sitting outside of the emergency room. I had been told that her kidneys were going to remain in Albuquerque and her liver was being flown to Tucson for transplant. That gave me some comfort as Sharon had attended the University of Arizona for a while. It seemed appropriate. However, as the family started toward our car, I could not leave the outdoor waiting area where I could see the helicopter. My husband begged me to leave but I told him that I could not leave until the helicopter actually left. Only then was she really gone. I know this was agonizing for him but I was fixated there. Eventually the helicopter did leave and I realized in that moment that my life had changed forever. How was I going to live without my oldest child and how would I reconcile what I suspected was major malpractice on the part of the physician and hospital?

After Sharon's death, on-going reminders of this horrific process plagued me. Shortly after we returned home, I was contacted by the patient safety officer from the hospital who happened to be a physician. She informed me that a series of devastating mistakes had occurred during Sharon's procedure and, unfortunately, those mistakes led to her death. She told me that there was a period of four hours where signs of pericardial bleeding occurred and Sharon could have been saved if she had been taken to the operating room. I again found myself sobbing on the floor of my office and thinking, How could this happen in this day and age? I commend this doctor for her honesty and compassion as she sobbed with me and said, "I am so sorry and cannot imagine how horrible this is to hear." She told me that I could call her anytime if I needed any more information. I did call her several times and she told me what she was allowed to but it left me without answers as to exactly what happened.

Secondly, the hospital repeatedly sent me a patient satisfaction questionnaire with questions about the food and was she happy with her stay. It seemed ludicrous to me that someone could not see that she had perished in their care and have the common decency not to send me these documents. Second, as I was driving home from work one day, I received a call from the budget office at the hospital. The call began, "Hi, I see that you are listed as the contact person for Sharon Fullilove. I guess she has decided to dodge paying her bill by changing her phone number and not answering our letters! So I need you to get hold of her for us." I nearly drove my car off the highway. I was shocked, infuriated, and distraught that this person was so callous and I started screaming at him. I am not sure I was even able to articulate my feelings. I think I was just screaming and crying. I pulled over as I could not see anything and told him that Sharon had passed away in their hospital and that is why they could not reach her. He continued to grill me about her insurance coverage and I was so angry, especially since I had been with her when we had accomplished all of that the day before surgery. He told me I would be responsible for the bill if I did not fix this and then he abruptly hung up. All I could think was, "Oh my god, all they care about is getting their money. Never mind they murdered (the word my son uses to describe these events) my daughter!" This same conversation happened two more times even though each time I provided them with the information from her insurance company. I kept thinking they could not even get this right, no wonder they couldn't take care of Sharon. During the last of these three calls, I hung up and contacted the Patient Safety Officer that had been so forthcoming all along. I told her of the calls and she immediately said, "You will never hear from them again—I will take care of it." I told her that if I had not ever planned on suing before, I was considering it now.

So much pain and distrust now surrounded the hospital, be it the one where we lost our daughter or the one where we worked. An invisible bubble surrounded it, an impenetrable dome I could no longer enter. I drove five miles out of the way to make sure I did not have to pass by the brick and mortar that had now become the enemy. The trust was never regained and forced my retirement as I no longer saw the hospital as a place of healing. Now it was a place of loss. Our life-world had been shattered.

REVIEW OF THE HOSPITAL RECORDS

I was so angry with everyone from the budget office to the physician that I felt these indignities needed to be exposed. We requested the medical record but were denied access which forced us to hire a lawyer to act as her personal representative. Once the chart was obtained and attorneys were able to view it, the following information was discovered.

On September 27, 2011, Sharon was admitted for an explantation and implantation (elective surgery) of a pacemaker by a well-known cardiologist. Evidence revealed that the cardiologist did not have the minimal number of procedures needing to be done annually to maintain his extraction skills. He had inadequately explained the risks of the procedure as they related to his skills and the equipment available at this particular facility. All of these variables increased the risk associated with this procedure. Furthermore, these deviations did not adhere to the standard of care. A consent form was presented and signed by Sharon for the wrong procedure which did not elucidate the real risks associated with performing the procedure.

The cardiologist did not anticipate or preclude eventual problems by ordering a type and crossmatch of Sharon's blood in the event a transfusion was required during surgery, as bleeding was a known complication of the procedure. Sharon was taken to the cardiac catheterization lab at about 8:36 a.m. with a blood pressure (BP) of 92/66 and a heart rate (HR) of 80. At some point during the pacemaker extraction, the cardiologist needed electrocautery lead extraction equipment which is the standard in the industry for lead extraction, but it was not available. A transporter was sent to another hospital to pick up electrocautery lead extraction equipment (hence, the man in the scrubs that ran past me in the waiting room). Despite not having the necessary equipment, the cardiologist continued with the extraction. At 11:15 a.m., Sharon's HR increased to over 100 beats per minute (BPM) for the first time and remained elevated until 11:40 a.m. when the transporter returned from a local hospital with the electrocautery lead extractor. Extraction continued and Sharon's heart rate remained over 110 BPM from 11:45 a.m. to 1:04 p.m. when the atrial lead was finally removed. The cardiologist noted Sharon was developing a pericardial effusion. He continued without calling for assistance or halting the procedure. At 1:22 p.m., the new pacemaker was placed. Vital signs were as follows: At 1:30 p.m., her BP was 105/58 and her HR was 110.

At 1:45 p.m., her BP was 93/53 and her HR rose to 122. Sometime before 1:50 p.m., the cardiologist realized Sharon's heart rate was increasing and her BP was decreasing and he called another cardiologist for a pericardial effusion consult. Once a pericardial effusion was suspected, the standards state that a thoracic surgeon should be consulted (Wilkoff et al., 2009). The second cardiologist requested a transesophageal echocardiogram (TEE) which per the standards, should be present throughout this procedure to carefully monitor for bleeding. The TEE was never obtained as it was a second piece of equipment not available at the facility along with the laser lead extractor. They determined she had a pericardial effusion and despite this determination, they chose not to call the surgeon and continued with the implantation. At about 2:00 p.m., Sharon's HR was 117 and her BP had dropped to 72/51. At 2:15 p.m., her BP was 77/48 and her HR had risen to 124. At the same time, her hemoglobin was found to be 6.1 gm/dL and her hematocrit was critically low at 18%. Again, the cardiologists did not call the thoracic surgeon, despite evidence of bleeding from a number of sources. At 2:22 p.m., the physician ordered two units of red blood cells "transfuse now" but failed to order the blood as an emergency release of uncrossmatched units. The lack of an appropriate type and crossmatch prior to surgery and failure to order the units as an emergency release breached the standard of care. She did not receive the blood. At 2:30 p.m., Sharon's BP was 64/47 and her HR was 108. At 2:33 p.m., the cardiologist submitted an order for a "type and screen." This was an inappropriate order as crossmatched blood was unavailable as an emergency release. The lack of a blood transfusion compromised Sharon's cardiovascular status. At 2:45 p.m., Sharon's BP was 46/27 and her HR was 90 with her oxygen saturation at 85%. At 2:47 p.m., the second cardiologist was at the bedside to perform a pericardiocentesis, but this should have been performed immediately upon determining she had a pericardial effusion. The effusion was severe by this time and could have been detected much earlier had the requisite TEE been available during the procedure. The second cardiologist removed approximately 200 cc of blood from around the heart and he stated in the chart that her blood pressure was in the 50s and she became "quite tachycardic." At 2:58 p.m., cardiopulmonary resuscitation (CPR) was started and finally the thoracic surgeon was called. The surgeon immediately assessed Sharon and made arrangements for transfer to the operating room. At 3:00 p.m., her heart rate was 77, her BP was 176/81 and her oxygen saturation was 78%. Two units of red blood cells were ordered "uncrossmatched now." At this point, Sharon had not received any blood or blood products despite having indications of a bleed for over an hour. At 3:06 p.m., the anesthesiologist put in an emergency transfusion request for uncrossmatched blood authorizing the release of uncrossmatched O negative units. At 3:10 p.m., Sharon was transferred to the operating room with CPR and bagging in progress. The over ten minutes required to transport Sharon to the OR was outside the window allowable via the standards. Sharon did not receive the packed red blood cells until 3:15 p.m. when she received 598 cc of red cells. At 3:15 p.m., Sharon's HR was 0 and her oxygen saturation was 38%. At 3:21 p.m., nearly 25 minutes after evaluating her, the surgeon started an exploratory sternotomy. He found a "large pericardial effusion" which was "bloody" and her heart at a complete standstill. He evacuated the blood and found a one-centimeter laceration at the junction of the superior vena cava and the right atrium on the lateral side. The surgeon was able to repair the laceration with two sutures. Several units of blood, platelets, and cryoprecipitate were ordered as a medical emergency once the chest had been opened. At 3:45 p.m., 4:00 p.m., 4:15 p.m., 4:30 p.m., and at 4:45 p.m., Sharon's heart rate was 0 presumably because she was on cardiopulmonary bypass. At 5:00 p.m., Sharon's surgery was complete and she was transferred to the post-anesthesia care unit with a HR of 104. She was in a coma and remained that way with an EEG showing electrocerebral silence. On September 30, 2011, Sharon remained neurologically non-responsive and a second EEG confirmed her brain death.

QUESTIONS FOR REFLECTION

The American College of Physicians' Charter on Medical Professionalism (2008) and the American Nurses Association Code of Ethics with Interpretive Statements (2015) both direct practitioners to uphold the values of their profession and place the interests of patients above those of the physician or nurse. Sharon's story most certainly permits us to pause and ponder some moral and ethical questions as we go about practicing our respective professions in health care. The following are presented for your thoughtful consideration and discussion.

1. What virtues and vices do you see present in Sharon's story?
2. Were there examples of moral complacency and/or moral courage?
3. What were the systems issues that contributed to Sharon's death? Could they have been foreseen or were they an unfortunate accident?
4. What were the stakeholder's motivations for doing the procedure and in their dealings with the family?

These and many more may resonate as you consider this case. At the very least, I hope to bring to the forefront the centrality of ethics in professional decision making within the context of health care.

REFERENCES

Allen, M. (2013). *How many die from medical mistakes in U.S. hospitals?* Retrieved from http://www.npr.org/blogs/health/2013/09/20/224507654/how-many-die-from-medical-mistakes-in-u-s-hospitals

American College of Physicians. (2008). Medical professionalism in the new millennium: A physician charter. *Annals of Internal Medicine, 136*(3), 243–246.

American Nurses Association. (2015). *Code of ethics for nurses with interpretive statements*. Silver Spring, MD: ANA, American Nurses Association.

Berlinger, N. (2005). *After harm: Medical error and the ethics of forgiveness*. Baltimore, MD: The Johns Hopkins University Press.

James, J. T. (2013). A new, evidence-based estimate of patient harms associated with hospital care. *Journal of Patient Safety, 9*(3), 122–128.

Wilkoff, B. L., Love, C. J., Byrd, C. L., Bonigorni, M. G., Carrillo, R. G., Crossley, G. H., et al. (2009). Transvenous lead extraction: Heart Rhythm Society expert consensus on facilities, training, indications, and patient management. *Heart Rhythm, 6*(7), 1085–1104.

CHAPTER 3

Family Impact of Military Mental Health Stigma

A Narrative Ethical Analysis

Susanne W. Gibbons and Edmund (Randy) Howe

ABSTRACT

Our past lessons from war trauma have taught us that mental health-care stigma and other issues surrounding mental health–seeking behaviors can negatively impact the healing trajectory and long-term function for service members and their families. It can take years to decades before a service member seeks professional help for psychological distress, if he or she seeks it at all. Unfortunately, signs of personal and family problems can be subtle, and consequences, such as suicide, tragic. In this chapter, we consider the story one military health-care provider submitted in response to a study solicitation that read: *Please provide your personal story telling me about any psychological distress you may have experienced after returning from deployment and your personal challenges accessing care and/or remaining in treatment.* This story is analyzed to explore the moral implications of his experience for the military and for other service members. The main points to be highlighted are that altruism can leave altruists more vulnerable, military mental health stigma may exacerbate this risk, and military families may profoundly be affected.

http://dx.doi.org/10.1891/0739-6686.34.35

INTRODUCTION

Health-care providers may have trouble finding the right words when patients are hurting. In these situations, when there are no words, silence may be better than speaking. Considering the problems health-care providers have at times when addressing their patient's distress, we wonder how difficult it might be for them to reveal their own pain and suffering. For military health-care providers who experience the horrors of war and often suffer quietly, remaining silent might be preferable to facing real or perceived mental health stigma from acknowledging they have a problem and seeking help. Perhaps this type of silence is a testimony to the culture they are a part of and the bond they share that comes about from the military brotherhood and the mission. This might explain why only one military health-care provider submitted a narrative in response to a study solicitation that read: *Please provide your personal story telling me about any psychological distress you may have experienced after returning from deployment and your personal challenges accessing care and/or remaining in treatment.*

The goal of this chapter is to use narrative ethical analysis, which is to interpret and gain insight from the story of this one participant who had the courage to reveal what was for him almost too awful for words; to compel, involve, and teach us about life as a health-care provider in the armed services; and to consider how the military health system might better meet the needs of all service members. Although one case study is useful from a pedagogical standpoint, it is not generalizable. Yet the lessons included in this manuscript may still be immensely valuable. Individuals in similar circumstances, facing similar challenges, may be able to apply some of the lessons learned. We begin by describing how the military is addressing mental health stigma and barriers to care, by presenting background on military mental health stigma and the impact of recent conflicts on military members and their families to develop the context for the analysis. Then, the research study design and methods are briefly described. After that, the narrative of one participant is presented, highlighting themes from his experiences using hermeneutic phenomenology, which means to contextually interpret the hidden and explicit meanings behind his story (Moustakas, 1994; Van Manen, 1990). The moral implications of the participant's actions and perceptions are also addressed. The main points that are highlighted are that altruism can leave altruists more vulnerable, military mental health stigma may exacerbate this risk, and military families may be profoundly affected.

BACKGROUND ON MILITARY MENTAL HEALTH-CARE STIGMA AND PERCEIVED BARRIERS TO CARE

Mental health stigma is of particular concern to the military because, together, individual and social stigmatizing beliefs and behaviors influence service members' willingness to seek professional help (Mojtabai, 2010; Vogel, Wade, &

Haake, 2006; Vogt, 2011). These stigmatizing beliefs can be adopted in a couple of ways. Individuals can enter the military with these beliefs or acquire them from the organization. Service members in need of mental health care can hopefully depend on support from family, friends, and leadership to guide them toward care that is accessible and affordable and offers the necessary privacy (Britt, Wright, & Moore, 2012; Warner, Appenzeller, Mullen, Warner, & Grieger, 2008; Wright et al., 2009). Privacy is often not guaranteed in the military because of mission needs. Those with mental health symptoms, who are most at risk, present the greatest concern since they are more likely to fail to seek treatment (Pietrzak, Johnson, Goldstein, Malley, & Southwick, 2009; Visco, 2009). In recent years, the military services have focused on dispelling the "myth" that a mental health problem means "weakness" and have encouraged service members to openly acknowledge the need for help so that service members look after one another (Gibbons, Migliore, Greiner, Convoy, & DeLeon, 2014).

All service members, regardless of occupation, are exposed to a similar set of values that include obedience; service; mission first; and never failing, quitting, or leaving another service member behind (Defense Health Board, 2015; Rondeau, 2011). Military health-care providers experience psychological problems similar to those seen in combat troops where stress, emotional instability, and family conflict are prominent upon return home (Jones et al., 2008; Kolkow, Spira, Morse, & Grieger, 2007; Milliken, Auchterlonie, & Hoge, 2007; Seal et al., 2009; Smith et al., 2008, Thomas et al., 2010). Even though over 75% of combat veterans recognize these problems, only 40% are interested in receiving help (Brown, Creel, Engel, Herrell, & Hoge, 2011). If not treated early, when treatment is necessary, significant posttraumatic stress symptomatology, poorer psychosocial functioning, and other psychological disorders can persist chronically or surface years later, resulting in long-term psychological distress (Gibbons, Hickling, & Watts, 2012; Kulka et al., 1990). It can take years to decades before a service member seeks professional help for psychological distress, if he or she seeks it at all. Our past lessons from war trauma have taught us that mental health-care stigma and other issues surrounding mental health-seeking behaviors can also negatively impact the healing trajectory and long-term function for service members and their families. Even if service members can get better over time, which many do, early intervention can profoundly help their families. An example that follows most sadly makes this point.

Unfortunately, signs of family problems can be subtle, and consequences, such as suicide, tragic (Nock et al., 2014; Sareen, 2014). Furthermore, the lives of military children are intertwined with those of their parents to such an extent that it is believed that health risks for these children often reflect those of their families (Cozza, 2015). Even though the literature has predominantly focused on service members, concern also has been raised that mental health problems are not adequately treated among military family members (Chandra et al., 2010; Lester et al., 2013). In the general community, there is evidence that adolescents, in particular, underutilize mental health services because of stigma, concerns about confidentiality, lack of accessibility, and because of the preference to rely on themselves only (Gulliver, Griffiths, & Christensen, 2010). The exaggerated belief that one must be self-reliant in all circumstances might also be more pronounced among military families, than others with teenagers, where a strong desire to solve problems without outside support is a point of exceptional pride, and thus in this context, seeking help is a hurdle to overcome (Becker, Swenson, Esposito-Smythers, Cataldo, & Spirito, 2014). A further contributory factor to these obstacles is cultural indoctrination that occurs in the military. Military members and their families experience a system of spoken and written beliefs, values, language, manners, customs, courtesies, traditions, and expected behaviors that shape who they are and how they handle themselves (Hall, 2011).

The maladaptive goal of always being self-reliant, and never owning up to a feeling such as fear, might be best understood through the following narrative account of one service member's experience of mental health stigma and access to care, seen through the eyes of an altruistic military physician who ignored his own needs. His story is marked by personal tragedy and by what the ancient Greeks referred to as *peripeteia*, the sudden change of fortune from good to bad and a turning point in a person's life (Bruner, 1990; Bury, 1982).

THE STUDY

The story for this analysis is from a study with the overarching goal of better understanding barriers to care experienced by military health-care providers. Narrative stories are representations of events and experiences, communicated by the teller, that reflect the narrator's culture, institutions, and political environments (Reissman, 2008). While these stories can serve many purposes, in this study, the written narratives of military health-care providers were bound around a single concept—military mental health stigma and perceived access to care—to better understand how these individuals may perceive or misperceive their past experiences, understand or misunderstand what these mean, and how they came about. This study was approved by the Uniformed Services University of the Health Sciences Institutional Review Board. Solicitations were through social networking sites, list serves for communities of service members, and pro bono mental health-care providers. Consent to publish ideas and verbatim segments of the narrative without participants' name or other identifying information was obtained through written consent. The military health-care providers invited to participate were asked to e-mail their narratives directly to the principal investigator. The narrative of one service member is presented in the next section. While reading and considering the story and the researcher's interpretations, the reader is encouraged to make his or her own additional interpretations of what may underlie this writer's narrative, but not be explicitly expressed, in trying to capture and infer some of the most significant underlying considerations (Van Manen, 1990).

NARRATIVE

I deployed to Saudi and Bosnia without hesitation early in my career. I knew deploying was part of being a soldier physician but was not prepared for the effects on myself and my family. I observed inequities in poor leadership support of our troops, lack of continuity in medical care from Garrison to Overseas and back, and unwillingness of Unit and Medical Commands to involve families in soldier mental health evaluation and treatment. My eyes were opened to what our troops and their families were going through; I decided they deserved better advocacy and stayed on active duty rather than join a civilian practice after seven years. I saw career soldiers with destroyed joints and spines still soldiering on, waiting until retirement to begin taking care of their health. They truly sacrificed all for the Army and their careers. When they suffered from what they witnessed while deployed, we sent them "to the rear," and administratively discharged them. Returning from deployment, I found my family had endured injuries and my relationship with my boys was changed, more distant. Events had occurred needing a husband and father for best resolution, and I wasn't there. In Bosnia, I witnessed families who had been torn apart by war, women and children in refugee camps devoid of males, as they had been killed en masse. All of this, unbeknownst to me, was taking a great toll on my own psyche over the years. I internalized all I saw and worked harder and harder to reverse it, to prevent it, by advocating intensely for Soldiers, Airmen, Sailors, Marines, and Coasties and their Families. I, and my fellow care givers, could not see the toll it was exacting on myself and my family members. Especially, with the Medical Corps, we do not follow the mantra, "Physician, heal thyself."

Ironically, and sadly, as my 20th year approached, while in my first Medical Command, at the pinnacle of my career, my youngest son succumbed to suicide days after being seen in one of our military clinics for depression, anxiety, and suicidal ideation. He was turned away with an inadequate standard of care, given an antidepressant but not allowed to see mental health providers as "We only have enough for Active Duty, not family members." He left the clinic and immediately began plans for death by shotgun to the heart 14 days later. As I sought to explore and identify what happened, why we didn't respond when he came to us for help "one last time," I began to see why we've been so ineffective in dealing with suicide, posttraumatic stress disorder (PTSD), and mental health evaluation and treatment for troops and family members over the past 20 years. The more I spoke out in alarm, the more I was ostracized and alienated. Being patronized (ironically), downplaying my concerns, was bringing out PTSD I had harbored for 20 years, unrecognized and untreated. I realized I, too, was in denial all this time, not able to deal with my stress and anxiety, especially regarding ability to effectively advocate for Service Members and Families.

I began to think of suicide myself. I asked for help and saw military mental health personnel (psychologist and psychiatrist). They responded automatically, ironically, with anti-depressants, before a true evaluation was complete, just as happened with my son. While I was able to access mental health consultants, being Active Duty, sadly, these sessions were ineffective where real issues were ignored. After six months I realized I was unable to get effective care from within the military system. The culture of the military makes us ineffective and reluctant to address deep-seated issues causing PTSD. They were unable to assist me in identifying long-term stress while advocating for military families against all odds throughout my life and career. Fears I lived with while deployed, carrying a 9-mm pistol, gas mask, and wearing Kevlar, even though I'd not been in live-fire combat, were unresolved and contributing to continued intensity and drive, taking its toll. I recognized my inability to receive help from within the system, so sought mental health care outside the Tricare Network. I found a civilian psychologist who specialized in men's grief therapy, but who didn't take Tricare, a "non-Network Provider." The request to be referred out was denied, despite being written by my Primary Care Manager Provider who agreed therapy from within was ineffective. I appealed, reminding decision makers adequate care for me was unavailable within the military Tricare sphere, and was finally allowed to see this person. Work with him was transformational and allowed me to begin to see the chronic stress I'd developed over my career, both while deployed and while back in Garrison supporting those deployed, especially during Operation Enduring Freedom (OEF) and Operation Iraqi Freedom (OIF). (I volunteered to deploy but was in high-level positions disallowing deployment.)

The suicide of my son at 20 years of age while in the hands of the very health-care system I was part of exponentially deepened and drew out my PTSD. I realized it was time for me to separate from the military if I was to address my conditions in a timely manner. The Veterans Administration (VA) separation psych evaluation confirmed chronic PTSD from intense anxiety and passionate advocacy for military Service Members and their Families, as well as my fellow medical employees, exponentially heightened with the recent traumatic suicide of my son. The Retirement VA Claim indicates moderate PTSD with disability. I continue to work on depression, PTSD, guilt, and anxiety through various modalities as a retiree.

HERMENEUTIC PHENOMENOLOGY: INTERPRETATION OF THE MEMORY OF LIVED EXPERIENCE

Stories such as this one express the perception of the narrator who in this case is the actor in his own story. He involves us personally by revealing private and sensitive details of his life, deepening our ability to try to make additional interpretive sense out of what we read. Through the narrator's self-reflection, the story acquires hermeneutic significance as he goes beyond simple description when he attaches meanings to people, actions, events, and objects (Van Manen, 1990). This is like phenomenology in that it seeks to capture the essence of a person's subjective experience but is hermeneutic because it allows one to imagine multiple meanings in light of current history and context contributing to these perspectives. Through this exceptional explanatory endeavor, the narrator carefully and skillfully crafts his story to share events in his life, and we use this technique so that we can better understand his personal experience with military mental health stigma and trouble accessing and remaining in mental health care.

As a phenomenologic research method oriented to a more subtle study of the intentions and latent meanings and driving factors behind what people perceive, this is a process that allows us to look behind appearances or "the told" so that the narrator's intention and meaning is more fully understood (Moustakas, 1994). The hermeneutic goal is to understand the author better than the author may understand himself. This is a cyclical process for the researcher who reads the texts, writes reflectively, and interprets and then does this again, until all possibilities have been fully considered. For the reader, who in this case is a dialogic partner by virtue of listening and thinking about the story, hermeneutics happens when we find ourselves in the world, along with the narrator and his story, trying to use our own intuition to understand (Malpas, 2014). Through this reflective process, the researcher analyzes underlying conditions, historical events, and other details and nuances of phenomena to go beyond the pure description of experience. The hermeneutic assumption is that we can never know exact meaning since all we have is interpretation, but we can create meaning and possibly a deeper sense of understanding.

According to Brody and Clark (2014), narrative ethics is inherently hermeneutic. Similar to phenomenologic interpretation where there is an attempt to get beneath the surface subjective experience, the researcher goes through a process of listening to what the text is saying. The researcher frees himself/herself of fixed perspectives so that new questions can be asked and a new gestalt is possible. The interpretive process is existential phenomenology in that the analyst sees the phenomena through a particular lens that embraces the view that being human involves shared feelings and responses, which includes being responsive to others. Narrative ethical analysis is dialogical, accepting and imagining multiple points of view, and considering how these are acted out and responded to, the whole time recognizing the narrator's basic good intentions (Frank, 2014). The ultimate goal of this is to discern what we can do better. Thus in the ethical analysis that follows, we are also interpreting segments of the narrative from an ethical perspective because the narrator has convinced us that despite his best effort to do the right thing for himself and others, something got in the way.

ETHICAL ANALYSIS OF NARRATIVE

This story of sacrifice, advocacy, biographical disruption, and transformation is written in a way that allows us to appreciate the particular life of a "soldier physician" while illuminating the universal experience of life's unintended tragedy. The story helps generate new understanding and start dialogues—particularly with regard to care for self, care for family, and care for country in the context and value system associated with being a service member (Frank, 2014). The military health-care provider's story is resequenced so that we can appreciate how his altruistic journey led to his vulnerability. First, he speaks of a health-care provider's role and responsibility in the military as a noncombatant who wore Kevlar, carried a 9-millimeter pistol and a gas mask, and although he was never involved in live fire, still experienced fear. Then, he describes the physical distance caused by deployment as an expected part of his job, and he acknowledges not being prepared for the emotional impact on his family and the changed relationships with his wife and his sons, who were emotionally distant when he returned home. Finally, he portrays his participation in military missions and commitment to the armed service members and to his country, but admits to being unaware of "the toll it was exacting on" him and on his fellow caregivers who served beside him. He tells us that in the Medical Corps, they do not follow the mantra "physician heal thyself." Through the first section of his narrative account, we sense the ambivalence he must have felt over where to place his allegiance since he clearly wanted to do the right thing, but as is often the case when considering ethical implications, his moral decision making at earlier points in his life, to remain in the military and to advocate for fellow service members and their families led to "trouble"—a complicating factor in the story (Bruner, 1990).

Virtue Ethics: Good Character

Our physician narrator sought to do the responsible and right thing for those he served. As a moral agent, he exemplifies goodness of character. His story describes a virtuous person who has lived his life in a way that contributes to the good of others. People are drawn to medicine, nursing, and other helping professions because the practice contributes to individual as well as the greater societal good (Grace, 2014). In the military, people self-select by joining and serving their country, and then often and when possible, they further self-select their occupation. For this military health-care provider, the self-selection process came at a price. Despite the best intentions, even virtuous individuals who live life in a way that contributes to the good of others can get lost along the way because some choices have risks that might lead to sadness, helplessness, and even tragedy as seen in this case (Frank, 2014). Helping others carries its own risk and also sometimes serves as a defense mechanism that obscures an individual's ability to see his or her own need for help.

Narrative Analysis: How Not Why

To interpret and understand the meaning of choices and decisions made by our military physician narrator, we need to see what Montello (2014) refers to as the "topography" or structure of what was important to him, his "mattering map." The structure of this narrative can be understood by considering several key pieces. First, the analyst determines the prominent voice and central character, which involves identifying whose perspective is presented, what is presented, and how this is accomplished. Then, the plot or circumstances that led to writing the story are considered. Finally, a possible or actual resolution to the problem faced by the main character in the story is addressed. By providing this type of structure, it is easier to illuminate details and seemingly trivial aspects within the narration and gain greater insight into the author's intent.

First: Who Is Speaking? Learning by Being a Soldier

The military physician who narrates is at the center of the story. He shares an insider's perspective on deployment and on leadership inequities, with regard to how service members with physical and mental health issues are handled. He offers his perspective on the suffering of service members and the effect on their families and also the suffering of people living in the war-torn countries where he served. He chose not to "join a civilian practice after seven years," but instead "soldiered on" to intensely advocate for "Soldiers, Airmen, Sailors, Marines, and [Coast Guard personnel] and their Families." His perspective is one of self-sacrifice and altruism; however, this sacrifice made him vulnerable, increasing his risk for developing mental health problems and negatively impacting his role as a father and husband.

We learn a lot about the narrator's mattering map when he speaks of his recently deceased son, another character in the story. We wonder what his son would have said about his father's occupation, the military culture, and whether or not these elements in the story influenced the son's emotional distress and his not seeking help. It is unclear who did not respond "one last time" when his son "came to [us] for help." As he wrote this, it is unclear whether he is referring to himself or to others. We imagine that his son perhaps came with a veiled or indirect plea for help—to the physician narrator, his wife, or other family members—or sought informal help from the broader community, of which he was also a part. This last highly speculative point illustrates this hermeneutic phenomenologic approach of seeking to illustrate hidden realities for our understanding. If the narrator was referring to himself as the one who did not respond, he might be at risk for profound survival guilt and is perhaps attempting to deflect or dilute the unbearable self-blame. There appear to be other factors contributing to the story, perhaps the broader military family for whom the narrator physician sacrificed his mental health, being pushed to the brink of what he could take, as he "began to think of suicide [himself]." He says that his own "distress was exponentially heightened" with the suicide of his son.

We recognize the narrator's vulnerability and his central emotion, chronic distress, from decades of advocacy role and military responsibilities. By not addressing his own mental health needs and by not being present for his own family, he finds himself in an extreme state of despair. We feel the unbelievable pain and grief in this narration. If our narrator had cared for himself, would his son have killed himself? We will never know, since all we have is "mimesis" or what we can imagine, and the physician narrator's imagination of how the death of his son was impacted by his military service and then how his son was improperly handled by the military health system who missed the fact that he was suicidal. However, those affected by mental health problems may distort facts, and this may be the case with our physician narrator. Mental illness increases perceptions of stigma and makes it harder for those who really need help to reach out for help, a phenomenon that is not unique to the military, but might be intensified by the military culture (Pietrzak et al., 2009; Visco, 2009).

Second: Feeling the Importance to Share! Learning by Being a Patient

The story can be interpreted as a part of this physician's healing journey from decades of "anxiety and passionate advocacy for military members and their families" and from resulting distress compounded by the recent traumatic suicide of his son by "shotgun to the heart." This sudden tragic event is similar to what Brody has described as a loss that ruptures a person's life story, and the plea that is heard, "My story is broken, please help me fix it" is reflected in the words of this service member, who sacrificed so much to ensure advocacy for his fellow soldiers (Brody & Clark, 2014). The physician narrator has become one of the service members who "suffered from what they witnessed while deployed . . . [being] 'sent to the rear,' and administratively discharged." Perhaps he is suffering from survivor guilt, that he did not do enough or that he did not recognize the signs in his own son. Because of the devastating loss of his son, everything he had consciously denied, or internalized, all of the unresolved issues "contributing to [his] intensity and drive," bubbled to the surface. He becomes a patient in the military health system.

As a patient, the narrator says that his eyes were opened to how mental health issues are handled by military mental health-care personnel who he says "responded automatically . . . with [an] anti-depressant" when he experienced thoughts of suicide. We know that this is often a treatment for PTSD but he seems to dismiss this, illustrating the possibility that his own emotional impairment has gotten in the way of his ability to perceive accurately. We listen to his concern that the "culture of the military makes [military health-care providers] ineffective and reluctant to address deep-seated issues causing PTSD" and that this might also be the reason why no one was able to help him see the impact of his "long-term stress while advocating for military families against all odds throughout [his] life and career." He has insight regarding what went on and how he got to where he is; however, considering from a hermeneutic standpoint, his thinking might reflect a new position, one of distrust and loss of faith in the military health-care system that led to his "inability to receive help from within the system so [he] sought mental health care outside the Tricare Network." The concurrent magnification of distress and suspicion are possibly symptoms of his current predicament. He is having trouble moving forward with his life. And this may, in part, be a function of his misperceptions, which may include his seeing himself as more blocked or helpless than he truly is.

Third: Resolution—Learning by Being a Casualty

We see him as one of many military members in similar circumstances, enduring hardships as a part of their military duty and accumulating stress in the process. We wonder if his impression of military health care and his interpretation of events surrounding his experience of mental health stigma and accessing and remaining in treatment reflect his deep, raw emotional wound from the suicide of his son, and the temporary inability to get on with his life. Early in his narrative, he speaks of "career soldiers with destroyed joints and spines still soldiering on, waiting until retirement to begin taking care of their health . . . truly [sacrificing] all for the Army and their careers." We wonder if this is how many other military members may feel, who respond all too often when called upon, to tend to the needs of others. Perhaps, they slowly become a casualty of the system, during active duty or possibly even after service, since this seems to be how the physician narrator feels his military career evolved. His wounds are not physical, they are emotional. He was at the "pinnacle of his career" when his son committed suicide and then his entire world collapsed.

The narrative reflects the physician's attempts at restoring integrity and wholeness to his life. He continues in search of resolution since his story has not come to an end, but he is progressing with his life. The meaning and purpose that he seeks is perhaps being found as he "continue(s) to work on depression, PTSD, guilt, and anxiety through various modalities as a retiree." He continues to search for this through other avenues, including this story, to advocate for military members and their families; however, it is possible that he questions his own efficacy at this point. Perhaps he is in the process of forgiving himself. He seems to recognize the limitations of individuals/patients themselves and of mental health providers within the military health system and the limitations of the system itself. Despite recently instituted peer support programs to empower and sensitize service members to their own mental health needs, our narrator was unable to be effective in this regard (Gibbons et al., 2014). He knows that he was an insider and perhaps also ignored the obvious in his own patients, as he ignored his own needs for decades. Eventually, he will hopefully come to terms with his internal dissonance and conflict about his military career and his son's suicide in order to find peace. The time has come for him to take care of his own health and well-being.

CONCLUSION

The military physician who provided us with his story had the courage to break the silence in this study about individual and social stigmatizing beliefs and behaviors that are imposed by the self and the organization, and as he believes, may be perpetuated by the very people who are supposed to be eliminating them. He wants us to see the size and complexity of the problem and its reach—not only to soldiers but also to military families and our military-connected youth who are negatively impacted with depression and suicidal ideation (Cederbaum et al., 2014; Mansfield, Kaufman, Engel, & Gaynes, 2011). This physician's study participation exemplifies moral courage since he stepped outside of the military culture, deliberately and carefully constructing his narrative, to include elements for us, as dialogical partners, for reflection and action. He is courageous because of his admirable initiative to help others as he continues to advocate for his peers by drawing us into his story. He continues to move forward in his role as advocate, also perhaps as a means to seek resolution, possibly because the meaning and purpose in his life have always been tied to his health-care and military roles.

This interpretive exploration of a single case can be best understood in the current context of military life and operations. The problem may begin at the individual level. The price of altruism combined with culture and stigma is a cost known to many service members but may not be as well recognized by those of us who have not traveled this road. Systems may change, but change is slow. The success of current antistigma campaigns and efforts by military leadership and military health system personnel depend on culture change. This story teaches us that the personal cost of military service can be great, but that systems and individuals should have the capacity to do better. Change is going to take time and, for this reason, we all need to be maximally sensitive to subtle signs of distress and work to improve the lives of service members and their families.

ACKNOWLEDGMENTS

I dedicate this chapter to my PhD students who not only gave me the encouragement to write it, but also provided their insights, as uniformed members, into the experiences of health-care providers who have served for decades, been deployed, and have families.

The views expressed are those of the authors and do not reflect the official policy or position of the Uniformed Services University of the Health Sciences, the Department of the Defense, or the United States government.

REFERENCES

Becker, S. J., Swenson, R., Esposito-Smythers, C., Cataldo, A., & Spirito, A. (2014). Barriers to seeking mental health services among adolescents in military families. *Professional Psychology: Research and Practice, 45*(6), 504–513.

Britt, T. W., Wright, K. M., & Moore, D. (2012). Leadership as a predictor of stigma and practical barriers toward receiving mental health treatment: A multilevel approach. *Psychological Services, 9*(1), 26–37.

Brody, H., & Clark, M. (2014). Narrative ethics: A narrative (Narrative ethics: The role of stories in bioethics, special report). *Hastings Center Report, 44*(S1), S7–S11.

Brown, M. C., Creel, A. H., Engel, C. C., Herrell, R. K., & Hoge, C. W. (2011). Factors associated with interest in receiving help for mental health problems in combat veterans returning from deployment to Iraq. *The Journal of Nervous and Mental Diseases, 199*(10), 797–801.

Bruner, J. (1990). *Acts of meaning*. Cambridge, MA: Harvard University Press.

Bury, M. (1982). Chronic illness as biographical disruption. *Sociology of Health and Illness, 4*(2), 137–169.

Cederbaum, J. A., Gilreath, T. D., Benbenishty, R., Astor, R. A., Pineda, D., DePedro, K. T., et al. (2014). Well-being and suicidal ideation of secondary school students from military families. *Journal of Adolescent Health, 54*(6), 672–677.

Chandra, A., Lara-Cinisomo, S., Jaycox, L. H., Tanielian, T., Burns, R. M., Ruder, T., et al. (2010). Children on the homefront: The experience of children from military families. *Pediatrics, 125*, 16–25.

Cozza, S. (2015). Meeting the intervention needs of military children and families. *Journal of the American Academy of Child and Adolescent Psychiatry, 54*(4), 247–248.

Defense Health Board. (2015). *Ethical guidelines and practices for U.S. Military Medical Professionals, Office of the Assistant Secretary of Defense Health Affairs*. Falls Church, VA: Author.

Frank, A. W. (2014). Narrative ethics as dialogical storytelling (Narrative ethics: The role of stories in bioethics, special report). *Hastings Center Report*, *44*(S1), S16–S20.

Gibbons, S. W., Hickling, E., & Watts, D. D. (2012). Combat stressors and PTSD in deployed military healthcare professionals: An integrative review. *Journal of Advanced Nursing, 68*(1), 3–21.

Gibbons, S. W., Migliore, L., Greiner, S., Convoy, S., & DeLeon, P. H. (2014). Military mental health stigma challenges: Policy and practice considerations. *The Journal for Nurse Practitioners, 10*(6), 365–372.

Grace, P. J. (2014). *Nursing ethics and professional responsibility in advanced practice* (2nd ed.). Burlington, MA: Jones and Bartlett Learning.

Gulliver, A., Griffiths, K. M., & Christensen, H. (2010). Perceived barriers and facilitators to mental health help-seeking in young people: A systematic review. *BioMed Central Psychiatry, 10*, 113.

Hall, L. K. (2011). The importance of understanding military culture. *Social Work in Health Care, 50*(4), 4–18.

Jones, M., Fear, N., Greenberg, N., Jones, N., Hull, S., Hotopf, M., et al. (2008). Do medical service personnel who deployed to Iraq war have worse mental health than other deployed personnel? *European Journal of Public Health*, *18*, 422–427.

Kolkow, T. T., Spira, J. L., Morse, J. S., & Grieger, T. A. (2007). Post-traumatic stress disorder and depression in health care providers returning from deployment to Iraq and Afghanistan. *Military Medicine*, *172*, 451–455.

Kulka, R. A., Schlenger, W. E., Fairbank, J. A., Hough, R. L., Jordan, B. K., Marmar, C. R., et al. (1990). *Trauma and the Vietnam War generation: Report of findings from the National Vietnam Veterans Readjustment Study.* New York, NY: Brunner/Mazel.

Lester, P., Stein, J. A., Saltzman, W., Woodward, K., MacDermid, S. W., Milburn, N., et al. (2013). Psychological health of military children: Longitudinal evaluation of a family-centered prevention program to enhance family resilience. *Military Medicine, 178*, 838–845.

Malpas, J. (2014, Winter). Hans-Georg Gadamer. *The Stanford Encyclopedia of Philosophy* (2014 ed.), E. N. Zalta (Ed.). Retrieved from http://plato.stanford.edu/archives/win2014/entries/gadamer/

Mansfield, A. J., Kaufman, J. S., Engel, C. C., & Gaynes, B. N. (2011). Deployment and mental health diagnoses among children of US army personnel. *Archives of Pediatric & Adolescent Medicine*, *165*(11), 999–1005.

Milliken, C. S., Auchterlonie, J. L., & Hoge, C. W. (2007). Longitudinal assessment of mental health problems among active and reserve component soldiers returning from the Iraq war. *The Journal of the American Medical Association, 298*, 2141–2148.

Mojtabai, R. (2010). Mental illness stigma and willingness to seek mental health care in the European union. *Sociology Psychiatry and Psychiatric Epidemiology, 45*, 705–712.

Montello, M. (2014). Narrative ethics: Narrative ethics (Narrative ethics: The role of stories in bioethics, special report). *Hastings Center Report, 44*(S1), S2–S6.

Moustakas, C. (1994). *Phenomenological research methods*. Thousand Oaks, CA: Sage Publications.

Nock, M. K., Stein, M. B., Heeringa, S. G., Ursano, R. J., Colpe, L. J., Fullerton, C. S., et al. (2014). Prevalence and correlates of suicidal behavior among soldiers: Results from the Army Study to Assess Risk and Resilience in Service members (Army STARRS). *Journal of the American Medical Association Psychiatry*, *71*(5), 514–522.

Pietrzak, R. H., Johnson, D. C., Goldstein, M. B., Malley, J. C., & Southwick, S. M. (2009). Perceived stigma and barriers to mental health care utilization among OEF-OIF veterans. *Psychiatric Services, 60*(8), 1118–1122.

Reissman, C. K. (2008). *Narrative methods for the human sciences*. Thousand Oaks, CA: Sage.

Rondeau, A. E. (2011). Identity in the profession of arms. *Joint Forces Quarterly*, *62*(3), 10–13.

Sareen, J. (2014). Posttraumatic stress disorder in adults: Impact, comorbidity, risk factors, and treatment. *Canadian Journal of Psychiatry*, *59*(9), 460–467.

Seal, K. H., Metzler, T. H., Gima, K. S., Bertenthal, D., Maguen, S., & Marmar, C. R. (2009). Trends and risk factors for mental health diagnoses among Iraq and Afghanistan veterans using Department of Veterans Affairs health care, 2002–2008. *American Journal of Public Health*, *99*, 1651–1658.

Smith, T. C., Ryan, M. A., Wingard, D. L., Slymen, D. J., Sallis, J. F., & Kritz-Silverstein, D. (2008). New onset and persistent symptoms of post-traumatic stress disorder self-reported after deployment and combat exposures: Prospective population based US military cohort study. *British Medical Journal, 336*, 366–371.

Thomas, J. L., Wilk, J. E., Lyndon, A., Riviere, L. A., McGurk, D., Castro, C. A., et al. (2010). Prevalence of mental health problems and functional impairment among active component and national guard soldiers 3 and 12 months following combat in Iraq. *Archives of General Psychiatry, 67*, 614–623.

Van Manen, M. (1990). *Researching lived experience: Human science for an action sensitive pedagogy* (2nd ed.). Albany, NY: State University of New York Press.

Visco, R. (2009). Post-deployment, self-reporting of mental health problems, and barriers to care. *Perspectives on Psychiatric Care, 45*(5), 240–253.

Vogel, D. L., Wade, N. G., & Haake, S. (2006). Measuring the self-stigma associated with seeking psychological help. *Journal of Counseling & Psychology*, *53*, 325–337.

Vogt, D. (2011). Mental health-related beliefs as barrier to service use for military personnel and veterans: A review. *Psychiatric Services, 62*(2), 136–142.

Warner, C. H., Appenzeller, G. N., Mullen, K., Warner, C. M., & Grieger, T. (2008). Soldiers attitudes toward mental health screening and seeking care upon return from combat. *Military Medicine, 173*(6), 563–569.

Wright, K. M., Cabrera, O. A., Bliese, P. D., Adler, A. B., Hoge, C. W., & Castro, C. A. (2009). Stigma and barriers to care in solders post-combat. *Psychological Services, 6*(2), 108–116.

CHAPTER 4

Ethical Analysis of a Qualitative Researcher's Unease in Encountering a Participant's Existential Ambivalence

Marìa Elisa Moreno-Fergusson and Pamela J. Grace

ABSTRACT

Gaining in-depth understanding of the experiences of persons who have suffered traumatic events with physical and psychological sequelae is important for building effective interventions. However, qualitative research of this kind can be emotionally difficult for the researcher whose research interests derive from practice experiences with the population studied. It may be difficult for the researcher to separate the role of inquirer from that of practitioner. We explore this issue using ethical analysis to differentiate the responsibilities of the researcher from those of the clinician. In the first part of the chapter, we provide some background on the population studied and traumatic spinal cord injury and its aftermath as context for the issues raised by the narrative. Then, we describe briefly the first author's research exploring the meaning of bodily changes and embodiment in persons who have suffered a traumatic spinal cord injury. We provide the part of Jack's story that most troubled the researcher and led her to discuss the situation with an ethics colleague. Finally, we use the tools of moral reasoning, ethical analysis, and principles of research ethics to explore the pertinent excerpt of the narrative. The

http://dx.doi.org/10.1891/0739-6686.34.51

resulting clarifications are laid out for the reader with the intent of assisting other qualitative researchers in determining the extent and limits of their obligations to participants of qualitative studies, especially those that explore sensitive issues.

INTRODUCTION AND RESEARCHER BACKGROUND

As a result of her extensive experiences as rehabilitation nurse, the first author (MEM-F) had many opportunities to care for people with spinal cord injury in acute and rehabilitation settings in Colombia, South America. She developed a deep admiration for people with this type of injury, who have to face so many challenges in coming to grips with the attendant, often devastating sequelae. It requires courage and perseverance to adapt to the condition (Alcedo-Rodríguez, García-Carenas, Fontanil-Gómez, Benito-Arias, & Aguado Díaz, 2014); yet amazingly, many succeed in achieving an acceptable quality of life. Her dissertation work aimed at better understanding the experiences of this population as a preparatory step toward adequately meeting their nursing and social care needs. In the course of her qualitative study of the experience of embodiment for patients with traumatic paraplegia, she encountered one patient in particular whose revelations troubled her. Jack's adaptation to his situation, even several years after the injury, was incomplete. He expressed ambivalent thoughts about his future including the fact that he had considered suicide as preferable to aging in his altered state and/or to being a burden to himself and his family members. This encounter gave rise to feelings of uncertainty and moral disquiet for the first author. She wondered what the boundaries are of a researcher's responsibilities to participants.

In the first part of the chapter, we provide some background on traumatic spinal cord injury and its aftermath as context for the issues raised by the narrative. Then, we describe briefly the first author's research exploring the meaning of bodily changes and embodiment in persons who have suffered a traumatic spinal cord injury. We provide the part of Jack's story that most troubled the researcher and led her to discuss the situation with an ethics colleague (PG). Finally, we use the tools of moral reasoning, ethical analysis, and principles of research ethics to explore the pertinent excerpt of the narrative. The resulting clarifications are laid out for the reader with the intent of assisting other qualitative researchers in determining the extent and limits of their obligations to participants of qualitative studies, especially those that explore sensitive issues.

BACKGROUND ON SPINAL CORD INJURY AND ITS SEQUELAE

Traumatic spinal cord injury is a global problem. Sequelae are often complex and severe with devastating consequences for the injured person and those close to them. The incidence and prevalence of spinal cord injury are not consistently reported within and across countries—leaving gaps in data. Cripps et al. (2011) conducted a literature review of the epidemiology of this kind of trauma and found that the reported global prevalence of spinal cord injury is between 236 and 1,009 per million, and the incidence is 40 per million in North America, 15 per million in Australia, 16 per million in Europe, and 19 per million in the Latin American Andean (Brazil). The cumulative incidence of spinal cord injury in older adults has increased in the United States, from 79.4 per million older adults in 2007 to 87.7 by the end of 2009 but remained steady among younger adults (Selvarajah et al., 2014). In Colombia, South America, these injuries occur most frequently in young people; the mean age is 35.8 years, with a sex distribution (male/female) of 4 : 1 (Henao-Lema & Pérez-Parra, 2010).

The principal causes of spinal cord injury were traffic accidents in North America (47%), in Western Europe (46%), and in Australia (46%); in Brazil, falls in elderly people (39%) exceeded traffic accidents (31%) as a cause. Violence is also a leading cause in some countries (The International Spinal Cord Society, 2011).

Due to the consequences of the injury, and depending on the severity of the damage to the spinal cord, a person suddenly loses all or most of his or her sensory ability and voluntary movement below the level of the injury, and this impairs associated limb and organ functionality (Figueiredo-Carvalho et al., 2014). Almost inevitably, persons also experience incontinence due to neurogenic bladder and bowel and sexual problems. Bowel incontinence is reported to cause great discomfort and is a barrier to social reintegration (Burns et al., 2014, p. 1). For example, reentering the workplace and participating in social activities are hindered. For individuals with spinal cord injury, getting control of bowel function is often seen as more important than being able to walk (Burns et al., 2014, p. 1). In Jack's narrative, lack of bladder control emerged as an ongoing irritant and embarrassment, which although at the time of the interview he has more control over, its return still looms as a future threat and is among the existential concerns that periodically causes him to question the value of continuing to live.

BODY FUNCTION, EMBODIMENT, SELF-CONCEPT, AND ADAPTATION

Besides the psychological effects of a traumatic event, any change in body function has the potential to affect people's self-concept, change their roles within both the family and society, change the way they relate to other people, and represent a disruption of their previous life. It also signifies a biographical disruption (Bourke, Hay-Smith, Snell, & DeJong, 2014), that is, there may be a radical change in one's sense of self as an embodied whole. One's sense of an integrated self may be shattered. Changes in control of bladder and bowels and sexual dysfunction are among the most dramatically challenging and can affect a person's perception of the meaning and purpose of his or her life (Angel, Kirkevold, & Pedersen, 2011). Research into how people with spinal cord injury deal with the challenges of aging highlights that adjustments are often made. For example, within several years of the accident, many people with spinal cord injury experience increased satisfaction with employment. However, it was also found that with aging, there may be a decrease in satisfaction with social and sexual life and health (Krause & Bozard, 2012). What is not as clear is to what extent dissatisfaction with embodiment associated with aging changes can be attributed to the injury rather than personal characteristics, other life events, or the general experience of aging with its attendant losses (friends, family members, work, etc.).

During the acute phase after an injury, persons often experience high expectations for their recovery. While these high expectations may be beneficial in the short term, spurring hope and encouraging rehabilitation efforts, unrealistic expectations may work against adaptation in the chronic phase (Cao, DiPiro, Xi, & Krause, 2014). Cao et al. (2014) found that most of the persons they studied with spinal cord injury had unmet expectations of adjustment, and this was associated with a higher level of depression. In turn, depression decreases quality of life, interrupts activities of daily living, leads to loss of social integration, and decreases self-appraisal of health (p. 313). They also found that ambulatory persons had a greater risk of depression than people with more severe lesions, for example, tetraplegia. Cao and colleagues cite other studies where this seems to be explained by the fact that many ambulatory patients nevertheless have high dependency needs and have to rely on others for assistance. The presence of pain is another major cause of depression. From the literature, we see that there is much more to be learned and this need to know more provided the impetus for the first author's study.

EXPLORING MEANINGS OF BODILY CHANGES AND EMBODIMENT FOR PEOPLE WITH PARAPLEGIA

A prior manuscript documents in depth the results of the first author's doctoral dissertation work studying the meanings of bodily changes and embodiment for people with traumatic paraplegia (Moreno-Fergusson & Amaya-Rey, 2011).

A grounded theory design was used (Corbin & Strauss, 2007). Twenty-two participants were recruited by snowball sampling via the rehabilitation program of a university hospital in Colombia. Twenty-five interviews in all were conducted.

Semistructured questions based on the main purpose of the research were used to describe the processes and meanings of the changes in body and embodiment of people with paraplegia. Examples of the questions used are: What do the changes in your body that you experienced after the accident mean to you? How have the changes in your body changed your life? What is it like for you to need a wheelchair, catheters, and other equipment? Have your emotions and personality changed since the injury? How do you think others perceive you now?

The process of analysis led to the identification of nine general categories. Four categories explain the meaning that the bodily changes hold for participants; the remaining five explain the meaning of embodiment for the participants. The categories are as follows: changing the way of moving around, dealing with incontinence, recognizing the new body, caring for the body, being dependent and recovering autonomy, changing self-image, establishing a new way of relating, discovering a different way of experiencing sexuality, and changing the course of life.

The findings of the grounded theory resulted in the core category: "Discovering a new normalcy with paraplegia." Five stages were identified throughout the process: (a) losing self-control, (b) experiencing a rupture with the lesion, (c) losing meaning to existence, (d) adapting to the condition, and (e) acquiring a new normalcy

The results show that people with paraplegia undergo a process of transformation of their lives. Eventually, they learn to recognize new patterns of expression and movement of their body, to develop new skills, to adapt themselves to the use of accessories, and to discover a new normalcy, when they assimilate the changes in their being and get to accept themselves with the disability.

The study added insights helpful for the care of this population and by extrapolation to other populations who have experienced serious long-term physiological disruptions. However, in exploring this sensitive issue, information was revealed that caused the researcher concern and uncertainty about the extent of her responsibility to help Jack resolve his existential ambivalence and to keep Jack safe.

JACK'S NARRATIVE (FIRST AUTHOR'S INTERVIEW, WITH SOME DETAILS ALTERED TO PRESERVE ANONYMITY)

I met Jack 10 years ago during a nursing rehabilitation consultation. He was 28 years old at the time and in an interdisciplinary rehabilitation program. He was the innocent victim of a gunshot wound resulting in a spinal cord injury at the thoracic

11–12 level. We came to know each other fairly well over the next 6 months. He required nursing services every other day for wound healing of a Grade III sacral decubitus ulcer. He also had several admissions for urinary tract infections.

Jack is an artist by occupation. During the study recruitment process, he recognized me and expressed a willingness to be interviewed. At his request, we met at the hospital instead of his house. During the interview, he told me that this past 10 years had been a very painful experience, which changed his perspective on life. He also told me that some people are bothered when he tries to describe his change of perspective—they become uncomfortable. This prompted me to ask about this change of perspective. The following is his response:

> See, I tell you M-E, there are moments in which I clearly think about suicide . . . I mean, I believe that I have been in the process of dying for over ten years, since I got shot I have been slowly dying. Sometimes, when I get infections, which is what bothers me worst of all, I say that it is not about being in a chair as such, but the part about the neurogenic bladder what has hurt me most because it has been difficult for me to live urinating all the time; to pee on the chair, to pee in the car, to pee on the bed, to pee when there is a visitor, to pee on everything. So that particular part has been really hard for me. . . . The catheterization process I have gotten over it and I have even come to view it as . . . let's say erotic. To do this, to do those urinary catheter insertions, to pass that catheter through the penis and all that, seems really normal now to me . . . but the thing about the bladder really gets to me; the thing about the infections, really gets to me. I have had years in which I have been admitted into the hospital four times and that is annoying. I am talking about suicide because there will come a time when. . . . I am 38 years old right now, and I function and I have been rehabilitated, I try to do everything without asking anyone for a favor. This is not about pride, but about knowing that I have to lead a normal life, that I cannot use the language of the little finger [direct translation from Spanish], like some other people with disabilities use. These people tend to use this little-finger language to have others reach things for them, take them where they want to go, to bring them back, to give them things and even to ask for money. So I have understood it in a different way. I do have my job, I do my own things and I develop my own life. There are things that are difficult, especially when I am not able to perform my own catheterization, on the one hand. And on the other hand, the part of defecation is also very hard for me. Maybe nowadays I am able to do this in a normal way, right? To do a feel or maybe an anal stimulation so that poop may come out easily, I do that now with pleasure. But in the moment when I can no longer do this myself, that my daughter or wife have to do this for

me, I think then I will say good-bye to all this. Because truly . . . right now, after ten years, I am a firm believer in a dignified euthanasia. Maybe the word suicide is a bit rough and it sounds a little . . . harsh because a morbid society has interpreted that way, that suicide is about hanging yourself up, or throwing yourself into a river, the Tequendama waterfall. But for me, I see it in a different way. I think there are many different ways of suicide, right? Many ways to die with dignity, of dying happily, which is what matters most, right? To die happy and not because of rage. . . . This is like the view I have . . . of life right now. But of course, my life has been developing in a world that I like. I have been a historian and that has helped me a lot. I think the fact of having a certain level of intellect helps you enormously to overcome the difficulties because there are things in life that I really like. I like the subject of global warming and I also like the world´s politics, right? I would not want to die without knowing first what might happen in this world, right? This at least fills me with life. It fills me with life to know that I am an ecologist, knowing that I have some trees, that I have some animals, that I take care of them and that they are for the production of future oxygen, for breathing. So I see myself as necessary in this world, and as such, I see it as beautiful, right? Not because of my problem maybe I see something, hating the world, noooo. There are spiritual things that are not easy, right? When you are faced with the misunderstandings that may arise, the difficulties and differences from parents to children, from children to parents, the politics of countries, the hatred among siblings, the hatred among religions. But I do believe that we are a necessary element in this world. I believe that we are important for God and it is nice that I am able to feel it that way. It is more or less the vision that I have of my life and of my situation in this world, right? Of who I am in this world (2011, code:006.1.2.1-29).

AN ETHICAL ANALYSIS OF JACK'S NARRATIVE: IMPLICATIONS FOR THE RESEARCHER

Ethical Analysis

Ethical analysis is a tool of applied ethics, which, in turn, is an offspring of moral philosophy. Ethical analysis of a health-care practice question or a research project involving human subjects is a process that is aimed at determining good (or the best-possible-under-the-circumstances) actions. The goals of the process are to explore the aspects and underlying assumptions of a case or situation in order to separate out details, determine the validity of assumptions, and reveal areas where there are gaps in information. Ethical analysis "uses theoretical understandings, reasoned assumptions, and proposals about what is the good for human beings and applies these theoretical explanations" (Grace, 2014, p. 13) to a case or situation where the right thing to do is not immediately clear.

In health-care practices, the service goals of the profession provide the focus for the analysis, disciplinary knowledge allows facts to be gathered, and ethical theory and principles permit the nuances and aspects of the situation to be uncovered. The goals of nursing, as these have become consolidated over the years, are to provide a good for individuals and society related to health and well-being or relief from suffering (Grace, 2001, 2014; ICN, 2012). This is a professional ethical imperative. It is a societal expectation that nurses can actually provide the services that are promised in their codes of ethics. Thus in a practice situation, the goals of ethical action are to promote the good for the patient who has sought help for unmet health needs. The nurse, along with other members of the health-care team, is responsible for understanding what this person's needs are and how to meet them.

Goals of Practice Versus Goals of Research: An Important Distinction

The goal of health-care research is different from, although allied to, the goals of practice. Health-care research is undertaken for the purposes of developing generalizable knowledge (National Institutes of Health, Office for Human Research Protections, 2004) in the interests of promoting health and remedying disease for populations and society more generally.

Successful health-care research endeavors facilitate a given profession, or health-care professions more generally, in meeting the service goals. By service goals, we mean the ends for which a profession exists. An expectation of a profession's scholars and researchers is that they use their education, experience, and abilities to advance knowledge related to their discipline's purposes and when these goals cannot be achieved without the assistance of related disciplines through collaborative efforts.

This distinction of purpose that *professional practice* aims to provide a good for a specific individual or perhaps a specific family or community, whereas *research projects* are aimed at gaining generalizable knowledge (at least eventually or accumulatively) and are not meant to benefit the participant as such is important to grasp for present purposes. The goal of research projects is not intended to be therapeutic for the participant per se, although there is emerging evidence that participants in qualitative research can receive therapeutic benefit (Berger & Malkinson, 2000; Morecroft, Cantrill, & Tully, 2004; Murray, 2003). Indeed, the notion that we are researching something means either that we do not know the answer to the research question or we do not know whether the benefits of an innovation in medical research outweigh the potential risks of that intervention (e.g., drug, genetic, or surgical intervention studies). Related to quantitative random controlled trials, this concept of genuinely not knowing whether a drug or other innovation will be of benefit is termed a state of equipoise (Freedman, 1987). In qualitative research, we do not know or we have inadequate knowledge about the participant's experience of a phenomenon. However, without more insights, participants are unlikely to have their needs adequately addressed as we have incomplete knowledge about them. Moreover, qualitative research is most often undertaken by a professional who has worked with patients experiencing a particular phenomenon and has become aware of or has uncovered knowledge gaps. Lack of knowledge, in turn, interferes with the designing and enactment of effective interventions or the adequate provision of resources. In the present case, prior acquaintance with Jack in a therapeutic relationship coupled with her knowledge of and concern for the struggles of this population have probably added to the researcher's uncertainty about her role and its boundaries. In the following section, we use a decision-making heuristic to explore the unease she experienced.

Decision-Making Guidance: A Heuristic

Several different frameworks exist in the literature to assist clinicians and researchers to determine what the best actions to take in a troubling situation likely are. They are all essentially aimed at deep reflection on a situation and the separating out of important factors. They rely on personal, experiential, and factual knowledge as well as ethical principles to clarify details and aspects of a problem. The second author has developed a synthesized framework of things to consider from her combined philosophy and nursing education, knowledge, and experiences (Grace, 2014, pp. 82–83). This heuristic is not linear and not all considerations are applicable for every situation. In the following analysis, we use applicable elements to explore the researcher responsibilities in the case of Jack: What is the major problem (what is causing the ethical uncertainty)? What ethical principles apply? What supporting evidence is needed to validate or invalidate assumptions? What are appropriate actions? What is the effect on the researcher?

Elucidating the Sources of Unease

In conducting the interviews, I (ME M-F) realized how important the depth of exploration was in gaining insights about the phenomenon. However, as discussed later, the interviews were not always easy. My purpose as a rehabilitation nurse was to provide the best care possible for these individuals now faced with a condition of disability. For a condition like spinal cord injury, the resulting bodily limitations are difficult to accept and impose many challenges for the person, as noted earlier. But as a nurse, one knows that one's role related to the person as patient is to use knowledge and skills to provide a good for that person. The ethical principle of beneficence is the guiding principle for all actions. For spinal cord injury patients, this means optimizing and individualizing their care, providing resources and putting them in the best position possible to adapt and heal.

The struggle for me in the role of researcher was how to think of my responsibilities. The relationship of researcher to voluntary participant is different than that of nurse to patient, but it was very difficult to change my orientation especially in light of the fact that telling stories of their process of recovery can bring participants' vulnerabilities to the surface and elicit an empathetic response in the listener. The empathetic response is likely heightened when the researcher has previously known and/or cared for the participant. In the case of Jack, he had been a patient several years prior, and the trust that had been built at that time, along with my willingness to hear about his change of perspective since the illness, perhaps allowed him to share more than he would have done otherwise. So the main source of unease for me was the disclosure Jack made about his periodic consideration of suicide as an option should his dependence on others grow to be unacceptable to him. How should I think of the revelations he made? What should I do or say to him? How likely or near is the risk to him of this unresolved issue? What were my ongoing responsibilities?

Principles of Research Ethics

Understanding the principles of research ethics as these have developed over the years since World War II can provide assistance in sorting through this problem. However, as with any ethically complex situation, there are no easy or concrete answers. Each situation has nuances that cannot be captured by a general rule. The Council for International Organizations of Medical Science (2012) and the Belmont Report (National Institutes of Health, 1979) rely on the same guiding principles. The principle of *respect for persons* relies on the argument from moral theory, perhaps most comprehensively laid out by Immanuel Kant (1967), that each individual is worthy of respect and should not be treated merely as a means to accomplishing someone else's purposes. The principle of *respect for persons* protects the right of autonomous decision-making for people with decision-making capacity who elect to participate in research involving human subjects. This principle also protects those who do not have decision-making capacity—by providing guidance for proxy decision-makers. The principle underpins the idea of informed consent to participate in studies and puts responsibilities on the researcher to clearly explain the research, what is entailed, risks and benefits in so far as these are able to be anticipated, rights to withdraw, and alternative treatments or possibilities should the person withdraw. Informed consent also makes clear the role of the researcher related to the participant and what is available to the participants if they experience problems in the course of the study.

The principle of *beneficence* in research acknowledges that research with human subjects is directed to providing a social good but can pose a risk for the participant. Researchers are responsible for minimizing the likely risks to a participant and maximizing benefits where benefits are possible. In health-care ethics generally, the principles of *beneficence* and *nonmaleficence* have been discussed as separate principles. Beneficence is about obligations of health-care professionals to provide a good, and nonmaleficence is the proscription against doing harm to the patient in the course of providing care (Beauchamp & Childress, 2009). However, in research ethics, the principle of beneficence means that maintaining the welfare of the subject or participant is a priority and that harm must be avoided or anticipated and minimized.

Finally, the principle of *justice* in research has two main purposes. It requires that no one is excluded arbitrarily from participating in research that is likely to provide knowledge that will benefit the population and that people are not sought for research because of convenience (e.g., prisoners or the disadvantaged who are offered irresistible inducements). Second, it requires that studies are rigorously developed and carried out by competent researchers. That is, the study in order to meet the demands of justice must be capable of achieving its knowledge development aims (Council for International Organizations of Medical Sciences, 2012; Grace, 2014; National Institutes of Health, 1979).

Facts and Supporting Evidence

During the ethical analysis, it is important to ask ourselves what we can gather from Jack's narrative and researcher knowledge that can help to clarify the researcher's responsibilities in this case. Since Jack has alluded to having thoughts of suicide periodically, it is important to question, "How high and how likely is the physical risk currently?" From the narrative, it is reasonably clear that Jack is not in imminent danger—although in debriefing we will need to validate this. If he is in immediate danger, then the researcher has ethical obligations to act (the specific actions will depend on local regulations and resources—where possible, these should be anticipated and ready at hand). He is an intelligent, articulate narrator who is willing to discuss the positives and negatives in his life. His previous acquaintance with the researcher may have permitted a level of trust that freed him to reveal more than he would otherwise. In the narrative, he actually says that people do not generally want to listen to how his perspective on life has changed and the researcher gave him permission to explore this in a safe environment. While Jack is articulate enough to express his worries clearly, it is likely that he is not alone in having these sorts of thoughts; thus his are important insights that can contribute to the richness of the study. Jack also has many positives in his life and it is fairly clear that the existential concerns he has are anticipatory. Jack's existential ambivalence—recognizing the good parts of his life while wondering if the negative parts outweigh the positives—is not uncommon for persons aging with a chronic disease and who fear dependency (Greene & Goodrich-Dunne, 2014). Certainly, in debriefing him after the interview, we can provide him with resources and information that we identify as a need for him. However, the researcher's responsibility is to make it clear through the informed consent process that this is not a nurse–patient relationship.

The goals of the study are not therapeutic; although as noted earlier, Jack may actually experience some therapeutic benefit (Berger & Malkinson, 2000; Morecroft et al., 2004; Murray, 2003). It is only by maintaining the boundaries of the researcher role that such studies can be effectively completed. This is a matter of justice. In asking people to take the time and energy to participate in a study that may have some emotional risk, it is a requirement of justice that the study can actually be completed. If researchers cannot separate the roles and the emotional investment in the participants, then the research process may well suffer.

It is not uncommon for researchers to have known participants prior to a qualitative study, as their interest in a phenomenon often stems from their practice. Indeed, qualitative researchers have a commitment to understanding the participant's perspective. "They must provide the view of the reality that is important for the participants" (Streubert-Speziale & Carpenter, 2007, p. 22). Qualitative researchers are "instruments" of the process. For qualitative research to portray as accurately as possible the participant's perspective, the researcher has to be aware of his or her own understandings, feelings, and prejudgments about the phenomenon and control for them in the process of "bracketing." The origins of the term bracketing are in contemporary philosophy and there is controversy about what is actually entailed or possible in bracketing (Tufford, 2012); however, at minimum, the researcher is charged with trying to hold in check his or her knowledge about the problem in order to better capture the participants' experience.

In turn, a way to strengthen the credibility of qualitative research is to share the findings with some of the participants to see if the emerging themes cohere with their experiences. In the case of Jack, once coding was completed, the researcher shared with him interpretations of existential ambivalence related to future dependency needs.

Appropriate Actions

In qualitative research about potentially sensitive issues that may become distressing, anticipation of the sorts of concerns that might arise is important. Having a plan for what will be done and knowing what resources are available is important. In the United States, for example, an effective institutional review board will ask the researcher to identify counseling or support services and to share these in the informed consent process. For example, had Jack become very emotional during the interview, he would be asked if he wanted to stop, his status would be evaluated, and resources provided. Also in the process of informed consent, the researcher would share what her responsibilities are if she believes Jack to be in imminent danger of harm. As noted earlier, sharing insights that have emerged during prior interviews or studies about existential ambivalence can lessen a sense of isolation for him. In the debriefing process after the interview is completed, the researcher can help him identify resources such as support groups or spiritual guidance that are acceptable to him.

In the longer term, justice requires that the themes and insights from the study are shared with participants and ultimately published so that they can inform future care of the population and influence health policies to improve resources for them.

Effects on the Researcher

From this study and others, we can appreciate the emotionally difficult work that qualitative researchers undertake. The effect on researchers should not be underestimated. They immerse themselves in participant narratives that can be very painful to hear. Researchers may find themselves in moral distress. Moral distress has been well described in the practice literature (Corley, 2002; Corley, Elswick, & Jacobs, 2005; Epstein & Hamric, 2009; Jameton, 1984). It is the term given for feelings of disequilibrium when one cannot provide what is needed for a patient. When people experience unabated moral distress from feeling helpless to act, they suffer physical and psychological consequences and become less effective as nurses. Researcher moral distress has not been as well studied. However, from this narrative and analysis and what we know about qualitative research into sensitive topics, we can infer similar consequences for qualitative researchers. Thus, it is important for researchers to anticipate the emotional consequences of immersion in participants' narratives and identify resources to help them resolve or manage their feelings. In this case, the researcher reached out to colleagues to help her sort out why she was feeling uneasy and to help her put the situation into perspective. This is not to say that putting the situation into perspective will eliminate all lingering feelings—it may not. However, researchers are often willing to take this risk so that their populations will, in the end, be able to reap the benefits.

CONCLUSION

Using the tools of ethical analysis permitted us to explore a qualitative researcher's unease and uncertainty related to a particular participant's narrative of existential ambivalence. Engaging in this kind of analysis is important in separating out different facets of a situation in order to gain clarity. The analysis exposed a tension between individual and social good. In practice, nurses are most often focused on the individual good of a patient or patients in their care. In research, the nurse scholar is focused on gaining broader insights that can eventually provide a more generalized benefit to a population of patients or even a society. Gaining clarity about the different roles of practice and research permitted a resolution of the tension and revealed how risks and benefits to participants, populations, and the researcher can be managed.

REFERENCES

Alcedo-Rodríguez, M. A., García-Carenas, L., Fontanil-Gómez, Y., Benito-Arias, B., & Aguado Díaz, A. L. (2014). Adaptation process in women with spinal cord injury: The relationship between psychological and sociodemographic variables. *Aquichan, 14*(2), 159–169.

Angel, S., Kirkevold, M., & Pedersen, B. D. (2011). Rehabilitation after spinal cord injury and the influence of the professional's support (or lack thereof). *Journal of Clinical Nursing, 20*(11–12), 1713–1722.

Beauchamp, T. L., & Childress, J. F. (2009). *Principles of biomedical ethics* (6th ed.). New York, NY: Oxford University Press.

Berger, R., & Malkinson, R. (2000). "Therapeutizing" research: The positive impact of family-focused research on participants. *Smith College Studies in Social Work, 70*(2), 307–314.

Bourke, J. A., Hay-Smith, E. J., Snell, D. L., & DeJong, G. (2014). Attending to biographical disruption: the experience of rehabilitation following tetraplegia due to spinal cord injury. *Disability and Rehabilitation, 14*, 1–8.

Burns, A. S., St-Germain, D., Connolly, M., Delparte, J. J., Guindon, A., Hitzig, S. L., et al. (2014). A phenomenological study of neurogenic bowel from the perspective of individuals living with spinal cord injury. *Archives of Physical Medicine and Rehabilitation, 96*(1), 49–55.

Cao, Y., DiPiro, N. D., Xi, J., & Krause, S. (2014). Unmet expectations of adjustment and depressive symptoms among people with chronic traumatic spinal cord injury. *Rehabilitation Psychology, 59*(3), 313–320. http://dx.doi.org/10.1037/a0036868

Corbin, J., & Strauss, A. (2007). *Basics of qualitative research: Techniques and procedures for developing grounded theory* (3rd ed.). Thousand Oaks, CA: Sage.

Corley, M. C. (2002). Nurse moral distress: A proposed theory and research agenda. *Nursing Ethics, 9*(6), 636–650.

Corley, M. C., Minick, P., Elswick, R. K., & Jacobs, M. (2005). Nurse moral distress and ethical work environment. *Nursing Ethics, 12*(4), 381–390.

Epstein, E. G., & Hamric, A. B. (2009). Moral distress, moral residue, and the crescendo effect. *Journal of Clinical Ethics, 20*(4), 330–342.

Council for International Organizations of Medical Science. (2012). Retrieved from http://www.cioms.ch

Cripps, R. A., Lee, B. B., Wing, P., Weerts, E., Mackay, J., & Brown, D. (2011). A global map for traumatic spinal cord injury epidemiology: Towards a living data repository for injury prevention. *Spinal Cord, 49*(4), 493–501. http://dx.doi.org/10.1038/sc.2010.146

Epstein, E. G., & Hamric, A. B. (2009). Moral distress, moral residue, and the crescendo effect. *Journal of Clinical Ethics*, *20*(4), 330–342.

Figueiredo-Carvalho, Z. M., Gomes-Machado, W., Araújo-Façanha, D. M., Rocha-Magalhães, S., Romero-Rodrigues, A. S., & Carvalho-e-Brito, A. M. (2014). Avaliação da funcionalidade de pessoas com lesão medular para atividades da vida diária. *Aquichan*, *14*(2), 148–158.

Freedman, B. (1987). Equipoise and the ethics of clinical research. *The New England Journal of Medicine*, *317*(3), 141–145.

Grace, P. J. (2001). Professional advocacy: Widening the scope of accountability. *Nursing Philosophy*, *2*(2), 151–162.

Grace, P. J. (2014). *Nursing ethics and professional responsibility in advanced practice* (2nd ed.). Sudbury, MA: Jones & Bartlett.

Greene, E., & Goodrich-Dunn, D. (2014). *The psychology of the body* (2nd ed.). Baltimore, MD: Wolters Kluwer/Lippincott, Williams & Wilkins.

Henao-Lema, C. P., & Pérez-Parra, J. E. (2010). Spinal cord injuries and disabilities: A review. *Aquichan*, *10*(2), 157–172.

International Council of Nursing (ICN). (2012). *Code of ethics for nurses*. Geneva, Switzerland: Author.

The International Spinal Cord Society. (2011). *SCI Global Mapping*. Retrieved November 9, 2014 from http://www.iscos.org.uk/sci-global-mapping

Jameton, A. (1984). *Nursing practice: The ethical issues*. Englewood Cliffs, NJ: Prentice-Hall.

Kant, I. (1967). Foundations of the metaphysics of morals. In A. I. Melden (Ed.). *Ethical theories: A book of readings* (pp. 316–366). Englewood Cliffs, NJ: Prentice-Hall (original work published in 1785).

Krause, J. S., & Bozard, J. L. (2012). Natural course of life changes after spinal cord injury: A 35-year longitudinal study. Spinal Cord, *50*(3), 227–231. http://dx.doi.org/10.1038/sc.2011.106

Morecroft, C., Cantrill, J., & Tully, M. P. (2004), Can in-depth research interviews have a 'therapeutic' effect for participants? *International Journal of Pharmacy Practice*, *12*, 247–254. http://dx.doi.org/10.1211/0022357015002

Moreno-Fergusson, M. E., & Amaya-Rey, P. (2011). *Cuerpo y corporalidad en las paraplejia: Una teoria de enfermeria/Body and embodiment with paraplegia: A nursing Theory* Unpublished Dissertation. Universidad Nacional de Colombia, School of Nursing, Bogotá. Retrieved from http://www.bdigital.unal.edu.co/4121/#sthash.661YTOgY.dpuf

Murray, B. L. (2003). Qualitative research interviews: Therapeutic benefits for the participants. *Journal of Psychiatric and Mental Health Nursing*, *10*(2), 233–236. http://dx.doi.org/10.1046/j.1365-2850.2003.00553.x

National Institute of Health, Office of Human Subjects Research. (1979). *The Belmont Report: Ethical principles and guidelines for the protection of human subjects of research*. Retrieved January 24, 2015 from http://www.hhs.gov/ohrp/humansubjects/guidance/belmont.html

National Institutes of Health, Office of Research Protections. (2004). *Title 45 Code of Federal Regulations, Part 46, 102(d)*. Retrieved from http://www.hhs.gov/ohrp/humansubjects/guidance/45cfr46.html

Selvarajah, S., Hammond, E. R., Haider, A. H., Abularrage, C. J., Becker, D., Dhiman, N., et al. (2014). The burden of acute traumatic spinal cord injury among adults in the United States: An update. *Journal of Neurotrauma*, *31*(3), 228–238. http://dx.doi.org/10.1089/neu.2013.3098

Tufford, L. (2012). Bracketing in qualitative research. *Qualitative Social Work*, *11*(1), 80–96.

World Medical Association. (2013). *Declaration of Helsinki: Ethical principles for medical research involving human subjects*. Amended by the 64th Annual Assembly, Fortaleza, Brazil. October 2013. Retrieved December 24, 2014 from http://www.wma.net/en/30publications/10policies/b3/

CHAPTER 5

Ethical Issues in Family Care Today

Patrick Barrett, Mary Butler, and Beatrice Hale

ABSTRACT

The abstract consideration of ethical questions in family and informal caregiving might rightly be criticized for ignoring the lived experience of people. This chapter seeks to avoid such oversight by reflecting on ethical issues in family care in a way that is based on careful social scientific inquiry into the well-being of caregivers. The chapter draws on our research and experience in working with family caregivers, both professionally and personally. We step back from a practical concern with policies to support the well-being of caregivers to consider ethical issues associated with their typically hidden role. The chapter begins by noting the growing reliance on family care today. It proceeds to outline the dynamic experience of moving into and out of the caregiver role, before discussing key ethical issues associated with family care. Many of these stem from the risk that caregivers can come to share in the reduced circumstances and vulnerability of those for whom they care. Critical ethical issues are related to the typically "unboundaried" responsibility of family caregivers for the well-being of the cared-for person, something that can be contrasted with the more boundaried and intermittent responsibility of formal caregivers. Additionally, all too often, family caregivers encounter situations where their responsibilities exceed their capacities, but where a choice to not provide care will result in harm to the

http://dx.doi.org/10.1891/0739-6686.34.67

cared-for person. In discussing these issues, this chapter seeks to make the case for developing more responsive forms of support that promote positive benefits for both caregivers and care recipients.

INTRODUCTION

Abstract philosophical inquiry into ethical questions concerning family and informal care might rightly be criticized for ignoring the social experience of people, pointing to the wider issue of the disjuncture between philosophical scholarship and social science research. This chapter endeavors to bridge that gap by bringing conclusions based on careful social scientific inquiry. Our research has focused on questions associated with the well-being of caregivers with a view toward considering the need for better formal care policies. It draws on research and experience in working with family caregivers, both professionally and personally. In this chapter, however, we step back from that practical concern to consider the ethical issues associated with the growing dependency on family and informal caregivers. The chapter begins by noting the reliance on family care today. Our identification of ethical issues is framed within the context of our previous research, which has studied the caregiver experience as a rite of passage to capture the dynamic experience of moving into and out of the carer role. It proceeds to discuss specific ethical issues and how they might be responded to.

The paradigm shift in caring for people with multiple and complex needs, which over the past 50 years has driven the shift in care from the residential institution to the community and home, has resulted in new expectations of many family and informal caregivers, raising new ethical issues. Caring for an ill or disabled family member has become an expected part of family life (Lim & Zebrack, 2004). This is all the more so, given that families today deal with the consequences of the policy changes that have driven the shift from institutional care to community or home-based care. Families have become more, rather than less, involved in caring for members with impairments at different stages right across the life course, whether they live in the family home or outside of it. The significance of family and informal caregiving is all the more important, given the tendency for the greater longevity of people with chronic illnesses and disabilities, along with structural and numeric population aging. With more care being provided in the community as either support in the family home or supported living elsewhere, family and informal carers have become the "linchpin" of care (Nolan, Davies, & Grant, 2001, p. 91). This introduces family members into new normative stages and roles in the family life course, and these raise new ethical issues. Such challenges revolve around the demands of the care responsibilities with other accepted life stage roles, tensions around the competing demands of paid employment and family work, and issues of carer "burden."

It leads to practical questions about costs to families and to the wider society, how such care might be supported by formal care services, and the ideal arrangements of social service systems to complement family and informal caregivers (Arksey & Glendinning, 2007; Fine, 2007; Phillips, 2007). Key ethical issues, then, are related to questions about how family and informal care is integrated with formal care systems, including the vexed issue of financial and practical support for family and informal caregivers; the practical issue of organizational support for informal carers and developing sensitive needs assessment practices and training; and the need for greater recognition of the informal care sector and the development of shared understanding of the issues faced by family and informal caregivers by all stakeholders (Marin, Leichsenring, Rodrigues, & Huber, 2009, p. 5). These are, essentially, issues that stem from the tension in the relationship between informal and formal care. This is not a new observation. Twigg's (1989) analysis observed that family and informal caregivers were marginalized in the care process when formal care workers were involved. She asserted that "carers are on . . . the 'out-there' against which agencies act." Furthermore, care researchers have observed that not only do informal caregivers experience marginalization in relation to formal care workers, but all too often they are seen as a cheap resource that can be utilized to "reduce the long-term fiscal costs of care related to potentially avoidable institutionalization and worsening of disabilities" (Singer, Biegel, & Ethridge, 2009, p. 97). Nolan et al. (2001) point out that the most common goal in supporting informal caregivers is to maintain them in their role and thus contain caregiving costs. Such a view, he suggests, "is essentially exploitative and not supportable on moral, ethical or even pragmatic grounds" (Nolan et al., 2001, p. 92). Cummins (2001, p. 83) actually suggests that "the forces that encourage family care are minimally concerned with family welfare." Both argue that formal care policies that conceive of family and informal care as a free resource with the potential to compensate for deficiencies in publicly funded care grossly misrepresent the contribution and significance of informal care (see also Marin et al., 2009, p. 14).

Greater reliance on family and informal care has been occurring within the context of changing family structures, higher labor force participation by middle-aged women, and the emergence of "sandwich" generation caregivers. The taken-for-granted nature of informal and family care—it is "what one does" as an expression of family and neighborly affection, responsibility, and duty—tends to hide the fact that, typically, caregivers are female and the caregiving role is typically seen as an extension of the domestic work role

(Waring, 1990). The fact is, many adult children who care for a parent, particularly daughters, are also recognized as facing "sandwich generation" issues—caring for individuals at both older and younger life stages. Changing work practices mean more women in their middle years are in employment, and balancing care work and employment is increasingly a challenge. Employment consequences for adult children caregivers include loss of income and difficulties in returning to the workforce if time is taken out for caring (Bourke, 2009; Cook, 2007; Raschick & Ingersoll-Dayton, 2004; Stoller, 1983). So while family and informal care today have come to play a critical role in social care systems, it presents significant risks for individual caregivers in terms of the consequences of carer stress and burden and significant social, economic, and personal costs.

WHEN FAMILY CAREGIVING BECOMES EXTRAORDINARY

The care relationship begins with the care recipient and caregiver, but it generally extends to encompass a much wider constellation of actors. Consequently, caregiving places the individual in a context in relation to others as well as the care recipient. This involves at least three separate layers:

1. The care recipient, and his or her level of need, life expectations, and reactions to the need for care
2. The social and family network including formal carers where present, and their expectations, level of involvement, and recognition of the contributions made by the primary caregiver
3. The social care system, the availability of services, and conditions attached to support, and recognition and support of both informal and formal caregivers

Despite growth in formal care services over the past 40 years, family and informal care remains the preferred option for people with chronic illness and disability, particularly those with significant disability (Marin et al., 2009, p. 14). It is family members who almost always provide hands-on care, while emotional support and assistance with instrumental activities are also often undertaken by neighbors and friends and less socially close connections such as club or church contacts. Care provided by family and community connections reflects the goodwill, commitment, and capacity of social networks, and these are not necessarily long-standing ties as Peek and Lin (1999) and van Tilburg (1998) suggest. Such commitment can become designated as "caregiving," a set of actions that differ from the usual normative social relationships in everyday life (Walker, Pratt, &

Eddy, 1995), when family and informal caregivers are asked to increase instrumental or social and emotional support for an individual who is dependent "for any activity essential for daily living" (van Groenou & van Tilburg, 1997; Walker et al., 1995, p. 403). These include instrumental activities of daily living (such as cleaning, laundry, and meal preparation) or activities of daily living (such as bathing or walking). It is the level of need that is important in determining whether care becomes nonnormative and extraordinary, rather than the actions and emotions of the caregiver. In situations where the extent of the need is such that caregivers cannot walk away from an expression of dependency, caregivers cannot be said to have choice. Moreover, it is the level of need that determines the frequency and amount of care that is given, and, more importantly, the meaning of that care.

Informal care is preferred because it is seen as an ordinary expression of love, help, and support within families and among neighbors. Caregiving is, as Hilary Graham (1983) defined, a "labour of love," comprising two indispensable elements: the physical work of caring and the emotional work. Kittay (2002, pp. 259–260) adds that it is "a labor, attitude and a virtue." Differentiating between the labor involved in care and the kinds of attitude with which it is carried out captures what is required for "good" care.

> As labor, it is the work of maintaining ourselves and others when we are in a condition of need. It is most noticed in its absence, most needed when it can be least reciprocated. As an attitude, caring denotes a positive, affective bond and investment in another's well-being. The labor can be done without the appropriate attitude. Yet without the attitude of care, the open responsiveness to another that is so essential to understanding what another requires is not possible. That is, the labor unaccompanied by the attitude of care cannot be good care. (Kittay, 2002, p. 259)

Family and informal care becomes extraordinary, given that it goes beyond normal or usual care within the family life course (Biegel, Sales, & Shulz, 1991). Caring for a family member with a chronic illness or disability presents distinctive challenges. This type of caregiving is a significant extension of what families normally do, it is extraordinary to the extent that it constrains the caregiving family member from leading a normal life. Informal caregiving is, therefore, both ordinary and extraordinary. It implies an ongoing need and an ongoing commitment by the caregiver beyond the usual family care situation. It can be seen as an extension of family or neighborly duty, one that has important consequences for care recipients and caregivers.

ETHICAL ISSUES AT DIFFERENT STAGES OF THE CAREGIVING CAREER

Ethical issues in caregiving are evident during the dynamic process of moving into a caregiving role. The dynamic nature of caregiving has been captured by researchers who emphasize transitions (Bury, 1982; Hirst, 2005; Janlov, Halberg, & Petersson, 2006; Nolan et al., 2001; Olaison & Cedersund, 2006; Williams, 2000). Individuals move into and out of caregiving at different stages of the life course, and just as the person in need of care will be influenced by his or her life course stage, so too will the needs and experience of the family and informal caregiver be affected.

Process-oriented methods for examining caregiving experiences focus on key stages in the caregiving cycle, particularly the transition points in terms of initial points of change and disruption, periods of liminality and doubt, and reconnections. Such an approach has illuminated the dynamic experience of upheaval and change associated with the adoption and relinquishment of informal caregiver roles. The different care situations, the nature of the need or disability, and its trajectory, all influence how the care role is accepted, how the activity of caring changes over time, and the way in which caring will come to an end, or as Wilson (1989) says, how the role is taken on, worked through, and ended. In the words of Janlov et al. (2006, p. 334), these transitions are "marked by a starting point of change, through a period of instability, discontinuity, confusion and distress to a new beginning or period of stability."

Subdividing the transition into three stages—separation from a current role and identity; liminality, the uncertainty brought by change; and a third stage of "reconnection," the re-entering of the social world in a new life stage—allows for a detailed examination of the process of change and issues that arise.

The model illuminates the experience of *becoming* a carer and captures both the individual and social aspects of transition. The framework allows attention to be given to the stage of liminality, an "in-between" stage characterized by an unsettledness. The third involves reincorporation and reconnection with the wider society, with a new set of rules, roles, and responsibilities, raising the question of "reconnections" and some of the key issues with achieving "reconnection." Other theorists who have applied this concept to secular situations include Teather (1999); Hugman (1999); Hallman (1999); Hockey and James (1993); Twigg (2000); Frank (2002); Hale, Barrett, and Gauld (2010); and Barrett, Hale, and Butler (2014).

Separation: The Beginning of Transition

Family and informal caring is a moral or ethical response to the need of a family member, friend, or neighbor. However, with the provision of care in the home and community now being an aspect of the public service sphere (Fine, 2007), there are other means of meeting that need. So when someone's increasing need moves him or her across a threshold, then, an exchange with health and allied care professionals is initiated. Although the implications of the process of assessment are underacknowledged, this is a significant moment in the lives of both the person in need and the family or informal caregiver (Hale et al., 2010; Janlov et al., 2006; Olaison & Cedersund, 2006; Richards, 2000). For informal caregivers, it is associated with the movement into a new social role and identity, that of caregiver.

The process involves an ordinary family caring situation being transformed into a type of patient–caregiver relation (Efraimsson, Hoglund, & Sandman, 2001, p. 813). Bury's (1982) term *biographical disruption* seems to us to capture the nature of the experience. Becoming an informal caregiver is a dynamic experience. It can occur as a "drift" or a "sharply punctuated event," with subtle changes of relationships, group memberships, and social participation, and equally subtle changes in the attitudes of others. What makes this change significant as an experience of separation is the way in which it involves a challenge to the normatively defined role of spouse, parent, child, or neighbor.

The defining experiences are an initial realization of responsibility for care, a personal decision to take it on, and meeting with formal care services or assessors in the development of care plans, where the carer is officially recognized as a part of the arrangements for care. Cameron and Gignac (2008) observe that such experiences comprise that point in time where the primary responsibility of the family member or friend as that of caregiver is clearly recognized and expanded to such an extent that caregiving begins to define the identity and life choices. Ducharme et al. (2011), in their study of care for a family member with dementia, capture the significance of this when they refer to the way the inclusion of a spouse, parent, child, or neighbor in "diagnostic disclosures" mark entry into the caregiver role. Keady and Nolan (2003, pp. 25–26) refer to this as "the confirming stage," this being

> a period of transition to the caregiver role during which time caregivers are inevitably faced with new responsibilities. They must learn to cope with the losses and the changes in the relative's behavior that characterize the [need for care] and to plan for future care needs. (Ducharme et al., 2011, p. 485)

Typically, it is needs assessments or diagnoses that provide the basis for the formal recognition of needs and brings the caregiver into contact with the formal care system. The situation and capacity of caregivers is usually assessed at this time as well. Care plans, for example, formally take account of what the primary caregiver can do and what support she or he is able to call on.

Interactions with formal service personnel expose carers to dominant discourses of care, framing their role in the caregiving process in relation to the norms that inform the formal sector, with the effect that the caregiver learns the accepted philosophy and rationale for the provision of formal support services, such as respite care or other forms of funded support. This interaction is characterized by the power of the assessor to determine eligibility for assistance. In these exchanges, the informal caregiver has a relative lack of power. Assessors are the gatekeepers of access to formal support and the information required to get that support (Olaison & Cedersund, 2006). Care plans that incorporate an assessment of what it is the family member can do are thus developed, and these assessments and plans both reflect and reinforce socially defined expectations of caregiving and might be thought of as providing a social script for carrying out informal caregiving. The caregiver becomes aware of the particular needs categories recognized by the formal sector and begins to see her or his situation as falling within these. The cared-for person's needs are a defining element, influencing how the caregiver is positioned in relationship with the formal sector, for example, taking full responsibility as in the case of children or assuming increasing responsibilities in the case of older people. Situations vary depending on the disability, the level of need, and the degree of autonomy and control that can be exercised by the care recipient.

Liminality

The rites of passage framework suggests that separation experiences are followed by a period of liminality. Liminality indicates discontinuity, a threshold between what has been and the future, a state of betwixt and between and, as such metaphors suggest, the emotions here are of anxiety, bewilderment, confusion, and fear. Our analysis of the reported experiences of people who become informal carers leads us to conclude that they too experience liminality following the assumption of the caregiver role. In fact, many caregiver experiences could well be described as liminal (see Pereira & Botelho, 2011). Family carers can also be said to be in a liminal position in that they are neither professional caregivers nor passive family members. Their situation is often one of responsibility without authority. Stoltz, Willman, and Udén (2006) observe that family caregivers do "'worry a great deal about the future" and there is "much despair." Wilson (1989) referred to the type of experience we describe as "living on the brink." For individuals who are becoming caregivers, their ambivalent status in medical environments is linked with the little recognition they receive from health professionals for their interest in and knowledge of what is needed. They are expected to assume more responsibility for making decisions or in persuading the cared-for person about decisions, but at the same time they report that they are excluded from decisions that affect the person they care for, or decisions are made without consideration of the implications for them as caregivers.

The experience of liminality, as Olaison and Cedersund (2006) suggest, is not only one of confusion, anxiety, and of searching for a way through bewildering new systems but also of learning to negotiate within these systems. There is an important stage of learning the game. This is, however, a game where the assessors are in charge, controlling the engagement with the recipient and, when included, the caregiver. The subsequent allocation of care responsibilities affects caregiver capacity to control the organization of daily lives, influences choices about housing and household organization, and constrains the capacity for social participation as an individual, couple, or family.

Reconnection

Many informal caregivers become disconnected as a consequence of taking on the caregiving role, and many remain in that state through their experience of caregiving. Liminality is seen in the rites of passage framework as a temporary phase in the transition process. It is followed by a phase of reconnection to the broader community with a newly recognized and valued social standing that is characterized by its own set of "rules, roles and obligations" (Hockey & James, 1993). Searching for meaning is a part of the liminal experience. Finding meaning and making sense of the care situation in terms of one's life story implies reconnection. While becoming an informal caregiver presents many difficulties and stresses, the capacity to make a "larger sense" of the situation, as Pearlin, Mullan, Semple, and Skaff (1990) observe, has been found to be an important factor in coping. The way caregivers see their situation and ascribe meaning to it is linked with their ability to cope. Meaning in this sense, as Rubinstein (1989) defines it, is "the often affectively laden array of significations and associations individuals attribute to the events they experience" (p. 119). Giuliano, Mitchell, Clark, Harlow, and Rosenbloom (1990, p. 2) define meaning in this context as "positive beliefs one holds about one's self and one's caregiving experience such that some benefits or gainful outcomes are construed from it."

Reconnections, however, are not assured, and much of the research into caregiving experiences suggests informal caregivers live in states of liminality. That is, many caregivers, despite aspiring to express their moral duty to help a spouse, parent, child, friend, or neighbor in a way that meets their needs, have experiences of continuing liminality. The aspiration to provide help to a family member, and the actual provision of such help, is not sufficient to move the carer beyond the liminal state. From our observations, for example, many find themselves expected to carry the responsibility for the well-being of the person in need of care, while having little authority to make key decisions about that care. This is particularly the case of adult children caring for once-independent older people. Those who live in the same house as the person they care for are faced, often, with their home becoming a space for the delivery of care. Private spaces become public, and home takes on new meanings, which are defined by the disability or need for care. The need to be present as caregivers ties them to their homes or places of care and limits their mobility. Caregivers thus find themselves losing control over the organization of their daily lives, how they use their time being defined by the needs of the care situation. This has a profound influence on their ability to maintain social connectedness, and social networks are thus modified, usually in the direction of becoming narrower. Many informal caregivers become disconnected as a consequence of taking on the caregiving role, and many remain in that state through their experience of caregiving.

Addressing disconnection and facilitating reconnection in a new and socially valued role is, therefore, critical. But what does it mean to say that a caregiver has become reconnected? Reconnection means the informal caregiver is not alone with the responsibility for the life and well-being of the person he or she cares for but is connected through lines of support that allow the expression of the basic human inclination to care for a family member or neighbor. Reconnection, thus, implies a social context—connection with others. Stoltz et al. (2006) have captured this sense of connection when they describe the experience of "togetherness with others" and "togetherness with oneself." Stoltz et al. (2006) have studied the experience of caregivers of older people at home with a view to understanding the meaning of support. Their findings are most helpful in making sense of the meaning of reconnection at this stage of life. They examined what support for family caregivers, in the form of day care services, respite care, telephone support, online support, and group sessions, meant to those receiving that support. Their analyses pointed to the importance of a sense of togetherness with others in the care tasks as a key to managing and coping. While they acknowledged that there was a large amount of evidence indicating that the "effectiveness of interventions for family carers is not convincingly strong," (Stoltz et al., 2006, p. 595) with much research focusing on the negative outcomes of caregiver burden and stress, they were concerned with understanding better what characterized positive outcomes.

The idea of being connected can be taken to imply not being alone in the caregiver role and being able to share the responsibility for decision making or the practical tasks of caring. It is this sharing of the role that provides caregivers an assurance in, as Stoltz et al. (2006, p. 595) state, the "resourcefulness of others." Being connected to support provides caregivers an assurance that others, be they health professionals, care workers, or wider family and friends, will ensure things work out well and that they will be "helped to help their loved one" (p. 595). It is having their needs recognized that provides reassurance, and this can be contrasted with the feelings of abandonment, of having care situations dismissed or unacknowledged, which occurs when support is not forthcoming.

Alongside a strong sense of assurance in the resourcefulness of others, Stoltz et al. (2006, p. 595), along with Scorgie and Sobsey (2000), identified confidence in the "resourcefulness within oneself," a sense of calm and confidence in knowing how to respond in caregiving situations and in where to turn for rightful help. Caregivers who felt this assurance of their own resourcefulness were said to be connected with themselves, their own strength or ability to cope, and their capacity to ensure their own needs were met within the caregiving situation.

Connectedness in caregiving, therefore, can be understood as meaning "togetherness with others" and a sense of "togetherness with oneself." When caregivers experience a sense of togetherness with others, they describe "feeling encircled by action potential . . . [a] sensing of a network that would step in, should they need it, . . . [this being] a great asset to them in the reassurance of honouring the promise that many had made to care for their relative at home" (Stoltz et al., 2006, p. 600). A strong sense of trust that someone else "could step in and take over caring, should the need arise" provided reassurance that family caregivers would be assisted in coping with the practical and felt demands of caregiving. It was a sense of shared responsibility and knowledge that someone else could step in if required that provided this assurance, and of not being "the sole accountable bearer of the wellbeing of their relative or for making decisions pertaining to the health of the person cared for" (Stoltz et al., 2006, p. 601).

The notion of "togetherness with oneself" refers to the increasing clinical competence of the caregiver, acquired through the trial and error of caregiving. That competence leads to a transition to a stage where family caregivers are able to have a sense of equality with the formal caregivers and allied health professions they work with. They get a degree of control within the process—and learn how to get the help that they need.

While these experiences imply reconnection, a lack of connection implies ongoing liminality—being alone with the responsibility, feeling overwhelmed by that responsibility and, as a consequence, feeling unsure and apprehensive. The feeling of having nowhere to turn, no one to turn to, is captured in the comments of one of their respondents:

> Because this was unbelievably tough, this was probably the toughest time when nobody listens, they listen to you and say certainly, right, sure we will

> do that, and then nothing happens. I think that is really bad because you should keep your promises. . . . You called: "No it's not our pigeon"; "No, it's not us"; "No, we have to have a referral from the physician" . . . so that it was, mmm, yeah five, six places before we got hold of someone who could help. (Stoltz et al., 2006, p. 601)

Having presented the family and informal caregiving experience as a dynamic process that presents many threats to the well-being of caregivers, the chapter now moves to address specific ethical issues that emerge within that process.

ETHICAL ISSUES IN FAMILY CAREGIVING TODAY

Many of the critical ethical issues in informal caregiving stem from the fact that caregivers can come to share in the reduced circumstances of the person with complex needs. Carers' needs tend to be unacknowledged, but both the person in need of care and the family caregiver are vulnerable to poor and negative outcomes. Unrecognized caregiver needs lead to shared vulnerability of care recipients, carers, and the wider family. The caregiver actually comes to share the dependency of the person cared for, during the lifetime of the cared-for person and afterward. In fact, the greater the need of the cared-for person, the greater the risk to the caregiver (Kittay, 2002). In effect, the complex need can become the circumstance for reducing the resources (we might characterize these as social capital) of the family group. The manner in which this can push a family to the edge of endurance has often been kept as a private matter. Affluent as well as poor families can find themselves overwhelmed with the responsibilities of care. It is easy to ignore the extraordinary stresses faced by families when they lack sufficient resources, financial, social, physical, or emotional. How these are negotiated has important implications for the well-being of the caregiver, the cared-for person, as well as wider family members.

The Absence of Boundaries for the Potential Response of Family Caregivers

Since informal care is given to single individuals who are connected in some way with the carer, this relationship is troubled from the outset by the fact that there are no boundaries for the potential response (Levinas, 1989). Formal care, by contrast, is constrained from the outset by organizational pressures in the direction of efficiency. Formal care is provided by a range of individuals, with a greater or lesser degree of training and skills from paid carers to health professionals. The degree of formality in the relationship varies considerably, depending on the bureaucratic context. It is, in Ignatieff's (1984) terms, society's response to the "needs of strangers." While informal care has a lower level of social recognition than paid or professional care, it typically requires a higher level of focus and responsibility across multiple domains. The degree of responsibility carried by informal carers tends to be constant and without borders, whereas professionals have a more boundaried responsibility. It is not possible for informal carers to avoid responsibility in the same way as formal caregivers. Their relationship is sustained over time in the sense that it is "continuing," whereas the typical response of the health professional is occasional. The differences in the temporal and spatial parameters of formal and informal care are compared in the following table. Table 5.1 also identifies the implications of each form of care for the degree of responsibility that lies with the caregiver and the implications for the relationship between the caregiver and the cared-for person.

The degree of formality, depicted in the left-hand column, has implications for the time spent caring, the place for the delivery of care, and the responsibility of care. Informal caregiving tends to be continuous and sustained, it is associated with a lack of mobility for both the cared-for person and the caregiver, and the responsibility for that care is constant. Formal paid care is much more episodic, formal caregivers move into and out of the caring space much more readily, they are not tied to the space for the delivery of care in the same way as informal caregivers, and the responsibility for care is intermittent. Care and oversight by professionals is, by comparison, irregular with defined temporal boundaries, occasional, and mobile and has, in general, much more clearly defined boundaries.

TABLE 5.1

The Relationship Between Care and the Degree of Formality and Informality of the Relationship

		Time	Place	Responsibility	Relationship
Degree of Formality	Informal	Sustained	Constrained	Constant	Thick
		⇩	⇩	⇩	⇩
	Formal paid carer	Episodic	Permeable	Intermittent	Less thick
		⇩	⇩	⇩	⇩
	Formal professional care	Occasional	Mobile	Boundaried	Thin

The quality of the relationships is obviously different and Margalit (2002) used the comparison of thick and thin to capture this distinction:

> Thick relations are grounded in attributes such as parent, friend, lover. . . . Thick relations are anchored in a shared past or moored in shared memory. Thin relations, on the other hand, are backed by the attribute of being human. Thin relations rely also on some aspects of being human, such as being a woman or being sick. Thick relations are in general our relations to the near and dear. Thin relations are in general our relations to the stranger and the remote. (p. 197)

Depicting the care relationship in this way emphasizes the particular challenges associated with the role of family and informal care. It is a constant responsibility that is sustained over time and one that places real constraints on the caregiver.

Need for Informed Choice

Being forced to take on responsibilities that exceed capacity, however, leads to situations of unsustainable carer burden. Being an active agent indicates the possibilities of choice, and choices include to not care, to care, to have help, to be in the workforce outside the home, and to recognize care at home in terms of work, rather than solely in terms of family duty, love, and affection. All too often, carers entering the care relationship feel that there are few or no choices. Featherstone (1980) described this when she likened the moment of choosing to care with the situation of saving someone from drowning. It would be hard to call this a choice, where inaction will result in harm, and action, conversely, has such a peculiarly urgent quality. For many it is a kind of Hobson's choice.

The issue of choice touches on the interconnectedness of the choices that are made by both the carer and the cared-for person. But there is a need to recognize the importance of informed choices in care, the need for adequate support and preparation, ongoing responsive support, and the provision of information, knowledge, and skills. Nolan et al. (2001, pp. 92–93) talk of many carers who "feel ill-prepared for their role, lacking essential information and basic caring skills" and describes Askham's call for carer support as interventions that assist carers to "take up (or not take up) the caring role; continue in the caring role; give up the caring role."

Support at the initial stage of the care process, therefore, is critical. Family caregivers at the initial stage of the caregiving process are often

> at a loss of what to do . . . feel confused about which services are available and from which institutions or agencies. . . . Not knowing what to do and

> feeling abandoned or alone with caregiving could be labelled as feeling unsupported, for although the family carers are in need of support, they are also expected, sometimes by others but also by themselves, to support the person they care for. (Stoltz et al., 2006, p. 603)

The sense of responsibility to meet the needs of the cared-for person alone can be overpowering. Within this context, the experience of engaging with health and care professionals is critical. The quality of service at the point of engagement is a critical factor in determining the extent to which caregivers have choice in their situation.

Decisional Autonomy and Independence in the Care Relationship

Within family and informal care exchanges, family caregivers are often expected to, and often do, take on greater decision responsibility leading to tensions around supporting the decisional autonomy and independence of the cared-for person. Within the context of the care relationship, family carers often play a role in persuading the cared-for person, for example, to accept decisions relating to his or her health care. This may involve persuading care recipients to have an assessment, to visit the doctor, to change or review medication, to go into hospital, to have an operation, or to accept formal help. Moreover, family carers are often expected by formal care workers to take responsibility for such decisions.

This points to changes that occur in the relationship between the family caregiver and cared-for person through the care process. For example, becoming a caregiver involves carrying out personal care tasks that can lead to challenges to the norms of spousal or parent–child relationships, such as showering or toileting. As one partner becomes dependent on the other for care, the structure of the relationship changes. Taking responsibility for physical safety and hygiene of another is a key part of this changing dynamic. In one sense, the relationship is a continuation of family care norms, yet, in another, it exceeds these norms and redefines the boundaries and content of the relationship. For example, the role change can involve an adult child becoming a parental caregiver carrying out the intimate work of toileting, showering, and "cleaning up" a parent's body. The change is often experienced as a tussle for authority. These may relate to the management of medication, the performance of domestic work, the preparation of meals, personal care, and house maintenance. Each of these can be a point of some resistance and opposition from the cared-for person. Caregivers cannot, however, be said to have authority over the cared-for person—this goes against the norms of reciprocity and compassion that are often the motivation for the caring role.

Power Dynamics in the Care Relationship

Questions over authority and control in the care relationship, however, have been a key concern of the disability movement (Kroger, 2009). Disability researchers have voiced the criticism that the historical practice of care has reinforced narratives and perceptions of care recipients as dependent, nonautonomous citizens. This has led to some harsh commentary from the most articulate disability researchers: "Care . . . has come to mean not caring about someone but caring for in the sense of taking responsibility for. People who are said to need caring for are assumed to be unable to exert choice and control" (Morris, 1997, p. 54).

The criticism draws attention to the way caregiving presents a fundamental threat to the ability of the cared-for person to be self-directing. It indicates the existence of conflicting interests between the carer and the cared-for person. Furthermore, leading spokespeople from within the disability movement have stressed that informal family care is the worst possible scenario since "enforced dependency on a relative or partner is the most exploitative of all forms of so-called care delivered in our society today for it exploits both the carer and the person receiving care" (Morris, 1997, p. 56). These arguments have informed strategies for individualized funding that challenge assumptions of dependency and promote greater choice and control.

The apparent polarity, however, does not appear to be so great when it is remembered that both the disability movement and the carer movement (through its feminist links) have a strong commitment to emancipatory aims (Watson, McKie, Hughes, Hopkins, & Gregory, 2004, p. 341). Williams (2001, p. 483) has suggested that there should be new dialogue between informal carers, formal carers, and those who receive care and support. The individualized funding movement, which seemed originally to exacerbate the divisions between caregiving and disability, has increasingly begun to articulate common aims. Caregivers require some form of recognition for the vulnerability that they share with their disabled family members; people with disability increasingly want to include family care among the range of possible options that are available to them. However, neither party wants to feel that this relationship is marked by the kind of exploitation described by Morris (1997) earlier.

Real choice, however, should include family and informal care:

> Some people will wish to have their support needs met through personal relationship, which means there will still be family members and friends involved in providing care. However, this must be something that both parties feel they have choice over and, where choices conflict, that they have some scope for negotiation. (Parker & Clarke, 2002, p. 357)

The development of a range of alternative concepts, such as "help" (Shakespeare, 2000), "support" (Finkelstein, 1998) or "assistance" emphasizes the contractual element of the relationship that began to arise around questions of individualized or personalized funding. In practice, these terms have been used as people with disability have moved into the market for employing personal assistants, rather than in relation to informal care. As this relationship has become more commonplace, there has been a tendency on the part of disability writers to return to the language of care (Morris, 2001; Shakespeare, 2006). At the root of these struggles is a tension about what is considered "good" care; Disability activists, working within a justice paradigm, emphasize rights, independence, choice, and control. Care scholars highlight the underlying collective interests between caregivers and those for whom they care (Kroger, 2009, p. 406).

Relationship With the Formal Care Sector: A Need for Greater Recognition

A central theme in research on informal caregiving addresses the extent to which formal care arrangements facilitate or frustrate the abilities of families to provide care to family members. The way we appreciate the significance of informal care is evident in the way it is seen as being linked in with the formal care sector. This is evident in the way informal care is conceptualized within the caregiving process. The role has been characterized for formal care workers as that of an "informant," a "therapy assistant," a "coclient," a "collaborator," and a "director" (Nolan et al., 2001, p. 94; see also Twigg, 1989). Each of these perspectives positions informal caregiving in relation to formal care, with the former tending to see it as a marginalized activity and the latter as central to the care process.

In becoming informal caregivers, individuals build up detailed knowledge about the cared-for person. Caregivers learn the skills of caring by doing—by the hands-on care, emotional and behavioral care, and coping with, for example, the difficulties of dementia. Some health professionals are meticulous in asking for caregiver input, acknowledging their expertise and knowledge. Recognizing caregivers as experts, however, can present a profound challenge to professionals and the formal care sector who are less able to recognize caregiver knowledge, and, in fact, may give very little time to become involved with the family care situation.

Practical Responses to Ethical Issues

Becoming a caregiver is increasingly an inevitable part of the life cycle and a likely life transition for family members. Positive outcomes are often disregarded in the caregiving literature (Jorgensen, Parsons, Jacobs, & Arksey, 2010), given the focus on highlighting the vulnerabilities of family caregivers. There is, however, an association between family caregiving and both high stress and high satisfaction (Walker et al., 1995, p. 404). Both can coexist. Caregiving can lead to lives that are rigidly scheduled, with less flexibility and a loss of privacy, but it can also lead to emotional satisfaction (Scorgie & Sobsey, 2000). Studies that identify positive outcomes for caregivers suggest it can be an enjoyable and a positive transformational experience. It can improve the quality of the relationship and, within the context of that relationship, can be an important form of social and emotional support to both the care recipient and the caregiver.

Reconnected caregivers are supported in their caring through, for example, opportunities for respite care, and they may be linked with formal support systems. Social recognition of the needs of carers implies being included in discussions with the cared-for person and professionals. Reconnection implies a social context that encourages positive meanings of the caregiver role and the support to sustain that. Reconnection is finding one's feet as a caregiver and being recognized and valued in that role. It means not being alone but being reintegrated into the wider community, sharing the burden of care, feeling assured in the resourcefulness of oneself as a caregiver, as well as feeling assured in the resourcefulness of others, be they formal care services or other members of a social network.

With much attention in policy and practice concentrated on ensuring that carers continue in the role, and less interest in why and how they take it up or how they move on afterward, informal caregiving continues to be poorly appreciated within formal health and social services, and, as a consequence, these have been less than responsive to the needs of informal carers. Formal care services, however, are the primary means for support of reconnected caregiving. They can complement the day-to-day, round-the-clock care of family caregivers by providing episodic support and more specialized care to the older person when required. Day care services, respite care, education, telephone support, online support, and group sessions for caregivers have potential to supplement and enhance informal care. Seen as something that complements rather than supplants informal care challenges views that suggest formal care services somehow weaken the incentives for family members to care for their own. Such views are influential among policy-makers who look for arguments to cut the costs of formal care, but they are not empirically supported and serve only to weaken the capacity and sustainability of family and informal caregiving. The resources of the formal care sector, in terms of information, expertise, and funding need to be seen as complementary to the resources of informal caregivers.

In contrast with the view that an active formal care sector weakens the incentives and inventiveness of the informal "community" sector, we assert that smart policy informed by a grounded knowledge of the needs of carers, particularly at key moments in the caring cycle, enhances the capacity of both sectors to provide quality care for those in need. If informal carers are to be supported effectively and if such care is to be sustained, there is a need for a greater awareness by formal care workers and health and social care professionals of the experiences of carers and the issues they face. The purpose of such awareness is, of course, to support the environments of home and community, so that carers are empowered and able to perform the practical and emotional work of caring in such a way as to facilitate quality care that respects and supports the dignity of the cared-for person. Support for caregiving families ought to be aimed at not only reducing stress and ameliorating distress but also promoting potential positive benefits to the caregiver and care receiver (Singer et al., 2009, p. 98). Such supports should be considered as a matter of justice, suggests Kittay (1999, p. 132), and carers should be treated "as if their work mattered (because it does) and as if they mattered (because they do)."

REFERENCES

Arksey, H., & Glendinning, C. (2007). Choice in the context of informal care-giving. *Health and Social Care in the Community*, *15*(2), 165–175.

Barrett, P., Hale, B., & Butler, M. (2014). *Family care and social capital: Transitions in informal care*. Dordrecht: Springer.

Biegel, D. E., Sales, E., & Schulz, R. (1991). Family caregiver in chronic illness: Alzheimer's disease, cancer, heart disease, mental illness and stroke. *Family Caregiver Applications Series*. Thousand Oaks, CA: Sage.

Bourke, J. (2009). *Elder care, self-employed women and work-family balance*. Palmerston North: Massey University.

Bury, M. (1982). Chronic illness as biographical disruption. *Sociology of Health and Illness*, *4*(2), 137–169.

Cameron, J., & Gignac, M. (2008). Timing it right: A conceptual framework for addressing the support needs of family caregivers to stroke survivors from the hospital to the home. *Patient Education and Counselling*, *70*(3), 305–314.

Cook, T. (2007). *The history of the carers' movement*. London: Carers U.K.

Cummins, R. A. (2001). The subjective well-being of people caring for a family member with a severe disability at home: A review. *Journal of Intellectual and Developmental Disability*, *26*(1), 83–100.

Ducharme, F. C., Lévesque, L. L., Lachance, L. M., Kergoat, M. J., Legault, A. J., Beaudet, L. M., et al. (2011). Learning to become a family caregiver. Efficacy of an intervention program for caregivers following diagnosis of dementia in a relative. *The Gerontologist*, *51*(4), 484–494.

Efraimsson, E., Hoglund, I., & Sandman, P. (2001). The everlasting trial of strength and patience: Transitions in home care nursing as narrated by patients and family members. *Journal of Clinical Nursing*, *10*, 813–819.

Featherstone, H. (1980). *A difference in the family*. New York, NY: Basic Books.

Fine, M. D. (2007). *A caring society? Care and the dilemmas of human service in the 21st century*. Basingstoke: Palgrave Macmillan.

Finkelstein, V. (1998). *Re-thinking care in a society providing equal opportunities for all.* (Discussion Paper prepared for the World Health Organization). Milton Keynes: Open University.

Frank, J. (2002). *The paradox of aging in place in assisted living.* Westport, CO: Bergin and Garvey.

Giuliano, A., Mitchell, R., Clark, P., Harlow, L., & Rosenbloom, D. (1990, June). *The meaning in caregiving scale: Factorial and conceptual dimensions.* Poster session presented at the meeting of the Second Annual Convention of the American Psychological Society, Dallas, Texas.

Graham, H. (1983). Caring: A labour of love. In J. Finch & D. Groves (Eds.), *A labour of love: Women, work and caring* (pp. 13–30). London: Routledge and Kegan Paul.

Hale, B., Barrett, P., & Gauld R. (2010). *The age of supported independence.* Dordrecht: Springer.

Hallman, B. (1999). The transition into eldercare—An uncelebrated passage. In E. K. Teather (Ed.), *Embodied geographies: Space, bodies and rites of passage* (pp. 208–223). London: Routledge.

Hirst, M. (2005). Carer distress: A prospective, population-based study. *Social Science & Medicine, 61*(3), 697–708.

Hockey, J., & James, A. (1993). *Growing up and growing old.* London: Sage.

Hugman, R. (1999). Embodying old age. In E. K. Teather (Ed.), *Embodied geographies: Space, bodies and rites of passage* (pp. 193–207). London: Routledge.

Ignatieff, M. (1984). *The needs of strangers.* London: Vintage.

Janlov, A., Hallberg, I., & Petersson, K. (2006). Older persons' Experience of being assessed for and receiving public home help: Do they have any influence over it? *Health and Social Care in the Community, 14*(1), 26–36.

Jorgensen, D., Parsons, M., Jacobs, S., & Arksey, H. (2010). The New Zealand informal care givers and their unmet needs. *New Zealand Medical Journal, 123*(1317), 9–16.

Keady, J., & Nolan, M. (2003). The dynamics of dementia: Working together, working separately, or working alone. In M. Nolan, U. Lundh, J. Keady, & G. Grant (Eds.), *Partnerships in family care* (pp. 15–32). Maidenhead: Open University Press.

Kittay, E. F. (1999). *Love's labor: Essays on women, equality and dependency.* Longon: Routledge.

Kittay, E. F. (2002). When caring is just and justice is caring: Justice and mental retardation. In E. F. Kittay & E. K. Feder (Eds.), *The subject of care: Feminist perspectives on dependency* (pp. 257–276). Oxford: Rowman and Littlefield.

Kroger, T. (2009). Care research and disability studies: Nothing in common? *Critical Social Policy, 29*, 398–420.

Levinas, E. (1989). Ethics as first philosophy. In *The Levinas reader* (pp. 75–87). Oxford: Blackwell.

Lim, J., & Zebrack, B. (2004). Caring for family members with chronic physical illness: A critical review of caregiver literature. *Health and Quality of Life Outcomes, 2*, 1–10.

Margalit, A. (2002). *The ethics of memory.* Cambridge, MA: Harvard University Press.

Marin, B., Leichsenring, K., Rodrigues, R., & Huber, M. (2009). *Who Cares? Care coordination and cooperation to enhance quality in elderly care in the European Union.* Vienna: European Centre for Social Welfare Policy and Research.

Morris, J. (1997). Care or empowerment? A disability rights perspective. *Social Policy and Administration, 31*(1), 54–60.

Morris, J. (2001). Impairment and disability: Constructing an ethics of care that promotes human rights. *Hypatia, 16*(4), 1–16.

Nolan, M., Davies, S., & Grant, G. (2001). *Working with older people and their families.* Buckingham: Open University Press.

Olaison, A., & Cedersund, E. (2006). Assessment for home care: Negotiating solutions for individual needs. *Journal of Aging Studies, 20*, 367–389.

Parker, G., & Clarke, H. (2002). Making the ends meet: Do carers and disabled People have a common agenda. *Policy and Politics, 30*(3), 347–359.

Pearlin, L. I., Mullan, J. T., Semple, S. J., & Skaff, M. M. (1990). Caregiving and the stress process: An overview of concepts and their measures. *The Gerontologist*, *30*(5), 583–594.

Peek, M., & Lin, N. (1999). Age differences in the effects of network composition on psychological distress. *Social Science and Medicine*, *49*, 621–636.

Pereira, H. R., & Botelho, R. (2011). Sudden informal caregivers: The lived experience of informal caregivers after an unexpected event. *Journal of Clinical Nursing*, *20*, 2488–2457.

Phillips, J. (2007). *Care*. Cambridge, MA: Polity Press.

Raschick, M., & Ingersoll-Dayton, B. (2004). The costs and rewards of caregiving among aging spouses and adult children. *Family Relations, 53*(3), 317–325.

Richards, S. (2000). Bridging the divide: Elders and the assessment process. *British Journal of Social Work*, *30*(1), 37–49.

Rubinstein, R. L. (1989). Themes in the meaning of caregiving. *Journal of Aging Studies*, *3*(2), 119–138.

Scorgie, K., & Sobsey, D. (2000). Transformational outcomes associated with parenting children who have disabilities. *Mental Retardation, 38*, 195–206.

Shakespeare, T. (2000). *Help*. Birmingham: Venture Press.

Shakespeare, T. (2006). *Disability rights and wrongs*. London: Routledge.

Singer, G. H., Biegel, D. E., & Ethridge, B. L. (2009). Toward a cross disability view of family support for caregiving families. *Journal of Family Social Work*, *12*(2), 97–118.

Stoller, E. P. (1983). Parental caregiving by adult children. *Journal of Marriage and the Family*, *45*(4), 851–858.

Stoltz, P., Willman, A., & Udén, G. (2006). The meaning of support as narrated by family carers who care for a senior relative at home. *Qualitative Health Research*, *16*(5), 594–610.

Teather, E. K. (Ed.). (1999). *Embodied geographies: Space, bodies and rites of passage*. London: Routledge.

Twigg, J. (1989). Models of carers: How do social care agencies conceptualise their relationship with informal carers? *Journal of Social Policy*, *18*(1), 53–66.

Twigg, J. (2000). *The body and community care*. London: Routledge.

van Groenou, M., & van Tilburg, T. (1997). Changes in the support networks of older adults in the Netherlands. *Journal of Cross-Cultural Gerontology*, *12*(1), 23–44.

van Tilburg, T. (1998). Losing and gaining in old age: Changes in personal network size and social support in a four-year longitudinal study. *Journal of Gerontology: Social Sciences*, *53B*(6), S313–S323.

Walker, A., Pratt, C., & Eddy, L. (1995). Informal caregiving to aging family members: A critical review. *Family Relations*, *44*, 402–411.

Waring, M. (1990). *Counting for nothing: What men value and what women are worth*. Wellington: Bridgette Williams Books.

Watson, N., McKie, L., Hughes, B., Hopkins, D., & Gregory, S. (2004). (Inter) Dependence, needs and care the potential for disability and feminist theorists to develop an emancipatory model. *Sociology*, *38*(2), 331–350.

Williams, F. (2001). In and beyond new labour: Towards a new political ethics of care. *Critical Social Policy*, *21*(4), 467–493.

Williams, S. (2000). Chronic illness as biographical disruption or biographical disruption as chronic illness? Reflections on a core concept. *Sociology of Health and Illness*, *22*(1), 40–67.

Wilson, H. S. (1989). Family caregiving for a relative with Alzheimer's dementia: Coping with negative choices. *Nursing Research, 38*(2), 94–98.

CHAPTER 6

Self-Neglect

Ethical Considerations

Mary Rose Day, Patricia Leahy-Warren, and Geraldine McCarthy

ABSTRACT

Self-neglect is a significant international public health issue. Estimates suggest that there may be over one million cases per year in the United States. Aging populations will put more people at risk of self-neglect. This chapter presents background literature, self-neglect definitions and policy context, risk factors, and a brief overview of research on perspectives of self-neglect from both clients and community health and social care professionals. A case study is presented from the perspective of an individual and is used to explore ethical issues therein. A person-centered assessment within a multidisciplinary team approach is required for building a therapeutic relationship with clients. Capacity is a central issue in the management of responses to self-neglect. Ethical considerations of importance for community health and social care professionals include beneficence and nonmaleficence, autonomy and capacity, and respect for people's rights and dignity. A model of ethical justification is presented to explain dilemmas, challenges, and actions. Competence of professionals, multidisciplinary team working, informed consent, privacy, confidentiality, and best interest are also critical considerations. Effective decision making by an interdisciplinary team of professionals needs to be person-centered and give due consideration to the

http://dx.doi.org/10.1891/0739-6686.34.89

best interest of self-neglecting clients. The purpose of this chapter is to provide an in-depth discussion and examination of ethical issues and challenges relating to self-neglecting clients.

BACKGROUND LITERATURE

Self-neglect is a complex multidimensional concept that was first identified in the 1950s. Historically, terminologies used to describe self-neglect have included senile breakdown, (McMillan & Shaw, 1966), senile recluse (Post, 1982), senile squalor syndrome (Clark, Mankikar, & Gray, 1975; Sheikh & Yesavage, 1986), Diogenes syndrome (Reyes-Ortiz, Burnett, Flores, Halphen, & Dyer, 2014), and domestic squalor (Snowdon, Halliday, & Banerjee, 2013). Self-neglect is defined as the behavior of a person that consequently threatens his or her health and safety (Dong et al., 2009). It can vary in presentation and severity but is mainly characterized by profound environmental neglect and cumulative diverse behaviors and deficits that can threaten the person's health, safety, and well-being (Day & McCarthy, 2015; Gibbons, Lauder, & Ludwick, 2006). A case study, illustrating self-neglect sets the context to critically analyze ethical considerations and practice responses to self-neglect.

There are many definitions of self-neglect, but there has been no consensus on a common definition. In addition, there is no one theory that can explain self-neglect. Conceptual models and frameworks have been used to portray self-neglect, for example, medical construct or disease model (Pavlou & Lachs, 2006) and the risk vulnerability model that focus on internal and external vulnerabilities (Paveza, VandeWeerd, & Laumann, 2008). A conceptual model of elder self-neglect captures the physical/psychosocial and environmental influences and embraces a wide array of individual and population-level determinants of health (Iris, Ridings, & Conrad, 2010). Gibbons (2009) theorized self-neglect from a behavioral perspective and differentiated between "intentional" and "nonintentional" self-neglect and key factors related to insight, readiness, coping, and ability of the person to meet complex health and social care factors.

Self-neglect is associated with depression, dementia, executive dysfunction, reduced physical function, old age, living alone, poor social networks, alcohol and substance abuse, economic decline, and poor coping (Gibbons, 2009; Pickens et al., 2013). Self-neglect can occur in younger and older people, but research has mainly focused on older people (Lauder, Roxburgh, Harris, & Law, 2009). Age-associated morbidities are largely absent in younger people, suggesting that it may be somewhat different in this age group (Iris et al., 2010). Younger people who displayed features of self-neglect portrayed fractured chaotic life histories, that is, alcohol/drug addictions, poor physical function, and health issues (Lauder et al., 2009). Traumatic life circumstances influenced the way younger and older people coped over time (Band-Winterstein, Doron, & Naim, 2012; Day, Leahy-Warren, & McCarthy, 2013). There is a connection between self-neglect, animal hoarding, animal cruelty, and social isolation (Devitt, Kelly, Blake, Hanlon, & More, 2014). Animal hoarding may be a symptom of a physical or psychological disorder (Patronek & Nathanson, 2009).

Self-neglect accounts for the highest number of referrals, approximately 1.2 million cases, to Adult Protective Services (APS) in the United States annually (O'Brien, 2011). Prevalence of self-neglect is expected to escalate as populations age. The prevalence of risk is reported to be higher in older black people (85+ years; 10.1%; Dong, Simon, & Evans, 2012a). Low income (≤USD 15,000) is associated with increased prevalence of risk in men (21.7%) and women (15.3%; Dong, Simon, & Evans, 2010a). Data from general practitioner caseloads in Scotland reported that prevalence rates varied from 166 to 211 per 100,000 populations (Lauder & Roxburgh, 2012), and to date, there is no available data in England. In Ireland, elder self-neglect cases account for 18%–20% of the referrals received by Senior Case Workers (SCWs). The criteria for referral to SCWs is people aged 65 years and above who are living in conditions of extreme self-neglect, which is not well defined (Health Service Executive, 2012). Approximately 59% of the referrals come from Public Health Nurses (Health Service Executive, 2013). These estimates do not reflect a true picture of the continuum of self-neglect across populations, and, furthermore, underreporting and nonengagement are issues in this population group. Self-neglect is a serious and understudied public health issue internationally. Vulnerabilities for self-neglect will increase as populations age and this will present unique complex challenges for both health-care and other professionals and society in general.

Self-neglect clients have significantly higher health-care costs compared with other similar client groups (Franzini & Dyer, 2008). The potentially serious adverse implications associated with self-neglect include significantly increased mortality (Reyes-Ortiz et al., 2014); hospice admission (Dong & Simon, 2013); nursing home placement (Lachs, Williams, O'Brien, & Pillemer, 2002); hospitalization (Dong, Simon, & Evans, 2012b); increased emergency department (ED) visits (Dong, Simon, & Evans, 2012c); caregiver neglect (Dong, Simon, & Evans, 2013); and emotional and financial abuse (Mardan, Jaehnichen, & Hamid, 2014). The question often asked is, does self-neglect arise as a consequence of elder abuse or does elder abuse lead to self-neglect? The cause and effect relationship between self-neglect and elder abuse is unclear and Professor

Desmond O'Neill (personal communication, January 31, 2014) contends that self-neglect is "occult elder abuse."

Self-neglect is an emerging, pervasive, complex, and challenging problem, and it is critical that decisions made by health and social care professionals are evidence and skills based and give due consideration to ethical, legal, and policy contexts (Day & McCarthy, 2015). This chapter provides an overview of self-neglect definitions and policy context of self-neglect, executive functioning (EF) and self-neglect, and explores perspectives and understanding of self-neglect from clients and health and social care professionals.

SELF-NEGLECT: DEFINITIONS AND POLICY CONTEXTS

Different definitions and policy contexts and different service approaches are used internationally in the safeguarding and protection of people who self-neglect (Department of Health, 2000, 2014; McDermott, 2010; Working Group on Elder Abuse, 2002). Self-neglect is included in the lexicon of elder abuse definitions in many states in the United States (Teaster, Dugar, Mendiondo, Abner, Cecil, & Otto, 2006) and some APS laws in, for example, Texas do not require distinction between self-neglect and neglect by others (Choi, Kim, & Asseff, 2009). In addition, the term *vulnerable adult* is often used in the context of self-neglect (Ohio Department of Job and Family Services, 2013). The Elder Justice Act (2010) statutorily defined self-neglect as "an adult's inability due to physical or mental impairment, or diminished capacity, to perform essential self-care tasks" (p. 4).

Central to this definition is inability due to cognitive or functional impairment to meet basic health and safety needs and finances. This definition excludes a mentally competent older person who understands the consequences of decisions. Poythress, Burnett, Naik, Pickens, and Dyer (2006) differentiate types of self-neglect by including "inability or unwillingness" in the definition of self-neglect (p. 7). Nurse researchers developed a nursing diagnosis and definition of self-neglect that differentiated intentional and unintentional self-neglect. This captures the choice factors as well as sociocultural influence of the behavior and potential of the negative impact for the individual, the family, and community (Gibbons et al., 2006). In the United States, legislation requires mandatory reporting of self-neglect to APS.

In contrast, Ireland, Scotland, United Kingdom, and Australia do not categorize self-neglect as a form of elder abuse and neglect, as it does not happen within a relationship (Health Service Executive, 2014a; Lauder, 1999; McDermott, 2010). In Ireland, *Protecting Our Future* policy document (Working Group on Elder Abuse, 2002) provided the framework and context for the establishment of elder abuse services and 32 specialist SCWs who are social workers were appointed in 2007. The complexity and uniqueness of the challenges of self-neglect cases present led to a national procedural policy for responding to "extreme self-neglect" cases in 2009 (Health Service Executive, 2012). The policy document *Safeguarding Vulnerable Persons at Risk of Abuse* has included "extreme self-neglect" as a dimension of self-neglect (Health Service Executive, 2014b). There is no mandatory reporting of elder abuse or self-neglect in Ireland, and self-neglect is not included in the definition of elder abuse.

There are divergent views as to whether self-neglect should be included in the definition of elder abuse (Lauder, Anderson, & Barclay, 2005). Some argue that inclusion in elder abuse is appropriate (O'Brien, 2011), while other researchers argue that it creates confusion and ambiguity (Doron, Band-Winterstein, & Naim, 2013). Nevertheless, self-neglect can present simultaneously with elder abuse (Health Service Executive, 2014a). The etiology of self-neglect is multifactorial, and determination of behavior is poorly defined in relation to underlying causes and effects (Dyer, Goodwin, Pickens-Pace, Burnett, & Kelly, 2007; Pickens, 2012). Many risk factors associated with self-neglect have the potential to adversely impact the capacity of individuals to live independently and remain connected with their community as they age. Details are presented in Table 6.1.

Executive Function and Self-Neglect

Self-neglect is associated with multiple comorbidities and many of these can lead to mental health issues, for example, depression and cognitive dysfunction

TABLE 6.1
Risk Factors

- Cognitive impairment (e.g., depression, dementia, executive dysfunction)
- Multiple morbidities (cardiovascular disease, hypertension, diabetes, malnutrition, etc.)
- Poor/reduced social networks, living alone
- Poverty, poor economic circumstances, deprivation
- Traumatic life history (e.g., abuse in early years, bereavement, divorce, chaotic lifestyles due to mental health issues, and drug or alcohol abuse)
- Poor coping
- Older age and mental status problems strongly associated with global neglect behaviors

Source: Bozinovski (2000); Burnett et al. (2014); Burnett et al. (2006); Choi et al. (2009); Gibbons (2009); Lauder et al. (2009).

(Abrams, Lachs, McAvay, Keohane, & Bruce, 2002; Dong, Simon, et al., 2010b; Dong, Wilson, Mendes de Leon, & Evans, 2010c). Greater self-neglect has been associated with poor performance in episodic memory, perceptual speed, and executive tasks (Dong, Simon, et al., 2010b). A decline in episodic memory and EF can be an indicator of early Alzheimer's disease. EF (frontal lobe function) is necessary for planning, initiation, organization, self-awareness, and execution of tasks and is critically important for protection and safety and independent living. Executive dysfunction inhibits appropriate decision making and problem solving (Hildebrand, Taylor, & Bradway, 2013). The perceptions of six clients living in squalor who had deficits in EF and impaired memory were examined by Gregory, Halliday, Hodges, and Snowdon (2011). Five individuals aptly comprehended and assessed photographs of squalor situations; four displayed concern for persons living in such circumstances but did not transfer concerns to their own physical and personal living situation. A decline in EF was associated with severity of self-neglect (Dong, Simon, et al., 2010b) and EF may be an important factor in older adults who self-neglect (Pickens et al., 2013). To identify EF in individuals with self-neglect, a battery of EF tests need to be administered and completed (Pickens et al., 2013). The Mini Mental State Examination (Folstein, Folstein, & McHugh, 1975) is the most widely used tool for assessment of cognition by community nurses but does not measure EF. Judgement and determination of capacity and understanding self-neglecting clients' views of their situation is critical.

Clients' Perspectives and Understanding of Self-Neglect

A dearth of research has captured the meaning and experiences of individuals who self-neglect, and their perspectives are particularly important for understanding self-neglect phenomena. Bozinovski (2000) used a constructivist grounded theory approach (Charmaz, 1991) to gain insight into perceptions, understanding, and feelings of older self-neglecting adults. The findings identified that self-neglecting participants continuously strove to maintain customary control within their everyday lives as they dealt with a range of threats and challenges. Participants did not see their behaviors as self-neglecting as they strove to maintain independence. However, behaviors were often dysfunctional as capacity started to fail. Individuals felt threatened and distrustful when people interfered. Bozinovski (2000) identified two social psychological processes, "preserving and protecting identity" and "maintaining customary control" as an explanation for much of the self-neglect behavior. The researcher maintained that the term "self-neglect" as currently applied is a misnomer (p. 54).

Kutame (2008) used a multiple case study design involving 12 individuals and noted that participants did not interpret their behavior as one of self-neglect and saw the problems as outside of their own control. They recounted that they strove to do their best to look after themselves and "make ends meet" but at times they had to "let other things go" (Kutame, 2008, p. 171). Band-Winterstein et al. (2012) described experiences and meaning of 16 self-neglecting individuals. Four key themes emerged: "I was unlucky"; "That is the way it is"; "They tell me that I am disabled"; and "My empire." Participants wished that people would recognize their attributes and look beyond the presenting external image. Self-neglect was not related solely to old age. Life history and narratives recounted traumatic sufferings (loss of family members, divorce, migration, violence, and traumatic life events), and this changed the way older people coped with life. Participants described their lives as normal, while professionals viewed their behaviors as "personal and medical neglect" (p. 6). Day et al. (2013) described a combination of comorbidities and social issues including alcohol abuse, grief, fear, helplessness, isolation, institutionalization, and childhood abuse among people who self-neglect. Participants' living and personal circumstances were diverse. These ranged from having no home, water, sanitation, or electricity to living in severe squalor, with varying degrees of hoarding, frugality, odors, unkempt appearance, and poor self-care. The majority of participants did not feel vulnerable or see any immediate problems similar to previous research (Band-Winterstein et al., 2012; Bozinovski, 2000; Kutame, 2008). The meaning and descriptions suggest that the alternative behaviors and choices adopted by participants named as "self-neglect" may be their way of trying to cope and survive. Similarly, Gibbons (2009) concluded that coping abilities and personal beliefs were factors in intentional self-neglect situations. The choices of people who self-neglect over a long period need to be viewed in the context of their lives and stories. The term *self-neglect* suggests the problem is with the individual and does not acknowledge the contextual issues, which can be problematic. Home care nurses in the United States believe that people who self-neglect see their situation as "normal" (O'Connell, 2015).

Health and Social Care Professionals' Perspectives of Self-Neglect

Community health and social care professionals, especially community nurses and social workers, have always played a key role in supporting vulnerable population groups. These include clients with multiple comorbidities, individuals living in poor neighborhoods, and those who are socially isolated, frail, and at risk for elder abuse and self-neglect. The concept of self-neglect is socially constructed and judgement of risk is socially and culturally defined (Bohl, 2010; Eisikovits, Koren, & Band-Winterstein, 2013; McDermott, 2010). The perspectives of professionals and their clients can differ significantly. Severe self-neglect cases are more often referred to specialist services, and responses are at the discretion of the formal system. Self-neglect cases pose particular challenges and if they are not categorized as extreme self-neglect, they are not prioritized by professionals due to demanding caseloads (O'Donnell et al., 2012).

Gunstone (2003) found some agreement among community mental health workers in relation to the classification of self-neglect but no agreement on the definition of severe self-neglect. Exploitation by others and financial and sexual abuse were elements of self-neglect identified. A critical component of risk assessment was building a therapeutic relationship, establishing if self-neglect was active or passive (competence), and ascertaining information on recent and past life story. Decision making was supported by team process, ongoing assessment, interagency policy and procedures, and individual supervision.

Dyer et al. (2006) examined perspectives of APS specialists (n = 24) of the indicators for validation of self-neglect. The participants identified 125 indicators of self-neglect and described them in terms of deficiencies in environment, personal hygiene, and cognition. Assessment of client's decision-making capacity was a concern, and training, experiences, and "gut feelings" supported validation of self-neglect. The term self-neglect was used infrequently by community organization professionals in Australia and was associated more with acute risks (noncompliance with medical treatment, falls, visible pressure sores, self-harm, and psychosis) that warranted intervention (McDermott, 2008). Squalor was used frequently to describe situations that involved extreme environmental uncleanliness that included "presence of vermin and animals, garbage and waste and resultant odours" (p. 239). Health-care providers readily declined involvement with environmental neglect situations, and this created tension and frustration among professionals in other organizations. Professional judgements on causes of self-neglect were based on formal health assessments and decisions were influenced by organizational background (McDermott, 2010). Poor nutrition, falls, visible sores, self-harm and psychosis were acute risks for self-neglect. Squalor was perceived to be more dangerous and mortality risk was higher and required an immediate response. Participants agreed that medical assessments were necessary to assess if people were legally capable of making decisions.

Bohl (2010) described how APS workers assess and treat elder self-neglect. Self-neglect was constructed and operationalized by ethical and legal considerations, largely due to their role. They articulated that assessment of decision-making was central and questions needed to relate to capacity; personal health and hygiene; housing; relationships; and finances (p. 131). Participants highlighted the importance of honoring people's self-determination and right to refuse services when they were assessed as competent. In many of the studies outlined in the preceding text, the assessment methods used were not articulated in publications, leading to a conclusion that a valid and reliable method of assessment of self-neglect is not available. The majority of SCWs in Ireland indicated that there was no self-neglect assessment tool in use and classification of "extreme self-neglect" was open to interpretation (Day, McCarthy, & Leahy-Warren, 2012). The complexity of cases presented many challenges, and lack of legislation in guardianship and capacity contributed to feelings of powerlessness among community health and social care professionals.

Doron et al. (2013) utilized a phenomenological approach to understand aspects of self-neglect from 14 SCWs in Israel. Participants had difficulty in conceptualizing and defining characteristics of self-neglect and linked it with abuse and neglect. Managing self-neglect cases raised contradictory feelings, that is, disgust and rejection, empathy, and burnout. Community responses that disregard clients' rights and choices including refusal to engage with services can create conflict. Encounters with self-neglecting clients present ethical, personal, and professional challenges with regard to duty to care, respecting clients' autonomy, and refusal of intervention. The complexities of self-neglect cases coupled with conflicting values, beliefs, and principles of clients, professionals, and communities on balancing risk and safety issues can create ethical dilemmas and influence response and interventions. A case study of self-neglect is presented that illuminates the complexity of ethical dilemmas and assessment and management challenges therein. The difficulties in responses for health and social care professionals are outlined.

THE CASE BASED ON A HOME VISIT (DAY ET AL., 2013)

Arthur (name and details changed) was a 71-year-old single man, housebound, who lived alone. Arthur's home was a single-story terraced house in a small rural town. The building was a solid structure but looked dilapidated, the windows were black with dirt, and there were no locks on inner doors that were held back with empty barrels. Arthur's living room and kitchen were very neglected and in need of considerable home maintenance, and there were no cooking facilities. The living room was cold with no home comforts, the open fire was full of rubbish, and the floor was barely visible underneath heaps of rubbish, empty bottles of alcohol, and empty fast-food containers. In the living room, Arthur had a bed with no bedding clothes and the mattress was bare, dirty, and discolored; this was where he spent his days and nights. His general appearance was slim and hardy with evidence of filthy personal appearance (lack of hygiene, ingrained dirt on skin, shoddy dirty clothing, bad odor, disheveled appearance, etc.). Arthur had four cats that were positioned among the mounds of rubbish in the living room, a young puppy was running around freely, and there was a nasty odor of animal excrement.

Arthur's Script

My name is Arthur and I am one of three sons born to an Irish mother and I never knew my father. I had no relationship with my mother and my memory of her is poor. I have very poor memories of my mother, I do not wish to talk about her, and I would describe her as a "loose woman," a "prostitute." It is enough to say that my very early memories were: I was often alone and hungry for long periods and my single mother was unable to care for me and my brothers. My two older brothers and I were taken from my mother and moved into institutional state care when I was four years old.

Growing up in the institution was very difficult and many things happened there that I do not want to talk about and did not talk about for many years. I lived for 14 years in an Industrial school and left there when I was 18 years old. I immigrated to another country but life skills did not prepare me for this new and strange world outside of an institution.

Unskilled, I worked wherever I could, labouring on farms and building sites. I had what could be described as a nomadic lifestyle. I had no fixed abode and lived in different places over the years. These included a tent, a ditch on the side of the road, farmers sheds, and sometimes I resided in lodgings or took a room at an inn. I had no friends and was disconnected from family, and I sought refuge in the evenings in the local inn or ale house. I became very fond of the drink and frequently got into arguments and fights due to my severe drinking. I was unable to relate to women or people and was unable to form any lasting friendships and felt inferior and was isolated. I never returned to Ireland during these chaotic years and I avoided seeking out information on my brothers and never made contact with my extended family.

In 2009, I returned to Ireland and I was aged 65 years. I did odd farm labouring jobs to survive, my transport was a push bike and I lived in a caravan that leaked water. I met up with my brothers and discovered that my two brothers and I were among the many children that had been victims of child sexual abuse while under the protection of the State in Ireland. I applied and received a settlement like many other survivors of abuse under the Redress Board or Court awards. This changed my financial circumstances and the court provided money for the purchase of my first home. I have no relationship with my brothers and my extended family and I have no need for one. My family are my surrogate pup and my four cats who I love dearly. My home is a palace.

Ethical Considerations

Many ethical conflicts arise in health and social care delivery systems, and safeguarding and protecting older people who self-neglect can present ethical dilemmas such as those profiled in the preceding subsection. A central s as his family. Arthur may view intervening as authoritative. nd autonomy may feel threatened and distrustful and is more e access to his home and reject future interventions.

esponsibility, and sensitivity to cultural differences are key cal professional practice. A relational response to vulnerable -neglect recognizes that people's experiences are shaped by nd social determinants of health (Doane & Varcoe, 2008). on of community nursing practice is nurse–client relation- erapeutic relationship with clients is a key factor (Gunstone, on of Arthur's vulnerability, continuing efforts by a commu- e with Arthur will potentially lead to long- or short-term Arthur's preferences. Self-neglect situations can evolve over high risk for change over time (Day, Mulcahy, Leahy-Warren, Ongoing assessment of capacity and evaluation of risk will Part of the challenge is knowing what to do and understand- rest is being met.

as defined by Beauchamp and Childress (2001), needs careful thur's case: "The intentional overriding of one's person known ns by another person, where the person who overrides justi- he goal of benefiting or avoiding harm" (p. 274).

h is not person-centered and does not respect Arthur's rights, utonomy, and self-determination. The rules of informed con- missed in consideration of his "best interest." Prevention in out empowering Arthur to make small changes and it is not rotective. State policy and laws on self-neglect are extremely for example, categories of abuse, definitions, eligibility, man- scope of services, penalties, and guardianship. Community are professionals need to be guided by the philosophies, safe- protocols, and clinical guidelines of their member states and Service Executive, 2014b; White, 2014). Effective best practice ernance structures, comprehensive procedural guidelines, col- aring of information, supportive supervision, and a person- h (Braye, Orr, Preston-Shoot, & Penhale, 2015). Paternalistic merge in the handling of self-neglect cases.

n, community health and social care professionals have a col- s part of the multidisciplinary team in enabling and supporting people like Arthur to live in dignity and safety in their own as possible. Effective decision making needs to balance choice, mination, independence, and well-being and requires sensitiv- l careful evaluation of all options. Ethical dilemmas arise when

principle in nursing ethics and core values central to the code of ethics of nurses and midwife professionals is respecting the uniqueness of each person and his or her choice, autonomy, and self-determination as a basic human right (American Nurses Assocciation, 2015; Nursing and Midwifery Board of Ireland, 2014).

Asking "How should I act?" in this case leads to finding an answer within the relationship. Realizing and respecting that it is Arthur's choice is one of the challenges. Mary, a neighbor, made telephone contact with the community nurses, as she was worried about Arthur's living circumstances. The community nurse did a home visit. The observed and assessed vulnerabilities based on a comprehensive holistic assessment included extreme environmental neglect, poor hygiene, reduced physical function, low physical activity, underweight, and bullying from teenage children. Arthur was dependent on two neighbors for all his shopping needs, and they had also informally taken responsibility for obtaining money from Arthur's bank account. While it was laudable of the neighbors to be helpful and concerned, Arthur was vulnerable. Assessment of self-neglect was subjective. Some authors support the use of standardized self-neglect assessment tools (Day, 2015; Day et al., 2013; McDermott, 2010; Naik, Teal, Pavlik, Dyer, & McCullough, 2008).

The community nurse asked Arthur to use his money to employ a cleaning service and a painter. Home help services were offered to Arthur, but he was very clear that he did not want people coming into his home and making any changes. The community nurse referred the case to the SCW, protection of older people services and also made contact with the general practitioner. After several home visits and a multidisciplinary team meeting, there were different views expressed on what decisions and responses were required. Two of the most significant deliberations in cases of self-neglect are determining (a) if the person is competent and (b) if the person is safe to live in these circumstances.

The model of ethical justification in a case of elder abuse (Linzer, 2004) was revised, and a new adapted version for the context of self-neglect is presented in Table 6.2. This seeks to understand values, rules, principles, actions, and ethical challenges of clients and community professionals. It is understood from the case presentation that independence and autonomy are values and principles acknowledged by Arthur. He values living independently in his own home where he feels safe. The question is whether he has the mental capacity to make an informed choice about his behavior and way of living. Does Arthur comprehend and understand the degree of risk and dangers involved in his current living situation? Many older people have diminished cognition and physical impairment, and elements that need to be evaluated are vulnerability, safety, and capacity for self-determination (Harnett & Greaney, 2008;

TABLE 6.2
Model of Ethical Justification in a Case of Self-Neglect

	Values	Rules	Principles	Actions
Client (self-neglect)	Being independent and living in his own home; Arthur's choice is to remain in current situation	Informed consent must be obtained for a home visit and before executing services	Respect for autonomy and self-determination	Seeks help for shopping and accessing money, accepts home visits, refuses any interventions or cleaning services
Community health and social care professionals	Therapeutic relationship between community health and social care professional and the client that is based on trust, understanding, compassion, and support serves to empower the client to make life choices Ensuring ethical practice of community nursing and social work is embedded in national and international codes of ethics Maintaining the highest standards of quality is foremost	Informed consent is necessary prior to intervention	Respect choice, autonomy, and self-determination. Resolve ambiguity in duty of care/best interest Social justice (challenging discrimination, recognizing diversity, working in solidarity with team members, and challenging unjust policies and practice)	Multidisciplinary team approach in management of risk: intervene/duty of care vs. do not intervene Whose best interest? What are the risks if we intervene? Wait for change in situation

perspectives differ. Arthur's case study portrays and describes how past and present social conditions were shaped biologically, psychologically, interpersonally, and culturally. Contextualizing risk and relationally entering into Arthur's situation and undertaking a comprehensive holistic assessment is a necessity. Multidisciplinary working is key, as is ongoing review and assessment of capacity and risk. Self-neglect can present significant demands and ethical challenges for health-care providers and professionals. Community health and social care professionals need training in self-neglect and risk assessment of clients. This is to ensure that they are reflective, knowledgeable, and skilled in safeguarding older people vulnerable for self-neglect. Empirical research into ethical issues including how community nursing and social workers conceptualize and handle ethical difficulties and self-neglect is required.

REFERENCES

Abrams, R. C., Lachs, M., McAvay, G., Keohane, D. J., & Bruce, M. L. (2002). Predictors of self-neglect in community-dwelling elders. *American Journal of Psychiatry, 159*(10), 1724–1730.

American Nurses Assocciation. (2015). *Code of ethics for nurses with interpretive statements.* Retrieved from http://www.nursingworld.org/MainMenuCategories/EthicsStandards/CodeofEthicsforNurses/Code-of-Ethics-For-Nurses.html

Band-Winterstein, T., Doron, I., & Naim, S. (2012). Elder self neglect: A geriatric syndrome or a life course story? *Journal of Aging Studies, 26*(2), 109–118.

Beauchamp, T., & Childress, J. (2001). *Principles of biomedical ethics.* Oxford: Oxford University Press.

Bohl, W. (2010). *Investigating elder self-neglect: Interviews with adult protective service workers* (Electronic Thesis or Dissertation). Retrieved from https://etd.ohiolink.edu/

Bozinovski, S. D. (2000). Older self-neglecters: Interpersonal problems and the maintenance of self-continuity. *Journal of Elder Abuse & Neglect, 12*(1), 37–56.

Braye, S., Orr, D., Preston-Shoot, M., & Penhale, B. (2015). Learning lessons about self-neglect? An Analysis of serious case reviews. *The Journal of Adult Protection, 17*(1), 3–18.

Burnett, J., Dyer, C. B., Halphen, J. M., Achenbaum, W. A., Green, C. E., Booker, J. G., et al. (2014). Four subtypes of self neglect in older adults: Results of a latent class analysis. *Journal of the American Geriatrics Society, 62*(6), 1127–1132.

Burnett, J., Regev, T., Pickens, S., Prati, L. L., Aung, K., Moore, J., et al. (2006). Social networks: A profile of the elderly who self-neglect. *Journal of Elder Abuse & Neglect, 18*(4), 35–49.

Charmaz, K. (Eds.). (1991). *Good days, bad days: The self in chronic illness and time.* New Brunswick, NJ: Rutgers University Press.

Choi, N. G., Kim, J., & Asseff, J. (2009). Self-neglect and neglect of vulnerable older adults: Reexamination of etiology. *Journal of Gerontological Social Work, 52*(2), 171–187.

Clark, A. N. G., Mankikar, G. D., & Gray, I. (1975). Diogenes syndrome clinical study of gross self-neglect in old age. *The Lancet, 1*(7903), 366–368.

Day, M. R. (2015). *Self-neglect: Development and evaluation of a self-neglect (SN-37) Measurment instrument.* Unpublished doctoral dissertation. University College Cork, Ireland.

Day, M. R., Leahy-Warren, P., & McCarthy, G. (2013). Perceptions and views of self-neglect: A client-centered perspective. *Journal of Elder Abuse & Neglect, 25*(1), 76–94.

Day, M. R., & McCarthy, G. (2015). A national cross sectional study of community nurses and social workers knowledge of self-neglect. *Age and Ageing, 44*, 717–720. Retrieved from http://ageing.oxfordjournals.org/content/early/2015/03/06/ageing.afv025.abstract

Day, M. R., McCarthy, G., & Leahy-Warren, P. (2012). Professional social workers' views on self-neglect: An exploratory study. *British Journal of Social Work, 42*(4), 725–743.

Day, M. R., Mulcahy, H., Leahy-Warren, P., & Downey, J. (2015). Self-neglect: A case study and implications for clinical practice. *British Journal of Community Nursing, 20*(3), 110, 112–115.

Department of Health. (2000). *No secrets*. London: Department of Health.

Department of Health. (2014). *Care act 2014*. Retrieved from http://www.legislation.gov.uk/ukpga/2014/23/contents/enacted

Devitt, C., Kelly, P., Blake, M., Hanlon, A., & More, S. J. (2014). Dilemmas experienced by government veterinarians when responding professionally to farm animal welfare incidents in Ireland. *Veterinary Record Open, 1*(1). Retrived from http://vetrecordopen.bmj.com/content/1/1/e000003.full

Doane, G. H., & Varcoe, C. (2008). Knowledge translation in everyday nursing: From evidence-based to inquiry-based practice. *Advances in Nursing Science, 31*(4), 283–295.

Dong, X., Fulmer, T., Simon, M., Mendes de Leon, C., Fulmer, T., Beck, T., et al. (2009). Elder selfneglect and abuse and mortality risk in a community-dwelling population. *Journal of the American Medical Association, 302*(5), 517–526.

Dong, X., & Simon, M. A. (2013). Association between elder self-neglect and hospice utilization in a community population. *Archives of Gerontology and Geriatrics, 56*(1), 192–198.

Dong, X., Simon, M. A., & Evans, D. A. (2012a). Prevalence of self-neglect across gender, race, and socioeconomic status: Findings from the Chicago Health and Aging Project. *Gerontology, 58*, 258–268.

Dong, X., Simon, M. A., & Evans, D. A. (2012b). Elder self-neglect and hospitalization: Findings from the Chicago Health and Aging Project. *Journal of the American Geriatrics Society, 60*(2), 202–209.

Dong, X., Simon, M. A., & Evans, D. A. (2012c). Prospective study of the elder self-neglect and ED use in a community population. *The American Journal of Emergency Medicine, 30*(4), 553–561.

Dong, X., Simon, M., A., & Evans, D. A. (2013). Elder self-neglect is associated with increased risk for elder abuse in a community-dwelling population: Findings from the Chicago Health and Aging Project. *Journal of Aging and Health, 25*(1), 80–96.

Dong, X., Simon, M. A., & Evans, D. A. (2010a). Cross-sectional study of the characteristics of reported elder self-neglect in a community-dwelling population: Findings from a population-based cohort. *Gerontology, 56*(3), 325–334.

Dong, X., Simon, M. A., Wilson, R. S., Mendes de Leon, C. F., Rajan, K. B., & Evans, D. A. (2010b). Decline in cognitive function and risk of elder self-neglect: Finding from the Chicago Health Aging Project. *Journal of the American Geriatrics Society, 58*(12), 2292–2299.

Dong, X., Wilson, R. S., Mendes de Leon, C. F., & Evans, D. A. (2010c). Self-neglect and cognitive function among community-dwelling older persons. *International Journal of Geriatric Psychiatry, 25*(8), 798–806.

Doron, I., Band-Winterstein, T., & Naim, S., (2013). The meaning of elder self-neglect: Social workers' perspective. *The International Journal of Aging and Human Development, 77*(1), 17–36.

Dyer, C. B., Goodwin, J. S., Pickens-Pace, S., Burnett, J., & Kelly, P. A. (2007). Self-neglect among the elderly: A model based on more than 500 patients seen by a geriatric medicine team. *American Journal of Public Health, 97*(9), 1671–1676.

Dyer, C. B., Toronjo, C., Cunningham, M., Festa, N. A., Pavlik, V. N., Hyman, D. J., et al. (2006). The key elements of elder neglect: A survey of adult protective service workers. *Journal of Elder Abuse & Neglect, 17*(4), 1–10.

Eisikovits, Z., Koren, C., & Band-Winterstein, T. (2013). The social construction of social problems: The case of elder abuse and neglect. *International Psychogeriatrics* (Special Issue), *25*(8), 1291–1298.

Elder Justice Act. (2010). Retrived from http://www.nlrc.aoa.gov/Legal_Issues/Elder_Abuse/Elder_Justice_Act.aspx

Folstein, M. F., Folstein, S. E., & McHugh, P. R. (1975). "Mini-mental state." A practical method for grading the cognitive state of patients for the clinician. *Journal of Psychiatric Research, 12*, 189–198.

Franzini, L., & Dyer, C. B. (2008). Healthcare costs and utilization of vulnerable elderly people reported to adult protective services for self-neglect. *Journal of the American Geriatrics Society, 56*(4), 667–676.

Gibbons, S. (2009). Theory synthesis for self-neglect: A health and social phenomenon. *Nursing Research, 58*(3), 194–200.

Gibbons, S., Lauder, W., & Ludwick, R. (2006). Self-neglect: A proposed new NANDA diagnosis. *International Journal of Nursing Terminologies and Classifications, 17*(1), 10–18.

Gregory, C., Halliday, G., Hodges, J., & Snowdon, J. (2011). Living in squalor: Neuropsychological function, emotional processing and squalor perception in patients found living in squalor. *International Psychogeriatrics, 23*(5), 724–731.

Gunstone, S. (2003). Risk assessment and management of patients whom self-neglect: A 'grey area' for mental health workers. *Journal of Psychiatric and Mental Health Nursing, 10*(3), 287–296.

Harnett, P. J., & Greaney, A. M. (2008). Operationalizing autonomy: Solutions for mental health nursing practice. *Journal of Psychiatric and Mental Health Nursing, 15*(1), 2–9.

Health Service Executive (2012). *Policy and procedures for responding to allegations of extreme self-neglect*. HSE, Dublin.

Health Service Executive. (2013). *Open your eyes there is no excuse for elder abuse*. Dublin, Ireland: Author.

Health Service Executive. (2014a). *Open your eyes there is no excuse for elder abuse*. Dublin, Ireland: Author.

Health Service Executive. (2014b). *Safeguarding vulnerable persons at risk of Abuse: National policy and procedures*. Dublin, Ireland: HSE, Social Care Division.

Hildebrand, C., Taylor, M., & Bradway, C. (2013). Elder self-neglect: The failure of coping because of cognitive and functional impairments. *Journal of the American Association of Nurse Practitioners, 26*(8), 452–462.

Iris, M., Ridings, J. W., & Conrad, K. J. (2010). The development of a conceptual model for understanding elder self-neglect. *The Gerontologist, 50*(3), 303–315.

Kutame, M. M. (2008). *Understanding self-neglect from the older person's perspective*. ProQuest Information & Learning, US. Retrieved from http://search.ebscohost.com/login.aspx?direct=true&db=psyh&AN=2008-99011-293&site=ehost-live Available from EBSCOhost psyh database

Lachs, M. S., Williams, C. S., O'Brien, S., & Pillemer, K. A. (2002). Adult protective service use and nursing home placement. *The Gerontologist, 42*(6), 734–739.

Lauder, W. (1999). Constructions of self-neglect: A multiple case study design. *Nursing Inquiry, 6*(1), 48–57.

Lauder, W., Anderson, I., & Barclay, A. (2005). Housing and self-neglect: The responses of health, social care and environmental health agencies. *Journal of Interprofessional Care, 19*(4), 317–325.

Lauder, W., & Roxburgh, M. (2012). Self-neglect consultation rates and comorbidities in primary care. *International Journal of Nursing Practice, 18*(5), 454–461.

Lauder, W., Roxburgh, M., Harris, J., & Law, J. (2009). Developing self-neglect theory: Analysis of related and atypical cases of people identified as self-neglecting. *Journal of Psychiatric and Mental Health Nursing, 16*(5), 447–454.

Lee, M., & Kropf, N. P. (2013). Capacity Evaluation Screen—Social Work (CES-SW): Development of a brief instrument. *Journal of Social Service Research, 39*(4), 1–9.

Linzer, N. (2004). An ethical dilemma in elder abuse. *Journal of Gerontological Social Work, 43*(2–3), 165–173.

MacLeod, H., & Stadnyk, R. L. (2015). Risk: 'I know it when I see it': How health and social practitioners defined and evaluated living at risk among community-dwelling older adults. *Health, Risk & Society, 17*(1), 46–63.

Mardan, H., Jaehnichen, G., & Hamid, T. A. (2014). Is self neglect associated with the emotional and financial abuse in community-dueling? *IOSR Journal of Nursing and Health Science (IOSR-JNHS), 3*(3), 51–56.

McDermott, S. (2008). The devil is in the details: Self-neglect in Australia. *Journal of Elder Abuse & Neglect, 20*(3), 231–250.

McDermott, S. (2010). Professional judgements of risk and capacity in situations of self-neglect among older people. *Ageing and Society, 30*(06), 1055–1072.

McMillan, D., & Shaw, P. (1966). Senile breakdown in standards of personal and environmental cleanliness. *British Medical Journal, 2*(5521), 1032–1037.

Naik, A. D., Teal, C. R., Pavlik, V. N., Dyer, C. B., & McCullough, L. B. (2008). Conceptual challenges and practical approaches to screening capacity for self-care and protection in vulnerable older adults. *Journal of the American Geriatrics Society, 56*, S266–S270.

Nursing and Midwifery Board of Ireland. (2014). *Code of professional conduct and ethics for registered nurses and registered midwifes.* Dublin: Nursing & Midwifery Board of Ireland.

O'Brien, J. G. (2011). Self-neglect in old age. *Aging Health, 7*(4), 573–581.

O'Connell, Y. J. (2015). Home care nurses' experiences with and perceptions of elder self-neglect. *Home Healthcare Now, 33*(1), 31–38.

O'Donnell, D., Treacy, M. P., Fealy, G., Lyons, I., Phelan, A., Lafferty, A., et al. (2012). *Managing elder abuse in Ireland: The senior case worker's experience*. Dublin, Ireland: UCD.

Ohio Department of Job and Family Services. (2013). *Adult protective services protocol 2013.* Retrived from http://jfs.ohio.gov/OFC/APSProtocol2013.stm

Patronek, G. J., & Nathanson, J. N. (2009). A theoretical perspective to inform assessment and treatment strategies for animal hoarders. *Clinical Psychology Review, 29*(3), 274–281.

Paveza, G., VandeWeerd, C., & Laumann, E. (2008). Elder self-neglect: A discussion of a social typology. *Journal of the American Geriatrics Society, 56*(Suppl 2), S271–S275.

Pavlou, M., & Lachs, M. (2006). Could self-neglect in older adults be a geriatric syndrome? *Journal of the American Geriatrics Society, 54*(5), 831–842.

Pickens, S. L. (2012). *Assessment of executive function before and after vitamin D replacement in vulnerable adults who self-neglect* (January 1, 2012). Paper presented at the meeting of the Texas Medical Center Dissertations, (via ProQuest). Paper AAI3528769. University of Texas School of Nursing, Houston, US. Retrived from http://digitalcommons.library.tmc.edu/dissertations/AAI3528769

Pickens, S., Ostwald, S. K., Pace, K. M., Diamond, P., Burnett, J., & Dyer, C. B. (2013). Assessing dimensions of executive function in community-dwelling older adults with self-neglect. *Clinical Nursing Studies, 2*(1). Retrieved from http://www.sciedupress.com/journal/index.php/cns/article/view/2354

Post, F. (1982). Functional disorders. In R. Levy & F. Post (Eds.), *The psychiatry of late life* (pp. 180–181). Oxford, UK: Blackwell Scientific Publications.

Poythress, E. L., Burnett, J., Naik, A. D., Pickens, S., & Dyer, C. B. (2006). Severe self-neglect: An epidemiological and historical perspective. *Journal of Elder Abuse & Neglect, 18*(4), 5–12.

Reyes-Ortiz, C. A., Burnett, J., Flores, D. V., Halphen, J. M., & Dyer, C. B. (2014). Medical implications of elder abuse: Self-neglect. *Clinics in Geriatric Medicine, 30*(4), 807–823.

Sheikh, J. I., & Yesavage, J. A. (1986). Geriatric Depression Scale (GDS): Recent evidence and development of a shorter version. *Clinical Gerontologist, 5*(1/2), 165–173.

Snowdon, J., Halliday, G., & Banerjee, S. (2013). Severe domestic squalor. *Psychiatry, Psychology and Law, 20*(1), 152–155.

Teaster, P. B., Dugar, T., Mendiondo, M., Abner, E. L., Cecil, K. A., & Otto, J. M. (2006). *The 2004 survey of adult protective services: Abuse of adults 60 years of age and older*. Washington, DC: The National Centre on Elder Abuse. Retrieved from http://www.ncea.aoa.gov/Resources/Publication/docs/2-14-06_FINAL_60_REPORT.pdf

White, W. (2014). Elder self-neglect and adult protective services: Ohio needs to do more. *Journal of Law and Health, 27*(107), 130.

Working Group on Elder Abuse. (2002). *Protecting our future*. Dublin, Ireland: Stationery Office.

CHAPTER 7

Military Serving at What Cost?

The Effects of Parental Service on the Well-Being of Our Youngest Military Members

Alicia Gill Rossiter, Rita D'Aoust, and Michaela R. Shafer

ABSTRACT

Since the onset of war in Iraq and Afghanistan in April 2002, much attention has been given to the effect of war on servicemen and servicewomen who have now been serving in combat for over thirteen years, the longest sustained war in American history. Many service members have served multiple tours in Iraq and Afghanistan and suffered from the visible and invisible wounds of war. Much work has been done in the Veterans Administration, the Department of Defense, and the civilian sector after observing the effects of multiple deployments and overall military service on the service member. A survey of the literature revealed that the ethics of conducting research on programs to assist these brave men and women is fraught with ethical concerns based on a military culture that often precludes autonomy and privacy. While strides have been made in developing strategies to assist service members deal with their military service issues, a serious lack of information exists on the impact of a parent's service on the health and well-being of military children. A discussion of current research on services for children is presented with an analysis of the ethical problems that have precluded adequate study of those who need society's help the most.

http://dx.doi.org/10.1891/0739-6686.34.109

BACKGROUND

Since the onset of military action in Iraq and Afghanistan, roughly 2.2 million Active Duty, National Guard, and Reserve members have been tasked for upward of 3.3 million deployments (Paley, Lester, & Mogil, 2013; White House, 2011). Nearly 40,000 Active Duty members are married to other service members, and there are nearly 75,000 single-parent military families (National Center for Infants, Toddlers, and Families, 2012). Approximately 58% of service members have families and approximately 40% have at least two children (Brendel, Maynard, Albright, & Bellomo, 2014; Flake, Davis, Johnson, & Middleton, 2009).

According to data compiled by the Sogomonyan and Cooper (2010), the majority of military children are in early and middle childhood—78% of the children of Active Duty parents are under the age of 11 years and 80% of reserve component children are under 15 years of age.

Since the onset of military action in Iraq and Afghanistan, more than 700,000 military children have had a parent deploy (Verdeli et al., 2011). With the increased operations tempo, the risk for abuse and neglect among military children has increased (Verdeli et al., 2011). The welfare of military children is directly impacted by the mental health status of the nondeployed parent, especially if the nondeployed parent suffers from depression (Verdeli et al., 2011). According to Johnson and Ling (2013), upward of 33% of military children have experienced maltreatment and/or abuse. Lastly, at least 19,000 children have experienced the wounding of a parent and over 2,200 have experienced the death of a parent secondary to military service in Iraq or Afghanistan, which can have long-term physical and psychological health implications for military children (Sogomonyan & Cooper, 2010).

Research pertaining to the long-term effects of parental deployment and the physical and psychological sequelae and educational ramifications on children is almost nonexistent. This article aims to look at what research is available regarding the children of service members to answer the question—Do we have a moral and ethical obligation to support the emotional and physical needs of military children?

METHODS

A literature search in PubMed was conducted using the key search terms "deployment," "redeployment," "military children," "military family," "resilience," "posttraumatic stress," and "soldier." Articles from this literature search focused on the family and the deployment cycle and the effects of deployment on the family. Highlights from this search revealed two major themes. First, profound effects of exposure to war during a deployment can adversely affect reunification of a service member with the family (Butera-Prinzi & Perlesz, 2004; Gewirtz, Plusny, Khaylis, Erbes & DeGarmo, 2010; Messinger, 2010). Second, a myriad of postcombat physical and psychological symptoms experienced by the service member may adversely affect interactions with the family (Gewirtz et al., 2010; Schell & Marshall, 2008).

Creech, Hadley, and Borsari (2014) conducted a systematic review on the effect of deployment on the relationship of parents and their children during the Iraqi and Afghan operations including Operation Iraqi Freedom, Operation New Dawn, and Operation Enduring Freedom. The systematic review examined research in the following areas: (a) the impact of deployment separation on parenting and children's emotional and behavioral health outcomes; (b) the impact of parental mental health symptoms during and after reintegration; and (c) current treatment approaches in veteran and military families. Several trends emerged. Findings indicate that across all age groups, deployment of a parent may be related to increased emotional and behavioral difficulties for children, including higher rates of health-care visits for psychological problems during deployment. Second, parental posttraumatic stress disorder (PTSD) and depression can lead to increased symptomatology in children as well as problems with parenting during and after reintegration. Third, while numerous treatments have been developed to meet the needs of military families, many have not yet been tested or are in the early stages of implementation and evaluation.

A second literature search in PubMed was conducted using the key search terms for moral distress, ethical dilemma, and ethical issues. However, none of the articles focused on the ethical or moral issues regarding military children specifically. A few articles described the moral dilemma or distress regarding military service and children in the field of operation, but not that of children of U.S. service members. However, some of the same ethical issues related to autonomy and privacy that affect military service members apply to military children.

DISCUSSION

Military service does not affect just the service member. The entire family becomes part of the military and the military culture. The impact of service, both positive and negative, and its associated stressors contribute to physical and psychosocial changes in military children.

Several studies on the effect on PTSD in children of Vietnam Veterans indicate that children are impacted by their parents' PTSD symptomology. Studies indicate these children are at a higher risk for social, academic, emotional, and behavioral problems as well as secondary traumatization such as developing PTSD symptoms that include depression, anxiety, nightmares, and difficulty in concentrating (Price, 2015).

While any deployment can be stressful, recent studies on the effect of multiple deployments in the case of children of Iraq and Afghanistan war service members correlated with the number of challenges faced by these children, which include emotional difficulties (James & Countryman, 2012). The behaviors that are part of development, particularly in early childhood, such as dependency, clinginess, crying, tantrums, and defiance, may become triggers for an already stressed military member or at-home parent (Matsakis, 1988). With a receptive and well-adjusted parent buffering the impact of repeated stressors, the child may attain optimal development. However, if a parent is struggling with the stress and distress of his or her experiences, this may well stunt the emotional growth of that child leading to maladaptive outcomes in relationships and in development (Galinsky, 2011; Huth-Bocks, Levendosky, Bogat, & von Eye, 2004; Lieberman & Van Horn, 2008; Osofsky & Lieberman, 2011).

In 2010, the Pentagon voiced concern about the rising divorce rate among women veterans in the military, which was three times higher than that of their male counterparts—among all women, the rate was 7.8%, among enlisted women, the rate was 9%, and among men, the rate was 3% (Stampler, 2011). The Pentagon cited theories such as women in the military being less traditional than their civilian counterparts and lack of support services for women veterans as causes for the higher divorce rate (Rossiter & Chandler, 2013; Stampler, 2013). In a study conducted by Rossiter and Chandler in 2012, 25% of the 27 participants reported undergoing a divorce while serving on Active Duty or in the Reserves. Factors contributing to the high divorce rate included deployment ($n = 5$), PTSD ($n = 4$), military sexual trauma ($n = 4$), temporary duty assignment ($n = 3$), spousal infidelity ($n = 5$), and stress assimilating back into the marriage and family issues ($n = 5$; Rossiter & Chandler, 2013). While divorce itself can negatively impact the physical and psychological well-being of a child, the addition of physical and/or psychological distress as well as lack of transitional support can adversely impact not only a military marriage but the lives of military children. To date, there are no studies examining the impact of marital relationship deterioration and divorce on military children.

"While the literature relating to relational trauma is expansive, there are few studies which examine the relationship between adult-occurring trauma and early childhood development" (Williams & Mulrooney, 2012, p. 52). These studies and the serious lack of information on how to help our youngest members of the military family warrant a serious look at how to study and develop programs that can ensure these children grow into happy and secure adults. To that end, the research will need to be conducted in an ethical manner to protect the inherent vulnerability of this population.

ETHICAL ANALYSIS

Military rules and requirements often have blurred lines that are very well delineated in civilian practice. It is essential to the ethical integrity of research on military children that sensitivity is maintained for the military mission and provisions are taken to ensure the best interest of the child and the family. When conducting counseling or research, it is imperative that counselors and researchers understand the specific ethical codes that are relevant to the military population. Three areas of ethical concern are presented in an article by Prosek and Holm (2014). They include confidentiality, multiple relationships, and cultural competence.

Confidentiality

The American Counseling Association in their Code of Ethics (2005) stated that informed consent must include a discussion of rights and responsibilities expected within the counseling relationship (Prosek & Holm, 2014). The confidentiality inherent in an informed consent has limitations and they include information that may suggest harm to self, harm to others, and illegal substance use. In the military setting, counselors may need to contemplate other limitations such as privacy regarding domestic violence (Reger, Etherage, Reger, & Gahm, 2008), harassment, criminal activity, and issues concerning fitness for duty (Kennedy & Johnson, 2009). While these do not, on the surface, appear to refer to military children, care within the military system that reveals this type of behavior on the part of the parent may require mandatory reporting. The fear of this type of discovery may preclude service members from seeking the necessary care for themselves or their family. Counselors must have training in the military culture to be able to effectively deal with the problems that may arise from counseling or research questions.

Multiple Relationships

The dilemma here concerns transfers that occur frequently in the military. Due to this fact, teams often provide care to the service member and/or the family. These teams require collaboration and exposure of certain behaviors that may be considered reportable by the military. It is also important that care plans are tailored and brief to ensure that the treatment is portable and effective. It is best to find care that does not reside within the military service member chain of command to prevent compromising privacy and confidentiality. In contrast, many studies have suggested that counseling in groups with persons experiencing similar traumas may be helpful. In this case, only other military children would be able to understand and help the child articulate the fear and anxiety. It is a fine line that must be walked in order to protect and ultimately help our military children.

Cultural Competence

The third ethical concern arises in that the military population has a unique "language, a code of manners, norms of behavior, belief systems, dress, and rituals" (Reger et al., 2008, p. 22). It is important that anyone who deals with this community understands the meaning of military rituals and words so that evaluating what is happening to both the parent and child is placed in context. Much like interactions with other underserved populations, professions that deal with military children face an ethical challenge regarding cultural competency (Flanagan, 2014). It is vitally important that DoD and civilian agencies that work with military children collaborate and educate each other regarding the unique needs of the children they are caring for, as it is well known that high numbers of military children are seen outside of the DoD health-care system. This topic also raises the question regarding the provision of services to veteran children within the VA and whether or not the physical and psychological impact of 14 years of war needs to be evaluated in military children. At a minimum, all health-care providers should be educated regarding the culture of the military and the unique health-care needs of service members, veterans, and their families to include the behavioral, physical, psychological, and educational needs specific to military children. To date, one state has adopted a continuing education requirement for nursing license recertification that requires a continuing education course specific to the unique health-care needs of veterans. Additionally, it is important that in any research effort, investigators use culturally sensitive measures. Military-specific cultural considerations, values, principles, and beliefs must be addressed to inform the responses of the service member and family to questions and events.

IMPLICATIONS

The effects of war extend well beyond the battlefield. While maintenance of a fit and fighting force is critical to the security of our nation, so is the maintenance of our military children. A resilient, physically and emotionally healthy child strengthens the military family and sustains the health and welfare of our servicemen and servicewomen. While there is no doubt that military parents struggle with moral and ethical dilemmas secondary to their service and the impact these have on the role as a parent(s), we are unsure as to the impact on military children. To date, there is limited research studying the impact experienced by this unique population. We do know that military children experience physical and psychological sequelae secondary to their parents' service. What we do not know is the impact these sequelae will have on the long-term physical and psychological well-being of the children of our latest generation of veterans. It is imperative that caregivers, educators, health-care providers, and researchers monitor and support military children throughout childhood and into adulthood to determine potential risks and benefits of military lifestyle and the impact on our youngest military members. In addition, much like other underserved populations in communities, health-care providers must be educated to meet the unique needs of military children and families to include screening for physical, psychological, and behavioral conditions related to parental military service and deployment.

The Joining Force campaign developed by First Lady Michelle Obama and Dr. Jill Biden challenged colleges of nursing around the country to work to improve the health care of our veterans. To date, 660 nursing programs in all 50 states have joined forces to include veteran-centric health-care issues into nursing and advanced practice nursing curriculum, with several colleges including specific needs of military families in their curriculum. With increased awareness should come an increase in funding to research the needs of military families, in particular, military children. While most research funding is geared toward our service members, lines of funding should be aimed at the needs of the military family and healing the entire family, not just one individual. "All of these combat related stresses—parental deployment, injury, post-combat health consequences, and death—can have profound effects on the military family, with young children being the most vulnerable" (Cozza & Lieberman, 2007, p. 27). This segment of the population has been left behind and may suffer from the collateral damage of war—the children of those who serve being in harm's way. We have a moral and ethical obligation to care for those who were drafted into service, by virtue of birth, and are equally, if not more, vulnerable to the aftermath of war than their parent(s).

REFERENCES

Brendel, K. E., Maynard, B. R., Albright, D. L., & Bellomo, M. (2014). Effects of school-based interventions with U.S. military connected children: A systematic review. *Research on Social Work Practice, 24*(6), 649–658.

Butera-Prinzi, F., & Perlesz, A. (2004). Through children's eyes: Children's experience of living with a parent with an acquired brain injury. *Brain Injury, 18*(1), 83–101.

Cozza, S. J., & Lieberman A. F. (2007). The young military child: Our modern Telemachus. *Zero to Three, 27*(6), 27–33.

Creech, S. K., Hadley, W., & Borsari, B. (2014). The impact of military deployment and reintegration on children and parenting: A systematic review. *Professional Psychology: Research and Practice, 45*(6), 452–464.

Flake, E. M., Davis, B. E., Johnson, P. L., & Middleton, L. S. (2009). The psychosocial effects of deployment on military children. *Journal of Developmental and Behavioral Pediatrics, 30*(4), 271–278.

Flanagan, A. Y. (2014). *76330: Working with military families: Impact of deployment*. Retrieved August 2, 2015, from http://www.netce.com/coursecontent.php?courseid=1040#chap.7

Galinsky, E. (2011, December 1). Trusting relationships are central to children's learning—lessons from Edward Tronick. *Huffington Post*. Retrieved August 9, 2015, from http://www.huffingtonpost.com/ellen-galinsky/trusting-relationships-ar_b_1123524.html

Gewirtz, A. H., Polusny, M. A., Khaylis, A., Erbes, C. R., & DeGarmo, D. S. (2010). Posttraumatic stress symptoms among National Guard soldiers deployed to Iraq: Associations with parenting behaviors and couple adjustment. *Journal of Consulting and Clinical Psychology, 78*(5), 599–610.

Huth-Bocks, A. C., Levendosky, A. A., Bogat, G. A., & von Eye, A. (2004). The impact of maternal characteristics and contextual variable on infant-mother attachment. *Child Development, 75*, 480–496.

James, T., & Countryman, J. (2012). Psychiatric effects of military deployment on children and families. *Innovations in Clinical Neuroscience*, 9(2), 16–20.

Johnson, H. L., & Ling, C. G. (2013). Caring for military children in the 21st century. *Journal of the American Association of Nurse Practitioners, 25*, 195–202.

Kennedy, C. H., & Johnson, W. B. (2009). Mixed agency in military psychology. Applying the American Psychological Association ethics code. *Psychological Services*, 6(1), 22–31.

Lieberman, A. F., & Van Horn, P. (2008). *Psychotherapy with infants and young children: Repairing the effects of stress and trauma on early attachment*. New York, NY: Guilford Press.

Matsakis, A. (1988). *Vietnam wives: Women and children surviving life with veterans suffering post-traumatic stress disorder*. Kensington, MD: Woodbine House.

Messinger, S. D. (2010). Rehabilitating time: Multiple temporalities among military clinicians and patients. *Medical Anthropology, 29*(2), 150–169.

National Center for Infants, Toddlers and Families. (2012). *Research and resilience: Recognizing the need to know more. Understanding the experiences of young children in military families in the context of deployment, reintegration, injury, or loss*. Retrieved August 29, 2015, from http://www.zerotothree.org/about-us/funded-projects/military-families/march30researchandresilience.pdf

Osofsky, J. D., & Lieberman, A. F. (2011). A call for integrating a mental health perspective into systems of care for abused and neglected infants and young children. *American Psychologist*, 66(2), 120–128.

Paley, B., Lester, P., & Mogil, C. (2013). Family systems and ecological perspectives on the impact of deployment on military families. *Clinical Child and Family Psychology Review, 16*, 245–265.

Price, J. L. (2015). *When a child's parent has PTSD*. Retrieved August 2, 2015, from http://www.ptsd.va.gov/professional/treatment/children/pro_child_parent_ptsd.asp

Prosek, E. A. & Holm, J. M. (2014). *Counselors and the military: When protocol and ethics conflict*. Retrieved August 9, 2015, from http://tpcjournal.nbcc.org/counselors-and-the-military-when-protocol-and-ethics-conflict/

Reger, M. A., Etherage, J. R., Reger, G. M., & Gahm, G. A. (2008). Civilian psychologists in an army culture: The ethical challenge of cultural competence. *Military Psychology, 20*, 21–35.

Rossiter, A. G., & Chandler, R. (2013). Women veterans and divorce: What are the contributing factors? *Nurse Leader 11*(5), 51–53.

Schell, T. L., & Marshall, G. N. (2008). Survey of individuals previously deployed for OEF/OIF. In T. Tanielian & L. H. Jaycox (Eds.), *Invisible wounds of war: Psychological and cognitive injuries their consequences, and services to assist recovery* (pp. 87–115). Santa Monica, CA: RAND Corporation. Retrieved August 9, 2015, from http://www.rand.org/pubs/monographs/2008/RAND_MG720.pdf

Sogomonyan, F., & Cooper, J. L. (2010). *Trauma faced by children of military families: What every policymaker should know.* New York, NY: National Center for Children in Poverty. Retrieved June 29, 2015, from http://www.nccp.org/publications/pub_938.html#12

Stampler, L. (2011). Divorce rate for women in military double that of men. *Huffington Post*. Retrieved February 20, 2013, from http://www.huffingtonpost.com/2011/04/12/divorce-rate-for-women-in military_n_848125.html

Verdeli, H., Baily, C., Vousoura, E., Besler, A., Singla, D., & Manos, G. (2011). The case for treating depression in military spouses. *Journal of Family Psychology, 25*(4), 488–496.

White House. (2011). *Strengthening our military families: Meeting America's commitment.* Retrieved June 29, 2015, from http://www.defense.gov/home/features/2011/0111_initiative/strengthening_our_military_january_2011.pdf

Williams, D. S., & Mulrooney, K. (2012). Research and resilience: Creating a research agenda for supporting military families with young children. *Zero to Three, 32*(4), 46–56.

CHAPTER 8

The Gene Pool

The Ethics of Genetics in Primary Care

Karen J. Whitt, McKenna Hughes, Elizabeth (Betsy) S. Hopkins, and Ann Maradiegue

ABSTRACT

Aim: The purpose of this integrative review is to critically analyze the research literature regarding ethical principles that surround the integration of genetics and genomics in primary care clinical practice. Background: Advanced practice nurses (APRNs) play an important role in the provision of primary care services, in the areas of obstetrics, pediatrics, family practice, and internal medicine. Advances in genetic and genomic science are infiltrating these day-to-day health-care systems and becoming an integral part of health-care delivery. It is imperative for primary care providers to understand the ethical, legal, and social implications of genetics and genomics. Methods: A comprehensive multistep search of CINAHL, MEDLINE, Academic Search Premier, PsycINFO, Web of Science, and Scopus databases was conducted to identify primary research articles published from 2003 to 2015 that evaluated ethical issues related to genetics and genomics in U.S. primary care practice. A sample of 26 primary research articles met the inclusion criteria. Whittemore and Knafl's (2005) revised framework for integrative reviews was used to guide the analysis and assess the quality of the

http://dx.doi.org/10.1891/0739-6686.34.119

studies. Key findings from the studies are discussed according to Beauchamp and Childress's (2009) ethical principles of autonomy, beneficence, nonmaleficence, and justice. Results: Research conducted to date is mainly qualitative and descriptive and the analysis revealed several ethical challenges to implementing genetics and genomics in primary care settings. Conclusion: The review suggests that there are several implications for research, education, and the development of primary care practice that support APRNs delivering genetic and genomic care while incorporating knowledge of ethical principles. More research needs to be conducted that evaluates the actual genetic/genomic ethical issues encountered by primary care providers.

INTRODUCTION

When sequencing of the human genome was completed, it was envisioned that genetic- and genomic-based approaches could be used to predict disease susceptibility and drug response in order to provide individualized medicine based on genetic profiles (Collins, Green, Guttmacher, & Guyer, 2003). It was postulated that genetic services would become part of routine medical care. In the past decade, rapid advances have taken place with regard to genetic technologies and the vision for personalized medicine is becoming more of a reality. Since sequencing of the human genome, science has moved beyond single-gene testing to examining the whole genome and panel testing for multiple genes. Genomic medicine is defined as the study of the function of all the nucleotide sequences present within the entire genome. Innovations in technology have highlighted the role of genomics in common conditions encountered in the primary care setting (Mikat-Stevens, Larson, & Tarini, 2014).

Personalized genomic medicine promises to improve clinical outcomes by providing a more informed process for providers, which can predict disease prior to symptoms, improve patient outcomes, and reduce health-care costs through earlier prediction of disease and individualized interventions that reduce adverse side effects (Lazaridis et al., 2014). Primary care settings, including obstetrics, pediatrics, family and internal medicine, provide entry-level health care for individuals making use of a person-centered approach rather than focusing on disease (Johns Hopkins Bloomberg School of Public Health, 2014).

Primary care was envisioned as the most likely setting for the delivery of many basic genetic services, with practitioners playing a seminal role in the assessment and management of genetic risk in routine practice (Green, Guyer, Manolio, & Peterson, 2011; Kirk, 2000). There are many times throughout the life span that patients and families may require genetic services (Fleck, 2014). It is believed that genomic technology will lead to the delivery of health care that is precise and personal. The promising aspect of incorporating genetic and genomic medicine into primary care poses many ethical considerations that practitioners should be aware of. An integrative review of the published research literature was conducted in order to evaluate the empirical evidence related to the ethical principles of autonomy, beneficence, nonmaleficence, and justice associated with the provision of genetic and genomic services in the primary care setting.

METHODS

Whittemore and Knalf's (2005) updated integrative review method guided the analysis. This is considered a rigorous method that is useful when there is a need to appraise studies of varying quality and design with diverse research methodologies. Studies were analyzed and grouped based on how the purpose and key findings aligned with Beauchamp and Childress's (2009) four principles of biomedical ethics, autonomy, beneficence, nonmaleficence, and justice.

Search Methods

We systematically searched CINAHL, MEDLINE, Academic Search Premier, PsycINFO, Web of Science, and Scopus databases for articles published between 2003 and 2015, to identify original research studies that evaluated ethical issues related to genetics and genomics in primary care practice. We used combinations of the keywords "genetic," "genomic," "ethic," "legal," "social implications," "primary health care," "family practice," "primary care," "general practice," "family medicine," "physician assistant," "nurse practitioner," and "advanced practice nursing." Original research articles that were conducted in the United States and published in peer-reviewed journals were included in our analysis if they evaluated ethical issues related to genetics or genomics in primary care practice. Nonresearch articles were excluded from our review. Research articles not written in English, not conducted in the United States, not published in peer-reviewed journals, and studies that discussed ethical issues that only applied to research, hospital, or specialty settings were excluded from our analysis (Table 8.1). Research not conducted in the United States was excluded because health-care systems in other countries vary and the impact of some ethical issues may be quite different.

Search Outcome

Our initial search yielded 358 articles. When duplicates were removed, there were 273 abstracts, which were reviewed by hand to identify 40 primary research articles. Each of these 40 research articles was reviewed according to our inclusion/exclusion criteria. Fourteen of the articles were excluded because they were

TABLE 8.1
Literature Inclusion and Exclusion Criteria

Inclusion Criteria	Exclusion Criteria
Original research	Reviews, opinion editorials
Conducted in the United States	Conducted outside of the United States
Published in peer-reviewed journal	Non-peer-reviewed articles, abstracts, dissertations
Evaluated ethical issues related to genetics/genomics in primary care	Studies that evaluated ethics of genetics/genomics in research, hospitals, or specialty settings
	Not written in English

studies conducted outside of the United States. We identified 26 studies that met the inclusion criteria. Each study was reviewed, evaluated for methodological rigor and relevance to topic, and grouped according to the ethical principles of autonomy, beneficence, nonmaleficence, and justice that were addressed in the key findings and purpose of the study (Figure 8.1).

Quality Appraisal

All studies were evaluated for methodological rigor using a 3-point scale (1 = low, 2 = moderate, 3 = high) based on qualitative criteria from the "Critical Review Form—Qualitative Studies Version 2" (Letts et al., 2007) and quantitative criteria from the "Quality Assessment Tool for Quantitative Studies" (National Collaborating Centre for Methods and Tools, 2008). Each study was evaluated for relevance to topic using a 3-point scale (1 = low, 2 = moderate, 3 = high) by three reviewers. Each score was determined by consensus of the reviewers. Table 8.2 shows the studies listed by year of publication with each study's relevance to topic and methodologic rigor scores. We included all 26 articles in our analysis since there were so few studies that met our inclusion criteria.

Synthesis

The goal of the synthesis phase was to group all of the data into subgroups in order to identify patterns and relationships among the data (Whittemore & Knafl, 2005). The studies were categorized according to Beauchamp and Childress's (2009) four principles of medical ethics as related to genetics and genomics in primary care and compiled into a matrix located in Table 8.3. The purpose and results of each study were analyzed to identify relationships between the principles of autonomy, beneficence, nonmaleficence, and justice. Analysis strategies

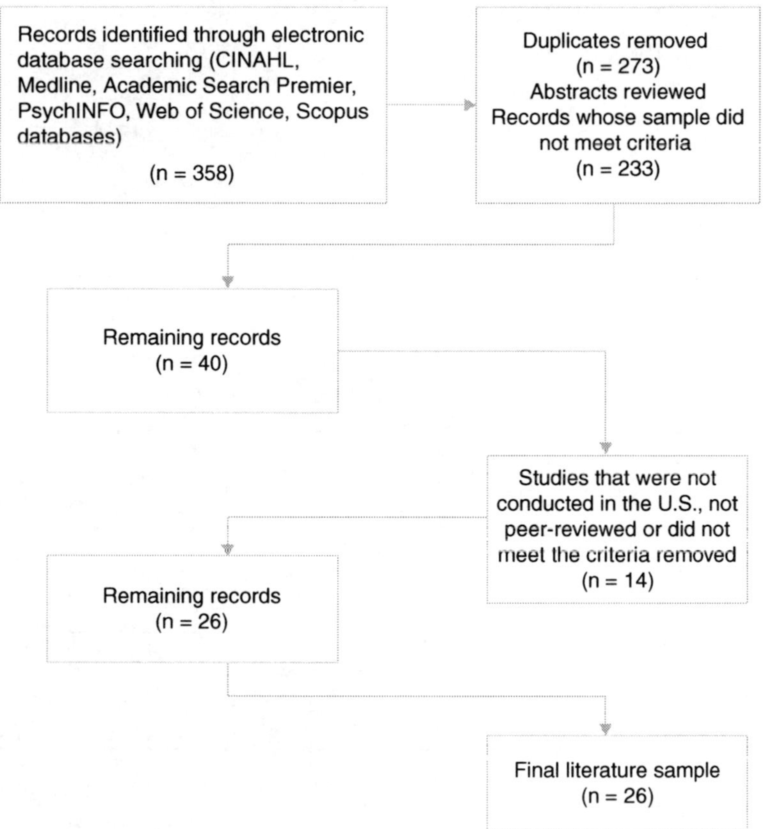

FIGURE 8.1 Search and inclusion process.

included noting intervening factors among the variables. The reorganized and synthesized data formed the basis for this review. Several implications related to ethical issues of genomics in the primary care setting were identified for APRNs, and areas for future research were revealed supported by the textual and numerical ratings.

RESULTS

We identified 26 primary research articles. There were 16 studies with quantitative designs that included mainly descriptive surveys and pretest and posttest designs, 9 studies with qualitative designs including interviews, focus groups, and content analysis of websites, and 1 study that utilized a mixed-method design. The purpose and findings of the studies revealed that 10 of the studies

TABLE 8.2

Quality and Relevance of Appraisal Criteria and Process

Criteria
A = methodological quality (MQ) judgement of overall quality (1, 2, 3)
B = topic relevance (TR) judgement of overall weight (1, 2, or 3)

Author (Year)	Ethical Principle	Design	MQ Score	TR Score	Overall Score
Bell et al. (2014)	Beneficence	Quantitative	1	2	2
Constantine, Allyse, Wall, Vries, and Rockwood (2014)	Autonomy	Quantitative	1	3	2
Goldenberg, Dodson, Davis, and Tarini (2014)	Autonomy	Quantitative	1	3	2
Strong, Zusevics, Bick, and Veith (2014)	Autonomy	Quantitative	1	3	2
Wasson, Cherny, Sanders, Hogan, and Helzlsouer (2014)	Nonmaleficence	Qualitative	1	3	2
Hunt and Kreiner (2013)	Justice	Qualitative	1	3	2
Klitzman et al. (2013a)	Nonmaleficence	Quantitative	1	2	2
Klitzman et al. (2013b)	Nonmaleficence, justice	Quantitative	1	2	2
Christianson et al. (2012)	Justice, beneficence	Qualitative	2	2	2
Haga, Tindall, and O'Daniel (2012)	Nonmaleficence	Qualitative	1	1	1
Hay et al. (2012)	Autonomy	Quantitative	2	1	2
Hurley et al. (2012)	Autonomy	Qualitative	1	2	1

Wasson, Hogan, Sanders, and Helzlsouer (2012)	Autonomy	Qualitative	1	3	2
Lewis, Treise, Hsu, Allen, and Kang (2011)	Autonomy	Qualitative	2	3	2
Srinivasan et al. (2011)	Nonmaleficence	Quantitative	2	3	2
Arar Seo, Abboud, Parchman, and Noel (2010)	Nonmaleficence	Qualitative	2	1	1
O'Neill et al. (2010)	Nonmaleficence	Quantitative	2	3	2
Hindorff et al. (2009)	Justice	Quantitative	1	2	2
Brandt, Ali, Sabel, McHugh, and Gilman (2008)	Nonmaleficence	Quantitative	1	2	1
Lowstuter et al. (2008)	Justice	Quantitative	2	3	2
Trinidad et al. (2008)	Nonmaleficence	Qualitative	1	1	1
Levy, Youatt, and Shields (2007)	Justice	Quantitative	2	2	2
Erde, McCormack, Steer, Ciervo, and McAbee (2006)	Nonmaleficence	Quantitative	2	3	3
Acheson, Stange, and Zyzanski (2005)	Justice	Mixed methods	1	3	2
Hall et al. (2005)	Justice	Quantitative	2	3	3
Maradiegue, Edwards, Seibert, Macri, and Sitzer (2005)	Beneficence	Quantitative	2	2	2

TABLE 8.3

Literature Characteristics

Author (Year)	Ethical Principles Addressed	Design	Sample	Purpose	Findings	Limitations
Acheson et al. (2005)	Justice	Descriptive survey; mixed methods	National random sample of 190 family physicians	Describe genetic issues encountered by family physicians in clinical practice	Most of the physicians reported discussing the genetics of common cancers, cardiovascular disease, and Alzheimer's disease with patients in the past year. 13% of the physicians made a referral for breast/ovarian cancer in the past year. 23% said access to genetic consultation is difficult to obtain particularly in rural areas. Some physicians felt that genetic tests were expensive and that the drawbacks of gaining information about genetics outweighed the benefits.	The researchers cited limitations in the survey instrument, since the survey was based on self-reported recollection of past experience and did not ask how many patients were actually referred for genetic consultation, which could introduce bias in the answers.

Arar et al. (2010)	Nonmaleficence	Qualitative, interviews	20 primary care providers from the Veterans Administration (VA)	Examine providers' intentions toward utilizing genomic services	Most providers thought that primary care plays an important role in genetics but that providers need more training regarding genetic testing and how to make referrals to genetic specialists.	Small sample size. Findings may not be generalizable to providers who do not work for the VA.
Bell et al. (2014)	Beneficence	Randomized controlled trial (RCT) with qualitative Transcripts coded for presence or absence of key topics discussed during a standardized patient encounter	121 community physicians	Evaluate the outcome of an interactive web-based curriculum vs. text curriculum for improving physician practice related to screening for breast cancer	The majority of the standardized patient encounters had inadequate discussion of ethical implications and inadequate history taking.	Possible selection bias. The physicians knew they were being evaluated during the standardized patient encounter. The outcome data collected was not quantitative, which is usually the type of data collected in RCTs.
Brandt et al. (2008)	Nonmaleficence	Descriptive survey	51 primary care and 31 specialist physicians	Provide insight about why, when, and to whom primary care physicians make a referral for cancer genetic testing	Primary care physicians were significantly less comfortable with identifying patients for referral and discussing genetics compared with specialists.	Small sample size. Survey used close-ended questions.

(*Continued*)

TABLE 8.3

Literature Characteristics (Continued)

Author (Year)	Ethical Principles Addressed	Design	Sample	Purpose	Findings	Limitations
Christianson et al. (2012)	Justice, beneficence	Qualitative, focus groups	16 primary care providers	Obtain input regarding incorporation of a family health history risk assessment tool in community practice	Identified several areas of concern regarding genetics in practice including provider's level of expertise, cost of preventive care based on genetics, genetic discrimination, reimbursement, clarity of follow-up guidelines	Self-selected, small sample. Researchers unable to reach qualitative saturation with the responses from the small sample
Constantine et al. (2014)	Autonomy	Descriptive survey	226 female prenatal patients	Evaluate patient's informed consent decision process for quad screen testing	Patients who consent to have the quad screen often lack an understanding about the reason for this test. Having the provider offer the test was viewed by the patient as an endorsement to have the testing done, which was an impediment to the informed consent process.	Possible selection bias, nonresponse error. Findings may not be generalizable because the sample was from one region in the United States.

Erde et al. (2006)	Nonmaleficence	Descriptive survey with hypothetical case studies	165 osteopathic family physicians	Evaluate osteopathic family physician's opinions about disclosing genetic test results to patient's family members	Most providers agreed that adult children should be told about genetic test results if the disease was treatable. Age played a role in disclosure of test results. Most providers agreed they would tell a 22-year-old, were unsure about telling a 17-year-old, and would not tell a person 12 or younger.	Findings may not be generalizable. All providers were from New Jersey, mostly White and male.
Goldenberg et al. (2014)	Autonomy	Descriptive survey	Nationally representative sample of 1,539 parents	Assess parents' interest in whole genome sequencing (WGS) of newborns	74% of the parents were interested in having WGS for newborn screening if it was offered by the state. 70% were interested in WGS if it was offered in a pediatric office. Test accuracy and the ability to prevent a disease from developing were rated as important information for making an informed decision about testing.	Survey asked hypothetical questions and may not represent decisions in actual situations. The researchers suggested that the participants may not have fully understood the benefits and limitations of WGS.

(*Continued*)

TABLE 8.3

Literature Characteristics (Continued)

Author (Year)	Ethical Principles Addressed	Design	Sample	Purpose	Findings	Limitations
Haga et al. (2012)	Nonmaleficence	Qualitative focus groups	21 primary care providers and genetics professionals	Assess attitudes about pharmacogenetic testing	Primary care providers had concerns regarding the impact of pharmacogenetic testing on delay of treatment, clinical utility, insurance coverage, and ability to interpret test results.	Small sample size from one region of the country, may not be representative of the greater population.
Hall et al. (2005)	Justice	Descriptive survey	Multiethnic sample of 86,859 adult primary care patients from 5 U.S. states and 1 Canadian province	Measure concern about insurance problems relating to genetic testing	40% of survey participants were concerned that genetic testing could lead to insurance discrimination.	Assessed insurance discrimination with a question that did not specify the type of insurance (i.e., life vs. health insurance). Participants had already agreed to undergo genetic screening; also does not represent the views of the general public.

Hay et al. (2012)	Autonomy	Descriptive telephone survey	1,772 multiethnic adults who were members of a health maintenance organization (HMO)	Determine if skin cancer awareness, family history, and health information seeking were related to perceived importance of learning about how genes affect health risk	Patients felt that learning about genetics and family history provided important information about health risks.	Self-report of genetic information–seeking behavior, not actual behavioral assessments.
Hindorff et al. (2009)	Justice	Descriptive survey	112 primary care physicians	Investigate primary care physicians' self-reported motivation for ordering Factor V Leiden genetic tests	Many of the physicians felt that lack of availability of genetic counseling services was a barrier that influenced their motivation to order genetic testing.	Self-report responses to hypothetical survey questions. The survey was long and could have introduced inaccurate responses.
Hunt & Kreiner (2013)	Justice	Qualitative interviews	58 primary care clinicians	Explore how pharmacogenetics is integrated in current practice	Pharmacogenetics has led to racial/ethnic profiling instead of individual genetic profiling.	Small sample size. Methods for data collection and analysis are not clearly articulated. Interview questions not provided or discussed in the article.

(*Continued*)

TABLE 8.3

Literature Characteristics (Continued)

Author (Year)	Ethical Principles Addressed	Design	Sample	Purpose	Findings	Limitations
Hurley et al. (2012)	Autonomy	Qualitative interviews	33 carriers of BRCA1/2 mutation	Determine BRCA1/2 carriers' preferences regarding preimplantation genetic diagnosis	Some participants preferred discussing preimplantation genetic diagnosis with a trusted primary care provider.	Small sample size. Results may not be generalizable. Males underrepresented in the study. Noncarrier partners were not interviewed.
Klitzman et al. (2013a)	Nonmaleficence	Descriptive survey	220 internists	Determine internists' views regarding preimplantation genetic diagnosis	Most of the providers felt that they had very little knowledge about preimplantation genetic diagnosis and did not feel comfortable answering patient's questions.	Internists from only two medical centers. Low response rate. High percentage of women in the sample
Klitzman et al. (2013b)	Nonmaleficence, justice	Descriptive survey	220 internists	Determine internists' utilization of genetic testing	The majority of internists surveyed felt that they needed more training about when to order tests and how to counsel patients. Less than 2% of the internists had patients who had testing and experienced genetic discrimination.	Sample not representative of the population of internists in the United States since there was a high percentage of women

Levy et al. (2007)	Justice	Descriptive survey	Random sample of 562 primary care physicians in the United States	Determine the importance of eight factors that influence whether to order a genetic test for smoking cessation treatment	The majority of participants felt that the most important factor influencing decision to order genetic test was if the test would improve cessation outcomes. If the test led to discrimination, this made the physicians less likely to order a test.	Survey was regarding a hypothetical test scenario, not actual patient encounter. Sample may not be representative due to response rate.
Lewis et al. (2011)	Autonomy	Qualitative content analysis of website data	25 direct-to-consumer (DTC) genetic testing company websites	Assess compliance of DTC companies with the American Society of Human Genetics (ASHG) transparency recommendations	The majority of DTC companies did not meet standards for compliance with transparency recommendations issued by ASHG. Most DTC companies did not disclose the limitations of genetic tests to consumers.	Could be some accuracy issues with the data influenced by the dates that the websites were accessed
Lowstuter et al. (2008)	Justice	Descriptive survey	1,181 nongenetic health-care providers	Describe nongenetic clinicians' perception and knowledge of cancer genetic testing and discrimination	The majority of providers felt that testing was of benefit, but believed genetic discrimination was an issue. The majority of providers were not aware of laws that protect against genetic discrimination.	91% of the respondents practiced in urban settings, which could influence survey results.

(*Continued*)

TABLE 8.3
Literature Characteristics (Continued)

Author (Year)	Ethical Principles Addressed	Design	Sample	Purpose	Findings	Limitations
Maradiegue et al. (2005)	Beneficence, nonmaleficence	Descriptive survey	46 advanced practice nursing students	Describe nurse practitioner students' knowledge of genetics	Students perceived that they had minimal knowledge of and training in medical genetics.	Small sample size, self-report
O'Neill et al. (2010)	Nonmaleficence	Descriptive survey	161 primary care providers	Assess primary care providers' willingness to order BRCA predictive testing for adolescents, given a hypothetical case scenario	31% of primary care providers would order BRCA genetic testing for an adolescent.	Small sample size; bias may be present because participants were attendees of a conference. Findings may not be generalizable. Using a hypothetical example does not reflect what may happen in actual clinical practice;
Srinivasan et al. (2011)	Nonmaleficence	Pretest–posttest ethical, legal, social efficacy scale	279 primary care residents	Assess effectiveness of a web-based program to increase knowledge and self-efficacy with genetic ethical, legal, and social implications (ELSI) issues	After participation in the web-based educational program, residents increased their self-efficacy with ELSI skills by 15%. Felt that they could apply content to the clinical setting	There were differences in the way the curriculum was implemented that were not assessed.

Strong et al. (2014)	Autonomy	Descriptive survey	258 primary care providers	Assess views of primary care providers regarding the return of incidental findings	About half of the providers surveyed felt that they would like to have their whole genome sequenced and more than one third would have their child's whole genome sequenced. A little over half of the participants would want to know incidental findings for diseases with no preventive treatment options. Many of the participants did not want to learn about incidental findings even if treatment or preventive actions are available.	The researchers mentioned that the survey was administered after a genetics presentation, which could have introduced biased answers. Sample may not be representative of primary care providers in the United States since the sample size was predominantly female.
Trinidad et al. (2008)	Nonmaleficence	Qualitative telephone interviews	24 primary care providers	Identify primary care providers attitudes toward genetic medicine and their educational needs	Providers were interested in learning more about when and how to order genetic testing and that they would like to have more resources to guide clinical decision making.	Small sample size

(*Continued*)

TABLE 8.3

Literature Characteristics (Continued)

Author (Year)	Ethical Principles Addressed	Design	Sample	Purpose	Findings	Limitations
Wasson et al. (2014)	Nonmaleficence	Qualitative interviews	20 primary care patients who had DTC genetic testing	Explore primary care patient's views, attitudes, and decision-making process related to DTC genetic testing	Most of the participants would disclose information about their genetic test results to their immediate family and less than half of the participants would disclose results to extended family.	Small sample size
Wasson et al. (2012)	Autonomy	Qualitative interviews	29 primary care patients	Explore decision-making process and ethical considerations of primary care patient who had DTC genetic testing	Patients were interested in DTC testing but were concerned about the accuracy and reliability of the testing and were concerned about risk regarding confidentiality of test results.	Small sample size, selection bias. Results are not generalizable.

were related to nonmaleficence, 7 were related to autonomy, 3 to beneficence, and 8 were related to justice. There were two studies that had findings related to two different ethical principles (Christianson et al., 2012; Klitzman et al., 2013b). Detailed characteristics of the literature sample are summarized in Table 8.3. A synthesis of the findings from each of the studies along with commentary for each of the four ethical principles of autonomy, beneficence, nonmaleficence, and justice as they relate to ethical issues of genetics/genomics faced by advanced practice nurses (APRNs) in primary care settings are provided in the following text.

Autonomy

Autonomy implies support for independent decision making by the patient (Beauchamp & Childress, 2009). There were seven studies that had either the purpose or a finding that evaluated aspects of autonomy related to genetics in primary care settings. These studies evaluated decision-making processes and informed consent. Four of the studies were descriptive surveys, two were qualitative interviews, and one study was a qualitative analysis of website content. Five of the studies evaluated patient viewpoints regarding informed consent and the decision-making process for genetic testing. One study evaluated websites of companies that offer direct-to-consumer (DTC) genetic testing to determine if enough information is provided for a consumer to make an informed decision. All of the studies had some methodologic limitations such as selection bias, low response rates, and self-report data. However, the findings from these studies are informative to APRN practice in primary care.

Decision-Making Processes

Studies reveal that there are some patients who are interested in exercising autonomy and seeking information about genetic risk and testing options. A survey of 1,772 patients who were interested in genetic testing and genetic health information concluded that individuals who autonomously seek genetic risk information may be more receptive to prevention and interventions that promote healthy lifestyles (Hay et al., 2012). Relationships with a trusted provider play a role in patient's decision process. A qualitative study of 33 carriers of the BRCA1/2 mutation that explored decisions regarding preimplantation genetic diagnosis reported that some of these patients preferred discussing genetic issues with a trusted primary care provider with whom they have a relationship as opposed to a specialist (Hurley et al., 2012).

It is difficult to separate the decision-making process from informed consent. One of the problems with the process of informed consent is that there are times when patients do not receive enough information to make an informed decision. A qualitative study of 29 primary care patients who participated in focus groups to discuss interest in DTC genetic testing reported that the patients were interested in testing but were also concerned about the accuracy and reliability of the testing and the risk regarding confidentiality of test results (Wasson, Hogan, Sanders, & Helzlsouer, 2012). Another qualitative study evaluated the websites of 25 companies that offered DTC genetic testing revealed that the majority of these websites did not include enough information to comply with transparency recommendations issued by the American Society of Human Genetics and most did not disclose the limitations of genetic tests (Lewis, Treise, Hsu, Allen, & Kang, 2011). This lack of information makes it difficult for consumers to make informed decisions regarding genetic testing. These findings illuminate the relationship between the decision-making process and the role of informed consent.

Informed Consent

The informed consent process can be inadequate for patients who are considering testing ordered by a primary care provider. An evaluation of the consent process for 226 women for quad screening, a first-trimester prenatal genetic test, concluded that women who underwent this type of testing often lacked understanding about the reason for this test. Findings from this study indicated that having a provider offer the test was viewed as an endorsement for genetic testing, regardless of the level of patient understanding for testing (Constantine, Allyse, Wall, Vries, & Rockwood, 2014). This was an impediment to the informed consent process.

New genomic testing technologies such as whole genome sequencing (WGS) and whole exome sequencing (WES) are increasingly replacing traditional genetic testing procedures and presenting a challenge to informed consent and autonomy. WGS analyzes an individual's entire genetic blueprint and generates data on approximately three billion base pairs. WES analyzes the exome or the 1% of DNA that codes for proteins (Bunnik, de Jong, Nijsingh, & de Wert, 2013). Three applications of WGS and WES technology that primary care providers may encounter are newborn screening, prenatal screening, and DTC personal genome testing. These new genomic technologies are at odds with the principle of respect for autonomy and challenge the process of informed consent because all of the information gained from testing is not immediately interpretable (Bunnik et al., 2013; Hogarth, Javitt, & Metzer, 2008). Therefore, patients may not have the necessary information to make an informed decision about testing because of the possibility of future, incidental findings that may become apparent as more research is conducted that correlates health conditions with these genetic markers.

Incidental findings are defined as likely pathogenic test results that are not apparently relevant to the diagnosis or initial reason for seeking testing. In many instances, it is unclear if these incidental findings are clinically significant and this leads to controversy about what providers should do with this information. In some cases, the significance of incidental findings is not known unless a detailed family history is obtained and additional family members are tested. Family members often need to participate in testing and surveillance in order to decide if incidental findings are significant, which is part of the informed consent process (Crawford, Foulds, Fenwick, Hallowell, & Lucassen, 2013). The ethical challenges of dealing with the large amount of data generated from WGS/WES and how clinicians will disseminate this information has been discussed by a number of authors (Ali-Khan, Daar, Shuman, Ray, & Scherer, 2009; Letendre & Godard, 2004; Sharp, 2011).

There are currently no electronic health records that have standardized protocols for storing and analyzing the vast amount of data or the incidental findings in order to allow for responsible and appropriate disclosure of this information to providers and patients (Hazin et al., 2013; Shoenbill, Fost, Tachinardi, & Mendonca, 2014). According to Biesecker (2012), the nature of WGS and WES is best considered as a health-care resource that can be utilized and interpreted over the patient's life span, rather than a one-time test, and should be written into the patient consent.

Since newborn screening is one of the suggested applications for WGS and WES, this raises the concern of what to do with incidental findings when children are the patients. A nationally representative survey of 1,539 parents to assess interest in WGS of newborns reported that 74% of the parents were interested in having WGS for newborn screening if it was offered by the state and 70% were interested in WGS if it was offered in a pediatric office. However, test accuracy and the ability to prevent a disease from developing were rated as important information in order to make an informed decision about WGS testing (Goldenberg, Dodson, Davis, & Tarini, 2014). The researchers who conducted this study suggested that the participants may not fully understand the benefits and limitations of WGS and that incidental findings may require future follow-up. Another study that assessed the views of 258 primary care providers regarding WGS testing and the return of incidental findings noted that about half of the providers surveyed felt that they would like to have WGS testing and more than one third would have WGS for their own child. Over half of those surveyed wanted to know incidental findings for diseases with no preventive or treatment options. In contrast, some of the participants did not want to learn about incidental findings even if there were treatment or preventive actions available (Strong, Zusevics, Bick, & Veith, 2014).

One way to deal with incidental findings in children is to offer families a choice of which incidental findings they receive during pretest counseling, limit the findings to conditions with childhood onset that have immediate medical interventions, and make findings for adult-onset disease with no preventive measures or carrier status optional (Clayton et al., 2014; Mulchandani et al., 2014). The ethical dilemma is allowing children who are not able to consent for themselves the right to an open future without knowledge of genetic predispositions versus the knowledge of genetic predisposition to disease that may or may not be preventable (Borry, Evers-Kiebooms, Cornel, & Clarke, 2009; Borry, Howard, Senecal, & Avard, 2010; Bush & Rothenberg, 2014).

Historically, responsible laboratory testing and screening have been based on the ethical criteria that a test needed to be meaningful and highly predictive, the condition screened for needed to be serious, and there were follow-up actions or interventions available (Bunnik et al., 2013). The Centers for Disease Control and Prevention (CDC) Office of Public Health Genomics developed the ACCE model for evaluating genetic tests. This model uses 44 targeted questions to evaluate genetic tests according to analytic validity, clinical validity, clinical utility, and ethical, legal, and social implications (ELSI; CDC, 2010). A vast amount of data is generated from WGS and WES, which leads to ethical issues for both practitioners and patients. Data from WGS and WES may not be entirely interpretable at the time of testing, with meaningful results becoming available years later as research reveals new correlations between genetic markers and health conditions. The prospect of incidental findings from WGS and WES has implications for informed consent and disclosure of information. Respecting autonomy would allow patients the right to know or not to know about incidental findings.

Some authorities suggest that practitioners have a duty to recontact patients about incidental findings in order to satisfy the principles of beneficence and nonmaleficence (Clift et al., 2015). The American College of Medical Genetics recommends that patients who have their own or their child's WGS or WES should be informed of incidental findings that are of medical value (Green et al., 2013). There are currently no national or international guidelines about when and how to recontact patients with incidental findings (Otten et al., 2015). Very few research studies have been published about this topic and the implications for primary care settings. The information from the few publications on this topic suggest that patients expect to be recontacted by their health-care provider with new information as it becomes available (Otten et al., 2015). The right not to know should be incorporated into the informed consent process for WGS testing (Hull & Berkman, 2014). Patients should be given control over future data use rather than a one-time consent process that does not accommodate privacy concerns or actively involve patients in relevant future results (Erlich et al., 2014).

Providers need to counsel patients on a case-by-case basis in order to come to an agreement about which incidental findings the patient would like to know. Compassion and advocacy are critically important during and after the genetic testing process.

Nonmaleficence

Nonmaleficence is the responsibility to minimize harm in the technology used (Beauchamp & Childress, 2009). We identified 10 studies with findings related to nonmaleficence, which included 6 descriptive survey studies, 2 qualitative studies, 1 study that utilized focus groups, and 1 study that included a pretest/posttest design. Studies that had findings that addressed issues of nonmaleficence were mainly related to providers' lack of knowledge about genetics/genomics (9 studies) and concerns about confidentiality of genetic test results (2 studies).

Provider's Lack of Knowledge

Although many support integrating genetic/genomic services into primary care, there is an ongoing debate as to whether primary care providers are prepared to provide genetic services. We identified several studies in our analysis that reported providers' lack of knowledge and skills related to the application of genetics in primary care practice. O'Neill et al. (2010) surveyed 161 primary care providers and reported that 31% would order genetic testing for BRCA1/2 for an adolescent. Providers who would order this testing had significantly higher patient volume and frequency of ordering tests. This suggests that primary care providers who are willing to order genetic tests for adolescents may not fully understand the risks and benefits regarding testing of minors for adult-onset diseases (Ross et al., 2013). Two qualitative studies of primary care providers concluded that the providers felt that they needed more education as to how to order genetic testing and when to make a referral to a genetic specialist (Arar, Seo, Abboud, Parchman, & Noel, 2010; Trinidad et al., 2008). A survey of 46 APRN students noted that the students perceived they had minimal knowledge of genetics (Maradiegue, Edwards, Seibert, Macri, & Sitzer, 2005). Similarly, two studies of 220 internists who practice in primary care settings noted that the majority surveyed felt they needed more training about when to order genetic tests and how to counsel patients regarding genetic conditions (Klitzman et al., 2013a, 2013b). Additionally, a survey that compared the comfort of 51 primary care and 31 specialist physicians with initiating a referral for cancer genetic testing reported that primary care physicians were significantly less comfortable making a referral and discussing genetics compared with specialists (Brandt, Ali, Sabel, McHugh, & Gilman, 2008).

It has been suggested that primary care practitioners are lacking in the theoretical knowledge and skills to provide genetic services and that they could provide information to patients that is misleading (Schmitz, 2010; Shoenbill et al., 2014). Busy clinicians who work in primary care settings may not have the time to adequately counsel patients about genetic testing causing additional distress (Mikat-Stevens et al., 2014). A recent review of case studies with adverse outcomes as a result of genetic testing and counseling provided by primary care practitioners identified that the adverse outcomes were related to wrong tests ordered, misinterpreted results, and unnecessary tests (Brierley et al., 2012). This review also reported lawsuits where practitioners were found to be negligent because insufficient family history was obtained, genetic tests were not ordered, appropriate referral to genetic specialists were not made, and suitable risk reduction options were not provided (Brierley et al., 2012). There are alternative learning methods that could aid with this dilemma. Srinivasan and colleagues (2011) found that a web-based course was effective for improving the self-efficacy of primary care medical residents with ethical issues related to genetics in clinical practice. Primary care providers have an obligation to be up-to-date in their practice and this includes advances in genetics (Badzek, Henaghan, Turner, & Monsen, 2013).

Another area of concern for primary care providers is the lack of knowledge about pharmacogenetics, which is becoming increasingly important for medication management. Qualitative focus groups that included 21 primary care and genetics professionals reported that providers expressed concerns and lack of knowledge about implementation of pharmacogenetic testing in clinical practice. Reasons providers gave for concerns about implementing pharmacogenetics in their practice included delay of treatment, limitations in clinical utility, insurance coverage and reimbursement issues, and inability to interpret test results (Haga, Trindall, & O'Daniel, 2012).

Part of the resistance providers have to implementing pharmacogenomics into practice is related to a lack of clinical decision support tools to guide clinicians to order the correct tests and use genetic data to prescribe medications effectively (Weitzel et al., 2014). Lack of pharmacogenomic knowledge by providers could lead to liability and adverse patient outcomes. For example, a case study reported that a breast-fed newborn who died from morphine poisoning was later genotyped for the cytochrome P450 2D6 genetic variant and found to be an "ultrarapid metabolizer" of codeine to morphine. The mother was taking codeine, which is a commonly prescribed pain medication in the postpartum period (Koren, Cairns, Chitayat, Gaedigk, & Leeder, 2006). In another case, an adult patient who was treated for a cough with codeine cough syrup developed life-threatening opioid intoxication even though only a small dose of medication was prescribed. Genotyping consequently revealed that the patient was an ultrarapid metabolizer of codeine (Gasche et al., 2004). While pharmacogenomic testing for the metabolization of opioids is not yet commonplace, there are several drugs that do require genetic testing prior to administration, and other drugs where genetic testing is available to prevent adverse outcomes (PharmGKB, 2015; U.S. Food and Drug Administration, 2014).

Confidentiality

Another ethical issue associated with nonmaleficence is confidentiality. Health-care providers are required to keep patient information confidential. This requirement raises ethical concerns with regard to genetic test results. Genetic test results are of significance to not only patients but also entire families, making it challenging for providers who may feel the need to inform family members who are at risk for a genetic condition. A qualitative evaluation of the disclosure decisions of 20 primary care patients who decided to have DTC genetic testing noted that most of the patients would want to disclose information about their genetic test results to their immediate family and less than half wanted to disclose to extended family (Wasson, Cherny, Sanders, Hogan, & Helzlsouer, 2014). This shows that patients would like to be able to have the choice about disclosure of sensitive genetic test results among family members.

An ethical dilemma exists as to whether a provider should breech individual confidentiality in order to provide information to family members who may be at risk for a life-threatening condition versus respecting patient confidentiality (Resnik, 2003). A survey of 165 osteopathic physicians in family practice settings regarding opinions about disclosing test results to patient's family members reported that the majority felt that adults should be told genetic test results but were unsure about disclosing results to teenagers and children (Erde, McCormack, Steer, Ciervo, & McAbee, 2006). This group of providers felt that they needed more guidance about when, how, and whether to disclose genetic testing information to family members. It is highly unlikely that a health-care provider would face legal charges because a family member was not warned (Badzek et al., 2013). Healthcare providers are not legally required to warn family members about genetic risk. They are only required to encourage a patient to inform family members about the results of genetic testing (Badzek et al., 2013). Genetic predispositions can be somewhat uncertain, can take quite a few years to develop into a condition, and the development is often influenced by environmental factors. However, there could be cases where a family member's health would be improved if they had knowledge of a genetic predisposition.

Health-care providers are not legally required to warn family members about genetic risk. They are only required to encourage a patient to inform family members about the results of genetic testing (Badzek et al., 2013). If patients do not object to informing relatives, there are no legal obstacles that prevent health-care providers from informing patients' relatives (Stol, Menko, Westerman, & Janssens, 2010).

Beneficence

Beneficence is defined as patient advocacy and compassion (Beauchamp & Childress, 2009). Few studies were located that evaluated the principle of beneficence as it relates to genetics/genomics in primary care practice. We identified three studies that had findings related to the principle of beneficence. One of these studies utilized videotaped physician–patient encounters that were qualitatively analyzed, one study utilized focus groups, and one study was a descriptive survey.

Patient Advocacy

The first study was a randomized controlled educational trial that evaluated the effects of web-based versus text-based educational programs on the abilities of 121 physicians to interact with a standardized patient who was at risk for inherited breast cancer (Bell et al., 2014). The standardized patient encounters were video-recorded and analyzed. The study found that the majority of the physician–standardized patient encounters had inadequate family history taking and little discussion about genetic testing and ethical implications regardless of the educational program the physicians were exposed to. These findings show a lack of attention to detail that is ethically important for patient advocacy to take place.

A second study of 16 primary care providers (14 physicians and two midlevel providers) who participated in focus groups to discuss integration of family health history and risk assessment in their practice reported several findings related to the principles of beneficence and justice (Christianson et al., 2012). All of the primary care providers in this study reported that they collected family health history information at initial offices visits, but the information collected varied widely with some providers using standardized questionnaires and others using verbal questions. The providers mainly asked patients about family history of breast, colon, and prostate cancer and reported that a positive family history of these disorders initiated different physical exam techniques and screening recommendations (Christianson et al., 2012). Providers in this study were concerned, because given these limitations, they did not know how to best advocate for their patients. Similarly, a third study of 46 APRN students found these students were not comfortable discussing treatment options with a family diagnosed with a genetic condition, nor were they comfortable collecting a family history (Maradiegue et al., 2005). These studies highlight the problem with a lack of standardization for the collection and discussion of family health history with patients in the clinical setting. This lack of attention to the patient's explanations about family health history diminishes the provider's ability for patient advocacy.

Compassion

Another area of ethical concern related to beneficence is how patients react to genetic/genomic information and the ability to empathize with the patient and family members. Considering the inclusion criteria for our review, few, if any, published research studies in the United States have evaluated the principle of beneficence as it relates to patient outcomes of personal genomic testing in primary care settings. What do patients do with the information from genetic tests? An individual who tests negative for an inherited disorder can have a variety of reactions including relief, survivor guilt, or concern over caregiving responsibilities for members of the family who are affected with the disease. Positive test results can lead to increased surveillance, prophylactic surgery, anxiety, and changes in life planning (Ormond, 2008). Some suggest that having knowledge from genetic testing does not necessarily translate into behavioral changes, while others argue that knowledge of genetic susceptibility to disease can actually reduce motivation to participate in preventive measures (Brower, 2004). Genetic testing results are not always informative and need to be interpreted carefully. In order to accurately interpret genetic test results, the individual medical history, family history, and type of genetic test all need to be considered. A negative test result often means that a change was not identified in the genetic material tested, thereby in singularity, not giving any useful information. Genetic testing is a complex process; negative results cannot always confirm or negate a diagnosis (Genetic Home Reference, 2015). The genetic testing process can cause additional problems for the individual and family members potentially leading to stigmatization, family discord, and psychological distress, which need to be dealt with in a compassionate manner (Nyrhinen, Hietala, Puukka, & Leino-Kilpi, 2007).

Justice

Justice includes the principles of impartial, equal, and fair distribution of resources and treatment (Beauchamp & Childress, 2009). We identified eight articles that had key findings or a purpose related to genetics/genomics in primary care practice and the principle of justice. Six of the studies utilized surveys and two of the studies were qualitative interviews. The studies were related to the issues of impartial treatment and access to genetic services.

Impartial Treatment

There is a national and international problem with genetic discrimination (Otlowski, Taylor, & Bombard, 2012). A study examining impartial treatment found the majority of 1,181 nongenetic health-care providers felt that genetic testing was of benefit for patients but thought that genetic discrimination was an issue that would cause patients to decline testing (Lowstuter et al., 2008). The majority of the providers surveyed were unaware of laws that were in place to prohibit genetic discrimination. This lack of awareness of laws was related to decreased comfort among providers for ordering genetic testing (Lowstuter et al., 2008). Similarly a qualitative study of 16 primary care providers reported that these physicians had concerns with ethical issues related to genetic discrimination and legal liability when ordering genetic tests (Christianson et al., 2012), though few patients have reported genetic discrimination during the testing process (Klitzman et al., 2013b). A random sample of 562 U.S. primary care physicians ranked test results actually leading to improved cessation outcomes as the most important factor for ordering a genetic test for smoking cessation; however, the physicians reported that they would be less likely to order the genetic test if test results led to genetic discrimination (Levy, Youatt, & Shields, 2007). Another survey with a large sample of 86,859 adults in primary care settings regarding their views toward genetic testing reported that 40% of the participants felt that genetic testing might create discrimination related to obtaining health insurance (Hall et al., 2005).

Some fear that the practice of personalized medicine could lead to genetic and racial profiling. For example, advances in pharmacogenetics allow providers to prescribe medications based on an individual patient's genotype results. However, it has been reported that some providers use racial profiling instead of the actual genotype as a basis for prescribing. Interviews of 58 primary care providers suggest that instead of pharmacogenetics leading to individualized medicine, it has led to racial profiling in health care. This is attributed to a lack of knowledge on the part of health-care providers (Hunt & Kreiner, 2013). Genomic scientists are finding that genetic groupings often do not correspond with racial categories. The overlap of socially contrived and genetically bound categories can undermine the potential of personalized medicine, which focuses on the care tailored to the individual based on the identification of genomic risks (Fujimara & Rajaglopalan, 2011). Another consideration in this age of WGS is the possibility that the self-identified race, ethnicity, or nationality of an individual may not represent the genetic ancestry. These factors must be considered when presenting research study results and genomic test results to individuals and families. The distribution of human diversity is complex; therefore, subtleties in race, ethnicity, and nationality are important considerations in the translation of genomic results.

Results of genetic and genomic tests are of interest to a variety of societal institutions and organizations. Employers and insurers have a particular interest in employees' health and genetic and genomic test results, which could potentially lead to discrimination against employees as these entities seek to make hiring decisions and maintain budgets. In the United States, the Genetic Information Nondiscrimination Act (GINA) of 2008 is a law to protect individuals from genetic discrimination by employers and health insurance companies. However, GINA is not entirely comprehensive since it is limited to the civilian population and does not apply to active members of the military, veterans, and Native Americans served by the Indian Health Service (Badzek et al., 2013). GINA only protects against genetic discrimination for health insurance, but not for life, disability, or long-term care insurance. The possibility for genetic discrimination exists regarding eligibility for these types of insurance. There is a need for additional legislation that protects individuals against genetic discrimination including regulatory and legislative protections for privacy of WGS/WES data to ensure ethical considerations are being upheld when evaluating genomic information (Ginsburg & Willard, 2009).

Access to Genetic Services

Two studies in our analysis reported findings that address the issue of access to genetic services. A survey of 498 family physicians reported that these providers routinely provide a variety of genetic services to patients including consulting for perinatal conditions and familial cancers (Acheson, Stange, & Zyzanski, 2005). In this same study, physicians practicing in rural settings reported that it was difficult to find genetic consultants. A group of 112 primary care physicians were surveyed regarding motivations and barriers associated with ordering genetic testing for Factor V Leiden. Many of the physicians felt that lack of the availability of genetic counseling services was a barrier that influenced their motivation to order genetic testing (Hindorff et al., 2009).

Cost also affects access to genetic services. Although it is projected that genomic discoveries and personalized care will provide cost savings, this is not always the case. As the genomic science moves ahead, there are significant pharmacogenomic discoveries; however, these discoveries often come with a stunning price tag. In an era of health-care policy calling for price controls, this poses roadblocks for educated consumers demanding access to the medications that can provide personalized treatments (Carlson, 2008). For example, the cost of crizotinib, a targeted therapy for non-small-cell lung cancer, is approximately $115,000.00 annually or $10,000.00 per month. Although crizotinib is considered a clinically effective treatment, the cost is prohibitive and insurers are rarely willing to cover the cost of this drug (Djalalov et al., 2014). Access to genetic treatment and services is not always available. In rural areas, there are a lack of available genetic services, which raises concerns about access for patients (Hawkins & Hayden, 2011).

CONCLUSIONS

Sparse research has been conducted on the actual ethical issues encountered by health-care providers in the primary care setting. The majority of research that addresses ethical issues related to genetics and genomics in primary care settings were descriptive surveys or qualitative designs with very few experimental or quasi-experimental designs. There were few studies where the main purpose was to evaluate the ethical issues related to genetics/genomics in primary care practice. Most of the studies included key findings that were pertinent to this topic but few were designed to exclusively evaluate ethical issues related to genomics in primary care practice. Many of the studies had various limitations including small sample sizes, bias associated with self-report data, and samples that were not representative of the general population. These limitations decrease the generalizability of the findings of these studies. Much of the research was based on opinions related to hypothetical case studies and situations presented in survey form. Very few studies have focused directly on the role of primary care providers with genetic and genomic services and the ethical issues faced by this group. It is interesting to note that when the studies are listed by date of publication and topic, more studies have been conducted regarding the topic of autonomy in the past 4 years. This may be influenced by the development of new genomic testing technologies. However, few studies to date have directly evaluated the ethical implications related to advanced technologies such as WGS and WES and their utilization in primary care settings. Little research has been conducted on the actual ethical issues encountered by health-care providers in the primary care setting. More research needs to be conducted that examines the actual experiences of primary care providers with ethical issues associated with genetics and genomics in clinical practice.

Implications for Primary Care Practice

Genomic science is infiltrating day-to-day health care practice and therefore is an integral part of the care delivered by primary care providers. ELSI issues that arise from this science are complex and are too important to be ignored (McCarthy, 2014). Often in the primary care setting, providers take a directive approach with the patient, rather than understanding the perspective and wishes of the patient that are critical to the decision-making process for informed genomic testing. A trusted partnership between patient and provider that is neither judgmental nor compulsory is important to having the patient make an informed choice that is ultimately his or her decision. The current primary care system allots minimal time for patient visits, whereas the time allotments required for pretest and posttest genomic counseling are an hour or longer, often require follow-up visits, and are integral to the management of genomic patient care and assisting with informed decisions. Innovative models of care that address these issues are required to meet the growing technology that is rapidly entering primary care (American Hospital Association, 2013).

On the horizon is the genomic health record containing WGS that will merge with data from the current electronic medical record actualizing the paradigm of personalized medicine (Fraser & Pai, 2014). Primary care providers including APRNs must understand genomic science and how it will be integrated into clinical practice as well as its impact on the ethical implications for individuals, families, and communities. This requires that primary care providers keep current on this rapidly changing field and integrate new evidence-based genomic information into practice at all levels of care. Medical schools and organizations are addressing the integration of personalized medicine into curricula, and nursing will require leadership skills to incorporate genetic technology into patient care (Demmer & Waggoner, 2014; Huston, 2013). ELSI matters that arise from the science of genetics and genomics are too important to be ignored and cannot be learned in the clinical setting alone. Continuing education regarding ELSI and genetic/genomic services should be a part of staff education using an interprofessional team approach to discuss genetic privacy, screening, and other issues that may impact the individual's care management.

REFERENCES

Acheson, L. S., Stange, K. C., & Zyzanski, S. (2005). Clinical genetics encountered by family physicians. *Genetics in Medicine, 7*(7), 501–508.

Ali-Khan, S. E., Daar, A. S., Shuman, C., Ray, P. N., & Scherer, S. W. (2009). Whole genome scanning: Resolving clinical diagnosis and management amidst complex data. *Pediatric Research, 66*(4), 357–363. http://dx.doi.org/10.1203/pdr.0b013e3181b0cbd8

American Hospital Association. (2013, January). *Workforce roles in a redesigned primary care model.* Retrieved from https://www.google.com/url?sa=t&rct=j&q=&esrc=s&source=web&cd=1&cad=rja&uact=8&ved=0CB0QFjAAahUKEwjk2urV2-XIAhVFFT4KHbe1C-Y&url=http%3A%2F%2Fwww.aha.org%2Fcontent%2F13%2F13-0110-wf-primary-care.pdf&usg=AFQjCNEBp01ohNhw5_E7OVYznpRQ5ZbaLw&sig2=Dd7pzQqmez-K9KrciOtfpw

Arar, N., Seo, J., Abboud, H. E., Parchman, M., & Noel, P. (2010). Providers' behavioral beliefs regarding the delivery of genomic medicine at the veterans health administration. *Personalized Medicine, 7*(5), 485–494.

Badzek, L., Henaghan, M., Turner, M., & Monsen, R. (2013). Ethical, legal, and social issues in the translation of genomics into health care. *Journal of Nursing Scholarship, 45*(1), 15–24.

Beauchamp, T. L., & Childress, J. F. (2009). *Principles of biomedical ethics* (6th ed.). New York, NY: Oxford University Press.

Bell, R. A., McDermott, H., Fancher, T. L., Green, M. J., Day, F. C., & Wilkes, M. S. (2015). Impact of a randomized controlled educational trial to improve physician practice behaviors around screening for inherited breast cancer. *Journal of General Internal Medicine, 30*(3), 334–341. http://dx.doi.org/10.1007/s11606-014-3113-5

Biesecker, L. G. (2012). Opportunities and challenges for the integration of massively parallel genomic sequencing into clinical practice: Lessons from the ClinSeq project. *Genetics in Medicine, 14*(4), 393–398.

Borry, P., Evers-Kiebooms, G., Cornel, M. C., & Clarke, A. (2009). Genetic testing in asymptomatic minors. *European Journal of Human Genetics, 17*, 711–719. http://dx.doi.org/10.1038/ejhg.2009.25

Borry, P., Howard, H. C., Senecal, K., & Avard, D. (2010). Health-related direct to consumer genetic testing: A review of companies policies with regard to genetic testing in minors. *Familial Cancer, 9*, 51–59.

Brandt, R., Ali, Z., Sabel, A., McHugh, T., & Gilman, P. (2008). Cancer genetics evaluation: Barriers to and improvements for referral. *Genetic Testing, 12*(1), 9–12.

Brierley, K. L., Blouch, E., Cogswell, W., Homer, J. P., Pencarinha, D., Stanislaw, C. L., et al. (2012). Adverse events in cancer genetic testing: Medical, ethical, legal, and financial implications. *The Cancer Journal, 18*(4), 303–309.

Brower, V. (2004). Genomics and health care. *European Molecular Biology Organization Reports, 5*(2), 131–133.

Bunnik, E. M., de Jong, A., Nijsingh, N., & de Wert, G. M. (2013). The new genetics and informed consent: Differentiating choice to preserve autonomy. *Bioethics, 27*(6), 348–355.

Bush, L. W., & Rothenberg, K. H. (2014, March). *The drama of DNA: Psychosocial, ethical, & policy implications for NBSeq.* Paper presented at the meeting of American College of Medical Genetics, Nashville, TN.

Carlson, R. (2008). Preemptive public policy for genomics. *Journal of Health Policy, Politics and Law, 33*(1), 39–51.

Centers for Disease Control. (2010). *ACCE model process for evaluating genetic tests.* Retrieved from http://www.cdc.gov/genomics/gtesting/ACCE/

Christianson, C. A., Powell, K. P., Hahn, S. E., Blanton, S. H., Bogacik, J., & Henrich, V. C. (2012). The use of a family history risk assessment tool within a community health care system: Views of primary care providers. *Journal of Genetic Counseling, 21*(5), 652–661.

Clayton, E. W., McCullough, L. B., Biesecker, L. G., Joffe, S., Ross, L. F., & Wolf, S. M. (2014). Addressing the ethical challenges in genetic testing and sequencing in children. *American Journal of Bioethics, 14*(3), 3–9.

Collins, F. S., Green, E. D., Guttmacher, A. E., & Guyer, M. S. (2003). A vision for the future of genomics research. *Nature, 422*, 835–847.

Constantine, M. L., Allyse, M., Wall, M., Vries, R. D., & Rockwood, T. H. (2014). Imperfect informed consent for prenatal screening: Lessons from the quad screen. *Clinical Ethics, 9*(1), 17–27. http://dx.doi.org/10.1177/1477750913511339

Clift, K., Halverson, C., Fiksdal, A., Kumbamu, A., Sharp, R., McCormick, J. (2015, March). Patients' views on incidental findings from clinical exome sequencing. *Applied & Translational Genomics, 4*, 38–43. Retreived from http://www.sciencedirect.com/science/article/pii/S2212066115000071

Crawford, G., Foulds, N., Fenwick, A., Hallowell, N., & Lucassen, A. (2013). Genetic medicine and incidental findings: It is more complicated than deciding whether to disclose or not. *Genetics in Medicine, 15*(11), 896–899.

Demmer, L. A., & Waggoner, D. J. (2014). Professional medical education and genomics. *Annual Review of Genomics and Human Genetics, 15*, 507–516. http://dx.doi.org/10.1146/annurev-genom-090413-025522

Djalalov, S., Beca, J., Hoch, J., Krahn, M., Tsao, M., Cutz, J., et al. (2014). Cost effectiveness of EML4-ALK fusion testing and first-line Crizotinib treatment for patients with advanced ALK-positive non-small-cell lung cancer. *Journal of Clinical Oncology*, 32, 1012–1019.

Erde, E. L., McCormack, M. K., Steer, R. A., Ciervo, C. A. Jr., & McAbee, G. N. (2006). Patient confidentiality vs disclosure of inheritable risk: A survey-based study. *The Journal of the American Osteopathic Association, 106*(10), 615–620.

Erlich, Y., Williams, J., Glazer, D., Yocum, K., Farahany, N., Olson, M., et al. (2014, November). Redefining genomic privacy: Trust and empowerment. *PLoS Biology, 12*(11), e1001983. Retrieved from http://www.plosbiology.org/article/info%3Adoi%2F10.1371%2Fjournal.pbio.1001983

Fleck, L. M. (2014). Personalized medicine: An introduction to the ethical challenges. *Urologic Oncology, 32*(2), 186.

Fraser, H., & Pai, A. (2014). The role of genomic medicine in transforming healthcare. *Health Policy and Technology, 3*, 223–225.

Fujimara, J., & Rajaglopalan, R. (2011). Different differences: The use of genetic ancestry versus race in biomedical genetic research. *Social Studies of Science, 41*(1), 5–30.

Gasche, Y., Daali, Y., Fathi, M., Chiappe, A., Cottini, S., Dayer, P., et al. (2004). Codeine intoxication associated with ultrarapid CYP2D6 metabolism. *New England Journal of Medicine, 351*(27), 2827–2831.

Genetic Home Reference. (2015, January). *What do the results of genetic tests mean?* Retrieved from http://ghr.nlm.nih.gov/handbook/testing/interpretingresults

Ginsburg, G. S., & Willard, H. F. (2009). Genomic and personalized medicine: Foundations and applications. *Translational Research, 154*(6), 277–287. http://dx.doi.org/10.1016/j.trsl.2009.09.005

Goldenberg, A. J., Dodson, D. S., Davis, M. M., & Tarini, B. A. (2014). Parents' interest in whole-genome sequencing of newborns. *Genetics in Medicine: Official Journal of the American College of Medical Genetics, 16*(1), 78–84. http://dx.doi.org/10.1038/gim.2013.76

Gornick, M. C., Fagerlin, A., Exe, N., Larkin, K., Magoc, E., & Zikmund-Fisher, B. J. (2014, March). *Failure of negative genetic test results to reassure both patients and clinicians in the context of family history.* Paper presented at the meeting of the American College of Medical Genetics, Nashville, TN.

Green, E., Guyer, M., Manolio, T. A., & Peterson, J. L. (2011). Charting a course in genomic medicine from base pairs to bedside. *Nature, 470*, 204–213. http://dx.doi.org/10.1038/nature09764

Green, R. C., Berg, J. S., Grody, W. W., Kalia, S. S. Korf, B. R., Martin, C. L., et al. (2013). ACMG recommendations for reporting of incidental findings in clinical exome and genome sequencing. *Genetics in Medicine, 15*(7), 565–574.

Haga, S. B., Tindall, G., & O'Daniel, J. M. (2012). Professional perspectives about pharmacogenetic testing and managing ancillary findings. *Genetic Testing and Molecular Biomarkers, 16*(1), 21–24. http://dx.doi.org/10.1089/gtmb.2011.0045

Hall, M. A., McEwen, J. E., Barton, J. C., Walker, A. P., Howe, E. G., Reiss, J. A., et al. (2005). Concerns in a primary care population about genetic discrimination by insurers. *Genetics in Medicine: Official Journal of the American College of Medical Genetics, 7*(5), 311–316.

Hawkins, A. K., & Hayden, M. R. (2011). A grand challenge: Providing benefits of clinical genetics to those in need. *Genetics in Medicine, 13*(3), 197–200.

Hay, J., Kaphingst, K. A., Baser, R., Li, Y., Hensley-Alford, S., & McBride, C. M. (2012). Skin cancer concerns and genetic risk information-seeking in primary care. *Public Health Genomics, 15*(2), 57–72. http://dx.doi.org/10.1159/000330403

Hazin, R., Brothers, K. B., Malin, B. A., Koenig, B. A., Sanderson, S. C., Rothstein, J. D., et al. (2013). Ethical, legal, and social implications of incorporating genomic information into electronic health records. *Genetics in Medicine, 15*(10), 810–816.

Hindorff, L. A., Burke, W., Laberge, A., Rice, K. M., Lumley, T., Leppig, K., et al. (2009). Motivating factors for physician ordering of factor V Leiden genetic tests. *Archives of Internal Medicine, 169*(1), 68–74.

Hogarth, S., Javitt, G., & Metzer, D. (2008). The current landscape for direct-to-consumer genetic testing: Legal, ethical, and policy issues. *Annual Review of Genomics and Human Genetics, 9*, 161–182.

Hull, S. C., & Berkman, B. E. (2014). Grappling with genomic incidental findings in the clinical realm. *Chest, 145*(2), 226–230.

Hunt, L. M., & Kreiner, M. J. (2013). Pharmacogenetics in primary care: The promise of personalized medicine and the reality of racial profiling. *Culture, Medicine, & Psychiatry, 37*(1), 226–235.

Hurley, K., Rubin, L. R., Werner-Lin, A., Sagi, M., Kemel, Y., Stern, R., et al. (2012). Incorporating information regarding preimplantation genetic diagnosis into discussions concerning testing and risk management for BRCA1/2 mutations. *Cancer (0008543X), 118*(24), 6270–6277. http://dx.doi.org/10.1002/cncr.27695

Huston, C. (2013). The impact of emerging technology on nursing care: Warp speed ahead. *The Online Journal of Issues in Nursing, 18*(2), Manuscript 1.

Johns Hopkins Bloomberg School of Public Health. (2014). *The Johns Hopkins Primary Care Policy Center*. Retrieved from http://www.jhsph.edu/research/centers-and-institutes/johns-hopkins-primary-care-policy-center/definitions.html

Kirk, M. (2000). Genetics, ethics, and education: Considering the issues for nurses and midwives. *Nursing Ethics, 7*(3), 215–226.

Klitzman, R., Chung, W., Marder, K., Shanmugham, A., Chin, L. J., Stark, M., et al. (2013a). Views of internists towards uses of PGD. *Reproductive BioMedicine Online, 26*(2), 142–147.

Klitzman, R., Chung, W., Marder, K., Shanmugham, A., Chin, L. J., Stark, M., et al. (2013b). Attitudes and practices among internists concerning genetic testing. *Journal of Genetic Counseling, 22*(1), 90–100. http://dx.doi.org/10.1007/s10897-012-9504-z

Koren, G., Cairns, J., Chitayat, D., Gaedigk, A., & Leeder, S. J. (2006). Pharmacogenetics of morphine poisoning in a breastfed neonate of a codeine-prescribed mother. *The Lancet, 368*, 704.

Lazaridis, K. N., McAllister, T. M., Babovic-Vuksanovic, D., Beck, S. A., Borad, M. J., Bryce, A. H., et al. (2014). Implementing individualized medicine into medical practice. *American Journal of Medical Genetics, 166C*, 15–23.

Letendre, M., & Godard, B. (2004). Expanding the physician's duty of care: A duty to recontact? *Medicine and Law, 23*(3), 531–539.

Letts, L., Wilkins, S., Law, M., Stewart, D., Bosch, J., & Westmoreland, M. (2007). *Critical review form—Qualitative studies (Version 2.0)*. Retrieved from http://srs-mcmaster.ca/wp-content/uploads/2015/04/Critical-Review-Form-Qualitative-Studies-Version-2.pdf

Levy, D. E., Youatt, E. J., & Shields, A. E. (2007). Primary care physicians' concerns about offering a genetic test to tailor smoking cessation treatment. *Genetics in Medicine, 9*(12), 842–849.

Lewis, N. P., Treise, D., Hsu, S. I., Allen, W. L., & Kang, H. (2011). DTC genetic testing companies fail transparency prescriptions. *New Genetics and Society, 30*(4), 291–307. http://dx.doi.org/10.1080/14636778.2011.600434

Lowstuter, K. J., Sand, S., Blazer, K. R., MacDonald, D. J., Banks, K. C., Lee, C. A., et al. (2008). Influence of genetic discrimination perceptions and knowledge on cancer genetics referral practice among clinicians. *Genetics in Medicine, 10*(9), 691–698. http://dx.doi.org/10.1097/gim.0b013e3181837246

Maradiegue, A., Edwards, Q. T., Seibert, D., Macri, C., & Sitzer, L. (2005). Knowledge, perceptions, and attitudes of advanced practice nursing students regarding medical genetics. *Journal of the American Academy of Nurse Practitioners, 17*(11), 472–479. http://dx.doi.org/10.1111/j.1745-7599.2005.00076.x

McCarthy, J. (2014, November). Driving personalized medicine forward: The who, what, when and how of educating the healthcare workforce. *Molecular Genomics and Genomic Medicine, 2*(6), 455–457.

Mikat-Stevens, N. A., Larson, I. A., & Tarini, B. A. (2014, September 11) Primary-care providers' perceived barriers to integration of genetics services: A systematic review of the literature. *Genetics in Medicine, 17*(3), 169–176. http://dx.doi.org/10.1038/gim.2014.101

Mulchandani, S., Dechene, E. T., Dulik, M. C., Conlin, L., Abrudan, J., Berhardt, B. A et al. (2014, March). *Lessons learned from utilizing an evidenced-based framework for incidental findings from exome sequencing in the pediatric setting.* Paper presented at the meeting of the American College of Medical Genetics, Nashville, TN.

National Collaborating Centre for Methods and Tools. (2008). *Quality assessment tool for quantitative studies.* Hamilton, ON: McMaster University (Updated 13 April, 2010). Retrieved from http://www.nccmt.ca/registry/view/eng/14.html

Nyrhinen, T., Hietala, M., Puukka, P., & Leino-Kilpi, H. (2007). Privacy and equality in diagnostic genetic testing. *Nursing Ethics, 14*(3), 295–308.

O'Neill, S. C., Peshkin, B. N., Luta, G., Abraham, A., Walker, L. R., & Tercyak, K. P. (2010). Primary care providers' willingness to recommend BRCA1/2 testing to adolescents. *Familial Cancer, 9*(1), 43–50. http://dx.doi.org/10.1007/s10689-009-9243-y

Ormond, K. E. (2008). Medical ethics for the genome world. *The Journal of Molecular diagnostics, 10*(5), 377–382.

Otten, E., Plantinga, M., Birnie, E., Verkerk, M., Lucassen, A., Ranchor, A., & Van Langen, I. (2015, August). *Genetics in Medicine, 17*(8), 668–678. doi:10.1038/gim.2014.173

Otlowski, M., Taylor, S., & Bombard, Y. (2012). Genetic discrimination: International perspectives. *Annual Review of Genomics and Human Genetics, 13,* 433–454.

PharmGKB. (2015). *Drug labels.* Retrieved from http://www.pharmgkb.org/view/drug-labels.do

Resnik, D. B. (2003). Genetic testing and primary care: A new ethic for a new setting. *New Genetics and Society, 22*(3), 245–256.

Ross, L., Saal, H., David, K., Anderson, R., American Academy of Pediatrics., & American College of Genetics and Genomics. (2013). Technical report: Ethical and policy issues in genetic testing and screening of children. *Genetics in Medicine, 15*(3), 234–245.

Schmitz, D. (2010). Exceptional know how? Possible pitfalls of routinizing genetic services. *Journal of Medical Ethics, 36*(9), 529–533.

Sharp, R. R. (2011). Downsizing genomic medicine: Approaching the ethical complexity of whole-genome sequencing by starting small. *Genetics in Medicine, 13*(3), 191–194.

Shoenbill, K., Fost, N., Tachinardi, U., & Mendonca, E. A. (2014). Genetic data and electronic health records: A discussion of ethical logistical and technological considerations. *Journal of the American Medical Informatics Association, 21*, 171–180.

Srinivasan, M., Day, F. C., Griffin, E., Tancredi, D. J., Burke, W., Pinsky, L., et al. (2011). Implementation outcomes of multi-institutional web-based ethical, legal, and social implications genetics curriculum for primary care residents in three specialties. *Genetics in Medicine, 13*(6), 553–562.

Stol, Y. H., Menko, F. H., Westerman, M. J., & Janssens, R. M. (2010). Informing family members about a hereditary predisposition to cancer: Attitudes and practices among clinical geneticists. *Journal of Medical Ethics, 36*(7), 391–395.

Strong, K. A., Zusevics, K. L., Bick, D., & Veith, R. (2014). Views of primary care providers regarding the return of genome sequencing incidental findings. *Clinical Genetics, 86*(5), 461–468. http://dx.doi.org/10.1111/cge.12390

Trinidad, S. B., Fryer-Edwards, K., Crest, A., Kyler, P., Lloyd-Puryear, M., & Burke, W. (2008). Educational needs in genetic medicine: Primary care perspectives. *Community Genetics, 11*(3), 160–165. http://dx.doi.org/10.1159/000113878

U.S. Food and Drug Administration. (2014, August). *Table for pharmacogenomics biomarkers in drug labeling.* Retrieved from http://www.fda.gov/drugs/scienceresearch/researchareas/pharmacogenetics/ucm083378.htm

Wasson, K., Cherny, S., Sanders, T. N., Hogan, N. S., & Helzlsouer, K. J. (2014). Who are you going to call? Primary care patients' disclosure decisions regarding direct-to-consumer genetic testing. *Narrative Inquiry in Bioethics, 4*(1), 53–68. http://dx.doi.org/10.1353/nib.2014.0026

Wasson, K., Hogan, N. S., Sanders, T. N., & Helzlsouer, K. J. (2012). Primary care patients' views, attitudes, and decision-making factors regarding direct-to-consumer personal genome testing: Results from a qualitative study. *AJOB Primary Research, 3*(2), 24–35. http://dx.doi.org/10.1080/21507716.2011.650344

Weitzel, K. W., Elsey, A. R., Langaee, T. Y., Burkley, B., Nessl, D. R., Obeng, A. O., et al. (2014). Clinical pharmacogenetics implementation: Approaches, successes, and challenges. *American Journal of Medical Genetics, 166C*, 56–67.

Whittemore, R., & Knafl, K. (2005). The integrative review: Updated methodology. *Journal of Advanced Nursing, 52*(5), 546–553.

CHAPTER 9

Ethical Considerations Regarding the Use of Smart Home Technologies for Older Adults

An Integrative Review

Jane Chung, George Demiris, and Hilaire J. Thompson

ABSTRACT

Problem: With the wide adoption and use of smart home applications, there is a need for examining ethical issues regarding smart home use at the intersection of aging, technology, and home environment. Purpose: The purpose of this review is to provide an overview of ethical considerations and the evidence on these ethical issues based on an integrative literature review with regard to the utilization of smart home technologies by older adults and their family members. Review Design and Methods: We conducted an integrative literature review of the scientific literature from indexed databases (e.g., MEDLINE, CINAHL, and PsycINFO). The framework guiding this review is derived from previous work on ethical considerations related to telehealth use for older adults and smart homes for palliative care. Key ethical issues of the framework include privacy, informed consent, autonomy, obtrusiveness, equal access, reduction in human touch, and usability. Results: Six hundred and thirty-five candidate articles were identified between the years 1990 and

http://dx.doi.org/10.1891/0739-6686.34.155

2014. Sixteen articles were included in the review. Privacy and obtrusiveness issues appear to be the most important factors that can affect smart home technology adoption. In addition, this article recommends that stigmatization and reliability and maintenance of the system are additional factors to consider. Implications: When smart home technology is used appropriately, it has the potential to improve quality of life and maintain safety among older adults, ultimately supporting the desire of older adults for aging in place. The ability to respond to potential ethical concerns will be critical to the future development and application of smart home technologies that aim to enhance safety and independence.

INTRODUCTION

There is a rapid growth in the number of older adults worldwide. According to projections by the U.S. Census Bureau (2014), the population of adults age 65 years and older will account for 15% in 2015 and is expected to reach about 24% by 2060 due to longer life spans and the aging baby boom generation. This situation presents many challenges for our health-care system due to conditions that come with aging, such as chronic diseases, sensory and cognitive impairments, physical disabilities, and isolation. These health challenges then place substantial social, psychological, and financial burden on older adults, their family caregivers, and society. As a result, there is increased need for high-quality, efficient, and accessible care. Especially critical are community-based solutions, as older adults have a desire to remain independent in their homes or in the community setting (Rantz et al., 2010; Rantz et al., 2013; Vasunilashorn, Steinman, Liebig, & Pynoos, 2012; Wild, Boise, Lundell, & Foucek, 2008). The use of technology applications in the home setting can be one of these solutions; yet there are ethical issues to be considered regarding their use. This article discusses ethical considerations and dilemmas arising from smart home implementations to support older adults and their family caregivers at home. Also we provide an integrative review of the literature on ethical issues regarding smart home technologies by analyzing and synthesizing the current state of smart home technology ethics. An ethical framework derived from the previous literature guides the review.

BACKGROUND

The emergence of novel home-based sensor technologies has introduced a new way of providing care for older adults and assistance to their family caregivers. Personal living spaces of older adults with embedded sensor technologies to promote independence and wellness are termed *smart homes* (Reeder, Meyer, et al., 2013). Smart home technologies are designed to support older adults or people with disabilities by monitoring their health and facilitating prevention of undesirable events. These technologies may allow for functional independence by assisting the elderly population to cope with various health issues such as falls, mobility limitations, cognitive impairment, or social isolation (Berke, Choudhury, Ali, & Rabbi, 2011; Scanaill, Garattini, Greene, & McGrath, 2011). Also, smart home applications have the potential to enable real-time, accessible, and minimally intrusive ways of monitoring health and delivering care to individuals who are in need.

There are two distinct smart home approaches, *distributed direct sensing* (DDS) and *infrastructure-mediated sensing* (IMS; Demiris, 2009). DDS refers to infrastructure with a new sensing network physically installed in the home to sense motion, presence, or other behavioral indicators. On the other hand, IMS indicates existing sensor-based residences through electrical or air conditioning systems with the aim of monitoring activities of the individual. There are various types of smart home applications, including, but not limited to, (a) activity monitoring system employing wireless motion sensors, refrigerator door sensor, toilet flush sensor, water consumption sensor, bed sensor, or pressure mats, (b) video monitoring system, or (c) home-based sensors for enhancing safety such as smoke detector, temperature sensor, door security system, and so forth (Alwan, 2009; Bruce, 2012; Kang et al., 2010). A smart home is viewed as a holistic and centrally controlled environment that enables interpretation of resident health needs and proactively responds to changes in health (Johnson, Davenport, Mann, & Otr, 2007). Passive monitoring features of smart homes do not require older adults to operate the device or use a computer. Therefore, these can benefit various populations of older adults with limited technological knowledge or those with cognitive impairment, while avoiding problems caused by incorrect or nonuse of a system (Alwan, 2009; Mahoney, 2011). Smart home applications were found to be useful for individuals with chronic conditions because the systems can be further applied to examination, diagnosis, and consultation of the person being monitored (Chan, Estève, Escriba, & Campo, 2008). However, the monitoring function depends on complex algorithms to interpret the data generated by the sensors.

Multiple forms of smart home applications are being developed and applied in the health-care sector to support aging in place (Figure 9.1). The pervasive use of smart home technologies requires thoughtful considerations on the complexity of ethical issues. Although smart homes have positively impacted patients, family caregivers, and health-care providers, there is a potential for harm and abuse that may result from privacy invasion, the breach of confidentiality, loss of

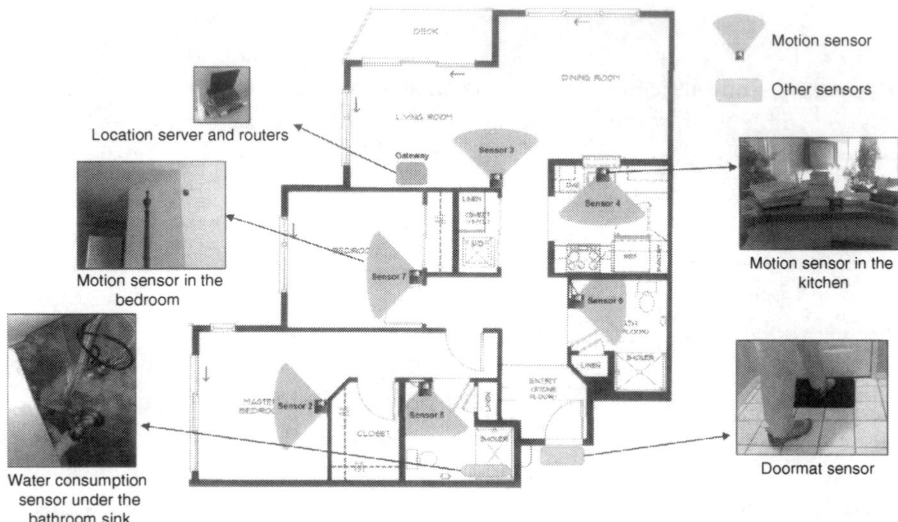

FIGURE 9.1 A sample floor plan and its sensor network. The simulated smart home system in this diagram consists of various types of home-based wireless sensors and a location server. These sensors are designed to monitor different types of activities such as movement from one location to another, water use, stepping out of the house, and so forth. Each sensor sends the signal to the local server, and the server sends the data to a central server so that engineers or data personnel download and analyze the data. Please note that there are different types of smart home applications and system architectures.

touch, or dehumanization. Also, ethical considerations arising for older adults may not be the same as ethical concerns for other age groups. They may have difficulty in technical understanding of the information they receive due to lack of technology experience or instruction as well as age-related capabilities. In order to ensure the optimal use of smart home applications, it is necessary to adequately address the ethical issues at the intersection of aging, technology, and home environment when considering the adoption of smart homes for supporting aging in place (Lorenzen-Huber, Boutain, Camp, Shankar, & Connelly, 2011). Addressing these issues can guide better design and help predict successful implementation of the technology.

METHODS

Whittemore and Knafl's methodology (2005) was used to guide the current review. Two researchers (JC & GD) discussed which ethical categories should be included for this review based on the previous studies on telehealth and smart home ethics. This integrative review includes qualitative, quantitative, and mixed methods studies and uses studies published in English between 1990 and August 2014. Computerized database searches were conducted by the first author (JC) using PubMed, CINAHL, and PsycINFO. Search terms included "smart home," "sensor," "sensor technology," "home-based health monitoring," "home-based health technology," "gerontechnology," and "gerotechnology" combined with "older adults," "elderly," and "community-dwelling."

Inclusion and exclusion criteria were developed by two authors (JC & GD). We did not exclude any studies based on study design or methodology because we wanted to cover all studies that examined ethical issues with actual or potential end users of smart home technologies. Titles and abstracts were reviewed by the first author (JC) and included if they met the following criteria: (a) The study examined ethical concerns of older adults or caregivers with regard to the utilization of smart homes using either a survey or an interview, (b) the study focused on home-based technologies to support older adults in residential settings with an aim of either monitoring activities or preventing adverse health outcomes, (c) the study sample included older adults or their informal or formal caregivers, and (d) the study was a quantitative or qualitative analysis of data. Studies were excluded if they focused on remote monitoring of health among older adults with a specific disease (e.g., diabetes). In total, 635 articles were returned from database searches and reference list reviews. During the full-text article review, another researcher (HT) independently reviewed three randomly selected articles from the downloaded full-text results and applied the inclusion and exclusion criteria for testing interrater reliability. The two researchers (JC & HT) discussed differences until agreement was reached about application of the inclusion and exclusion criteria. Initial agreement before reconciliation was 67%, and agreement after reconciliation was 100%. Figure 9.2 shows literature identification and screening processes, indicating that from the initial 635 publications, finally, 16 articles were selected for this review.

ETHICAL FRAMEWORK GUIDING THE REVIEW

In order to successfully implement smart sensor projects for older adults, an ethical framework is important to guide the design, development, and evaluation of smart home technologies. Such a framework better informs the application of smart home technologies and delivery of care through those technologies. The framework for ethical dimensions in this review is based on previous

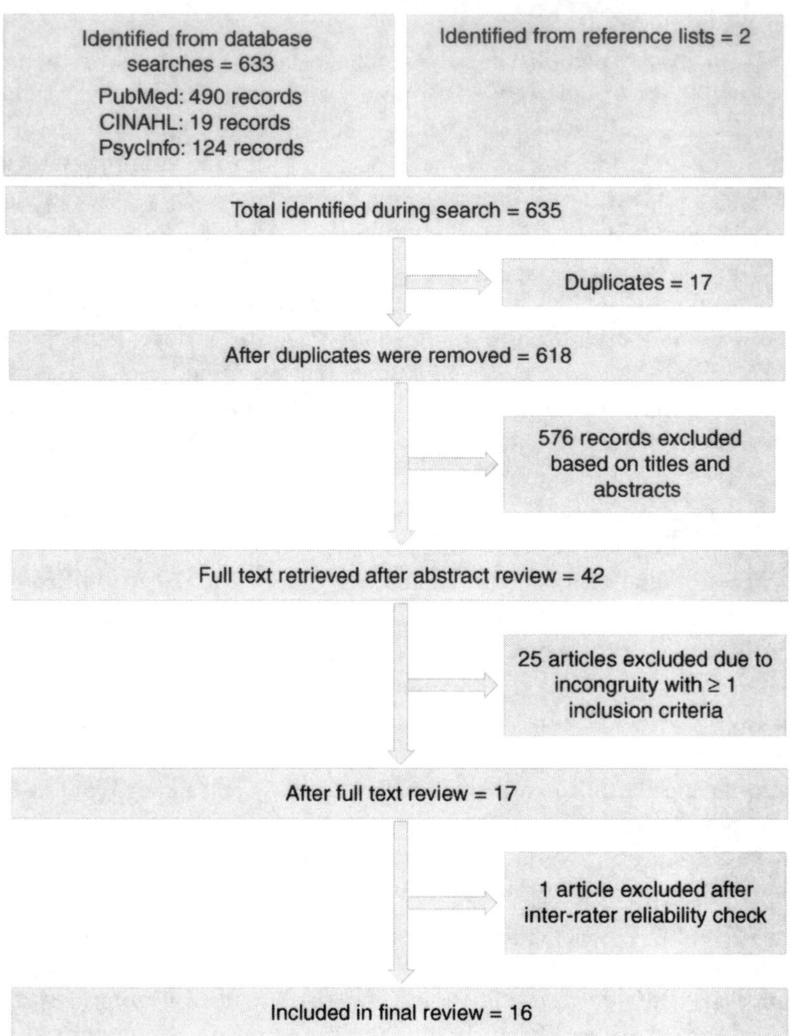

FIGURE 9.2 Flow chart of selection process with search results.

work on ethical considerations in the use of telehealth technologies for older adults (Demiris, Doorenbos, & Towle, 2009) and smart homes for palliative care (Demiris & Hensel, 2009). Key ethical factors that form the framework in this chapter include privacy, informed consent, autonomy, obtrusiveness, equal access, reduction in human contact, and usability (Table 9.1).

TABLE 9.1

Categories of an Ethical Framework for the Use of Smart Home Technologies and Their Theoretical and Operational Definitions

Category	Theoretical Definition	Operational Definition
Privacy	The control and management of personal space around one's body (physical), cognitive and affective processes related to formation of values, personal identity, self-esteem, or agency (psychological), social contacts (social), and personal information use and dissemination (informational) (Hughes, 2004)	In the context of smart homes, the concept of privacy is discussed primarily in terms of *informational privacy* that refers to an individual's right to control the access to personal data (Demiris, Oliver, & Courtney, 2006). On the other hand, *confidentiality* is an act of respecting an individual's right to make a decision with regard to sharing information with others (Fleming, Edison, & Pak, 2009).
Informed consent	An individual's agreement to give permission for a medical procedure or participation in a clinical intervention or research (Demiris & Hensel, 2009)	A formal statement that describes the purposes of the research, procedures to be followed, and all potential benefits and risks related to the in-home use of technologies. Informed consent could be used in a way that assists an individual to comprehend and evaluate information to make an informed choice about what information will be disseminated or kept private (Bruce, 2012).
Autonomy	The capacity of an individual to make a choice without coercion or external influence (Le, Di Mascolo, Gouin, & Noury, 2007; Mallers, Claver, & Lares, 2014)	A sense of empowerment and independence obtained by becoming involved in the health-care plan based on the automation of the technology (Demiris et al., 2006)

(Continued)

TABLE 9.1

Categories of an Ethical Framework for the Use of Smart Home Technologies and Their Theoretical and Operational Definitions (Continued)

Category	Theoretical Definition	Operational Definition
Obtrusiveness	The characteristic of being prominent or noticeable in an unpleasant way (Hensel, Demiris, & Courtney, 2006)	A user's evaluation based on features of the technology that are perceived as physically and psychologically noticeable (Hensel et al., 2006)
Equity of access	Equal and fair access to information and necessary resources (Fleming et al., 2009)	Universal access to necessary health information and means for monitoring of health and safety (Demiris et al., 2006)
Reduction in human contact	Deprivation of the chance to have therapeutic human touch (Demiris et al., 2009)	An individual's dependence on virtual visits or remote monitoring without meaningful interaction between an individual and health-care provider (Chan et al., 2008)
Usability	An attribute of products or systems that is assessed by the degree of ease and usefulness (Nielsen, 2012)	The extent to which the technology is used by specified users to perform tasks in a defined environment (Yen & Bakken, 2012)

RESULTS

Study Characteristics

Among the 16 articles included in this review, 8 were part of a technology trial where participants were involved in smart home projects while 8 studies were conducted to form evidence related to ethical issue identification (Table 9.2). Typically, an interview approach to data collection was used (*n* = 15) to explore attitudes and perceptions concerning the ethical use of smart home applications among older adults or stakeholders (caregivers, service managers, or policy advocates). The number of study participants ranged from 7 to 119. Types of smart home technologies included for field test or inquiry were various sensors (motion, bed, stove, door, etc.). The majority of the studies were conducted in the United States (*n* = 14), while one study was performed in the Netherlands (Nijhof, van Gemert-Pijnen, Woolrych, & Sixsmith, 2013) and another in Canada (Mihailidis, Cockburn, Longley, & Boger, 2008).

Ethical Issues Addressed in the Reviewed Studies

We discuss ethical considerations according to the framework and then provide the evidence for each ethical issue from the selected studies on the use of smart home technologies.

Privacy

Technological advances in the health-care sector have brought a widespread concern about the privacy of the health information of patients. Especially, with the implementation and evaluation of smart home technologies, the right to privacy is recognized as a core issue that should be discussed in order to appropriately perform gerontechnology research and practice. The violation of privacy can be manifested in two ways: sharing one's information without permission and obtaining personal information against one's will (Leino-Kilpi et al., 2001). Smart home applications are designed to collect information about resident health in the *home* setting to enhance functional health, quality of life, security, and safety. However, information about the home environment may also be accessible, so technologies installed at home can be a challenge to the perception of privacy in many ways.

There should be a precaution to ensure that personal data recorded through home monitoring sensors are protected in every step, for instance, gathering, storage, and retrieval of files, tapes, or images on behavioral or physiological data (Demiris, Oliver et al., 2006; Mahoney et al., 2007). There are other possible sources of privacy violations with regard to electronic transmission of information such as communication over phone lines, satellite, or wireless Internet. Confidentiality often cannot be ensured with the presence of technical staff who

TABLE 9.2

Description of All Identified Studies

Author (Year)	Study Design	Technologies	Participants	Purpose of the Study
Boise et al. (2013)	Descriptive study, technology trial	Motion sensor, door sensor, and refrigerator sensor	119 older adults	Evaluated participant willingness to share sensor data with others and privacy or security concerns of monitoring technology implemented over 1 year in community settings
Chung et al. (2014)	Descriptive study, technology trial	Motion sensor–based monitoring technology	7 older adults	Explored older adults' perceptions of informed decision making regarding sensors installed in their homes
Coughlin, D'Ambrosio, Reimer, and Pratt (2007)	Descriptive study	Smart home technologies	30 aging services leaders and policy advocates	Assessed participant perceptions of smart home technology to better inform the design of the technology
Courtney (2008)	Descriptive study	Bed sensor, motion sensor, kitchen sensor, and fall detection sensor	14 older adults	Explored factors affecting the decision to adopt a smart home technology among community-dwelling older adults
Courtney Demiris, Rantz, and Skubic (2008)	Descriptive study	Smart home technologies	14 older adults	Assessed older adults' willingness to accept smart home technology

Demiris et al. (2004)	Descriptive study, technology trial	Smart home technologies	15 older adults	Evaluated participant perceptions of smart home technologies installed in a retirement community for older adults
Demiris, Hensel, Skubic, and Rantz (2008)	Descriptive study, technology trial	Motion sensor, bed sensor, gait monitor, stove temperature sensor, and video sensor	14 older adults	Evaluated smart home residents' perceptions of in-home sensors from an ongoing longitudinal study
Demiris, Oliver, Dickey, Skubic, and Rantz (2008)	Descriptive study, technology trial	Motion sensor, sensor mat, stove temperature sensor, door sensor, gait monitor, and bed sensor	9 older adults	Assessed participants' perceptions of smart home applications installed in their homes
Demiris (2009)	Descriptive study	Two smart home approaches (distributed direct sensing vs. infrastructure-mediated sensing)	20 older adults and 14 informal caregivers	Assessed older adults' and caregivers' acceptance of two smart home approaches
Johnson et al. (2007)	Descriptive study	Tracking system, remote monitoring, voice activation, smart wave, smart mailbox, smart front door, cueing system to remind washing hands, and security system	18 older adults	Assessed older adult perceptions of smart home applications among participants who received demonstration of a lab-based single-family smart home

(*Continued*)

TABLE 9.2

Description of All Identified Studies (Continued)

Author (Year)	Study Design	Technologies	Participants	Purpose of the Study
Mihailidis et al. (2008)	Descriptive study	Home-based monitoring technologies	15 baby boomers and 15 older adults	Evaluated participant willingness to accept home monitoring technologies
Nijhof et al. (2013)	Descriptive study, technology trial, feasibility testing	ADLife comprising a gateway and sensors	14 older adults with dementia and 14 caregivers (formal/informal)	Evaluated the feasibility of home-based sensor system for activity monitoring over 9 months
Reder, Ambler, Philipose, and Hedrick (2010)	Descriptive study, technology trial, feasibility testing	Wireless shake sensors	12 older adults, 12 family and/or paid caregivers, and 2 service managers	Pilot study implemented over 1 year to test sensor technology for remote monitoring of activities
Reeder, Meyer, et al. (2013)	Descriptive study, technology trial, feasibility testing	Motion sensors for monitoring mobility	8 older adults	Evaluated participant perceptions of home-based sensor technology installed for 6 months in a retirement community

Steggell, Hooker, Bowman, Choun, and Kim (2010)	Descriptive study	Video communication device, emergency-monitoring device, sleep monitor, and medication reminder/dispenser	32 older women	Investigated perceptions of Korean and Hispanic older women living in the United States regarding monitoring technology designed to promote aging in place
Wild et al. (2008)	Descriptive study	Home monitoring technologies	23 older adults and 16 family members/friends	Explored attitudes and concerns of older adults and their family members or friends regarding unobtrusive home monitoring technologies

provide assistance in transmitting data from one site to another and maintaining Web portals containing individual health information (Demiris et al., 2006). It is necessary to ensure safe and secure communication to safeguard access to data obtained from home monitoring technologies. To do so, encryption or security systems must be in place for transmitting messages or identifiable patient information especially through the Internet (Chan et al., 2008; Fleming et al., 2009).

Review Results. Based on the review, it became apparent that privacy is the most critical factor affecting older adults' willingness to participate in smart home projects. Twelve out of 16 studies address the issues of privacy and confidentiality (Table 9.3). This is the case for smart home residents as well as individuals who have not been exposed to smart home applications. For example, older adults were concerned about potential judgment of their activity patterns through sensor data, or they simply did not want others to know when specific activities were done, such as toilet use (Demiris et al., 2008; Reeder, Chung, Lazar, Demiris, & Thompson, 2013). Also the perception of privacy invasion was related to the extent of detailed data the technology collects, for example, motion detection as compared to sound or image capturing. However, as long as technology meets the needs of older adults for maintaining independence in their homes, privacy issue is no longer an important concern for older adults (Courtney et al., 2008; Steggell et al., 2010; Wild et al., 2008).

Informed Consent

Informed consent is an important tool for protecting the autonomy, dignity, and well-being of older adults (Fleming et al., 2009). Informed consent emphasizes three bioethics principles: (a) nonmaleficence (prohibition of doing harm to an individual), (b) beneficence (an act of doing good), and (c) autonomy (a person's own right of making a decision) (Beauchamp & Childress, 2012). Despite potential benefits of smart home technologies, it is often difficult for older adults to make a decision about accepting or refusing smart home technologies, especially if they do not have sufficient information (Bruce, 2012). If an older adult faces cognitive decline related to dementia or other neurodegenerative diseases, this individual's ability to comprehend and evaluate information and to make a reasonable choice may be compromised.

Effective clinical interactions rely largely upon respect and trust in a patient–provider relationship. The provider's respect for patient rights can be manifested through informed consent. The use of consent allows an opportunity through which older adults can make an informed decision whether or not to participate in a technology trial. In the context of smart home technologies, informed consent needs to be pursued during the process of technology interventions, because clinical interactions are presented continuously through

TABLE 9.3

Ethical Issues Identified in the Reviewed Studies

Author (Year)	Method for Addressing Ethical Issues	Ethical Framework							Other Ethical Issues
		Privacy	Informed Consent	Autonomy	Obtrusiveness	Equal Access	Reduction in Human Contact	Usability	
Boise et al. (2013)	Survey	X		X					Security risks
Chung et al. (2014)	Semistructured individual interviews	X	X		X				
Coughlin et al. (2007)	Focus group interviews	X				X		X	Reliability of technology
Courtney (2008)	Focus group and individual interviews	X		X					
Courtney et al. (2008)	Focus group and individual interviews	X							
Demiris et al. (2004)	Focus group interviews	X			X	X		X	

(*Continued*)

TABLE 9.3

Ethical Issues Identified in the Reviewed Studies (Continued)

Author (Year)	Method for Addressing Ethical Issues	Ethical Framework							Other Ethical Issues
		Privacy	Informed Consent	Autonomy	Obtrusiveness	Equal Access	Reduction in Human Contact	Usability	
Demiris, Hensel et al. (2008)	Focus group interviews	X		X					Stigmatization, reliability of technology
Demiris, Oliver, et al. (2008)	Individual interviews				X				
Demiris (2009)	Individual interviews	X		X	X				Stigmatization
Johnson et al. (2007)	Focus group interviews			X		X			
Mihailidis et al. (2008)	Survey and interviews	X					X		

Nijhof et al. (2013)	Semistructured individual interview				X			X	Reliability and accuracy of technology
Reder et al. (2010)	Individual interviews			X		X	X		Reliability of technology
Reeder, Chung, et al. (2013)	Semistructured individual interviews	X	X	X					Data security
Steggell et al. (2010)	Focus group interviews	X		X		X		X	Maintenance of the system
Wild et al. (2008)	Focus group interviews	X		X					

ongoing monitoring or communications via technology applications (Demiris et al., 2009; Fleming et al., 2009). Also, consenting as a procedural tool provides older adults with an opportunity to discuss their preferences, lifestyles, and any changes in health status.

Some people may argue that there is not a significant difference in ethical considerations regarding the use of technologies between older and younger adults. However, because many older adults are not familiar with the mechanism of information gathering and sharing through technologies and may have a lack of technical understanding, they might not be well aware of the importance of protecting private information (Lorenzen-Huber et al., 2011). There is also a possibility that potential risks or discomforts related to the use of technology are not fully explained to older adult participants. This may hinder older adults from making an appropriate decision.

According to gerontechnology research, all families or informal caregivers residing with the older adults should be aware of all possible impacts of the technology on themselves as well as their own exposure to the technology. Multiple consents in this case should be obtained from all stakeholders who are involved in the use of technology, such as an individual's family or legal guardian. Then they should be given an opportunity to approve the installation (Demiris et al., 2009).

Review Results. The importance of informed consent or informed decision making was addressed in two studies. One study reported that despite the information provided during the recruitment as well as study enrollment sessions, misperceptions were found among a few participants regarding technology functionality (Reeder, Chung, et al., 2013). In a study by Chung et al. (2014), older adults expressed a need for information about potential benefits and harms of smart home technologies in order to ensure voluntary participation in smart home projects. However, unlike literature findings, older adults were less interested in system functionality than in the purpose of the technology. Importantly, there was an emphasis on the role of health-care professionals in conveying knowledge and information about smart home applications to older adults in order to facilitate their understanding of the technology as part of encouraging informed decision making.

Autonomy

The aims of smart home technologies are extended to generating datasets that enable detection of abnormal patterns and proactively responding to potential risks beyond monitoring of residents. Therefore, smart homes can contribute to gaining a sense of empowerment and independence among older adults and family caregivers (Demiris et al., 2006). However, despite the focus on enhancing autonomy, some people are concerned about the possibility that they might become overly dependent on those technologies (Bruce, 2012). Such a situation may result in human touch being traded for technology-based interactions (Demiris & Hensel, 2009). Moreover, the passive monitoring feature may keep end users away from being actively involved in operation and management of the system. Physicians, nurses, social workers, or case managers need to provide older individuals and their families with practical recommendations in order to engage them in care process planning based on data collected by smart home applications.

Review Results. The desire of older adults to have control over who will be granted access to data was identified in several studies with regard to potential privacy concerns. Generally, older adults are willing to share information collected through technology with family, friends, or health-care providers, but at different levels of sharing. For example, participants were not concerned if activity data could be viewed by anyone (Boise et al., 2013), while reluctance was observed with regard to information sharing with anyone other than health-care providers (Wild et al., 2008) or unauthorized third parties (Demiris, 2009). This was further amplified by individuals who indicated the need for control over the amount and frequency of information sharing (Demiris, Hensel, et al., 2008). On the other hand, Johnson et al. (2007) reported participant concern about losing control. Study participants had a tour of a smart home equipped with smart floor, voice activation, smart microwave, smart mailbox, smart front door, cueing system, and security system, and were encouraged to express their expectations and concerns about living in a smart home environment. While older adults had a desire that the technology performs tasks they cannot do, they did not want the system to take over the role for fear that they would be overly relying on the system.

Obtrusiveness

The perception of obtrusiveness is subjective and varies from person to person (Courtney, Demiris, & Hensel, 2007). Eight dimensions of user perception of obtrusiveness were identified with regard to technologies installed in the home setting, such as physical, usability, privacy, function, human interaction, self-concept, routine, and sustainability (Hensel et al., 2006). For example, physical considerations such as physical discomfort or strain, excessive noise, and aesthetic incongruence associated with the technology, or functional factors including malfunction or inaccurate measurement may contribute to users' perception of obtrusiveness. Because smart home technologies are installed in private residences, researchers should be aware of the possibility of obtrusiveness concerns associated with the technology. It is also essential to develop nonobtrusive technologies to maximize technology adoption among older adults.

Review Results. In reviewed studies, smart home residents indicated the importance of nonobtrusive technology because of the effect on their privacy concerns (Chung et al., 2014; Demiris, Oliver, et al., 2008), but this was not observed among participants of the studies that did not involve technology installation. Also obtrusiveness issues were associated with installation locations (e.g., bedroom or bathroom) or types and size of technologies. For instance, older adults perceive that a video camera installed in a home would become a major source of privacy violation (Demiris, 2009; Demiris et al., 2004). Importantly, physical aspects of sensors, such as noises or flickering lights from the system, would become a nuisance or even a source of anxiety among smart home residents and caregivers (Nijhof et al., 2013).

Equal Access

Universal access to necessary health information technologies is the first step to supporting older adults to benefit from those technologies. The term *digital divide* refers to the gap in access to and usage of information and communication technologies between those who have access to the technology and those who do not, because of age, income, education, community type, disability, or other factors (Pew Research Center, 2013; Shrewsbury, 2002). Despite the fact that the population of older adults is the fastest growing group using the Internet, those who are older, who are in low socioeconomic status, or who live in rural or urban underserved areas are more likely to lag behind in technology use (Olson, O'Brien, Rogers, & Charness, 2011; Pew Research Center, 2014). Moreover, lack of access to appropriate health care among ethnic minority older adults is becoming a central issue in the U.S. health-care delivery system, which also has implications for the deployment of smart home technologies. Considering long-standing mistrust of the health-care system among individuals from underserved groups, it may be challenging to develop specifics of home-based technologies tailored to the needs of older adults in low-access settings (Fleming et al., 2009).

In addition to efforts to extend access to infrastructure such as computers, wireless Internet, or even electricity, there is an ongoing challenge revolving around the issue of health literacy and customized Web content for the elderly with low literacy and sociocultural barriers.

The cost of implementing technology is another of the widely recognized barriers to health resources and opportunities for innovative technologies. In most cases, technology installation at the initial stage should require expenditure to acquire or purchase equipment, which is often charged to the user or provider, rather than the insurer (Goldwater & Harris, 2011). If the technology needs to be connected to the Internet or Web portal, then the user may be required to pay for a monthly fee or subscription. Because insurance companies usually do not cover the cost, and only a small number of older adults can afford the devices and services, these fees can be a barrier to the access to the technology. If family caregivers are responsible for monetary support for the elderly, the perceived cost of technology for the family should be discussed because it depends on the family's income and resources.

Review Results. In five studies (Coughlin et al., 2007; Demiris et al., 2004; Johnson et al., 2007; Reder et al., 2010; Steggell et al., 2010), older adults were concerned about the cost of purchasing and maintaining the device, which could be a potential barrier to technology adoption. Also, among a group of older adults who have limited English proficiency, instructions written only in English were found to prevent them from accessing necessary technology solutions (Steggell et al., 2010).

Reduction in Human Contact

The loss of human touch resulting from smart sensor adoption is a significant concern among older adults, because the technology may be used in ways that replace face-to-face contact. Technology may deprive the chance of therapeutic interactions between older adults and their formal caregivers or clinicians, while making older adults solely dependent on virtual visits or remote monitoring (Chan et al., 2008). Therefore, reduced number of actual visits is often expected as a main outcome of the technology use. Older adults and their families who agree to live in smart homes should be aware of such possibilities.

Cost reduction is one of the main interests among patients, families, and health-care managers. Many home-based monitoring technologies are being adopted in the hope of achieving cost-effectiveness resulting from saving of time and avoidance of travel (Ratliff & Forch, 2005). However, if the focus of utilizing technologies is solely on cost cutting, the importance of the therapeutic touch in patient–provider relationship might be ignored. Thus, it is necessary to emphasize that technology is not a substitute for skilled health-care professionals or caregivers but a supplement to traditional face-to-face care (Demiris et al., 2006; Fleming et al., 2009; Kang et al., 2010).

Review Results. In a sensor-based monitoring technology implementation, Reder et al. (2010) found that older adults did not want a situation in which technology could replace human touch when they are in need of social interaction. Similarly, in a study by Mihailidis et al. (2008), older adults preferred a sensor system that encourages human contact, which ultimately leads to a high adoption rate.

Usability

There has been increasing attention to the usability issue related to home-based health information technologies. Usability influences people's decision as to whether the technology is useful and acceptable to them. While usability is a critical factor in the adoption and use of technologies, the issues of usability have not been fully addressed in the context of smart home environments for older adults. Technologies that are designed poorly and do not meet the needs of older adults are likely to be refused. So far, heuristics and cognitive functioning associated with human-technology interaction have been largely discussed for a wide range of consumer groups of health information technologies, but it has not been fully discussed for the population of older adults. Often the design of technology fails to address age-related constraints and lack of experience in using technology among seniors (Joe, Chaudhuri, Chung, Thompson, & Demiris, 2014). Specifically, reduced sensory function associated with normal aging as well as possible cognitive impairment or mobility limitations may cause older adults to be less adept at fully implementing smart home environments (Cashen, Dykes, & Gerber, 2004; Demiris et al., 2009). For instance, even simply switching the system on or off is challenging, especially if the individual experiences vision loss or cognitive decline. Therefore, it is necessary to examine important usability aspects of smart homes and home-based sensor technologies. Also training and user education need to be developed to meet older adults' needs in order to maximize the usability that ultimately leads to the increased acceptance of technology among older adults (Mei, Marquard, Jacelon, & Defeo, 2013).

Review results. In four studies, older adults and their caregivers voiced the opinion that the user-friendly feature of technologies is critical for wide adoption and use. There were some suggestions for improving usability in terms of training sessions, manuals, readability, and data visualization techniques (Coughlin et al., 2007; Demiris et al., 2004; Nijhof et al., 2013; Steggell et al., 2010), all of which can contribute to the perceived ease of use of the technologies and data for both older adults and their families. Also, it becomes apparent that the design of interface or manuals should meet the needs of older adults who have not been exposed to technologies previously or who have difficulty comprehending information.

DISCUSSION

The use of smart homes and home-based sensors is becoming prevalent in health-care service and delivery for older adults to support independence, safety, and security. Technology development and advances should be beneficial to end users and useful for stakeholders. However, the introduction of technology in the home setting inevitably brings challenges and ethical issues. This article provides the first integrative review on ethical issues with regard to the adoption and use of smart home technologies for older adults. The majority were qualitative studies that examined older adults' attitudes and perceptions about smart home applications in the preimplementation stage or in small-sized feasibility testing. Among them, only four studies had a main purpose of examining ethical issues related to smart home applications, such as privacy and informed decision-making (Boise et al., 2013; Chung et al., 2014; Courtney, 2008; Demiris, 2009), while others were originally focused on the acceptability of smart sensor systems.

The current ethical review suggests that technologies should be accessible, affordable, easy to use, and helpful for maintaining autonomy in order to increase adoption. More importantly, studies have shown that older adults want to live in smart homes in which their privacy is not invaded and which are not intrusive. However, privacy was not a major concern in some older adults or they were willing to use the technology in spite of a privacy risk if the technology provided a critical function (Demiris, Oliver et al., 2008; Reder et al., 2010; Wild et al., 2008). Similarly, in three studies, participants mentioned obtrusiveness issues related to technologies installed in homes, but it worked for older adults in a positive way (e.g., avoiding a lazy lifestyle or increasing physical activity) or was simply not a significant concern (Reder et al., 2010; Reeder, Chung, et al., 2013; Wild et al., 2008).

Besides the seven dimensions of the framework, we identified two other ethical issues that need further attention. First, older adults were concerned about social stigma after adopting the system because living in smart homes may be viewed as a loss of the ability to be independent (Demiris, Hensel, et al., 2008; Demiris, 2009). Kang et al. (2010) provides recommendations in order to prevent a situation in which older adults feel stigmatized, such as using invisible sensors or employing technology before the onset of functional decline. Second, older adults were favorable to devices that are reliable and do not require maintenance efforts to have a greater sense of security. When considering adoption of technology solutions into older adults' residences, reliability or maintenance issues of the technology may be overlooked including hardware or software glitches, incompatibility, power outages, or abrupt shutdown (Kang et al., 2010). Therefore, when home-based technology is introduced, researchers or clinicians must rigorously validate and test the system whether it is robust and secure. Technical staff should be ready in case of a need for troubleshooting, and the question of who will pay for the maintenance and service costs should be discussed prior to the technology implementation (Scanaill et al., 2011). Moreover, end users should be well informed about the possibility of technical problems in order to avoid excessive dependence on such technology (Mahoney et al., 2007).

When smart home technology is correctly used, it can increase the sense of well-being and quality of life and ultimately support older adults' desire for remaining in their homes as long as possible. To effectively employ the benefits of the technology and to support the successful integration of the technology with traditional care, the development and applications of technology innovations for older adults should be carried out with strict ethical standards that aim to ensure an individual's safety and independence. Professionals who are interested in the application of technology are required to have moral principles that lead to efforts to mitigate all possible risks and to maximize benefits for older adults. Ethical issues identified in this review need to be thoroughly examined by professional groups who consider using smart home technologies.

REFERENCES

Alwan, M. (2009). Passive in-home health and wellness monitoring: Overview, value and examples. In *31st Annual International Conference of the IEEE Engineering in Medicine and Biology Society* (2009/12/08 ed., Vol. 2009, pp. 4307–4310). http://dx.doi.org/10.1109/iembs.2009.5333799

Beauchamp, T. L., & Childress, J. F. (2012). *Principles of biomedical ethics* (7th ed.). Oxford: Oxford University Press.

Berke, E. M., Choudhury, T., Ali, S., & Rabbi, M. (2011). Objective measurement of sociability and activity: Mobile sensing in the community. *The Annals of Family Medicine*, *9*(4), 344–350. http://dx.doi.org/10.1370/afm.1266

Boise, L., Wild, K., Mattek, N., Ruhl, M., Dodge, H. H., & Kaye, J. (2013). Willingness of older adults to share data and privacy concerns after exposure to unobtrusive in-home monitoring. *Gerontechnology*, *11*(3), 428–435. http://dx.doi.org/10.4017/gt.2013.11.3.001.00

Bruce, C. R. (2012). Informed decision making for in-home use of motion sensor-based monitoring technologies. *The Gerontologist*, *52*(3), 317–324. http://dx.doi.org/10.1093/geront/gnr124

Cashen, M. S., Dykes, P., & Gerber, B. (2004). eHealth technology and internet resources: Barriers for vulnerable populations. *Journal of Cardiovascular Nursing*, *19*(3), 206–209.

Chan, M., Estève, D., Escriba, C., & Campo, E. (2008). A review of smart homes—Present state and future challenges. *Computer Methods and Programs in Biomedicine*, *91*(1), 55–81. http://dx.doi.org/10.1016/j.cmpb.2008.02.001

Chung, J., Reeder, B., Lazar, A., Joe, J., Demiris, G., & Thompson, H. J. (2014). Exploring an informed decision-making framework using in-home sensors: Older adults' perceptions. *Informatics in Primary Care*, *21*(2), 73–77. http://dx.doi.org/10.14236/jhi.v21i2.53

Coughlin, J., D'Ambrosio, L. A., Reimer, B., & Pratt, M. R. (2007). Older adult perceptions of smart home technologies: Implications for research, policy & market innovations in healthcare. In *29th Annual International Conference of the IEEE Proceedings of the Engineering in Medicine and Biology Annual Conference* (2007/11/16 ed., Vol. 2007, pp. 1810–1815). http://dx.doi.org/10.1109/iembs.2007.4352665

Courtney, K. L. (2008). Privacy and senior willingness to adopt smart home information technology in residential care facilities. *Methods of Information in Medicine*, *47*(1), 76–81. http://dx.doi.org/10.3414/me9104

Courtney, K. L., Demiris, G., & Hensel, B. K. (2007). Obtrusiveness of information-based assistive technologies as perceived by older adults in residential care facilities: A secondary analysis. *Medical Informatics and the Internet in Medicine*, *32*(3), 241–249. http://dx.doi.org/10.1080/14639230701447735

Courtney, K. L., Demiris, G., Rantz, M. J., & Skubic, M. (2008). Needing smart home technologies: The perspectives of older adults in continuing care retirement communities. *Informatics in Primary Care*, *16*(3), 195–201.

Demiris, G. (2009). *Privacy and social implications of distinct sensing approaches to implementing smart homes for older adults* (pp. 4311–4314). Paper presented at the meeting of the 31st Annual International Conference of the IEEE Engineering in Medicine and Biology Society, Minneapolis, MN.

Demiris, G., Doorenbos, A. Z., & Towle, C. (2009). Ethical considerations regarding the use of technology for older adults: The case of telehealth. *Research in Gerontological Nursing*, *2*(2), 128–136. http://dx.doi.org/10.3928/19404921-20090401-02

Demiris, G., & Hensel, B. (2009). "Smart Homes" for patients at the end of life. *Journal of Housing for the Elderly*, *23*(1–2), 106–115. http://dx.doi.org/10.1080/02763890802665049

Demiris, G., Hensel, B. K., Skubic, M., & Rantz, M. (2008). Senior residents' perceived need of and preferences for "smart home" sensor technologies. *International Journal of Technology Assessment in Health Care*, *24*(1), 120–124. http://dx.doi.org/10.1017/s0266462307080154

Demiris, G., Oliver, D. P., & Courtney, K. L. (2006). Ethical considerations for the utilization of tele-health technologies in home and hospice care by the nursing profession. *Nursing Administration Quarterly*, *30*(1), 56–66. Retrieved from http://ovidsp.tx.ovid.com

Demiris, G., Oliver, D. P., Dickey, G., Skubic, M., & Rantz, M. (2008). Findings from a participatory evaluation of a smart home application for older adults. *Technology and Health Care*, *16*(2), 111–118. Retrieved from http://www.ncbi.nlm.nih.gov/pubmed/18487857

Demiris, G., Rantz, M., Aud, M., Marek, K., Tyrer, H., Skubic, M., et al. (2004). Older adults' attitudes towards and perceptions of 'smart home' technologies: A pilot study. *Medical Informatics and the Internet in Medicine*, *29*(2), 87–94. http://dx.doi.org/10.1080/14639230410001684387

Fleming, D. A., Edison, K. E., & Pak, H. (2009). Telehealth ethics. *Telemedicine Journal and E-Health*, *15*(8), 797–803. http://dx.doi.org/10.1089/tmj.2009.0035

Goldwater, J., & Harris, Y. (2011). Using technology to enhance the aging experience: A market analysis of existing technologies. *Ageing International*, *36*(1), 5–28. http://dx.doi.org/10.1007/s12126-010-9071-2

Hensel, B. K., Demiris, G., & Courtney, K. L. (2006). Defining obtrusiveness in home telehealth technologies: A conceptual framework. *Journal of the American Medical Informatics Association*, *13*, 428–431. http://dx.doi.org/10.1197/jamia.m2026

Hughes, M. (2004). Privacy in aged care. *Australasian Journal on Ageing*, *23*(3), 110–114. http://dx.doi.org/10.1111/j.1741-6612.2004.00033.x

Joe, J., Chaudhuri, S., Chung, J., Thompson, H., & Demiris, G. (2014). Older adults' attitudes and preferences regarding a multifunctional wellness tool: A pilot study. *Informatics for Health and Social Care*, 1–16. http://dx.doi.org/10.3109/17538157.2014.965305

Johnson, J. L., Davenport, R., Mann, W. C., & Otr, L. (2007). Consumer feedback on smart home applications. *Topics in Geriatric Rehabilitation*, *23*(1), 60–72. Retrieved from http://offcampus.lib.washington.edu/login?url=http://search.ebscohost.com/login.aspx?direct=true&db=rzh&AN=2009524822&site=ehost-live

Kang, H. G., Mahoney, D. F., Hoenig, H., Hirth, V. A., Bonato, P., Hajjar, I., et al. (2010). In situ monitoring of health in older adults: Technologies and issues. *Journal of the American Geriatrics Society*, *58*(8), 1579–1586. http://dx.doi.org/10.1111/j.1532-5415.2010.02959.x

Le, X. H. B., Di Mascolo, M., Gouin, A., & Noury, N. (2007). *Health smart home: Towards an assistant tool for automatic assessment of the dependence of elders* (Vol. 2007, pp. 3806–3809). Paper presented at the meeting of the 29th Annual International Conference of the IEEE Engineering in Medicine and Biology Society, Lyon. http://dx.doi.org/10.1109/iembs.2007.4353161

Leino-Kilpi, H., Välimäki, M., Dassen, T., Gasull, M., Lemonidou, C., Scott, A., et al. (2001). Privacy: A review of the literature. *International Journal of Nursing Studies*, *38*(6), 663–671. http://dx.doi.org/10.1016/s0020-7489(00)00111-5

Lorenzen-Huber, L., Boutain, M., Camp, L. J., Shankar, K., & Connelly, K. H. (2011). Privacy, technology, and aging: A proposed framework. *Ageing International*, *36*(2), 232–252. http://dx.doi.org/10.1007/s12126-010-9083-y

Mahoney, D. F. (2011). An evidence-based adoption of technology model for remote monitoring of elders' daily activities. *Ageing International*, *36*(1), 66–81. http://dx.doi.org/10.1007/s12126-010-9073-0

Mahoney, D. F., Purtilo, R. B., Webbe, F. M., Alwan, M., Bharucha, A. J., Adlam, T. D., et al. (2007). In-home monitoring of persons with dementia: Ethical guidelines for technology research and development. *Alzheimer's and Dementia*, *3*(3), 217–226. http://dx.doi.org/10.1016/j.jalz.2007.04.388

Mallers, M. H., Claver, M., & Lares, L. A. (2014). Perceived control in the lives of older adults: The influence of Langer and Rodin's work on gerontological theory, policy, and practice. *The Gerontologist*, *54*(1), 67–74. http://dx.doi.org/10.1093/geront/gnt051

Mei, Y. Y., Marquard, J., Jacelon, C., & Defeo, A. L. (2013). Designing and evaluating an electronic patient falls reporting system: Perspectives for the implementation of health information technology in long-term residential care facilities. *International Journal of Medical Informatics*, *82*(11), e294–e306. http://dx.doi.org/10.1016/j.ijmedinf.2011.03.008

Mihailidis, A., Cockburn, A., Longley, C., & Boger, J. (2008). The acceptability of home monitoring technology among community-dwelling older adults and baby boomers. *Assistive Technology*, *20*(1), 1–12. http://dx.doi.org/10.1080/10400435.2008.10131927

Nielsen, J. (2012). *Thinking aloud: The #1 usability tool*. Retrieved March 5, 2014 from http://www.nngroup.com/articles/thinking-aloud-the-1-usability-tool/

Nijhof, N., van Gemert-Pijnen, L. J., Woolrych, R., & Sixsmith, A. (2013). An evaluation of preventive sensor technology for dementia care. *Journal of Telemedicine and Telecare*, *19*(2), 95–100. http://dx.doi.org/10.1258/jtt.2012.120605

Olson, K., O'Brien, M., Rogers, W., & Charness, N. (2011). Diffusion of technology: Frequency of use for younger and older adults. *Ageing International*, *36*(1), 123–145. http://dx.doi.org/10.1007/s12126-010-9077-9

Pew Research Center. (2013). *The state of digital divides*. Retrieved January 29, 2015 from http://www.pewinternet.org/2013/11/05/the-state-of-digital-divides-video-slides/

Pew Research Center. (2014). *Older adults and technology use: Pew Research Center's Internet and American Life Project*. Retrieved January 29, 2015 from http://www.pewinternet.org/2014/04/03/older-adults-and-technology-use/

Rantz, M. J., Skubic, M., Alexander, G., Popescu, M., Aud, M. A., Wakefield, B. J., et al. (2010). Developing a comprehensive electronic health record to enhance nursing care coordination, use of technology, and research. *Journal of Gerontological Nursing*, *36*(1), 13–17. http://dx.doi.org/10.3928/00989134-20091204-02

Rantz, M. J., Skubic, M., Miller, S. J., Galambos, C., Alexander, G., Keller, J., et al. (2013). Sensor technology to support aging in place. *Journal of the American Medical Directors Association*, *14*(6), 386–391. http://dx.doi.org/10.1016/j.jamda.2013.02.018

Ratliff, C. R., & Forch, W. (2005). Telehealth for wound management in long-term care. *Ostomy/Wound Management*, *51*(9), 40–45.

Reder, S., Ambler, G., Philipose, M., & Hedrick, S. (2010). Technology and Long-term Care (TLC): A pilot evaluation of remote monitoring of elders. *Gerontechnology*, *9*(1), 18–31. http://dx.doi.org/10.4017/gt.2010.09.01.002.00

Reeder, B., Chung, J., Lazar, A., Joe, J., Demiris, G., & Thompson, H. J. (2013). Testing a theory-based mobility monitoring protocol using in-home sensors: A feasibility study. *Research in Gerontological Nursing*, *6*(4), 253–263. http://dx.doi.org/10.3928/19404921-20130729-02

Reeder, B., Meyer, E., Lazar, A., Chaudhuri, S., Thompson, H. J., & Demiris, G. (2013). Framing the evidence for health smart homes and home-based consumer health technologies as a public health intervention for independent aging: A systematic review. *International Journal of Medical Informatics*, *82*(7), 565–579. http://dx.doi.org/10.1016/j.ijmedinf.2013.03.007

Scanaill, C. N., Garattini, C., Greene, B. R., & McGrath, M. J. (2011). Technology innovation enabling falls risk assessment in a community setting. *Ageing International*, *36*(2), 217–231. http://dx.doi.org/10.1007/s12126-010-9087-7

Shrewsbury, C. M. (2002). Information technology issues in an era of greater state responsibilities. *Journal of Aging and Social Policy*, *14*(3–4), 195–209. http://dx.doi.org/10.1300/j031v14n03_11

Steggell, C. D., Hooker, K., Bowman, S., Choun, S., & Kim, S. J. (2010). The role of technology for healthy aging among Korean and Hispanic women in the United States: A pilot study. *Gerontechnology*, *9*(4), 433–449. http://dx.doi.org/10.4017/gt.2010.09.04.007.00

United States Census Bureau. (2014). *2014 National population projections*. Retrieved February 11, 2015 from http://www.census.gov/population/projections/data/national/2014/summary-tables.html

Vasunilashorn, S., Steinman, B. A., Liebig, P. S., & Pynoos, J. (2012). Aging in place: Evolution of a research topic whose time has come. *Journal of Aging Research*, *2012*, 120952. http://dx.doi.org/10.1155/2012/120952

Whittemore, R., & Knafl, K. (2005). The integrative review. Updated methodology. *Journal of Advanced Nursing*, *52*(5), 546–553. http://dx.doi.org/10.1111/j.1365-2648.2005.03621.x

Wild, K., Boise, L., Lundell, J., & Foucek, A. (2008). Unobtrusive in-home monitoring of cognitive and physical health eactions and perceptions of older adults. *Journal of Applied Gerontology*, *27*(2), 181–200. http://dx.doi.org/10.1177/0733464807311435

Yen, P. Y., & Bakken, S. (2012). Review of health information technology usability study methodologies. *Journal of the American Medical Informatics Association*, *19*(3), 413–422. http://dx.doi.org/10.1136/amiajnl-2010-000020

CHAPTER 10

No Need to Object

Ethical Obligations for Interprofessional Collaboration in Emergency Department Discharge Planning

Laura Bentley Webster and Jamie L. Shirley

ABSTRACT

Emergency departments (EDs) serve a wide range of patient needs. A crucial aspect of safe and effective care in the ED is to appropriately transition patients to the next level of care. In most EDs, this disposition planning is done exclusively by physicians, which has the potential to result in unacceptable harm. A virtue ethics approach demonstrates the need for explicit inclusion of nurses in disposition planning. In utilizing this approach, it is necessary to examine four focal virtues as they relate to the work of disposition planning and the moral character of the nurse. The virtues of prudence, trustworthiness, vigilance, and courage show that interprofessional collaboration is needed during disposition planning to promote patient safety, facilitate interprofessional relationships, and prevent moral distress. The majority of literature on disposition planning is empirical in nature; this chapter adds a normative argument and a motive for policy reform.

http://dx.doi.org/10.1891/0739-6686.34.183

INTRODUCTION

Emergency departments (EDs) are serving as an ever-expanding safety net for Americans with patients presenting at higher acuities than ever before. Given the limited availability of primary care providers, patients will continue to utilize local EDs even as more patients have health insurance through the Affordable Care Act. Patients in the ED are generally in need of rapid assessments and a swift plan of action. A coordinated interprofessional team of professionals blends its skills and knowledge to ensure safe and quality interventions. Yet one of the most critical aspects of a patient's emergency stay, disposition planning, continues to be exclusive to a single discipline. Most EDs support the physician, or physician team, to determine whether and where the patient will receive ongoing care. Nurses are assumed to be in agreement with the plan unless they object. Their objections are then offered only in reaction to the already formed plan. Significantly, however, one of the key elements in planning disposition is the level of nursing care the patient will require. This chapter provides a virtue ethics analysis of this practice and argues for the inclusion of bedside nurses during ED disposition planning, in the interest of averting harm to patient safety, preserving or strengthening interprofessional relationships, and avoiding moral distress. This chapter is not arguing that one clinician's recommendation should trump that of another member of the team. Rather, it is advocating for an inclusive interprofessional policy in the disposition process.

DISPOSITION PLANNING

Disposition planning is the process of deciding what care patients require and where they can best receive that care after being stabilized in the ED (Perimal-Lewis, Hakendorf, & Thompson, 2015). For some patients, the plan is for discharge home. For others, the plan will be admission to a unit within the same hospital or to an outside facility for specialized care. The ED team's disposition decision determines the type, intensity, and location of the patient's subsequent care.

Determining the appropriate frequency and intensity of nursing assessments is critical to ensuring safe patient disposition. Patients with minimal or no nursing care needs are considered safe for discharge to their homes where they can care for themselves or receive assistance from their families. (Some of these patients may be discharged to residential facilities where different levels of skilled nursing care are available.) Patients who require professional nursing care are admitted to one of several units within the hospital: the intensive care unit (ICU), a step-down unit, a telemetry unit, or the acute care floor. Their destination is based on a match between their level of acuity and the availability of nursing care. In the ICU, nurses continuously monitor and assess patients. In contrast, patients on an acute care floor receive less frequently scheduled assessments and more shared care between registered nurses (RNs) and assistants. Step-down and telemetry units usually offer less frequent assessments than ICUs, but more than acute care floors. Hospital units are also differentiated by nurse–patient ratios, availability of technology, and access to other professional services.

Although the disposition determination process varies among hospitals, the potential for adverse events when the wrong disposition is selected is ubiquitous (Calder et al., 2012; Horwitz et al., 2009; Kennedy, Joyce, Howell, Mottley, & Shapiro, 2010). In the ED, a preventable adverse event is two times more likely to occur than in any other inpatient area (Fordyce et al., 2003). Patients arrive without a schedule and are in need of emergent care. As a consequence, clinicians in the ED have relatively limited experience with a particular patient and are often rushed, trying to move people out of the ED quickly and efficiently to make room for new patients. One study showed that over half of patients discharged home from the ED prematurely experienced preventable adverse advents (Calder et al., 2015). Similarly, ED patients admitted to the wrong level of care within the hospital make up one quarter of all rapid response activations within their first 24 hours and are at risk for delayed intensive interventions (Considine, Charlesworth, & Currey, 2014). By contrast, transfers to an inappropriately intensive setting can result in both increased costs and poor allocation of health-care resources, intensive care unit beds, and unnecessary tests and treatments (Calder et al., 2015; Considine et al., 2014).

IMPORTANCE OF NURSING CONTRIBUTION

Given the importance of nursing care for the determination of disposition, it is surprising that nurses are not systematically involved in the process. Nurses can offer valuable assessment and knowledge of institutional practices, but they are often constrained in their participation in disposition planning due to structural hierarchies.

Assessment skills are fundamental to nursing practice, referred to as "patient surveillance" by the Institute of Medicine, and one of only three components consistently tied to lower patient mortality (Page, 2003). The nursing assessment collects valuable information, both implicitly and explicitly, about the patient's physical, psychological, spiritual, and sociological status. A nursing assessment begins implicitly, noticing the particulars of a patient from across the room, from a patient's ability to sit in a chair and hold a spoon correctly to the pattern of breathing and tactile features of the skin. An explicit nursing assessment includes monitoring vital signs, the sounds of a patient's heart and lung, and a countless other formal examinations. There is no substitute for the nurse's expertise.

Nurses are often holders of institutional knowledge, in part due to their longevity and consistency in the hospital. In teaching hospitals, physicians rotate through the ED on an intermittent basis. Even in community hospitals with a more stable physician population, physicians often see their primary location as their office or other community setting. Nurses then have a heightened knowledge of patterns of disposition, treating like cases alike. They are likely to know the institutional issues related to departmental specialties, staffing, and acuity, which affect disposition beyond the particulars of the patient case.

Nurses' relative lack of institutional power, however, can make it difficult to contribute these elements of assessment and knowledge during disposition planning. Structural hierarchical relationships limit the ability or willingness of the nurse to collaborate in the interprofessional planning of care. Explicitly empowering nurses, through policy or system change, would facilitate the shared goal of patient well-being.

BRIEF OVERVIEW OF VIRTUE ETHICS

Virtue ethics focuses on a person's habits and character traits that tend to guide him or her to right action. The word *virtue* comes from an ancient Greek word *arête*, which translates as "an excellence of character." Aristotle claimed that virtues are states of character, separated into intellectual and moral virtues. Intellectual virtues are taught through instruction. Moral virtues are habitual, acquired only through practice and discipline (Armstrong, 2006; Timmons, 2006).

As defined by Aristotle:

> Excellence is an art won by training and habituation. We do not act rightly because we have virtue or excellence, but we rather have those because we have acted rightly. We are what we repeatedly do. Excellence, then, is not an act but a habit. (as cited in Durant, 2006, p. 98)

Virtues in health care are the expression of a collective understanding of the moral obligations of clinicians for the patients in their care. Virtues are important not only to the moral agent who acts in accordance with them, but also to the profession itself and to the patients who benefit from the providers' virtuous actions. Each profession is responsible for defining the relevant virtues and for guiding its members toward the development of these virtues.

The Society of Academic Emergency Medicine (SAEM) endorses a set of virtues physicians should embrace. Prudence, courage, temperance, justice, unconditional positive regard, charity, compassion, trustworthiness, and vigilance are considered "vital" to the practice of emergency medicine (SAEM, 1996). Emergency nurses should be guided equally by these virtues to promote the shared goal of patient health and welfare (Armstrong, 2006; Gardiner, 2003; Meyer & Lavin, 2005). Although all are important, disposition planning requires four virtues in particular: prudence, trustworthiness, vigilance, and courage.

Prudence is the ability to weigh virtues and vices in order to discern the wise choice in a particular situation. Aristotle called this virtue *phronesis* or practical wisdom. This virtue is considered the necessary prerequisite used to weigh other virtues (Larkin et al., 2009). Virtues are always held in tension with one another, and choosing the prudent action can be difficult. Clinicians' prudence is a form of expert clinical decision making. It facilitates their ability to see what is important, to be aware of what is missing, and to attend to potential biases in order to arrive at a morally sound and reasoned course of action (Dhaliwal, 2011).

According to Potter as cited by McLeod (2014), a clinician who is trustworthy is "one who can be counted on, as a matter of the sort of person he or she is, to take care of those things that others entrust to one" ("The Nature of Trust and Trustworthiness," para. 23). Clinicians enact trustworthiness and earn their patients' confidence through the development and maintenance of skills, honesty, and stalwart attention to patients' needs. Trustworthiness allows for vulnerable patients to receive treatment knowing they will be cared for, not exploited (Pellegrino & Thomasma, 1993). Clinicians who reduce their relationships with patients to a financial or legal enterprise are not trustworthy and jeopardize the very foundation of the therapeutic relationship (Larkin et al., 2009).

Vigilance is "a state of watchful attention, of maximal physiological and psychological readiness to act, and of having the ability to detect and react to danger" (Hirter & Van Nest, 1995, p. 96). Although some definitions of vigilance focus on the detection of enemies and the physical states that contribute to or detract from one's ability to be vigilant, in the health-care setting, this virtue is primarily interpreted as diligent watchfulness (Kooken & Haase, 2014).

Virtuous clinicians attempt to do what is right by being thorough and attentive to the obligations of their role. They protect their patients by foreseeing and avoiding or preventing potential harm, and by managing and overcoming adverse events (Kooken & Haase, 2014). Vigilance is necessary to respond to the directive of *primum non nocere* or "first do no harm."

Clinicians express moral courage when they speak up to ensure patient safety, are present even when it is difficult, and step in when needed. Moral courage is the "fortitude to do what is required, what is right, in the face of unpleasant or adverse conditions" (Larkin et al., 2009, p. 53). Clinicians who evade difficult situations, surrender to fear, or choose their course of action based merely on what is easy are not courageous (Larkin et al., 2009). Established hierarchies and institutional barriers to collaborative communication require, sometimes unreasonably, clinicians to have moral courage when caring for patients (Gordon & Hamric, 2006).

These four virtues are critical to the practice of disposition planning in the ED. The clinicians' shared goal to promote a safe discharge of their patients drives their commitment to habitually practice these virtues. In the chaotic environment of the ED, clinicians must be vigilant and prudent to efficiently discern the appropriate course of care. In order for the shared goal of patient well-being and safety to be achieved, all must be trustworthy and have their trustworthiness recognized by others. In this setting, courage is often called for by the traumatic nature of the patient presentation. Unfortunately, the current policies do not include nurses as a stakeholder, undermining the nurses' trustworthiness and requiring additional courage to participate.

PATIENT SAFETY RISKS

Patients' safe passage through their hospital stay depends critically on the work of virtuous clinicians to guide their journey. Incorrect patient disposition jeopardizes their safety and is linked to increased patient mortality and avoidable adverse events (Metcalfe, Sloggett, & McPherson, 1997; Trinkle & Flabouris, 2011; Vlayen et al., 2012). A noninclusive disposition process limits a clinician's ability to practice virtues and thus risks the virtues themselves. Similarly, a noninclusive disposition process may result in harm to the clinician on whom patients depend.

Nurses practice the virtue of vigilance through the nursing assessment. Some describe the nursing assessment as evidence of the presence of vigilance (Kooken & Haase, 2014; Meyer & Lavin, 2005). Experienced nurses refine their assessment skills through pattern recognition and have an accelerated development of clinical intuition, most likely due to the sheer number of hours they spend at the bedside of patients (Hurst, 2010; Odell, Victor, & Oliver, 2009). Pattern recognition is an unconscious assessment expressed through a clinician's intuition, often referred to as a *gut feeling*, which clinicians then learn to trust over time (English, 1993; Hathaway, 1956; Lyneham, Parkinson, & Denholm, 2008; Odell et al., 2009; Pretz & Folse, 2011; Ruter, Marcille, Sprekeler, Gerstner, & Herzog, 2012; Smith, 2009; Truman, 2003).

When experienced clinicians use intuition in patient care, it reflects both clinical and moral wisdom; both are developed through habit and time. As novices, everyone needs rules and procedures to guide correct behavior (Dreyfus & Dreyfus, 1986). Over time, clinicians develop their own expertise and vigilance. Just as they develop moral wisdom, so too they develop clinical intuition to respond to subtle situational clues with deep knowledge and instinctive behavioral responses (Kooken & Haase, 2014). For instance, in emergent situations, experienced clinicians will often rely on their clinical intuition first to guide interventions and treatments, rather than a formal explicit patient assessment (Bjork & Hamilton, 2011; Dhaliwal, 2011). The subtle signs and symptoms of clinical deterioration can be detected through clinical intuition long before there are perceived changes in lab values or vital signs (Bjork & Hamilton, 2011; English, 1993; Luntley, 2011; Lyneham et al., 2008; Odell et al., 2009). Expert nurses may be able to articulate, immediately, the objective details they are noticing through intuition, but many nurses cannot. Osler once remarked that "there is no more difficult art to acquire than the art of observation, and for some men it is quite as difficult to record an observation in brief and plain language" (Osler & Silverman, 2003, p. 99).

A nurse's relative lack of institutional power often makes it difficult to contribute his or her intuition to patient care decisions. During all patient–nurse interactions, from the moment the nurse sees the patient, they are continuously assessing the patient for potential threats. Once a threat of harm is identified, nurses diligently attend to this threat to prevent patient harm (Kooken & Haase, 2014). However when their intuitive knowledge is dismissed, ignored, or silenced, they must call upon moral courage to make their concerns heard (Kooken & Haase, 2014).

Expression of nurses' clinical intuition can be supported through institutional structures. Rapid response teams (RRTs) were developed to protect patients from harm, provide an immediate responses to all requests, and to increase patient safety through early recognition of a deteriorating patient (Bristow et al., 2000; Chaboyer, Thalib, Foster, Ball, & Richards, 2008; Chan, Jain, Nallmothu, Berg, & Sasson, 2010; Chan et al., 2008; Hughes & Clancy, 2005; Trinkle & Flabouris, 2011; Vlayen et al., 2012). Nurses are the primary users of RRTs, with the highest call origination, which suggests they are the first to recognize when a patient might be at risk for harm (Wynn, Engelke, & Swanson, 2009). The RRT system allows for nurses to identify clinical warning signs presenting through clinical intuition *without* having to articulate or identify specific clinical symptoms, challenge the hospital's hierarchy, or rely on trustworthiness between clinicians. RRTs are triggered 39% of the time by the categories of "worried" or "intuition" (Chen, Bellomo, Hillman, Flabouris, & Finfer, 2010). Retrospective chart reviews showed other triggers such as "respiratory problem" could have been selected instead of "worried" or "intuition" that support the creation of these seemingly ambiguous categories (Chen et al., 2010).

This example illustrates a policy, which affirms that the trustworthiness of nursing clinical intuition has been instituted successfully in other clinical areas.

Creating similar policies in the ED to include nurses in disposition planning would facilitate the practice of nursing vigilance and prudence. Full expression of these critical virtues will foster the goal of patient safety.

DAMAGE TO INTERPROFESSIONAL COHERENCE

The structure of high-functioning teams is a focus of patient safety literature, with particular attention to the need to promote clinicians' shared virtues as well as the welfare of patients (Storch & Kenny, 2007). Good teamwork and effective interprofessional communication increases patient safety and improves patient outcomes (DeJoy et al., 2011; Manser, 2009; Storch & Kenny, 2007). However, the coherence of the interprofessional team is at risk when clinicians are unable to fully express their professional recommendations.

Interprofessional trustworthiness is essential to the goals of health care and clinicians typically see all members of the health-care team as trustworthy; yet it is still very difficult to establish trustworthiness as habitual in health care. Recognizing trustworthiness in another person requires a strong correlating relationship (McLeod, 2014). The development of relationships over time is not always possible in the clinical setting, and often there is a member of the health-care team who is new to the unit or floor. This is especially true in academic teaching hospitals and in organizations that utilize agency per diem clinicians. When such clinicians attempt to go beyond their predefined roles to provide input, team members use prudence to decide whether the unknown clinician's assessment should be valued.

A fundamental element of clinical judgment is to determine the value of all presented information. This task is complicated by the perceived trustworthiness of the presenter. Not identifying someone as trustworthy when he or she acts outside of the role means valuable information is lost. By contrast, uncritically accepting recommendations based on established trustworthiness of a colleague risks overvaluing possible faulty information (Marshall, West, & Aitken, 2013). Whether a clinician is identified as trustworthy or not does not change the obligation of clinicians to value and assess all information presented to them (Dhaliwal, 2011; Marshall et al., 2013).

Although trustworthiness is generally understood as individually earned, a respect for trustworthiness can be mandated through policy. For example, advanced cardiovascular life support guidelines promote a shared team mentality to promote the perception of trustworthiness in other team members. This is seen as so fundamental to safe practice that an entire chapter is dedicated to "Effective Resuscitation Team Dynamics" in the 2010 guidelines (American Heart Association, 2011). Although during cardiac resuscitation, every team member is assigned a specific role, all members are also seen as trustworthy to provide input on any aspect of the code. The team promotes knowledge sharing and monitoring of one another. All clinicians are stakeholders in the decisional process, even when outside their defined role, because it promotes the team's shared goal.

The absence of an institutional policy explicitly including nurses in the disposition planning process leaves clinicians to question trustworthiness in others. This uncertainty has repercussions for patients and clinicians. Patients do not receive the benefit of the full range of available clinical knowledge. Additionally, to maintain virtues, clinicians must be able to practice them and consistently have them affirmed as valuable and meaningful. When they are not perceived as trustworthy, nurses are denied the opportunity to practice the virtue of trustworthiness. A policy explicitly including nursing in disposition planning would improve interprofessional function for the benefit of patient welfare.

MORAL DISTRESS

Moral distress was first defined by Jameton as "the painful psychological disequilibrium that results from recognizing the ethically appropriate action, yet not taking it, because of such obstacles as lack of time, supervisory reluctance, and inhibiting health care power structure, institutional policy, or legal considerations" (Jameton, 1984, p. 6). More recently, moral distress has been further refined as "the experience of being seriously compromised as a moral agent in practicing in accordance with accepted professional values and standards. It is a relational experience shaped by multiple contexts, including the socio-political and cultural context of the workplace environment" (Varcoe, Pauly, Webster, & Storch, 2012, p. 59). This latter definition takes into account professional values and standards that are compromised due to numerous constraints, most of which involve a blend of virtues clinicians must have to care for patients.

There are many practical reasons why health-care institutions should be concerned about moral distress and work to manage it. Moral distress has been found to endanger the retention of nurses, as many cite it as a reason for a nurse to leave a position (Bell & Breslin, 2008). Moral distress also carries a high financial cost for employers as it costs approximately eighty thousand dollars to train a new nurse (Boyle & Miller, 2008; Jones, 2008). Moral distress can also cause physical or emotional distress and result in moral residue or moral blunting (Austin, 2012; Austin, Rankel, Kagan, Bergum, & Lemermeyer, 2005; Bell & Breslin, 2008; Corley, Elswick, Gorman, & Clor, 2001; Corley & Minick, 2002; Kalvemark, Hoglund, Hansson, Westerholm, & Arnetz, 2004; Pauly, Varcoe, & Storch, 2012; Pavlish, Brown-Saltzman, Hersh, Shirk, & Rounkle, 2011; Rice,

Rady, Hamrick, Verheijde, & Pendergast, 2008). Moral residue is what is left after moral distress, when a person has been seriously compromised; it can shape future events and attitudes and can even damage or end a career (Epstein & Hamric, 2009). Moral blunting is similar to the well-known terms *professional burnout* and *compassion fatigue* and results in a muted conscience allowing the virtues to be compromised without the associated distress (Hanna, 2004).

One solution is the establishment of institutional systems that affirm nursing credibility, limiting the need for nurses to act with courage and affirming them when they do. One effort in this direction is hospitals becoming accredited to Magnet status. Magnet status is awarded by the American Nurses' Credentialing Center for excellence in nursing and addresses moral distress through the creation of inclusive system processes. There are many reasons hospitals strive to gain Magnet status: Nurses in Magnet hospitals yield better patient outcomes, work in a healthier environment, and are more productive (Kramer, Maguire, & Brewer, 2011). Magnet hospitals emphasize structural empowerment, which seeks to examine and reform the processes of accomplishing shared goals and desired outcomes (Kramer et al., 2011). Structural empowerment simultaneously tackles moral distress through including and valuing nursing input.

The practice of excluding nurses from patient disposition can inhibit nurses from being able to meet the standards held by the profession of nursing. When nurses are either unable to be courageous or are courageous and then unsuccessful, they may become unable to see themselves as "good" nurses. This is moral distress in action. The resulting moral residue or blunting can lead to erosion of the nurses' ability to care for their patients. Nurses may become silenced and no longer courageous, ineffective in their role, or leave their position. Moral distress is not completely avoidable but can be managed through policies, like inclusion in disposition planning, which promote virtues vital to the profession.

OVERCOMING OBJECTIONS

Although explicitly including nurses in disposition planning has the potential to improve patient safety, facilitate team cohesion, and prevent moral distress, it would be a significant change in current practice. Like any change, including nursing assessment and intuition in the planning of patient disposition could face a range of objections. Key among these would be the unreliability of nursing intuition and the increased time necessary to complete the process. While both of these are important considerations, neither is sufficient to override the benefits of the inclusion of nursing in disposition planning.

Nursing intuition and assessment ought not to trump other sources of data and the evaluations of other health-care providers. However, much, if not most, of the information used for clinical decision making is imperfect. Discernment is required even for applying data commonly considered "objective." For example, many lab tests have both false-positive and false-negative findings that must be accounted for in determining their meaning and relevance. The D-dimer blood test, which assesses for the presence of a clot or embolism in the body, is one such example. If the test is negative, it is very accurate for ruling out a clot in the lungs or legs. However, a positive result is more difficult to interpret. A recent study found that out of 237 people who tested positive, only 11 had an embolism (Vossen, Albrektson, Sensarma, & Williams, 2012). Nursing contributions can be similarly evaluated. If nursing judgments align with those of other providers, this would be a confirmation of the disposition plan. However, a judgment at odds with other assessments would call for further consideration.

Nurses are well equipped to participate in disposition planning. Nurses are already routinely involved in assessing discharge readiness in other clinical areas. Nursing expertise contributes to both decreasing length of stay (Gotz, Thompson, & Jones, 2014) and predicting the likelihood of 30-day readmission (Pace et al., 2014). The predictive value of combined physician and nurse assessment are likely to yield higher accuracy than either alone (Brabrand, Hallas, & Knudsen, 2014). The other key objection to the inclusion of nursing in disposition planning is the time required to consult with additional providers. Historically, the involvement of nurses has actually lowered the cost and time spent on patient care (Der, 2009; Durbin, 2006; Gonzalo, Masters, Simons, & Chuang, 2009; O'Leary et al., 2011; O'Leary et al., 2010; Sehgal & Auerbach, 2011). In the past decade, similar concerns where raised when ICUs began including the bedside nurse in patient care decisions. Team rounds actually reduced time spent on communication, decreased the length of stay, and increased patient safety, team morale, and interprofessional communication (Der, 2009; Durbin, 2006; Gonzalo et al., 2009; O'Leary et al., 2011; O'Leary et al., 2010; Sehgal & Auerbach, 2011).

CONCLUSION

Hospital policies should not only ensure patient health and welfare but also promote professional virtues and inspire collaborative practice. In the current structure, individual nurses may be valued as trustworthy—or may act with courage to intervene in an established plan—but their professional role in the process is not acknowledged. Routinely including nursing in disposition planning would facilitate the expression of their virtues of prudence, trustworthiness, courage, and vigilance. As these are virtues that are shared among all clinicians, honoring them in nurses would also facilitate their habitual practice by all team members.

The current practice of patient disposition planning in EDs carries high ethical hazards by not explicitly including the bedside nurse and results in unacceptable harm. Admittedly, there will challenges to implementing a structure such as the ones being proposed. Establishing good interprofessional communication, overcoming historical behavior patterns, and concern about added time and resources need to be addressed. As ambassadors of health, we must continue to improve our system to support our shared goal to increase the ethical quality of in-hospital patient care.

ACKNOWLEDGMENTS

We would like to thank Denise Dudzinski, PhD MTS, who improved this article with her advice and thoughtful comments.

REFERENCES

American Heart Association. (2011). *Advanced Cardiovascular Life Support Provider Manual*. Dallas, TX: Author.

Armstrong, A. E. (2006). Towards a strong virtue ethics for nursing practice. *Nursing Philosophy, 7*(3), 110–124. http://dx.doi.org/10.1111/j.1466-769x.2006.00268.x

Austin, W. (2012). Moral distress and the contemporary plight of health professionals. *HEC Forum, 24*(1), 27–38. http://dx.doi.org/10.1007/s10730-012-9179-8

Austin, W., Rankel, M., Kagan, L., Bergum, V., & Lemermeyer, G. (2005). To stay or to go, to speak or stay silent, to act or not to act: Moral distress as experienced by psychologists. *Ethics & Behavior, 15*(3), 197–212. http://dx.doi.org/10.1207/s15327019eb1503_1

Bell, J., & Breslin, J. M. (2008). Healthcare provider moral distress as a leadership challenge. *JONAS Healthcare Law, Ethics and Regulation, 10*(4), 94–97. http://dx.doi.org/10.1097/nhl.0b013e31818ede46

Bjork, I. T., & Hamilton, G. A. (2011). Clinical decision making of nurses working in hospital settings. *Nursing Research and Practice, 2011*, 1–8. http://dx.doi.org/10.1155/2011/524918

Boyle, D. K., & Miller, P. A. (2008). Focus on nursing turnover: A system-centered performance measure. *Nursing Management, 39*(6), 16, 18–20. http://dx.doi.org/10.1097/01.numa.0000320633.81435.75

Brabrand, M., Hallas, J., & Knudsen, T. (2014). Nurses and physicians in a medical admission unit can accurately predict mortality of acutely admitted patients: A prospective cohort study. *PLoS One, 9*(7), e101739. http://dx.doi.org/10.1371/journal.pone.0101739

Bristow, P. J., Hillman, K. M., Chey, T., Daffurn, K., Jacques, T. C., Norman, S. L., et al. (2000). Rates of in-hospital arrests, deaths and intensive care admissions: The effect of a medical emergency team. *The Medical Journal of Australia, 173*(5), 236–240.

Calder, L. A., Arnason, T., Vaillancourt, C., Perry, J. J., Stiell, I. G., & Forster, A. J. (2015). How do emergency physicians make discharge decisions? *Emergency Medical Journal, 32*(1), 9–14. http://dx.doi.org/10.1136/emermed-2013-202421

Calder, L. A., Forster, A. J., Stiell, I. G., Carr, L. K., Perry, J. J., Vaillancourt, C., et al. (2012). Mapping out the emergency department disposition decision for high-acuity patients. *Annals of Emergency Medicine, 60*(5), 567–576. http://dx.doi.org/10.1016/j.annemergmed.2012.04.013

Calder, L. A., Pozgay, A., Riff, S., Rothwell, D., Youngson, E., Mojaverian, N., et al. (2015). Adverse events in patients with return emergency department visits. *BMJ Quality & Safety, 24*, 142–148.

Chaboyer, W., Thalib, L., Foster, M., Ball, C., & Richards, B. (2008). Predictors of adverse events in patients after discharge from the intensive care unit. *American Journal of Critical Care, 17*(3), 255–264.

Chen, J., Bellomo, R., Hillman, K., Flabouris, A., & Finfer, S. (2010). Triggers for emergency team activation: A multicenter assessment. *Journal of Critical Care, 25*(2), 359.e1–359.e7. http://dx.doi.org/10.1016/j.jcrc.2009.12.011

Chan, P. S., Jain, R., Nallmothu, B. K., Berg, R. A., & Sasson, C. (2010). Rapid response teams: A systematic review and meta-analysis. *Archives of Internal Medicine, 170*(1), 18–26. http://dx.doi.org/10.1001/archinternmed.2009.424

Chan, P. S., Khalid, A., Longmore, L. S., Berg, R. A., Kosiborod, M., & Spertus, J. A. (2008). Hospital-wide code rates and mortality before and after implementation of a rapid response team. *Journal of American Medical Association, 300*(21), 2506–2513. http://dx.doi.org/10.1001/jama.2008.715

Considine, J., Charlesworth, D., & Currey, J. (2014). Characteristics and outcomes of patients requiring rapid response system activation within hours of emergency admission. *Critical Care and Resuscitation, 16*(3), 184–189.

Corley, M. C., Elswick, R. K., Gorman, M., & Clor, T. (2001). Development and evaluation of a moral distress scale. *Journal of Advanced Nursing, 33*(2), 250–256.

Corley, M. C., & Minick, P. (2002). Moral distress or moral comfort. *Bioethics Forum, 18*(1–2), 7–14.

DeJoy, S., Burkman, R. T., Graves, B. W., Grow, D., Sankey, H. Z., Delk, C., et al. (2011). Making it work: Successful collaborative practice. *Obstetrics and Gynecology, 118*(3), 683–686. http://dx.doi.org/10.1097/aog.0b013e318229e0bf

Der, Y. (2009). Multidisciplinary rounds in our ICU: Improved collaboration and patient outcomes. *Critical Care Nurse, 29*(4), 83–84. http://dx.doi.org/10.4037/ccn2009792

Dhaliwal, G. (2011). Going with your gut. *Journal of General Internal Medicine, 26*(2), 107–109. http://dx.doi.org/10.1007/s11606-010-1578-4

Dreyfus, H., & Dreyfus, S. (1986). *Mind over machine: The power of human intuition and expertise in the era of the computer.* Oxford: Blackwell.

Durant, W. (2006). *The Story of philosophy: The lives and opinions of the world's greatest philosophers.* New York, NY: Simon & Schuster, Inc.

Durbin, C. G. (2006). Team model: Advocating for the optimal method of care delivery in the intensive care unit. *Critical Care Medicine, 34*(3), S12–S17.

English, I. (1993). Intuition as a function of the expert nurse: A critique of Benner's novice to expert model. *Journal of Advanced Nursing, 18*(3), 387–393.

Epstein, E. G., & Hamric, A. B. (2009). Moral distress, moral residue, and the crescendo effect. *The Journal of Clinical Ethics, 20*(4), 330–342.

Fordyce, J., Blank, F. S., Pekow, P., Smithline, H. A., Ritter, G., Gehlbach, S., et al. (2003). Errors in a busy emergency department. *Annals of Emergency Medicine, 42*, 324–333.

Gardiner, P. (2003). A virtue ethics approach to moral dilemmas in medicine. *Journal of Medical Ethics, 29*(5), 297–302.

Gonzalo, J. D., Masters, P. A., Simons, R. J., & Chuang, C. H. (2009). Attending rounds and bedside case presentations: Medical student and medicine resident experiences and attitudes. *Teaching and Learning in Medicine, 21*(2), 105–110. http://dx.doi.org/10.1080/10401330902791156

Gordon, E. J., & Hamric, A. B. (2006). The courage to stand up: The cultural politics of nurses' access to ethics consultation. *The Journal of Clinical Ethics, 17*(3), 231–254.

Gotz, V. N., Thompson, A., & Jones, K. (2014). Developing and evaluating nurse led discharge in acute medicine. *Acute Medicine, 13*(4), 159–162.

Hanna, D. R. (2004). Moral distress: The state of the science. *Research and Theory for Nursing Practice, 18*(1), 73–93.

Hathaway, S. R. (1956). Clinical intuition and inferential accuracy. *Journal of Personality, 24*(3), 223–250.

Hirter, J., & Van Nest, R. L. (1995). Vigilance: A concept and a reality. *CRNA: The Clinical Forum for Nurse Anesthetists, 6*(2), 96–98.

Horwitz, L. I., Meredith, T., Schuur, J. D., Shah, N. R., Kulkarni, R. G., & Jenq, G. Y. (2009). Dropping the baton: A qualitative analysis of failures during the transition from emergency department to inpatient care. *Annals of Emergency Medicine, 53*, 701–710.

Hughes, R. G., & Clancy, C. M. (2005). Working conditions that support patient safety. *Journal of Nursing Care Quality, 20*(4), 289–292.

Hurst, K. (2010). How much time do nurses spend at the bedside? *Nursing Standard, 24*(52), 14.

Jameton, A. (1984). *Nursing practice: The ethical issues.* Englewood Cliffs, NJ: Prentice-Hall.

Jones, C. B. (2008). Revisiting nurse turnover costs: Adjusting for inflation. *The Journal of Nursing Administration, 38*(1), 11–18. http://dx.doi.org/10.1097/01.nna.0000295636.03216.6f

Kalvemark, S., Hoglund, A. T., Hansson, M. G., Westerholm, P., & Arnetz, B. (2004). Living with conflicts-ethical dilemmas and moral distress in the health care system. *Social Science & Medicine, 58*(6), 1075–1084.

Kennedy, M., Joyce, N., Howell, M. D., Mottley, L. J., & Shapiro, N. I. (2010). Identifying infected emergency department patients admitted to the hospital ward at risk of clinical deterioration and intensive care unit transfer. *Academic Emergency Medicine, 17*(10), 1080–1085. http://dx.doi.org/10.1111/j.1553-2712.2010.00872.x

Kooken, W. C., & Haase, J. E. (2014). A big word for something we do all the time: Oncology nurses lived experience of vigilance. *Cancer Nursing, 37*(6), E15–E24. http://dx.doi.org/10.1097/ncc.0000000000000113

Kramer, M., Maguire, P., & Brewer, B. B. (2011). Clinical nurses in magnet hospitals confirm productive, healthy unit work environments. *Journal of Nursing Management, 19*(1), 5–17. http://dx.doi.org/10.1111/j.1365-2834.2010.01211.x

Larkin, G. L., Iserson, K., Kassutto, Z., Freas, G., Delaney, K., Krimm, J., et al. (2009). Virtue in emergency medicine. *Academic Emergency Medicine 16*(1), 51–55.

Luntley, M. (2011). What do nurses know? *Nursing Philosophy, 12*(1), 22–33. http://dx.doi.org/10.1111/j.1466-769x.2010.00466.x

Lyneham, J., Parkinson, C., & Denholm, C. (2008). Explicating Benner's concept of expert practice: Intuition in emergency nursing. *Journal of Advanced Nursing, 64*(4), 380–387. http://dx.doi.org/10.1111/j.1365-2648.2008.04799.x

Manser, T. (2009). Teamwork and patient safety in dynamic domains of healthcare: A review of the literature. *Acta Anaesthesiologia Scandinavica, 53*(2), 143–151. http://dx.doi.org/10.1111/j.1399-6576.2008.01717.x

Marshall, A. P., West, S. H., & Aitken, L. M. (2013). Clinical credibility and trustworthiness are key characteristics used to identify colleagues from whom to seek information. *Journal of Clinical Nursing, 22*(9–10), 1424–1433. http://dx.doi.org/10.1111/jocn.12070

McLeod, C. (2014). Trust. *The Stanford Encyclopedia of Philosophy.* Retrieved March 29, 2015 from http://plato.stanford.edu/archives/sum2014/entries/trust/

Metcalfe, M. A., Sloggett, A., & McPherson, K. (1997). Mortality among appropriately referred patients refused admission to intensive-care units. *The Lancet, 350*(9070), 7–11. http://dx.doi.org/10.1016/s0140-6736(96)10018-0

Meyer, G., & Lavin, M. A. (2005). Vigilance: The essence of nursing. *Online Journal of Issues in Nursing, 10*(3), 8.

Odell, M., Victor, C., & Oliver, D. (2009). Nurses' role in detecting deterioration in ward patients: Systematic literature review. *Journal of Advanced Nursing, 65*(10), 1992–2006.

O'Leary, K. J., Buck, R., Fligiel, H. M., Haviley, C., Slade, M. E., Landler, M. P., et al. (2011). Structured interdisciplinary rounds in a medical teaching unit: Improving patient safety. *Archives of Internal Medicine, 171*(7), 678–684. http://dx.doi.org/10.1001/archinternmed.2011.128

O'Leary, K. J., Wayne, D. B., Haviley, C., Slade, M. E., Lee, J., & Williams, M. V. (2010). Improving teamwork: Impact of structured interdisciplinary rounds on a medical teaching unit. *Journal of General Internal Medicine, 25*(8), 826–832. http://dx.doi.org/10.1007/s11606-010-1345-6

Osler, W., & Silverman, M. (2003). The Quotable Osler. United States: American College of Physicians—American Society of Internal Medicine.

Pace, R., Spevack, R., Menendez, C., Kouriambalis, M., Green, L., & Jayaraman, D. (2014). Ability of nurse clinicians to predict unplanned returns to hospital within thirty days of discharge. *Hospital Practice, 42*(5), 62–68. http://dx.doi.org/10.3810/hp.2014.12.1159

Page, A. (Eds.). (2003). *Keeping patients safe transforming the work environment of nurses.* Washington, DC: Institute of Medicine, The National Academies Press. Retrieved from http://books.nap.edu/openbook.php?record_id=10851

Pauly, B. M., Varcoe, C., & Storch, J. (2012). Framing the issues: Moral distress in health care. *HEC Forum, 24*(2), 1–11. http://dx.doi.org/10.1007/s10730-012-9176-y

Pavlish, C., Brown-Saltzman, K., Hersh, M., Shirk, M., & Rounkle, A. M. (2011). Nursing priorities, actions, and regrets for ethical situations in clinical practice. *Journal of Nursing Scholarship, 43*(4), 385–395. http://dx.doi.org/10.1111/j.1547-5069.2011.01422.x

Pellegrino, E. D., & Thomasma, D. C. (1993). *The virtues in medical practice.* New York, NY: Oxford University Press.

Perimal-Lewis, L., Hakendorf, P. H., & Thompson, C. H. (2015). Characteristics favouring a delayed disposition decision in the emergency department. *Internal Medicine Journal, 45*(2), 155–159. http://dx.doi.org/10.1111/imj.12618

Pretz, J. E., & Folse, V. N. (2011). Nursing experience and preference for intuition in decision making. *Journal of Clinical Nursing, 20*(19–20), 2878–2889. http://dx.doi.org/10.1111/j.1365-2702.2011.03705.x

Rice, E. M., Rady, M. Y., Hamrick, A., Verheijde, J. L., & Pendergast, D. K. (2008). Determinants of moral distress in medical and surgical nurses at an adult acute tertiary care hospital. *Journal of Nursing Management, 16*(3), 360–373. http://dx.doi.org/10.1111/j.1365-2834.2007.00798.x

Ruter, J., Marcille, N., Sprekeler, H., Gerstner, W., & Herzog, M. H. (2012). Paradoxical evidence integration in rapid decision processes. *PLoS Computational Biology, 8*(2), e1002382. http://dx.doi.org/10.1371/journal.pcbi.1002382

Sehgal, N. L., & Auerbach, A. A. (2011). Communication failures and a call for new systems to promote patient safety: Comment on "Structured interdisciplinary rounds in a medical teaching unit." *Archives of Internal Medicine, 171*(7), 684–685. http://dx.doi.org/10.1001/archinternmed.2011.129

Smith, A. (2009). Exploring the legitimacy of intuition as a form of nursing knowledge. *Nursing Standard, 23*(40), 35–40.

Society of Academic Emergency Medicine Ethics Committee. (1996). Virtue in emergency medicine. *Academic Emergency Medicine, 3*(10), 961–966. http://dx.doi.org/10.1111/j.1553-2712.1996.tb03329.x

Storch, J. L., & Kenny, N. (2007). Shared moral work of nurses and physicians. *Nursing Ethics, 14*(4), 478–491. http://dx.doi.org/10.1177/0969733007077882

Timmons, M. (2006). *Conduct and character reading in moral theory* (5th ed.). Belmont, CA: Thomson Wadsworth.

Trinkle, R. M., & Flabouris, A. (2011). Medical reviews before cardiac arrest, medical emergency call or unanticipated intensive care unit admission: Their nature and impact on patient outcome. *Critical Care and Resuscitation, 13*(3), 175–180.

Truman, P. (2003). Intuition and practice. *Nursing Standard, 18*(7), 42–43.

Varcoe, C., Pauly, B., Webster, G., & Storch, J. (2012). Moral distress: Tensions as springboards for action. *HEC Forum, 24*(1), 51–62. http://dx.doi.org/10.1007/s10730-012-9180-2

Vlayen, A., Verelst, S., Bekkering, G. E., Schrooten, W., Hellings, J., & Claes, N. (2012). Incidence and preventability of adverse events requiring intensive care admission: A systematic review. *Journal of Evaluation in Clinical Practice, 18*(2), 485–497. http://dx.doi.org/10.1111/j.1365-2753.2010.01612.x

Vossen, J. A., Albrektson, J., Sensarma, A., & Williams, S. C. (2012). Clinical usefulness of adjusted D-dimer cut-off values to exclude pulmonary embolism in a community hospital emergency department patient population. *Acta Radiologica, 53*(7), 765–768.

Wynn, J. D., Engelke, M. K., & Swanson, M. (2009). The front line of patient safety: Staff nurses and rapid response team calls. *Quality Management in Health Care, 18*(1), 40–47.

CHAPTER 11

Postdeployment Reintegration

The Ethics of Embodied Personal Presence and the Formation of Military Meaning

E. Ann Jeschke

ABSTRACT

In 2014, the Institute of Medicine published a meta-analysis on current military reintegration programs, suggesting they have failed to improve postdeployment behavioral health. In this chapter, I explore some of the issues associated with the two paradigm reintegration programs supported by the Department of Defense (DoD), namely, BATTLEMIND postdeployment debriefings and Master Resilience Training. My discussion will be located within a subpopulation of military personnel I call warriors, particularly those men who have been exposed to combat. In performing a normative analysis of current reintegration programs, I rely on an ethics of embodied personal presence as a derivative locus of both nursing ethics and the just war tradition. Using an interdisciplinary approach to evaluate warriors' experiences of training across the military life cycle illustrates how reintegration challenges have been construed as potential pathology because disembodied reintegration programs do not consider the influence of military training and lifestyle in the development of certain health behaviors. When compared to the warrior's lived experience, a broader set of reintegration challenges emerge that cannot be fully captured by the symptoms of posttraumatic stress. Therefore, new reintegration programs need to be developed.

http://dx.doi.org/10.1891/0739-6686.34.199

Although I do not provide explicit details concerning what these reintegration programs should look at, I suggest that the DoD turn to something akin to the Healthy People campaign.

BACKGROUND

Postdeployment reintegration of military personnel has become a hot-button topic for the U.S. military as the conflicts in Iraq and Afghanistan wind down. Over 2.4 million military personnel have been deployed during the Global War on Terror (GWOT), many, multiple times. As the military moves forward into a state of peace and restoration, the topic of helping deployed military personnel readjust to civilian life after deployment is a salient one not just for the military, but also for the public health and social stability. In 2010, the Institute of Medicine (IOM) performed an initial meta-analysis to evaluate the ongoing needs of military personnel returning from deployment. This original meta-analysis suggested that "the depth and breadth of challenges faced by returning military service members" was the "result of a complex interplay of factors" (National Research Council, 2010, p. 5). Thereafter, a 2013 follow-up report found that in spite of military efforts, 44% of military personnel continued to face ongoing difficulties readjusting to life after deployment (IOM, 2013). In response, the military has implemented various programs to abate the increasing postdeployment rates of suicide, posttraumatic stress disorder (PTSD), anxiety disorders, depression, and alcohol use among the ranks of military personnel.

TOPIC

In this chapter, I will explore some of the issues associated with the two paradigm reintegration programs supported by the Department of Defense (DoD), namely, BATTLEMIND postdeployment debriefings and Master Resilience Training (MRT). These reintegration programs are meant to reduce negative postdeployment behavioral health outcomes, primarily by addressing the symptoms of posttraumatic stress (PTS). Unfortunately, on February 20, 2014, the IOM published an updated meta-analysis suggesting that BATTLEMIND and MRT failed to improve postdeployment behavioral health. In specific, the report suggested that the rates of anxiety and PTSD actually increased in returning military personnel by 62% after their implementation (Wang, 2014). David Rudd, a panelist on the IOM meta-analysis, said there was no evidence that these reintegration programs will have any enduring impact on the long-term postdeployment behavioral health of military personnel (Zoroya, 2014).

The IOM report suggested that there are two interconnected reasons that reintegration programs have failed. First, they were developed by a civilian research group and never tested on a military population. Therefore, reintegration programs encourage the improvement of health behavior in only a narrow set of outcomes (IOM, 2014). Put differently, reintegration programs are framed in such a way that they might not capture the complex set of reintegration challenges. Second, reintegration programs were implemented before there was solid quantitative evidence to establish that they would effectively mitigate negative behavioral health outcomes. Pilot tests were never performed, research failed to control for important confounding variables, and there were serious problems with the data analysis methods used. Although it seems clear that current reintegration programs have not produced positive behavioral health outcomes, the military did not take the IOM's advice, which was to develop a new understanding of reintegration challenges by relying on qualitative research (Slomski, 2014).

My discussion will be located within a subpopulation of military personnel I call warriors, particularly those men who have been exposed to combat. Therefore, my chapter will consistently use masculine pronouns. In performing a normative analysis of current reintegration programs, I will rely on an ethics of embodied personal presence as a derivative focus of both nursing ethics and the just war tradition by looking at warriors' experience of training and habit formation across the military life cycle. By embodiment, I mean how an individual, quite literally, comes to inhabit particular meanings in his body and expresses these meanings through his actions and behaviors in a communal setting. Often embodiment is referred to as a mind–body connection; however, I have chosen to avoid such language as it implicitly hints at a dualism wherein the mind and body are separate from the onset and must be brought together. Instead, I am working from the premise that the human being starts as an integral whole and behavior emerges as an indivisible union of body and mind.

An interdisciplinary assessment of current programs will illustrate how the current disembodied understanding of behavioral health construes reintegration challenges as potential pathology because reintegration programs have not considered the way in which military training and lifestyle influence the formation of habits. These health behaviors embody certain meanings attendant to the military community and do not always translate into appropriate behavior in the civilian community. When looking at reintegration challenges within this new framework, it becomes apparent that new reintegration programs need to be developed. Although I will not be able to provide explicit details about new reintegration resources, I suggest that the DoD turn to something akin to the Healthy People campaign. The original initiative was launched in 1979 to determine various areas of behavioral health that needed to be improved in an effort to advance the collective health of the United States. The Healthy People initiative continues to monitor outcomes, reassess targets, and evaluate the collective effects of various health promotion research, strategies, and resources (Koh, 2010). Similarly, the DoD could establish baseline areas of health behavior that impede reintegration and develop training programs that help reorient particular military habits as well as monitor outcomes, reassess challenges, and evaluate the long-term effectiveness of helping warriors reintegrate into civilian society.

OUTLINE OF ARGUMENT

To begin, I will describe my normative framework, which relies on the moral duty to bear witness to a patient, and which emerges from nursing ethics' and the just war tradition's understanding of *post bellum* (postwar) social rehabilitation. While the former focuses on an intersubjective encounter with another human being and the importance of personal accounts, the latter focuses on the individual as an embodied subject of care. Taken together, nursing ethics and the just war tradition provide a space for the embodied personal account of the warrior to emerge as a means of defining reintegration challenges. Thereafter, I will briefly describe the two main reintegration programs currently promoted by the DoD in order to establish that they are focused on mitigating the symptoms of combat trauma in the form of PTS by providing disembodied cognitive skills training that exclusively aims at changing the warrior's thought processes. After briefly highlighting key philosophical concepts taken from Edmund Husserl and Maurice Merleau-Ponty, I will describe my qualitative research on the warrior's embodied experience of transitioning across the military life cycle. Highlighting five reintegration challenges related to a warrior's health behavior will illustrate how certain habits have been formed through military training and how they impede the warrior's ability to effectively transition into the civilian society after deployment. These behaviors can be taken as baseline challenges that could be developed into a broader reintegration-training program.

NORMATIVE FRAMEWORK

As previously mentioned, my normative framework relies on literature from both the nursing ethics and the just war tradition. Rahel Naef has argued for a nursing ethic grounded in duty to bear witness to the patient. She suggests that "bearing witness is a moral way of engaging in the nurse-person relationship" (Naef, 2006, p. 147). First and foremost, bearing witness is about staying true to and being respectful of another human being's personal experience when caring for a patient. It is a way in which someone is present to another by beholding, revering, honoring, acknowledging, and integrating the private and intimate experiences. In reference to the topic of discussion, I am concerned with bearing witness to the warrior's personal experience of military training and habit formation when considering reintegration challenges. Relying on Naef's understanding of personal presence allows me to place the primary emphasis on the warrior's personal account when understanding reintegration challenges. Correspondingly, reintegration programs that uphold an ethic of personal presence will be built upon serious consideration of warriors' experiences, priorities, hopes, and dreams (Naef, 2006).

The just war tradition argues that it is unethical to engage in armed conflict and, thereafter, fail to rehabilitate the social, ecological, and individual damage brought about by the violence in which the state has engaged. Although just war scholars have not spent a great deal of time focusing on the question regarding what type of programs are owed to returning warriors, in arguing for the necessity of *jus post bellum* criterion, authors Tobias Winright and Mark Allman bring to light the plight of the returning warrior as an important aspect of social rehabilitation. They say: "When a nation sends its citizens to war, it turns ordinary men and women into potential killers. In so doing, nations should assume the responsibility to assist warriors in their transition to civilian life once the fighting has ended" (Allman & Winright, 2010, p. 164). Furthermore, as Rear Admiral Louis V. Iasiello suggested, *post bellum* social rehabilitation insists that warriors not be treated as disembodied "machines" or "mere weapons to be placed in combat against the enemy's weapons of war. Warriors are persons" (Iasiello, 2004, p. 48). In other words, Rear Admiral Iasiello's statement implies that upon returning home, warriors should not be approached as mere thinking beings with an attached mechanical body that is used for the purpose of executing combat missions. Instead, warriors are to be understood within an integrated, embodied appreciation of the human being.

Together with nursing ethics' emphasis on bearing witness, the *post bellum* emphasis on embodiment suggests that reintegration programs need to affirm how meaning animates the warrior's personhood as an integral aspect of his action in the world. I will use the ethics of embodied personal presence as a normative framework with which to evaluate current reintegration programs. Next, I turn to a brief description of the current reintegration programs to show that they are not only ineffective but also give primacy to the symptoms of PTS over the warrior's personal account as well as rely on disembodied cognitive skills training as a means of assisting the warrior's reintegration into the civilian community.

DESCRIPTION OF CURRENT REINTEGRATION PROGRAMS

As previously mentioned, the two main reintegration programs promoted by the DoD are the BATTLEMIND debriefing and MRT programs. Both seek to encourage a warrior's reintegration into family and social life during the postdeployment period by minimizing symptoms of PTS. BATTLEMIND is a psychoeducational de-briefing immediately provided to warriors upon returning home from deployment. This debriefing describes how PTS symptoms can become impediments to their postdeployment reintegration and eventually develop into chronic crystalized PTSD. These mandatory debriefings, generally given by a civilian psychologist, make use of PowerPoint slides and handouts to provide warning signs of PTS symptoms. The didactic session lasts approximately one-and-a-half hours and relies on military language as a means of normalizing combat trauma (Orsingher, Lopez, & Rinchart, 2007).

Battlemind

The BATTLEMIND acronym represents the warrior skills necessary to function in combat, particularly, buddies (cohesion), accountability, targeted aggression, tactical awareness, lethally armed, emotional control, mission operational security, individual responsibility, nondefensive combat driving, and discipline. Next to the BATTLEMIND acronym, PowerPoint slides and handouts list the most common symptoms of PTS: guilt, overcontrolling attitude, hyperarousal, hypervigilance, excessive anger, numbness, and detachment. The debriefing stresses that the cognitive thought processes associated with a battlemind are necessary for high performance in combat, but when applied in the civilian setting, they produce maladaptive thinking and behaviors. In other words, if warriors operate out of their battlemind in the civilian society, they will be at risk of developing the symptoms of PTS (Castro et al., 2006). The debriefing suggests that a warrior should regularly stop and check his thoughts to see whether they emerge from his battlemind or civilian mind. Unfortunately, the BATTLEMIND debriefing spends minimal time discussing what kind of thoughts are appropriate for engaging the civilian society. In fact, the debriefing simply says that warriors should shift into a civilian mind by slowing down their thought processes (Adler, Bliese, McGurk, Hoge, & Castro, 2011; Adler, Castro, & McGurk, 2007).

BATTLEMIND's understanding of reintegration challenges is descriptively structured around PTS symptoms that have not been validated according to the warrior's experience. Furthermore, reintegration challenges are coupled with maladaptive thinking that will impede the warrior's ability to reintegrate into the civilian community. Although BATTLEMIND describes the warrior's combat skills, it does not explore his predeployment training or habit formation within the military community. As such, BATTLEMIND exclusively describes a warrior's combat skills and postdeployment reintegration behavior in relationship to his thought processes. Therefore, BATTLEMIND maintains a disembodied understanding of warrior habits and behavior by approaching the warrior as merely a thinking thing without reference to his body, training, or community.

Master Resilience Training

MRT is provided in the form of ongoing resilience training that seeks to increase the number of warriors "who complete combat tours without pathology, and to decrease the number of warriors who develop stress pathologies" after deployment (Cornum, Matthews, & Seligman, 2011, p. 6). It is a form of higher order cognitive training that attempts to teach the warrior to focus on positive thoughts instead of negative ones (Reivich, Seligman, & McBride, 2011, pp. 27–29). More specifically, resilience training seeks to help the warrior increase his self-awareness, self-regulation, optimism, mental agility, character strengths, and connection to others by exploring how counterproductive thought processes about oneself, one's current circumstance, others, and the world lead to maladaptive behaviors. Thereafter, resilience training explores how positive thinking regulates negative impulses, emotions, and behaviors in order to achieve personal goals. The primary goal of resilience training is to help the warrior develop an optimistic orientation toward life through regulation of thoughts. First, a warrior should notice his thoughts and focus only on good thoughts in relationship to self and others. Second, he should focus on keeping his thoughts wedded to reality. Third, he should eliminate counterproductive thoughts that lead to negative interactions with other people. As such, the resilience module attempts to train a warrior to engage in positive thought processes that are meant to establish strong relationships within the warrior's military community and family (Reivich et al., 2011).

Similar to the BATTLEMIND debriefing, MRT is explicitly aimed at mitigating PTS symptoms through the use of disembodied cognitive training. Both of these reintegration programs describe behavior in terms of the warrior's thoughts. Moreover, they assume that reintegration challenges directly relate to combat trauma and emerge as symptoms of PTS without reference to the warrior's personal experience or a perception of the warrior as a human being whose military training and community have caused him to inhabit particular meanings that animate his behavior. As such, they both fail to uphold an ethic of embodied personal presence. Before turning directly to a qualitative research study, I will first develop a new understanding of embodied behaviors that allows communal meaning to be incarnate in the warrior's corporeal experience. To do so, I rely on key concepts from the philosophy of Edmund Husserl and Maurice Merleau-Ponty.

RECLAIMING COMMUNAL CONTEXT, PERSONAL ACCOUNTS, AND EMBODIED BEHAVIORS: A PHENOMENOLOGICAL PERSPECTIVE

Relying on the phenomenological tradition will help to illustrate the importance of situational context, personal accounts, and embodied behaviors in designing a qualitative study. Edmund Husserl, the philosophical father of phenomenology, was famous for proposing the idea that philosophers should "go back to the things themselves" (Husserl, 1965, p. 97). According to Husserl, the purpose of philosophy was to draw our "attention back to ideas and accomplishments" that have been taken for granted, overlooked, remained anonymous, or concealed by the human being's subjective and objective experience of the world. In returning to the things themselves, Husserl concentrated his exploration of meaning development on the immediate communal context in which the human being operated (Frierson, 2013, p. 260). Husserl named this context a *Lebenswelt* (lifeworld) when explaining that specific meanings attendant to behavior develop and emerge within a particular context (Dorfman, 2009). Lived experience was also a central concept in Husserl's phenomenological project. This term specifically refers to direct engagement with the world in everyday life before a human being has reflected on or theorized about it (Dorfman, 2009). Accordingly, a human being's lived experience is shaped by his lifeworld. These two Husserlian concepts suggest that a warrior's personal account of his lived experience within a communal context will be pivotal in understanding reintegration challenges.

Maurice Merleau-Ponty's notion of bodily intentionality allows me to move forward with an embodied notion of behavior. Bodily intentionality deals with how human action unfolds within a lifeworld. Merleau-Ponty suggested that bodily intentionality is composed of two distinct layers of corporeal interaction with the world, namely, the habitual and the present body. The habitual body is developed through experiential understanding that is infused into the body as a unique set of habits. In turn, these habits become practical ways of relating to the specific lifeworld. The present body is a readiness to incorporate new experiences into the habitual body by moving toward an entity, touching it, manipulating it, or using it to accomplish a particular task. In other words, the habitual body is the human being's background familiarity with the particular meanings associated with various behaviors in a specific lifeworld, while the present body exists toward tasks that are being performed in the moment. The habitual body and present body come together in an integrated body schema that is constantly operating to allow the human being to optimally and effectively navigate a known lifeworld, while also adapting to changes, ambiguity, and new circumstances that occur in real time (Merleau-Ponty, 2002).

Accordingly, bodily intentionality is not the outcome of cognitive consciousness. It is implicit understanding structured into the body. There is a unique form of body memory that holds precognitive, nonconceptual/representational awareness within the habitual body. For example, the experience of smelling a pie baking in the oven is immediately apprehended and the body moves toward the pie before thinking, "I smell a pie. I will stand up, walk into the kitchen, and see if it is baking in the oven." The immediate perception engages my bodily knowing before my reflective thoughts. In other words, reflective consciousness emerges from within and is integrated into the habitual body's understanding in the lifeworld. As such, Merleau-Ponty's conceptualization of the intentional body provides me with an integrated understanding of the human being wherein behavior is not relegated primarily to thought processes but is galvanized from within a body that is animated, sensing, knowing, and directed toward a project (Carman, 2008; Casey, 1985; Merleau-Ponty, 2002; Smith, 2007).

The habitual body is also the foundation of embodied behaviors that are developed through the ongoing practice of particular habits. As such, movement, not thought, becomes the scaffolding of behavior. Through constant performance of specific habits, movement imbues behaviors with a complex and integrated set of meanings that come to "inhabit" the body. Merleau-Ponty's theory of habit formation through ongoing practice also allows me to investigate the importance of military training to the infusion of meaning within a particular lifeworld.

RESEARCH DESIGN AND METHODOLOGY

My qualitative research was approved by the St. Louis University institutional review board on March 4, 2014. This chapter is a secondary study that emerged from within a larger dissertation project, which sought to gain a more robust understanding of reintegration challenges by exploring the phenomenon of transition as warriors moved across the military life cycle and back into the civilian community. My analysis was guided by hermeneutic phenomenology, which stresses that the researcher's personal experiences and assumptions are to be brought into the process of data analysis as a means of uncovering deeper shared meaning. Additionally, this method is built on the presupposition that interpretation is ongoing and not limited to the analysis presented in this chapter. Furthermore, it relies on the researcher as the instrument and an emergent design wherein the basic design of the project can be altered in light of new developments that arise during data collection.

During analysis, interpretive summaries for each warrior were constructed. These summaries included a broad description of each warrior followed by the specific codes that were discovered in the data. Block quotes from the individual interviews were placed under each code in order to track the particular warrior's narrative. Codes were established by looking at the data for common or contrasting words, themes, and experiences. Finally, my own interpretive commentary was written below each section of block quotes in order to capture how my personal interpretation of meaning developed in association with each code.

The original study limited participation to men—enlisted or officer—who actively participated in ground combat in support of GWOT. Combat participation was defined as directly experiencing enemy fire or direct exposure to the detonation of an improvised explosive device (IED) used by the enemy. Although women have involved in ground combat, the original study focused solely on men in order to limit the study population, as women warriors would be difficult to recruit. My original study excluded those warriors who had sustained major physical or psychological injury requiring ongoing treatment due to participation in combat activities. Since traumatized warriors would present with various comorbidities that might influence their experience of reintegration, I started with those who had not been severely injured in combat. Participants were recruited through a snowball method using both a recruitment e-mail and a recruitment flyer, which were sent to the leaders of various veteran organizations throughout the United States.

The informed consent process occurred during the first interview session, wherein warriors were informed of the study aims, risks, and benefits of research participation and asked to sign an official informed consent document before starting the first interview. During the informed consent process, participants were told that they were not obliged to participate, they were not required to answer any questions that made them uncomfortable, and they were free to drop out of the study at any time. A detailed explanation of how their personal information would be deidentified was provided. All personal names and identifying locations were eliminated from the data and replaced with pseudonyms and alternative locations to mask the identity of the participants as well as those individuals discussed in the interview session.

While the original data were collected during three sets of interviews with 16 warriors, this particular chapter comes from data solicited during the first interview session, which focused on the warrior's training and daily activities as he moved through the military life cycle into the civilian community. The goal was to better understand how the warrior came to inhabit particular military meaning in his behavior as well as whether or not military meaning embodied in the warrior's behavior interfered with his ability to reintegrate into the civilian community after deployment. This interview relied on the following four questions:

- Could you please walk me through your experience of meeting a recruiter through basic training?
- Could you please walk me through your specialized combat training?
- Could you please walk me through your ongoing training in deployment?
- Could you please walk me through your experience of reintegration training?

Probes were aimed at drawing out further details or clarifying narratives and included questions such as:

- What did you like?
- What did you not like?
- What was difficult?
- What was exciting?
- What was funny?
- What was unexpected?

Interviews took place in a private conference room on the St. Louis University medical school campus and were recorded on an MP3 device. Raw data were transferred to a password-protected computer and immediately deleted from the recording device. After the audio files were transcribed, corrected, and all information deidentified, the MP3 files were deleted from the computer. Electronic versions of the transcriptions were also saved in a password-protected location on the computer. All recording devices, computers containing data, and printed data remained in a locked office.

HABIT FORMATION AND EMBODIED MEANING ACROSS THE MILITARY LIFE CYCLE

Originally, I hypothesized that warriors needed to function in two lifeworlds, namely, civilian and military. As a result, I suspected that there would be two sets of habits formed in each lifeworld and it would be the difference in habits that gave rise to reintegration challenges. I also suspected that as warriors transitioned across the military life cycle, they would develop a set of adaptive habits that could be used as a means to bridge the transition from the military lifeworld to the civilian lifeworld after deployment. During data analysis, it became clear that warriors needed to effectively perform in three lifeworlds: military, deployment, and civilian. Honing in on the question of reintegration challenges, I found that most habits were actually common to all three lifeworlds. Figure 11.1 highlights how common habits exist across all three lifeworlds, but military meaning was formed through the practice of particular habits across the military life cycle that aimed at the goal of achieving optimal combat performance.

In the civilian lifeworld, there were sundry goals at which a habit could be aimed. When the warrior returned to the civilian lifeworld and acted in a precognitive fashion, he expressed the military meaning associated with combat performance, which did not always transfer into the civilian lifeworld except for within combat veterans' groups. Therefore, it was not the habit that was problematic but the embodied meaning.

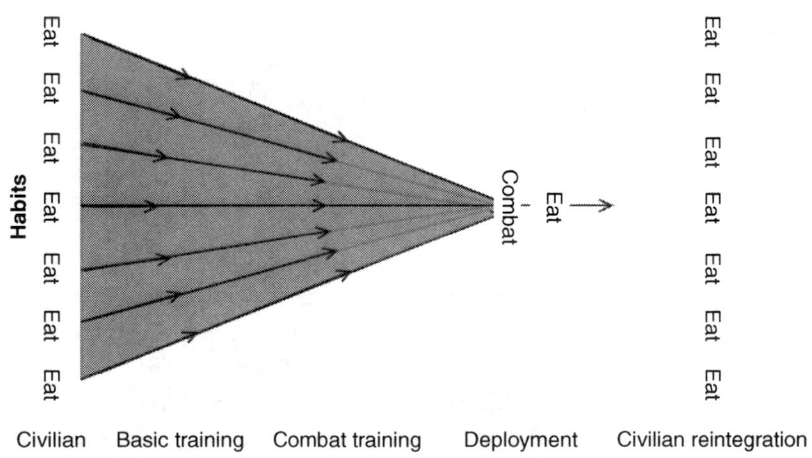

FIGURE 11.1 Warrior-embodied habits.

Ten common habits were identified: hydration, organization, alcohol, punctuality, sleeping, eating, thoroughness, language, humor, and friendship. In two instances—hydration and organization—meaning transferred across all three lifeworlds. One common habit did not have an end goal of combat performance, namely, socializing around alcohol. I will now present the narratives associated with five of the aforementioned common habits that relate more specifically to health behaviors: hydration, alcohol, eating, thoroughness, and sleeping. The following narratives will show that some health behaviors such as hydration do transfer into the civilian lifeworld without causing reintegration challenges. However, other health behaviors do not and cannot always be connected to the symptoms of PTS when describing reintegration challenges. Even when some of these health behaviors, such as thoroughness, mimic PTS symptomology, construing them as pathology might be an inappropriate way to frame the reintegration challenges. Finally, these narratives help to establish that reintegration challenge in the form of health behaviors cannot simply be addressed through didactic lectures or cognitive training that encourages positive thinking.

They Forced Us to Drink a Lot of Water: Hydration Habits

The development of military meaning associated with hydration health behaviors begin immediately in basic training. Rituals associated with the military formation of this habit were not pleasantly remembered by Daniel Scott:

> The worst memories I have from basic training are due to the fact that they make you chug tons of water and don't let you go to the restroom very often. They give you two minutes to drink a two quart jug of water. If you don't finish everyone was forced to do push-ups for a half an hour. Then they make you fill up again. All that water's got to go somewhere. Some people are throwing up. Inevitably you've got to go to the bathroom, but you're in the middle of some training. So grown men are peeing on themselves because they can't physically hold it anymore. You would be running to get to the bathrooms at every opportunity they gave you because you were so uncomfortable from chugging so much water. (Scott, 2014a, lines 149–162)

While forced hydration seemed undignified in basic training, Jacob Rogers illustrated the essential need for hydration habits during combat missions.

> We were walking around, but it was not a typical Sunday walk in the park. We were moving at a good pace, trying to cover ground. Then at times we had to stand on the side of the road where we would just

> bake and wait. I was sweating profusely and drinking tons of water. Just as I got to the bottom I started to get a mushy, cotton mouth, and stopped thinking clearly. I mean, my feet became heavy and it was hard to breathe because my mouth wasn't moist anymore. At that point, people start wearing down noticeably even though we were all stud athletes. Dehydration wears on you faster than I thought it would. (Rogers, 2014, lines 473–489)

Upon coming home, warriors continued to express this habit in a military fashion. Joseph Walker said: "I continue to drink a lot of water. I just slam water all the time" (Walker, 2014b, line 1048).

Most found this line of questioning comical; it seemed obvious that everyone needs to drink water. Samson Craig, however, connected the entire trajectory of how hydrating had become embodied in his health behaviors and realized that the military meaning carried into the civilian lifeworld:

> I drink a ridiculous amount of water, a crap load at one time. I don't sip on it throughout the day, I gulp tons of it. I always have water. When I don't have it, I get parched really easily. I mean it's good to have water all the time, but I drink so fast, because we had drinking sessions in boot camp where we chugged a ton. Naturally, we were wondering why we were chugging all of this water. If I'm thirsty in five minutes I'll have more, but they were like, "NO, chug it all now!" So I got in this habit of constantly chugging tons of water. So now I always have it with me. I'll walk straight into a business meeting where everyone's in suits and ties, and I'll slap this water bottle on the desk and I'm ready to go. I mean nobody asks questions, everyone has them. (Craig, 2014b, lines 51–72)

Military hydration habits expressed an embodied military meaning that transferred into the civilian lifeworld without any challenge or confusion. However, the next four common habits do not transfer meaning into the civilian lifeworld. I will begin by describing a challenge usually viewed in isolation from the broader context of military life cycle wherein habits develop particular military meaning, particularly, socializing around alcohol.

We Were All Wasted and Hung Over: Alcohol Habits

Since there was no alcohol allowed in basic training, alcohol habits started when warriors first left basic training. For the enlisted members, this habit was developed in day-to-day military recreational activities. Walker explained how the daily routine of living in the barracks included drinking copious amounts of alcohol:

> Barracks' life is such a different culture. . . . You train the way you want to go and fight. So we were blowing stuff up or shooting these guns all day and night for days or weeks on end. Then you would go back to the barracks and drink your ass off while playing X-Box. . . . Day in, day out . . . if we weren't in the field training, we would get up at 5:30 in the morning every single day, go out and PT, which sucked because we were all wasted and hung over. So you're out there running around, it's still dark outside, you got your little silkies on, and you're trying not to throw up. Somehow, amazingly, you're able to run. You do this every single day, and eventually my body was just conditioned to the routine. (Walker, 2014a, lines 1802–1827)

When warriors were not in the field training, they were training their bodies to be acclimated to drinking large volumes of alcohol. It just became a normal habit after coming home from field training and was associated with relaxed socialization after a long day of work.

Fascinatingly, almost every other enlisted warrior shared similar stories. Adam Taylor topped Walker's description of running while hung-over:

> Literally, we'd pop our first couple of beers at work. I usually worked out after work, so I'd already be 5-6 beers deep. Then I would go to the gym with my buddies, go shower up and have a few more beers. Then drink a few beers with dinner. Afterwards, we might go down to the combatives room and fight for a little while, play some beer pong, play some video games, drinking the whole time. I mean we lived our lives just drinking the whole time . . . it was a cultural thing. (Taylor, 2014b, lines 1578–1584)

Taylor was also encouraged to drink during the workday. In his particular company area, there was a full-fledged bar that was stocked with kegs and bottled beer. Taylor's narrative did mention the negative consequences of having so much beer around the workplace, but not due to the warrior's performance degradation. Instead, he mentioned that it took up viable work space.

In further elucidating alcohol habits, Taylor explained he could have been kicked out of his unit for failure to adapt to the military lifeworld had he been unwilling to participate in daily drinking habits:

> When I was a private I had team leaders knocking on my door forcing me to drink. I had one guy that was hammered drunk and angry. He came to my door with a gun and said, "If you don't come out I'm gonna shoot my way in," and then he made me drink. They drug me out of my room. I could be in bed trying to go to sleep, getting ready for the next day, but because I was a private and they were like, "Nope, you're coming out and

> drinking." Then they would force us to drink and because I wanted to do good, I did what they said. . . . People would probably get kicked out for failure to adapt to our culture, because that's part of our culture is drinking. . . . As a private you don't say, "Oh, I'm just having one." The team leaders and squad leaders say, "Drink this beer! Drink more!" You don't get an option. (Taylor, 2014b, lines 1593–1605)

Unfortunately, the *esprit de corps* surrounding alcohol created intense pressure and made Taylor feel that he would not have succeeded in the military lifeworld had he not participated in these hazing rituals, which he compared to games played in fraternity houses.

The case could be made that the military did not explicitly train such behaviors, but it did encourage it as part of the broader military communal context. Many warriors, both officer and enlisted, shared stories of the military command not only sanctioning the use of alcohol but also encouraging warriors to drink to excess. The mantra was not to drink less but to drink responsibly, which meant not driving while intoxicated according to Solomon Clark:

> Have you heard about a dining in? It's coordinated upper enlisted, officer drinking fest. . . . There are a bunch of ceremonies and a lot of tradition that goes along with it. The point is to build an *esprit de corps*, but there's a punch bowl of the most vile, evil alcoholic beverage in the world in front of you, and part of the ceremony is drinking from this vile, evil punch bowl. I was the junior officer when I went to my first dining in, and I was legless drunk by the end of the night. I mean bad drunk. It was assumed that I was going to be so drunk that I didn't drive myself there. It was assumed that there was no way I was going to be able to drive home so make sure, like my battalion commander told me, "Make sure you get a ride to the event." (Clark, 2014b, lines 164–175)

Obviously, the point was to encourage, not discourage, heavy drinking habits as a means to increase camaraderie. Not only were officers involved in these intense drinking sprees, but the chain of command was aware of the events. The simple advice offered to Clark was: "Don't drink and drive" (Clark, 2014b, line 185).

Joshua Hines provided a similar story about how drinking was an institutionalized military habit that began immediately upon finishing officer training:

> The first things you do, whether you're army, air force, it doesn't really matter; you always go to an initial school, once you come on active duty. Ours was six weeks long and the only people on base are essentially

> officers. In fact, the first weekend we showed up at the officers club, it was a required event. You're not required to drink, but it was like, "Show up! Oh, and by the way, the colonel is paying for pitchers of beer!" So you've got this second lieutenant, straight out of college, it's like one giant party. Do you really get anything out of it professionally? I mean the whole six weeks, it's worthless. (Hines, 2014b, lines 311–319)

Alcohol was a social lubricant for officers and enlisted alike. Furthermore, it became a natural habit that was reinforced by the structure of military activities, which centered on drinking. The deployment lifeworld should have been a dry environment, as alcohol was not permitted in the Middle East; however, warriors found ingenious ways to procure alcohol. Esau Austin shared a clever trick concerning the proper method to ship liquor without being detected:

> Alcohol was sent all the time. People would get Listerine bottles full of it. . . . You would get Tequila and put it in a Listerine bottle because it was the same color. Once the bottle was filled up, put the cap on tight, and then someone got really creative with it, because they had to put that protective seal back on. So people would take a hairdryer or something like that re-melt the seal enough to hold. . . . That way when it got inspected by our sergeants they would look at it and see a protective seal on the bottle and give it back to us. Then we'd go and take little shots and stuff like that. I mean by no means did we get hammered like we did back home. . . . We didn't go out drunk. . . . When we knew that we were gonna have a couple of hours of down time. We'd sit there and watch movies on my computer and whatever else, and everybody would take a shot or two. (Austin, 2014, lines 1088–1102)

Most warriors had similar stories and felt that drinking during deployment boosted morale. It was a way to relax and socialize. Even if warriors were drinking less in the deployment lifeworld and this habit was not directly aimed at combat performance, they continued to develop the military meaning associated with alcohol.

Upon coming home and interacting with the civilian lifeworld, warriors continued to drink to excess. Unfortunately, in the civilian lifeworld, the military meaning associated with developing *esprit de corps* was lost. More often than not, warriors' drinking was understood to be an out-of-control behavior in the civilian lifeworld. This negative health behavior expressed some sort of a need to self-medicate symptoms of PTS or combat trauma; it was not interpreted as a habit formed across the military life cycle that had potent military meaning. As Craig said, "Everyone in the military understood that we drank until we were under the table and so what? It was not a big deal; whereas it's different in the civilian world. They thought there was a problem" (Craig, 2014a, lines 2217–2218).

Jeremiah Allen agreed with Craig's assessment but suggested that the only place in the civilian lifeworld where a warrior could drink without it being viewed as a self-medicating health behavior was with fellow military friends or at the Veterans of Foreign Wars. In both situations, drinking a large amount of alcohol was not seen as inappropriate behavior:

> There are times where getting inappropriately drunk and saying inappropriate things would've been totally acceptable amongst like my military friends, either when we were in the military or even when we go out today. The goal was just to reconnect and have a good time. But those extreme behaviors are really not acceptable in civilian society. They're really not okay unless there is something wrong with you. (Allen, 2014c, lines 512–516)

Considering the common habit of drinking alcohol, which exists in all three lifeworlds, it is starting to become clear not only how military meaning is formed through social interactions and behaviors across the military life cycle, but also how this unique military meaning that is embodied in a warrior's health behavior does not transfer into the civilian lifeworld outside of veterans' groups. That is not to say that extreme drinking habits formed across the military life cycle are a productive way to increase *esprit de corps*; however, viewed from this new approach, the drinking to excess is no longer directly connected to a warrior's need to medicate his combat trauma but is instead a habit that was formed with particular meaning across the military life cycle. The next challenge associated with embodied skill formation was the first one that introduced me to the interpretation of skills as common across three lifeworlds.

Throw Whatever You Can Into Your Mouth: Eating Habits

The stories surrounding the development of health behaviors associated with eating habits are highly entertaining but are also insightful when considering how military training instills military meaning in countless behaviors through the systematic development as well as reinforcement of particular habits across the military life cycle. In basic training, the warrior was required to take in as much food as he could in a very short amount of time. As Craig explained, "They encouraged us to eat tons, but the question was whether or not we had time. . . . You could put as much stuff on your plate as you want, but they gave you anywhere from 30 seconds to 2 minutes to eat it all" (Craig, 2014a, lines 138–141). Practicing how to scarf as much food as possible fostered some fascinating eating habits. As Rogers said, "I would grab a slice of bread, pasta, veggies and as much crap as I could jam it into that bread and shove it down my mouth without choking myself. Then I was done eating" (Rogers, 2014, lines 2155–2158). The jury was out on whether or not the food tasted very good because as Walker said, "You didn't have time to taste it" (Walker, 2014a, line 597). However, everyone agreed that it was filling and provided enough calories to stay active.

In describing the gastronomic glories of Meals Ready to Eat, prepackaged food developed for combat missions, Scott shared how military eating habits were reinforced in the deployment lifeworld:

> They're just awful, they blocked me up and produced a chemical reaction to thoroughly dry out my mouth so it was completely parched. . . . I was only eating to sustain life. My only goal was to put calories down in my belly. So, I would open the biggest food packet. Let's say I had the chicken and salsa. I poured out the cheese, crumbled the crackers, and put the grape jelly in for shits and giggles. It got to the point where I didn't even use utensils. I'd break up the pouch, cut the corner off, squeeze it in my mouth like toothpaste, and swallow it, DONE! Move on. Half the time I didn't even have any time to eat it anyway. (Scott, 2014b, lines 3042–3053)

Not only was Scott forced to shovel his food due to the lack of taste, but eating in such a manner also supported his ability to function in the deployment lifeworld because it was faster than taking the time to attend to manners. The military habit of quickly nourishing continued to hold potent military meaning for Allen when he returned to the civilian lifeworld:

> For years after I got out of the military, I would eat much quicker than everyone else. It was not even about wanting to eat fast, but I felt hungry when I would sit down to a meal. It was as if my body said "It's time to eat!" I mean, I magically had an empty stomach and felt as if I needed to eat everything right now. (Allen, 2014b, lines 217–221)

Astutely, Craig's father, who had also served in the military, informed him that military eating habits might be challenging to reintegration. This tip caused Craig to try and be conscientious of how he ate in social settings outside of a military group:

> It has actually been a bit difficult. I've tried to force myself to slow down over the past couple of years because eating that fast is not normal. Other people don't eat that fast. I love food, so I try to enjoy it now, but the

> biggest problem is manners. When you are eating in the military no one cares. They don't give a shit. You can be a total slob, but when you get out people don't eat like that. Now I'm very particular. I cut my food and then I put my knife down to slow me down. It helps so that I don't shovel it, but I still eat fast and take big bites. It's just a habit. (Craig, 2014a, lines 145–153)

The previous example illustrates how military meaning associated with achieving optimal combat performance is formed across the military life cycle and does not transfer into the civilian lifeworld. Additionally, the BATTLEMIND and MRT programs cannot address this health behavior as it does not fit neatly into any of the symptoms of PTS. The next skill appears to parallel one of the most common symptoms of PTS, namely, hypervigilance. However, thoroughness will no longer be directly associated with traumatic exposure when evaluated within the framework of habits that develop into behaviors that embody specific military meaning.

Keep Your Head on Swivel: Thoroughness Habits

One of the most important habits a warrior develops in training is the skill of paying attention to his surroundings, which is better known in military terminology as situational awareness. This habit allows him to function in and more likely survive combat. Caleb Franks provided an excellent example of how military meaning began to be explicitly formed in basic training:

> When we were picking up expended cartridges after shooting on the range, we were trained to always look for things that were out of place, such as small brass cartridges in a field of grass. It was really stressed during our training that our eyes were getting used to always being on the look-out for things like booby traps, explosives, or roadside bombs. Those things would not be clearly visible in combat. The idea was to reinforce that we had to be looking around and aware of all things, at all times. (Franks, 2014d, p. 1)

Taylor not only confirmed Franks's explanation of learning to observe for IEDs in basic training but also explained how it carried through to all of his combat training as well as his social life in the military:

> Situational awareness [SA] was emphasized in our free time too. I remember having safety briefs where we were told to keep good SA when we went downtown. In somewhat of a joking manner, we were told to know where all the exits were in case things got hairy. For instance, we were supposed to know if a girl we were talking to had a boyfriend and was ready to kick

> your ass. We were also told to know where the other warriors were in the bar so they could be at your side in a fight. (Taylor, 2014c, p. 1)

Clark provided a somewhat amusing example of the intensity with which warriors practiced situational awareness in the deployment lifeworld. Even if a warrior was not in an intense firefight or engaged in action, he was always checking to see if something was out of place:

> When it had been quiet for a while, I would think, "It's been quiet for a while, and I'm in a crowded market!" I mean, a naked Victoria's Secret model could have been dancing around me and I would have been oblivious to that because I was constantly looking for someone with a puffy vest or anything that seemed out of place. We were keeping tight perimeters; I was checking where every one of my guys was. We would go 800 meters in one direction. If something was funny, I'd say, "What the fuck is that, is that a fucking IED? No, the wind just picked it up; it's a piece of garbage, keep going." (Clark, 2014a, lines 1666–1677)

Ironically, Clark's commentary fails to note that a naked Victoria's Secret model would have been very out of place in a Middle Eastern city. However, his point was that nothing, not even a gorgeous woman, could have diverted his attention from the nitty-gritty details within his tight perimeter.

Franks explained that warriors were not simply focusing on every detail at random but able to discern between friend and foe because they were thoroughly briefed about the local terrain and population before going out on missions. Thus, warriors were able to tell what was out of place:

> When we went into a village of, maybe 100 people, we had to be able to instantly size everybody up and assess them as a threat or not a threat as well as note what things seem out of place. It was a survival skill. If I saw a fat guy in the skinny crowd, I took mental note or the clean guy in the dirty crowd, or vice versa, whatever. You have to be a detective, and when you sit down with the locals, you have to very quickly pick up on who's full of shit and who's not. (Franks, 2014c, lines 481–479)

These snapshot assessments were not built on paranoia or being judgmental; they were a necessity of the job. The point of situational awareness was to intercept a potential hazard before it occurred or to quickly respond when things went wrong.

Upon coming home, this "super instinctive behavior" became overwhelming because there were no briefings to describe the environment into which Franks was entering (Franks, 2014c, line 703). Trying to negotiate commonplace activities in the civilian lifeworld was a challenge when he first came back from the deployment lifeworld:

> There were a lot of subtle things I did. Like someone just wearing a long jacket on a warm day, or anything that looked out of place, I would get nervous because in combat that's the kind of key information we were looking for. I definitely took that into the civilian world. . . . For instance, if there were no cars within 20 miles and all of a sudden some guy came driving up in a van. I was like, "Well he doesn't belong here, what's up?" It was just what we did all the time in combat. (Franks, 2014b, lines 1672–1687)

Constantly observing and analyzing his surroundings came as an enormous impediment when Franks attempted to ride the train to school. In fact, he suggested that he felt more anxiety riding the train in the United States than he felt in combat because on the train he never knew who or what to expect.

Many warriors, including Franks, were aware that this essential combat skill translated to a health behavior that was interpreted as hypervigilant upon entering the civilian lifeworld. Nonetheless, Allen portrayed situational awareness as an important habit:

> I don't know that I entirely decompressed or that I want to honestly. . . . I'm less focused on things, but I still focus on what's going on around me. . . . However, I view that skill as a plus. It's like "Hey, don't let your guard down, don't get too comfortable" I know that's part of PTSD the hyper alertness, but I don't want to lose my edge. (Allen, 2014a, lines 1768–1775)

Allen desired to maintain this keenly formed skill upon leaving the military in spite of the civilian interpretation of his behavior as hypervigilant. He considered it important to be able to meticulously attend to the details in his surroundings. Again, military meaning associated with thoroughness as situational awareness does not translate into the civilian lifeworld. Although this reintegration challenge is addressed in the BATTLEMIND and MRT programs, teaching warriors to check their thoughts is not sufficient even if they did wish to reshape the meaning associated with this particular health behavior.

I Was Having Hallucinations: Sleep Habits

When discussing sleep in basic training, most warriors talked about being so physically exhausted that they immediately went to sleep and did not wake until the next morning. As Rogers said, "I slept like a baby, every night" (Rogers, 2014, line 2329). In the next breath, however, he went on to describe a training activity that set in motion unique sleep patterns:

> The only time I didn't really get sleep was if I was doing fire watch. You get woke up in the middle of the night, handed a flash light and a watch, and told to guard the door for an hour, and then you wake up that guy. So that was always at least an hour and a half of wasted sleep every night, because you get woken up and you've got to be ready in ten minutes. Then you're awake, you're ready, you go stand in your post, and when your turn is over you have to wake the other guy up three times before you can crawl in bed. Then you've got to turn your brain back off and go back to sleep. So yeah, that sucked. (Rogers, 2014, lines 2329–2335)

Rogers's experience of getting great sleep in basic training was echoed by everyone. Most people were too tired to think after such a full day of physical exercise. Walker said, "My body just shut down at the end of the day" (Walker, 2014c, line 921). However, Rogers's experience of performing fire watch provides an intimation of what will continue throughout military life cycle, namely, training warriors to effectively manage and operate on little or no sleep.

Moving on to discuss specialized combat training will show how sleep habits quickly shift away from a standard 8 hours of sleep a night to varying amounts of time, in various locations, at various times of day. As Franks said, "It's a life of extremes. You're going 100 mph when you're training . . . and might not sleep for 2–3 days straight. Then you have four days off and you try to make up for those three days of training" (Franks, 2014a, lines 414–417). Warriors all concurred with Franks's story about sleep cycles during combat training. As Kelley said, even if he did sleep, "we were always soaking wet when we were in the field. They make it as miserable as physically possible . . . I just got used to it" (Kelley, 2014, lines 633–635).

Certain combat training intentionally deprived warriors of sleep in order to inure them to the hardships of combat. Hines provided a narrative related to sleep deprivation training:

> There were plenty of times when we were staring in the woods at some house or something, for two days. . . . Then you rotate back half a mile to this patrol base where you pretend to sleep in the middle of these woods . . . but there's no good sleep. . . . I remember one time. . . . We were trying to get back and we got caught up in these thorn bushes, it was me and this other guy . . . we got to the point, *now this is not an exaggeration*, where one guy would lie down on the thorns, the other guy would walk over. Then he'd fall down, the other guy would get up, because it was so thick. So you don't get any sleep, you're cold, you're wet, but you just keep doing it. (Hines, 2014a, lines 727–740)

Obviously, Hines and his comrade did not get 8 solid hours of uninterrupted sleep during intense training cycles. To some, this sort of training may sound masochistic, but as Hines explained, it allowed him to "run through every aspect of an operation" (Hines, 2014a, line 726).

In the deployment lifeworld, every warrior unilaterally agreed that sleep deprivation was a consistent reality. Franks shared a story that illustrated sleeping conditions under which warriors were operating:

> The problem was we were sleeping in beds that were four feet away from each other. So say I came back from my guard shift at 2:00 am, took off all my stuff, and slammed it down, I just woke up the guy next to me and he wakes up the guy next to him. Every two hours someone's trudging through with their boots and their machine gun, and you're just getting woken up, there's no getting away from it. . . I went a little bit crazy. I could feel the changes in my body, my speech was different, I was having hallucinations, and I finally went to the medic and said "I haven't slept in almost three months. I need a night's sleep. Give me just one night's sleep." She said, "You're not the only one, here are some pills, talk to sergeant so and so." Funny, nobody ever talked about it. We never talked amongst ourselves or said that we were slowing down, or that we weren't sharp. It was never discussed in the open. (Franks, 2014a, lines 1070–1091)

Everyone had to function with no more than 3–4 hours of sleep a day. Furthermore, these few hours may not have been consecutive. Bad sleeping conditions was not something that warriors fully adjusted to in the deployment lifeworld. However, they became embodied sleep habits that eventually carried forward into the civilian lifeworld.

Immediately, upon returning home from the deployment lifeworld, Franks rejoiced in his ability to sleep. The first thing he wanted to do after getting home was "to go to bed at 10:00 p.m. and sleep till noon" (Franks, 2014a, line 1467). A common adjective that described the sleeping conditions warriors had immediately upon returning home was "glorious." Most, like Franks, tried to make up for lost sleep by staying in bed all morning. Unfortunately, this ability to sleep for long hours quickly ended, and military sleep habits formed throughout the military life cycle returned. It was not simply that warriors slept significantly less than 8 hours a night; it was also that they continued to have restless sleep even if they did get 5–6 hours. Hines was the first to attribute his postdeployment sleep habits to the training and formation he received across the military life cycle:

> I have trouble falling asleep now . . . I go to bed at like 10:30 and then I'll think about something until 1:00. Did I really fall asleep in that time? No.

> In fact, I'll get hot and kick the covers off then I get cold. Then I think, "Why the hell am I doing this, why don't I go read?" But I don't want to read because I want to fall asleep. Then I watch a movie, and it's 2:00 in the morning. I didn't have that before training. (Hines, 2014a, lines 706–716)

Even if there are various ways of appropriately sleeping in the civilian lifeworld, it seems fair to say that military sleep habits give rise to a negative health behavior when a warrior is no longer attempting to train for combat in the civilian lifeworld. Hines did contemplate whether or not his current difficulties sleeping had to do with the stress, which is a meaningful way to explain this negative health behavior in the civilian lifeworld. Restless sleep is also associated with PTS. However, when viewed through the lens of training and formation of military meaning across the military life cycle, Hines's experience appears to be related to a military meaning that was formed to reinforce combat effectiveness. Again, this negative health behavior is not refashioned by simply provided information in the form of PowerPoint presentations or positive thinking.

IMPLICATIONS FOR FUTURE RESEARCH AND DEVELOPMENT OF NEW REINTEGRATION PROGRAMS

Having explored reintegration challenges from an ethics of embodied personal presence, a new interpretation of reintegration challenges places an emphasis on the formation of military meaning through the practice of specific habits aimed at combat and de-emphasizes the role of combat trauma. Nonetheless, my research was limited in that it only addressed warriors and not all military personnel. Future research will need to be performed in order to compare and contrast the lived experience of reintegration challenges for all deployed support personnel. Additionally, in order to limit the scope of my research, women were not asked to participate. It is likely that they have unique reintegration challenges. Finally, I was unable to recruit warriors who served in the Navy, National Guard, or Reserves. The latter two groups are particularly important in that they do not return to a military lifeworld after they go through the military reintegration process, but immediately return to the civilian lifeworld. Therefore, further research into the aforementioned populations will allow for a richer understanding of reintegration challenges and develop more meaningful programs. Having determined that combat exposure is not the singular catalyst of all reintegration challenges, it is critical to perform similar studies on the military support personnel population. As Taylor noted, "Reintegration is a challenge for anyone who has deployed, regardless of whether or not she/he saw combat" (Taylor, 2014a, p. 1).

The realization that military training and lifestyle give rise to a broad set of habits, which develop into health behaviors, suggests that with ongoing research, more habits could be discovered that have both transferrable and nontransferrable military meaning. Viewing reintegration challenges from within this new framework would allow the DoD to develop new reintegration programs similar to the Healthy People initiative. In particular, researchers could establish a baseline set of common habits that exist within both the military and civilian communities. Thereafter, they could explore how these habits develop into health behaviors with specific military meaning attendant to unique military cohorts. Habits with transferrable military meaning, such as hydration, could be promoted and used as a foundation upon which ongoing reintegration training would operate. In some instances, when considering certain habits, such as alcohol, it may be necessary to redefine the military meaning from the onset, as it is not simply a matter of reorienting this health behavior to a broader set of civilian goals. In other instances, such as eating, the goal would be to expand the military meaning associated with that habit in order to allow military personnel to embody a variety of meanings so as to act in a way appropriate to either the military or the civilian setting.

This new framework does not need to reject the value of providing information about PTS or integrate cognitive training that focuses on how various thought processes can help to moderate one's appreciation of the immediate circumstances. However, if the military is hoping to construct more effective reintegration programs that reduce the number of negative postdeployment health-care outcomes, it will be important to heed the experience of those who have attempted to reintegrate into the civilian community after deployment.

REFERENCES

Adler, A., Castro, C., & McGurk, D. (2007). *Battlemind psychological debriefings*. US Army Medical Research Unit—Europe, Walter Reed Army Institute of Research, Report 2007-001. Retrieved from http://usamru-e.amedd.army.mil/assets/docs/publications/adler_et_al_2007_report_2007-001_battlemind_procedures.pdf

Adler, A. B., Bliese, P. D., McGurk, D., Hoge, C. W., & Castro, C. A. (2011). Battlemind debriefing and battlemind training as early interventions with soldiers returning from Iraq: Randomization by platoon. *Sport, Exercise, and Performance Psychology*, *1*, 66–83.

Allen, J. (2014a, June 20). Interview One.

Allen, J. (2014b, July 16). Interview Two.

Allen, J. (2014c, August 4). Interview Three.

Allman, M. J., & Winright, T. L. (2010). *After the smoke clears: The just war tradition and post war justice*. New York, NY: Orbis Books.

Austin, E. (2014, April 15). Interview One.

Carman, T. (2008). *Merleau-Ponty* (1st ed.). London: Routledge.

Casey, E. S. (1985). Habitual body and memory in Merleau-Ponty. In *Phenomenology and the human sciences* (pp. 39–57). New York, NY: Springer.

Castro, C. A., Hoge, C. W., Milliken, C. W., McGurk, D., Adler, A. B., Cox, A., et al. (2006). *Battlemind training: Transitioning home from combat* (DTIC document). Silver Spring, MD: Walter Reed Army Institute of Research. Retrieved from http://oai.dtic.mil/oai/oai?verb=getRecord&metadataPrefix=html&identifier=ADA481083

Clark, S. (2014a, October 30). Interview One.

Clark, S. (2014b, November 13). Interview Two.

Cornum, R., Matthews, M. D., & Seligman, M. E. (2011). Comprehensive soldier fitness: Building resilience in a challenging institutional context. *American Psychologist, 66*, 4–9.

Craig, S. (2014a, October 24). Interview One.

Craig, S. (2014b, November 5). Interview Two.

Dorfman, E. (2009). History of the lifeworld: From Husserl to Merleau-Ponty. *Philosophy Today, 53*, 294–303.

Franks, C. (2014a, April 12). Interview One.

Franks, C. (2014b, April 29). Interview Two.

Franks, C. (2014c, May 29). Interview Three.

Franks, C. (2014d, December 17). Dissertation Research Email.

Frierson, P. R. (2013). *What is the human being?* New York, NY: Routledge.

Hines, J. (2014a, October 23). Interview Two.

Hines, J. (2014b, November 20). Interview Three.

Husserl, E. (1965). *Phenomenology and the crisis of philosophy* (Q. Lauer, Trans.). New York, NY: Harper and Row.

Iasiello, L. V. (2004). Jus post bellum: The moral responsibilities of victors in war. *Naval War College Review, 57*, 33–52.

Institute of Medicine. (2013). *Returning home from Iraq and Afghanistan: Assessment of readjustment needs of veterans, service members, and their families.* Washington, DC: The National Academies Press.

Institute of Medicine. (2014). *Findings from returning home from Iraq and Afghanistan and preventing psychological disorders in service members and their families.* Washington, DC: The National Academies Press.

Kelley, S. (2014, August 18). Interview Three.

Koh, H. K. (2010). A 2020 vision for healthy people. *New England Journal of Medicine, 362*, 1653–1656.

Merleau-Ponty, M. (2002). *Phenomenology of perception* (2nd ed.). London: Routledge.

Naef, R. (2006). Bearing witness: A moral way of engaging in the nurse–person relationship. *Nursing Philosophy, 7*, 146–156.

National Research Council. (2010). *Returning home from Iraq and Afghanistan: Preliminary assessment of readjustment needs of veterans, service members, and their families* (Consensus Report). Washington, DC: The National Academy Press. Retrieved from http://www.nap.edu/catalog.php?record_id=12812

Orsingher, J. M., Lopez, A. T., & Rinchart, M. E. (2007). Battlemind training system: "Armor for your mind." *U.S. Army Medical Department Journal*, 66–71.

Reivich, K. J., Seligman, M. E., & McBride, S. (2011). Master resilience training in the US Army. *American Psychologist, 66*, 25–34.

Rogers, J. (2014, July 29). Interview Two.

Scott, D. (2014a, April 9). Interview One.

Scott, D. (2014b, June 3). Interview Three.

Slomski, A. (2014). IOM: Military psychological interventions lack evidence. *Journal of the American Medical Association, 311*, 1487–1488.

Smith, A. D. (2007). The flesh of perception. In T. Baldwin (Ed.), *Reading Merleau-Ponty: On phenomenology of perception* (pp. 1–22). London: Routledge.

Taylor, A. (2014a, Demeber). Dissertation Research.

Taylor, A. (2014b, July 10). Interview Two.

Taylor, A. (2014c, December 18). Dissertation Research Email.

Walker, J. (2014a, August 22). Interview One.

Walker, J. (2014b, September 18). Interview Two.

Walker, J. (2014c, October 7). Interview Three.

Wang, S. S. (2014, July 8). Military's mental-health efforts are ineffective, Report finds. *The Wall Street Journal*. Retrieved from http://online.wsj.com/news/articles/SB10001424052702304914204579394941039669728

Zoroya, G. (2014, February 20). *Report: Military efforts to prevent mental illness ineffective*. Retrieved from http://www.usatoday.com/story/news/nation/2014/02/20/institute-study-prevention-military-ptsd-programs/5637987/

CHAPTER 12

Ethical Issues Encountered by Military Nurses During Wartime

Janice Agazio, Petra Goodman, Oluwakemi Opanubi, and Patricia McMullen

ABSTRACT

Military nurses encounter similar issues as civilian nurses in daily practice situations; however, wartime and humanitarian missions may bring unique and difficult ethical dilemmas. While nursing has the American Nurses Association code of ethics to provide a framework to guide ethical practice decisions, conflicts may arise from the unique aspects of nursing within a wartime environment. Understanding those conflicts occuring within the military wartime scenario can provide nurses with experiential examples from which to derive strategies for personal coping and professional behavior and decision making. This chapter describes the research that has focused upon the identification of these issues, the effects from uresolved issues, and those directions for future research to better prepare miltiary nurses before and during deployment.

INTRODUCTION

The War on Terrorism, beginning in 2001 with Operation Enduring Freedom (OEF) and continuing with Operation Iraqi Freedom (OIF) in 2003, has exposed nurses to situations and challenges for which many report feeling unprepared,

http://dx.doi.org/10.1891/0739-6686.34.227

particularly in terms of caring for those with multi-trauma injuries and devastating wounds suffered by military troops and civilians alike (Agazio, 2010; Middleton, 2009). Feeling unprepared and, in some circumstances, conflicted regarding treatment decisions, may lead to feelings of moral distress for nurses particularly if the situation was ethically challenging. These conflicts are not new for military nurses, or in wartime scenarios, but due to the length of the recent, and ongoing, conflicts, they were accentuated through repeated and extended deployments. Many nurses report that their nursing experiences during OEF and OIF have left an indelible mark on their practice (Agazio, 2010; Griffiths & Jasper, 2007; Middleton, 2009). Through understanding the types of situations and conflicts faced by military nurses, and importantly, how best the services can prepare their forces in anticipating and managing the issues, military nurses will be more prepared and at less risk for sequelae such as moral distress, posttraumatic stress disorder (PTSD), and burnout, than their predecessors.

Early in the war, military nurses were faced with injured individuals and mass casualty situations that challenged their experience and expertise. These injuries were primarily the result of motor vehicle accidents, grenades, and bullet wounds. However, in the second phase of the war, more injuries were a consequence of improvised explosive devices planted by insurgents resulting in extensive and high-acuity polytrauma requiring numerous complex surgical and medical interventions. The care of such injuries challenged the nurses' competency in the provision of care for complex polytrauma. However, in addition to the challenges to ensure quality care, the nurses, some for the first time in their nursing experiences, were also confronted with ethical issues for which they were ill-prepared. Due to limited resources and personnel, nurses were confronted with the need to triage care and resources. The admission of insurgents for receipt of care required that nurses provide care for combatants despite conflicting feelings and thoughts regarding care of the enemy. The nurses felt confused, uncertain, hopeless, angry, discouraged, and distressed as they coped with these issues, some of which directly affected morbidity and mortality. The nurses had not received any training on how to manage such issues and felt ill-prepared and forced to engage, despite personal beliefs.

The purpose of this chapter is to describe the research conducted to delineate the ethical situations faced by military nurses during wartime practice. The chapter begins with an overview of research in ethical issues experienced by civilian nurses as a background for differences in these issues in military nursing practice. Ethical issues specific to military nursing practice are discussed; in particular, research conducted regarding ethical issues emerging from wartime nursing is presented with specific attention to those studies conducted by nurses. Finally, the effects of unresolved ethical issues are discussed in some detail as this area has received extensive study within the context of military nursing practice. The chapter concludes with recommendations for needed research and education that are especially targeted to the management of ethical dilemmas and detection/prevention of moral distress.

ETHICAL CONDUCT EXPECTED IN NURSING PRACTICE

In the United States, nurses use a national code of ethics to guide their practice. Early in basic undergraduate nursing education, nurses are introduced to the American Nurses Association (ANA) *Code of Ethics for Nurses with Interpretive Statements* (2015), most recently revised and adopted in 2015, which guides practice, both military and civilian. The *Code* details the obligations and duties nurses have for their patients and families and also designates what is considered ethical conduct in the nursing profession. The International Council of Nurses (ICN) also denotes ethical standards for nurses worldwide in the *ICN Code of Ethics for Nurses* (2012). This document outlines four fundamental responsibilities for nurses: "to promote health, to prevent illness, to restore health, and to alleviate suffering." Further, the code details four principal elements that outline the standards of ethical conduct:

1. Nurses and people: The nurse's primary professional responsibility is to people requiring nursing care.
2. Nurses and practice: The nurse carries personal responsibility and accountability for nursing practice, and for maintaining competence by continual learning.
3. Nurses and the profession: The nurse assumes the major role in determining and implementing acceptable standards of clinical nursing practice, management, research and education.
4. Nurses and co-workers: The nurse sustains a cooperative relationship with co-workers. . . . and takes appropriate action to safeguard individuals when their health is endangered by a co-worker or any other person. (p. 4)

These universal ethical standards for nurses do not differentiate based on time or place such as wartime, disasters, peacekeeping operations, or stateside care delivery. Absent from these guidelines, however, is how nurses may resolve their personal feelings in ethically ambiguous conditions and any directed action for "solving" an ethical dilemma other than adhering to the principal elements.

ETHICAL ISSUES' RESEARCH IN NURSING PRACTICE

Ethical issues are encountered by nurses in every facet of practice (Redman & Fry, 2000; Ulrich, Taylor, Soeken, O'Donnell, & Farrar, 2010). Nurses are expected to provide competent and quality care to their patients and to act as their advocates. Early research has focused on (a) the ways in which ethical decisions are made; (b) attitudes and beliefs regarding ethical issues; (c) differences between nurses' and physicians' approaches to ethical situations; and (d) specific clinical issues with an ethical overlay (Harris, 2000). An example of a broad ethical issues research project was that of Grove (1996) in which he surveyed 573 nurses regarding ethical issues they confronted in practice, past education related to ethics, the resources they used to address ethical issues, how they rated their competencies related to the management of ethical issues, and barriers to the implementation of decisions (related to ethical dilemmas they encountered). The most common issues, ranked in order of frequency from the highest to the lowest, included issues with pain management, patient confidentiality, end of life, allocation of resources, organ donation, and fertility or abortion (Table 12.1). Patient autonomy; professional practice; patient noncompliance; housing and discharge; parenting skills; family conflicts; neonatal, cultural, religious, and quality of life issues were less frequent (Grove, 1996).

The majority of the nurses who participated in the Grove study (1996) indicated that they had not taken a formal ethics class in their undergraduate training. Those who had, reported that they felt better prepared for the management of ethical issues. Moreover, the majority indicated that they had taken continuing education classes on ethics since graduation. In terms of resources that helped the nurses address ethical issues, the majority indicated that work-rated resources (role models, staff meetings, and physician, supervisor, and peer consultations) were used most frequently. However, the nurses also used professional resources (journal articles and books) and personal resources (church). Resources that were employed less frequently included family discussions, interactions with institutional ethical committees, and personal experiences (experiences with illnesses themselves, with illness and death among family members and friends, and prior patient experiences). The majority of the nurses rated their skills in specific competencies related to handling ethical dilemmas as excellent or good. They indicated that they were good or excellent in (a) applying state or federal laws governing nursing practice in reference to an ethical issue, (b) using the ANA nursing code of ethics to guide their actions, (c) using an ethical framework to assist in the assessment and resolution of a dilemma, (d) identifying the moral aspects of nursing care, (e) identifying and using interdisciplinary resources to assist in the clarification and resolution of a dilemma, (f) gathering relevant facts regarding a dilemma, (g) clarifying and applying values in assessing and resolving dilemmas, (h) proposing alternative actions for resolving dilemmas, (i) actively participating in the resolution of a dilemma, (j) choosing and acting on a plan for resolution, and (k) applying ethical theories and principles

TABLE 12.1
Ethical Issues

Ethical Issues	Focus of Concern
Pain management	Withholding of medication for fear of adverse effects and a hastened death, addiction, drug abuse, or drug seeking behaviors
Patient confidentiality	Determination when a patient's health problems affects others and notification of others who may be harmed
Allocation of scarce resources	Distribution of expensive treatment for patients at the end-of-life
Organ donation	Process for identification of appropriate donors and recipients
Fertility issues	Ownership of frozen or unused embryos
Patient autonomy	Patient choices in terms of right to die, right to refuse treatment, and right to being fully informed regarding care
Professional practice issues	Teamwork, respect, privacy, communication, and physician-assisted suicide
Patient noncompliance	Reluctance to continue costly treatments for noncompliant patients, particularly patients with self-induced medical problems, especially if those problems were not congruent with societal norms, such as illicit drugs or alcohol abuse
Lifestyle issues	Homeless patients for whom there was a lack of community resources for shelter and income; nursing home placements and family conflicts; parenting issues largely centered on drug-abusing mothers, abusive mothers, and teenage mothers

Source: Grove, 1996.

when addressing a dilemma. Barriers to the implementation of an action related to an ethical dilemma included patient, family, or physician preferences, institutional factors, and legal regulations.

Similarly, Gold, Chambers, and Dvorak (1995) used semistructured interviews with 12 nurses to identify ethical issues emerging from direct patient care in acute, long-term, and home care practice settings. Using thematic analysis, these researchers identified four areas in which the majority of ethical situations occurred: (a) withholding of information and truth-telling; (b) unequal access or inequalities in care; (c) differences between business and professional values; and (d) breaking and reporting rules.

Verena Tschudin, founding codirector of the International Centre for Nursing Ethics and founding editor of the journal *Nursing Ethics,* has published several articles reviewing directions in nursing ethics research. She synthesized the last decade of research on ethical issues in nursing in her 2010 article stating that the understanding of ethical issues has been extended into international dimensions with cross-cultural comparisons of ethical orientation; the emergence of moral distress as a concept of interest; and a better understanding of the impact of ethics on the work environment, relationships, and quality and delivery of care.

The study of military nursing in peacetime demonstrates that military nurses experience similar ethical issues. However, due to the military culture, some of the issues may be unique even in a peacetime setting. Gilchrist (2000) completed a master's thesis considering ethical issues of Air Force Nurse Practitioners (AFNPs) in clinical practice. She interviewed seven AFNPs using narrative accounts of situations that they had encountered in clinical practice. Analysis involved categorizing the issues according to the ethical principles of autonomy, nonmaleficence, beneficence, and justice. Issues such as fairness in accessing appointments and referrals in a managed care environment; inequity in allocation of resources; insuring confidentiality in test results such as for HIV; potential harm to patients due to being short-staffed; and time constraints in addressing all of the patients' needs were not unique to a military environment. Some of the unique aspects related to military nursing practice included prohibitions in providing care to retirees in some settings due to the implementation of Tricare, which is an insurance program for retirees and their families, and rules of confidentiality not being sacrosanct in an environment where commanders could require release of information such as HIV status or psychiatric care. Her recommendations included a need for more education and research with this focus.

However, war and humanitarian situations present numerous other ethical dilemmas for nursing. Ethical situations differ based on the patient care demands, combatant care, cultural differences, and resource allocation requirements.

MILITARY NURSING ETHICAL ISSUES IN COMBAT AND HUMANITARIAN ENVIRONMENTS

Research considering military nurses' experiences with ethical situations has been conducted both directly and peripherally through studies of nursing practice for humanitarian missions and conflicts dating from previous wars through the current conflicts. In 2002, Harris delineated issues military nurses had in common with civilian nurses and the distinctive challenges faced by those engaged in army nursing practice. The purpose of the project was to describe the types and levels of distress caused by ethical issues and ethical education needs for both Department of the Army civilian and military nurses (Harris, 2000). This study included nurses who participated in operations in Kosovo, Bosnia, and Somalia. For data collection, Harris modified the Ethical Issues Scale (Fry & Damrosch, 1994) to be applicable for military nurses. The final report for this study is not available, but a portion of the project was published by nurse anesthetist students who extracted a subset of the data in order to analyze the responses of certified registered nurse anesthetists who participated in the survey. These respondents noted the nurses' desire for more education and preparation in the ethics of triage and the expected behavior of a health professional as a prisoner of war (POW) as the most concerning issues pre-OEF/pre-OIF (Jenkins, Elliott, & Harris, 2006). The most disturbing ethical issues noted by these respondents were related to conflicts with physicians in treatment decisions, working with impaired or incompetent colleagues, and staffing patterns. More applicable to wartime concerns, however, was their need to protect patient rights and dignity and risks to their own health in patient care delivery.

In 2000, Foley, Minick, and Kee explored the engagement in, and application of, nursing advocacy by military nurses deployed in Operation Joint Endeavor in Bosnia and Hungary in the 1990s. Using Heideggerian hermeneutic phenomenology, the team interviewed 24 nurses 3 months after their return to Germany. This operation was a peacekeeping mission, and nurses did not experience the same intensity or issues as in OEF/OIF, even though they also rendered care to the civilian populace during these missions. The authors noted that the learning of advocacy behaviors was somewhat haphazard and situational. They determined one overall pattern of safeguarding that included four themes of advocacy: for protection; for holistic care; for support of personhood; and for supporting the patient's voice. These themes echo the ethical principles, namely, autonomy, beneficence, and nonmaleficence in the advocacy activities described by their participants. The researchers also reiterated the need for more education, especially for new nurses, in learning and practicing patient advocacy. This team extended their project in 2001 to examine how nurses develop skills in advocacy. Advocacy was inherent in their definition of self and in their upbringing. Advocacy, in other words, was a core value participants brought with them into nursing. Advocacy was further developed as nurses worked with and watched other nurses' advocacy behaviors and by practicing advocacy that was supported by colleagues and supervisors. This led to increased confidence in choosing appropriate actions in helping their patients. Investigators recommended follow-on work to provide examples and stories that other nurses could use in defining and learning effective advocacy skills (Foley, Minick, & Kee, 2000).

Similarly, Almonte (2009) used grounded theory methods to identify ethical issues and subsequent moral distress in Navy nurses who were deployed on the USNS *Comfort* in response to the 2004 tsunami in the Indian Ocean. Focused upon humanitarian missions rather than wartime experiences, 11 Navy nurses were asked to explain nursing practice aboard the U.S. Naval Hospital ship *Mercy*, which had been deployed to provide relief to Indonesia, Dili, East Timor, Nias Island, and Papua New Guinea over a 5-month period following tsunami and earthquake natural disasters in the region. For these participants, having to deny care because of mission constraints and the sheer volume of need left them with no other choice but to say "no" to many and to defer definitive care. Many felt they were unprepared to deal with the heartbreak of not being able to provide what they assessed as an appropriate level of care and that they needed more preparation for these situations. Alamonte encouraged further examination of the situations these nurses encountered while providing care to the indigenous people in the region and the ramifications for education and intervention for nurses experiencing distress as they realized limitations in terms of providing definitive and sustainable treatment.

Related Ethical Issues Identified in Military Physician Research

Based on evidence delineating the types of ethical issues encountered by military nurses, the literature does present some discussion of dilemmas encountered by medical officers and some ethical discussions directed toward exploring the principles involved and the actions taken to resolve these conflicts (Beam, 2003). Probably the most controversial discussion has been in response to Gross's article in which he asserts that military medical ethics are built more upon the expediency of returning soldiers to battle rather than on treating those most injured, meaning that the priority is to return soldiers to duty rather than to provide care to the seriously wounded. This article has garnered several counterarguments from other authors seeking to clarify the triage system process necessitated by battlefield conditions (Gatliff, 2008; Gross, 2008; Repine, Lisagor, & Cohen, 2005).

In his response, Edmund Howe (2008), longtime chair of the institutional review board at the Uniformed Services University of the Health Sciences, acknowledged that no matter whether one agrees or disagrees with Gross, he raises questions that need to be, at the very least, heard and debated. Triage is, and will continue to be, a controversial issue in situations during deployment where casualties overwhelm resource availability and choices need to be made in prioritizing care. According to Repine et al. (2005), battlefield triage can assume basically two forms. The first is when the number and type of injuries do not exceed the capabilities of the unit and, in such situations, those with the worst injuries are cared for first. In the alternative situation, where the number and types of injuries exceed the capabilities of the medical unit, those with the most life-threatening injuries and those who are most resource demanding, may need to wait for definitive care until those with less severe injuries are treated. These authors find that in such situations, resources should be distributed to maximize the greatest good—to care for as many as can be helped with what is available. Further, they note that beneficence may also need to be sacrificed for one patient in order to provide care for many others. Patients and staff may find such choices difficult to accept, since the process of triage can require hard choices and demanding decisions in order to distribute care fairly in combat situations.

Other controversial issues in the medical literature consider the issue of dual loyalty: the obligations of medical officers in their duty to heal but also their sworn duty to support "the Constitution against all enemies foreign and domestic" that translates potentially into a conflict when physicians are asked to support military objectives (Army.mil, n.d.). London, Rubenstein, Baldwin-Ragaven, and Van Es (2006) noted that this dual loyalty can lead potentially to human rights violations, for example, when physicians become involved in interrogation techniques such as sleep deprivation or when they turn a blind eye to overly aggressive procedures. Benetar and Upshur (2008) discussed the fine line military physicians may face when caring for enemy POWs. Holmes and Perron (2007) and Singh (2007) directly accused health professionals of actual collusion with interrogators providing health information that could be used to design interrogation strategies and of engaging in unethical behaviors. Ritchie and Mott (2002), studying mental health and preventive medicine physicians, provided a historical perspective of ethical issues that emerged from Vietnam, Somalia, Rwanda, and Haiti. Primarily in this descriptive account, medical rules of engagement were discussed in terms of the balance that needs to be achieved between security requirements and provision of care and utilization of resources. For example, one incident they related concerned a man in Haiti who set fire to a woman in which he was injured following the attack. His medical costs for operations and postoperative care were estimated at $300,000. The staff had difficulty understanding the high-resource use for this individual, especially since he was abusive to members of the health-care team. In this situation, as in many of the countries in which humanitarian care is provided, the opportunity to transfer him to Haitian facilities was not an option because the infrastructure could not support his care. Thus, the ethical dilemma was situated between the need for careful resource allocation and care commitment.

ETHICAL ISSUES IN WARTIME MILITARY NURSING

Several publications by Army nurses who served at Abu Ghraib have tried to describe their efforts to treat detainees and enemy prisoners of war with respect and dignity, but clearly the issue is a "hot-button" one as evidenced by discussions in the medical literature. Many anecdotal accounts detail first-person accounts of military health-care providers' experiences. De La Rosa and Goke (2007) described the mental health mission within the team at Abu Ghraib internment facility. The ethical situations they encountered stemmed from cultural differences related to mental health care and some of the cultural biases that emerged during such encounters. Thompson and Mastel-Smith (2012) provided a descriptive account of deployment culled from multiple first-person accounts in the literature for the purpose of defining caring within the wartime setting. As with the previous article, they found that military nurses working with injured insurgents challenged "the ethical mandate to build a caring nurse-patient relationship" (p. 24). Emotional responses such as anger, fear, resentment, hatred, and prejudice conflicted with the ethical mandates of nursing. Many were able to move past the detainees' actions and view them as fellow human beings; however, many felt conflicting loyalties viewing those individuals as the enemy and perhaps the cause for harm to "friendly" forces (Germain & Lounsbury, 2007).

Haynes-Smith (2010) described the moral and ethical challenges she encountered while caring for Iraqi detainees during a deployment to Iraq in 2005. As she noted, "I was constantly aware that these detainees would harm or kill any member of my unit if given an opportunity. At the same time, I was bound by the rules of the Geneva Convention to provide the highest-quality care" (p. 31). She, like others, also struggled with stopping life-sustaining treatments to the detainees. As she described, "because of the fear of being accused of abusing detainees, my colleagues and I had to be extraordinarily careful" when there was a decision being made about a dying detainee (p. 31) that "added to the stress and strain of life in the combat zone." Kraemer (2008) also reported similar issues in the account of her experiences in Iraq. Further, she found it was difficult to reconcile the loss of life and what she perceived as the futility of treatment in many cases where every effort had been made to save life, limb, or eyesight.

Most often, insights into ethical dilemmas experienced by military nurses have emerged incidental to studies with a focus upon military nursing practice or reintegration issues. Using qualitative descriptive techniques, Mark et al. (2009) explored the deployment experiences of Army Medical Department personnel during 11 focus groups and 1 individual interview with 101 redeployed medical personnel from OIF/OEF. Some of the issues delineated by the participants reflected ethical issues that have been more clearly defined in more recent studies. These participants identified resource allocation to be challenging in the care of the friendly forces and confusion related to caring for civilian casualties. They were unsure of how and when to transition foreign combatants to their own health-care system. They also were unexpectedly faced with treatment requirements for military personnel deployed with chronic conditions, which strained the ability to allocate resources. Ross et al. (2008) also identified ethical issues as part of their mixed-method qualitative study utilizing focus groups to interview 72 military nurses. Additionally, in this study, e-mailed surveys were distributed to commanders of deployed medical facilities to query participants about the content of the after-action reports that were completed at the end of their deployments. The purpose of the study was to qualitatively extract and analyze the content of after-action reports and the utility of using these reports for improving and directing training for future deployments. While the focus of the project was on the content of the after-action reports, ethical dilemmas were also compared to those in existing research. Participants commented upon the risky nature of caring for enemy POWs; the difficulties they experienced while caring for foreign national civilian casualties; resupply problems; and the scope of practice role and expectations as posing ethical conflicts. Rushton, Scott, and Callister (2008) collected accounts of nurses' experiences in the Gulf War as part of a larger project, Nurses At War, which was directed more at nursing practice than specifically at ethical issues. In their interviews of 11 participants, the authors noted that life/death issues were mentioned by the nurses as presenting ethical conflicts in the wartime environment.

Lang, Patrician, and Steele (2012) did not specifically study ethical situations in their comparison of nurse burnout and the practice environment among 105 medical personnel who had been assigned to a combat support hospital in Iraq. They found that, across all different levels of personnel, exhaustion and burnout were present. They hypothesized that in addition to perceiving lack of support by leadership and the stress from the practice environment, some of the ethical situations the personnel encountered could have increased feelings of depersonalization that, in turn, may have led to burnout. Similarly, Scannell-Desch and Doherty (2010) detailed multiple ethical issues in their phenomenological study that included 37 military nurses from all services who participated in individual interviews querying them on their experiences in both Iraq and Afghanistan between 2003 and 2009. As with so many of the studies, nurses in this particular sample commented on the difficulties caring for both the U.S. military personnel and the insurgents who injured them, at the same time. Similar to the participants in the study of Ross and her colleagues, these participants also found it challenging to care for the insurgents because of the potential danger they represented.

Comparably, Goodman, Edge, Agazio, and Prue-Owens (2013) conducted a qualitative study to describe the cultural factors that had an impact on military nursing care for Iraqi patients. The sample consisted of military registered nurses and licensed practical nurses who were assigned to a military combat support hospital in Iraq. The cultural differences identified in the study between the military nurses and the Iraqi patients contributed to ethical dilemmas. Findings revealed that the nurses expressed difficulty encountering cultural norms that conflicted with the provision of care. Gender issues resulted in differences in the care, and expectations, of female patients. Based on the dominant role of men, men were the primary decision makers and could dictate the provision or withholding of care to female members or children in the family. In addition, cultural customs in the context of social, political, and economic factors in Iraq impacted the provision of care. Patients expressed fatalistic views and exhibited dependent behaviors, which may be secondary to years of economic sanctions, repression, and scarce resources. Patients would not actively participate in care, which may include lack of participation in prescribed activities such as ambulation, incentive spirometry, and other activities. Findings indicated that the nurses felt ill-prepared to deal with these challenges.

Interestingly, nurse researchers collaborating with coalition forces have also conducted studies among their military nurse colleagues to discern ethical issues in recent military conflicts. Specific to a wartime environment, Griffiths and Jasper (2007), British nursing faculty, identified some ethical concerns in their grounded theory study conducted from 1999 to 2002. The research was conducted in part during the start of the war in Afghanistan and explored the effects of war on the nursing role. Using a grounded theory design, the investigators interviewed 24 British military nurses. Nurses reported experiencing moral distress due to the loss of their respect and humane caring for combatants who displayed hatred toward them. The participants also reported ambivalence regarding the duality of the role of being both a nurse and a military member, resulting in a conflict in their beliefs regarding the provision of care. The core category identified in this study was named "caring for war: transition to warrior" a concept that captured the duality of the two positions and emphasizes the ethos between the codes and values espoused in both roles. Dual loyalties have been discussed by physicians as well. As noted by Olsthoorn, Bollen, and Beeres (2013), in some situations, the call to provide care may conflict with the purpose of the mission or with available resources. For example, the Hippocratic oath requires that physicians provide care and relieve suffering, but at times they may not be able to provide that care as it would deplete the supplies needed for coalition forces.

Similarly, Finnegan et al. (2015) considered British nursing practice in Afghanistan. Their study consisted of interviews with 18 nurses who had served at Camp Bastion in 2013. Taking primarily an educational focus, the issues in this study were focused on the principle of beneficence. The nurses who participated in this research reported they felt unprepared to care for children who experienced severe traumatic injuries. They worried that their lack of education or skill in pediatric trauma might prevent their "doing good" and their ability to "avoid harm" when providing nursing care. By compiling the experiences of these nurses, the intent was to use the lessons learned to improve the predeployment preparation given to military nurses.

Lundberg, Kjellstrom, Jonsson, and Sandman (2014) qualitatively explored the experience of Swedish medical personnel participating in an international military mission from 2009 to 2012. While the majority of the 20 participants were nurses and most had been assigned to Afghanistan, the study included physicians and combat lifesavers who had completed assignments in Africa and the Balkans that were primarily peacekeeping missions. As with their American counterparts, the participants reported difficulties in caring for the enemy and concerns with prioritizing the allocation of resources toward their own forces, while balancing the care extended to the host nation's ill and injured. They also expressed concerns about the lack of infrastructure in the host nation, resulting in the inability to provide follow-up for those for whom they had provided care. Interestingly, these participants expressed role concerns and probable international humanitarian law violations for acting in the role of medical care providers while needing to complete military duties such as always being prepared to engage in hostile actions. This conflict was not evident in studies with American military nurses.

Most recently, and comprehensively, Agazio et al. (2011) were funded by the Triservice Nursing Research Program, to explore the management of ethical issues by military nurses during the conflicts in Iraq and Afghanistan (OIF/OEF/Operation New Dawn [OND]). This project emerged from an earlier study describing Army nursing practice in wartime and operations other than war. While describing the competencies needed in wartime conflicts, Army nurses in the earlier study related ethical difficulties in providing care to enemy detainees and host nation civilian casualties; participating in triage decisions; monitoring the use of resources in mass casualty situations when resupply was difficult; and caring for patients with multiple amputations or facing imminent death (Agazio, 2010). Ethically, the nurses were also concerned that the assignment of young nurses who were not ready to practice in an operational environment could pose a risk to patient care and consequently led to the provision of ongoing in-service education for the younger officers and corpsmen assigned to their units. In the more contemporary, extensive, and ongoing study, Agazio and colleagues have preliminarily detailed ethical issues that can be categorized according to the ethical principles of beneficence, autonomy, and justice. Many echo those previously detailed in the earlier and related studies. Hopefully the findings from this study will be published soon as the study is completed in 2015.

EFFECTS OF UNRESOLVED ETHICAL SITUATIONS OR DILEMMAS

Researchers have considered what happens in situations where nurses experienced conflict between what their conscience and understanding of ethical behavior dictated should be done and what actually occurred. Redman and Fry (2000) completed a systematic review of five studies conducted with nurses from four specialties to consider situations where nurses were prevented from acting from their sense of moral principles, where the moral values conflicted with those of other health-care providers concerning the morally defensible action to be taken in a situation. In many instances, the research team found that the conflicts were less likely to be experienced as moral uncertainty (not knowing which principles were in conflict), but more often moral distress, where the nurse knows which choice is the right choice to make, but where organizational or institutional constraints prevent this action being chosen. Perhaps this situation is one that military nurses also face in the deployed environment, with courses of action possibly influenced by considerations of equitable distribution of resources, institutional policies, command structure, or environmental constraints.

In 2002, Fry, Harvey, Hurley, and Foley interviewed 13 Army Nurse Corps officers, who participated in Vietnam, the Persian Gulf War, or humanitarian missions, to develop a model of moral distress in military nursing (Fry, Harvey, Hurley, & Foley, 2002). These researchers recognized the unique environment in which military nurses practice and sought to validate if indeed moral distress could be identified, and if so, whether the characteristics were different than their civilian counterparts. The dangerous environment and field conditions, coupled with atypical patient conditions and application of military triage principles, were found to place military nurses at risk for moral distress. Specific situations that were the most bothersome included not being able to treat patients because of resource demands or availability; not being able to provide definitive care for non-life-threatening problems or chronic conditions; and behaviors of other team members that were not ethically congruent. The team found that once military nurses identified a need for ethical decision making and encountered a barrier to the "desired moral action," moral distress occurred. The nurses related implementing advocacy behaviors, but if these were ineffective, the moral distress persisted, which had both short- and long-term effects on nurses and consequences for their nursing practice. Similarly, studies conducted with civilian nurses have also linked the consequences of moral distress to negative impact upon nurses.

Following this study, Harvey led members of this same team to engage in a subsequent study of 34 military nurses who had deployed in a military crisis situation. These nurses had either deployed after 1990 or served in Vietnam. Stories of moral distress were elicited using an interview guide, and content analysis was used to identify aspects of moral distress in the stories. These findings further helped to develop and validate the dimensions of moral distress experienced after a military deployment (Harvey, Fry, Hurley, & Foley, 2000).

More recently, Bradshaw (2010) developed a Moral Distress Model based on the results of a grounded theory study of 10 military nurses deployed by the Canadian Forces. The theory addressed the processes involved in the development of moral distress as a result of the deliberation and moral impact processes. Moral deliberation was initiated when the nurses considered two or more moral options and ended when a single option was chosen. Moral options were compared to each other by assessing which option may be the most morally correct and/or which option held more benefits than risks. Moral distress occurred when the choice was blocked or the nurses underestimated the impact of their inaction, particularly when their decisions were based upon experience, core values and beliefs, and bioethical principles. Throughout the deliberation process, each nurse was influenced by perception, external influencers, and environmental aspects. Perceptions referred to the opinions and views of the nurses that influenced their consideration of issues such as collegial and chain-of-command support and impact on their career and the team and were based on their personal experiences, observations, assessment of the situation, and their thoughts of how other people might possibly react to their moral action choice. External influences (e.g., decisional power, team/intraprofessional dynamics, mandates and regulations, and daily challenges) and internal influences (e.g., commitment to one's core values and beliefs, fortitude, tolerance, and resources) were also considered. Finally, definition of the environment included such aspects as the presence of danger, atypical patient conditions, and finite resources that also influenced the process.

Within the environmental aspects, Bradshaw (2010) identified several factors that contributed to developing moral distress: (a) issues around patient care delivery, (b) chain of command, (c) lack of moral preparation and training in moral dilemmas, and (d) lack of professionalism. Issues around patient care delivery largely related to the type of patient and the resources available. Finite resources and resupply resulted in the prioritization of care, the manner in which care was provided, and the length of time care could be provided or sustained. Provision of care was based on the type of patient. Medical rules of eligibility or entitlement to care and the country's poor or nonexistent health-care infrastructure were factors that influenced the delivery of care to civilians. Chain-of-command issues were related to the failure of senior leadership to act equitably, in a timely fashion, and in a manner consistent with the maintenance of good order and discipline of subordinates. Lack of moral preparation and training in moral dilemmas referred to lack of knowledge of how to address and cope with moral dilemmas, such as disobeying an order, reporting of infractions, fraternization, and medical decision making. Lack of professionalism referred to the lack of respect and recognition between physicians and nurses and between officers and enlisted/noncommissioned officers. The nurses expressed feelings of marginalization, the absence of professional recognition, and physicians' lack of respect for nurses' input.

Within her study, Bradshaw (2010) found that when the impact of the decision was negative, the result for the nurses included feelings of guilt, regret, self-loathing, emotional withdrawal, self-blame, and self-doubt. Situational resolution and self-reflection were used to help the nurses achieve acceptance, reconciliation, self-protection, and the ability to cope with the outcomes. When this resolution was not possible, the results could lead nurses to implement drastic actions such as changing and/or compromising personal core values and beliefs, leaving the nursing profession, leaving the military, and/or losing their sense of self.

It is important to understand the cause and effect of moral distress for nurses and, for that matter, other health professions as well, since moral distress has been associated with burnout, dissatisfaction with and leaving the nursing profession, compassion fatigue, and disinterest in the provision of quality patient care (Corley, 2002; Corley, Minick, Elswick, & Jacobs, 2005). It is premature at this time to definitively declare that OEF/OIF nurses are experiencing moral distress, but it appears that they may be at risk since many have experienced ethical situations that have yet to be explored and described. It is important to understand the sources and types of ethical dilemmas faced by military nurses in wartime situations as well as their reactions and management of those situations. Ideally, nurses should be prepared ahead of time for the situations and dilemmas that may confront them and also receive education as to courses of action. Researchers have found that those who are more involved in participating and determining courses of action in ethical dilemmas have been found to feel less dissatisfied with the resolution decision and, as a consequence, perhaps experience less moral distress and/or sequelae (Corley, 2002; Corley et al., 2005; Sundin-Huard & Fahy, 1999).

MILITARY NURSES' PSYCHOLOGICAL RESPONSES TO ETHICAL ISSUES

Several nurse researchers have also identified the adjustments necessitated during reintegration after the intense experience of being in the wartime environment. Gibbons, Hickling, and Watts (2012) conducted an extensive systematic review of factors influencing stress response and postdeployment adjustments. They compiled studies that included Vietnam health-care professionals through the current conflicts. A major finding was that moral issues related to patient care decisions contributed to stress during and after deployment. Particularly bothersome issues were not delineated, as this was not the purpose of the integrated review. Comparably, Rivers, Gordon, Speraw, and Reese (2013) and Owen and Wanzer (2014) both identified moral issues occurring in more contemporary conflicts as factors in postdeployment adjustments. Psychological distress experienced upon return was related to a perception that there was a lack of understanding by stateside colleagues in relation to their adjustment after the deployment. While not specifically detailing the situations that may have precipitated the distress, previous work in the area of moral distress has been linked to feelings of stress during the readjustment period.

CONCLUSIONS AND RECOMMENDATIONS

To date, the majority of research on ethical issues experienced by military nurses in wartime has emerged from a limited number of qualitative studies and related research considering reintegration adjustments and from humanitarian missions. The consensus from these studies has identified ethical dilemmas emerging from the provision of care to enemy detainees and host nation civilian casualties; triage, polytrauma, and death/dying care provided to American forces; and utilization/allocation of resources. More research is needed that utilizes larger samples and quantitative research methods to elicit issues across all services in order to delineate, as in Fry's earlier studies, the frequency, types, and levels of distress associated with the ethical issues encountered during wartime. From this information, educational interventions could be structured to better prepare nurses to anticipate these situations and equip them with potential management strategies to assess and address these issues in wartime situations. Work such as that by Agazio and her team will identify some of those strategies to assist nurses who deploy for future conflicts.

Retention of military nurses has been an ongoing challenge (Zangaro & Kelley, 2010). Previous research has demonstrated that military nurses experience emotional and moral distress during reintegration as a consequence of unresolved ethical situations that they experienced during wartime deployments. Moral distress, in turn, can potentially contribute to PTSD, burnout, and retention issues in the military and/or nursing practice. The better we equip military nurses to successfully negotiate the ethical situations they encounter in wartime environments, the better the chance for improved patient care quality and outcomes and for protecting the well-being of nurses and other military medical personnel.

REFERENCES

Agazio, J. (2010). Army nursing practice challenges in humanitarian and wartime missions. *International Journal of Nursing Practice, 16* (2), 166–175.

Agazio, J., Goodman, P., Padden, D., Nayback, A., Throop, M., Steffan, N., et al. (2011). *Management of ethical issues by military nurses during wartime*. Retrieved from http://www.resourcenter.net/images/SNRS/Files/2014/AnnMtg/AbstractProceedings/data/papers/C2-1.html

Almonte, A. L. C. (2009). Humanitarian nursing challenges: A grounded theory study. *Military Medicine, 174*(5), 479–485.

American Nurses Association. (2015). *ANA code of ethics with interpretative statements*. Retrieved from http://www.nursingworld.org/MainMenuCategories/EthicsStandards/CodeofEthicsforNurses/Code-of-Ethics-For-Nurses.html

Army.mil. (n.d.). *Oath of commissioned officers*. Retrieved from http://www.army.mil/values/officers.html

Beam, T. E. (2003). Medical ethics on the battlefield: The crucible of military medical ethics. In T. E. Beam & L. R. Sparacino (Eds.), *Military medical ethics* (Vol. 2, pp. 369–402.) Washington, DC: Borden Institute.

Benetar, S. R., & Upshur, R. E. G. (2008). Dual loyalty of physicians in the military and in civilian life. *American Journal of Public Health, 98*(12), 2161–2167.

Bradshaw, T. (2010). *Canadian forces military nursing officers and moral distress: A grounded theory approach*. Available from ProQuest Dissertations & Theses Full Text (Order No. MR74172), (871631516). Retrieved from http://search.proquest.com/docview/871631516?accountid=9940

Corley, M. C. (2002). Nurse moral distress: A proposed theory and research agenda. *Nursing Ethics, 9*(6), 636–50. http://dx.doi.org/10.1191/0969733002ne557oa

Corley, M. C., Minick, P., Elswick, R. K., & Jacobs, M. (2005). Nurse moral distress and ethical work environment. *Nursing Ethics, 12*(4), 381–390.

De La Rosa, R., & Goke, K. (2007). Reflections on suffering and culture in Iraq: An Army Nurse perspective. *International Journal of Human Caring, 11*(2), 53–58.

Finnegan, A., Finnegan, S., Bates, D., Ritsperis, D., McCourt, K., & Thomas, M. (2015). Preparing British military nurses to deliver nursing care on deployment. An Afghanistan study. *Nurse Education Today, 35*(1), 104–112. http://dx.doi.org/10.1016/j.nedt.2014.07.008

Foley, B. J., Minick, P., & Kee, C. (2000). Nursing advocacy during a military operation. *Western Journal of Nursing Research, 22*(4), 492–507.

Fry, S. R., Harvey, R. M., Hurley, A. C., & Foley, B. J. (2002). Development of a model of moral distress in military nursing. *Nursing Ethics, 9*(4), 373–387.

Fry, S. T., & Damrosch, S. (1994). Ethics and human rights issues in nursing practice: A survey of Maryland nurses. *The Maryland Nurse, 13*(7), 11–12.

Gatliff, J. (2008). Principle of salvage: A mischaracterization of military medicine. *American Journal of Bioethics, 8,* 17–18.

Germain, D., & Lounsbury, C. (2007). *Reaching past the wire: A nurse at Abu Ghraib*. St Paul, MN: Borealis Books.

Gibbons, S. W., Hickling, E. J., & Watts, D. D. (2012). Combat stressors and post-traumatic stress in deployed military healthcare professionals: An integrative review. *Journal of Advanced Nursing, 68*(1), 3–21.

Gilchrist, C. L. (2000). *Ethical issues of air force nurse practitioners in clinical practice*. Available from ProQuest Dissertations & Theses Full Text (Order No. 1399511), ProQuest Dissertations & Theses Global (230787866). Retrieved from http://search.proquest.com/docview/230787866?accountid=9940

Gold, C., Chambers, J., & Dvorak, E. M. (1995). Ethical dilemmas in the lived experience of nursing practice. *Nursing Ethics, 2*(2), 131–142.

Goodman, P., Edge, B., Agazio, J., & Prue-Owens, K. (2013). Military nursing care of Iraqi patients. *Military Medicine, 178*(9), 1010–1015.

Griffiths, L., & Jasper, M. (2007). Warrior nurse: Duality and complementarily of the role in the operational environment. *Journal of Advanced Nursing, 61*(1), 92–99.

Gross, M. L. (2008). Why treat the wounded? Warrior care, military salvage, and national health. *The American Journal of Bioethics, 8*(2), 3–12.

Grove, T. P. (1996). *Nursing ethics in the 90s: Issues nurses face and how education can address them*. Available from ProQuest Dissertations & Theses Full Text (Order No. 9635651), (304326402). Retrieved from http://search.proquest.com/docview/304326402?accountid=9940

Harris, J. (Henry Jackson Foundation). (2000). *Ethical Issues in Department of Army Nursing Practice*. Unpublished grant proposal submitted to the Triservice Nursing Research Program.

Harvey, R. M., Fry, S. T., Hurley, A., & Foley, B. J. (2000). *The dimensions of moral distress experienced by nurses deployed in military crisis situations*. Retrieved April 27, 2015 from http://www.bc.edu/bc_org/avp/son/ethics/pdf/research_abstracts.pdf

Haynes-Smith, G. (2010). Nursing in the sandbox: A lived experience. *Creative Nursing, 16*(1), 29–32.

Holmes, D., & Perron, A. (2007). Violating ethics: Unlawful combatants, national security and health professionals. *Journal of Medical Ethics, 33*, 143–145.

Howe, E. G. (2008). Review of Michael L Gross. Bioethics and armed conflict: Moral dilemmas of medicine and war. *The American Journal of Bioethics*, 8(10), 82–85.

International Council of Nurses. (2012). *The ICN code of ethics for nurses*. Retrieved from http://www.icn.ch/images/stories/documents/about/icncode_english.pdf

Jenkins, C. L., Elliott, A. R., & Harris, J. R. (2006). Identifying ethical issues of the Department of the Army civilian and Army Nurse Corps certified registered nurse anesthetists. *Military Medicine, 171*(8), 762–769.

Kraemer, L. C. (2008). A military twist to the profession of nursing. *Medsurg Nursing: Official Journal of the Academy of Medical-Surgical Nurses, 17*(4), 275–277.

Lang, G. M., Patrician, P., & Steele, N. (2012). Comparison of nurse burnout across army hospital practice environments. *Journal of Nursing Scholarship*, 43(2), 274–283.

London, L., Rubenstein, L. S., Baldwin-Ragaven, L., & Van Es, A. (2006). Dual loyalty among military health professionals: Human rights and ethics in times of armed conflict. *Cambridge Quarterly of Healthcare Ethics, 15*, 381–391.

Lundberg, K., Kjellström, S., Jonsson, A., & Sandman, L. (2014). Experiences of swedish military medical personnel in combat zones: Adapting to competing loyalties. *Military Medicine, 179*(8), 821–826.

Mark, D. D., Connelly, L. M., Hardy, M. D., Robison, J., Jones, C. C., & Streett, T. A. (2009). Exploring deployment experiences of Army Medical Department personnel. Military Medicine, 174, 631–636.

Middleton, T. A. (2009, September 1). The ethics of care under fire. *EMS magazine*, 46–48.

Olsthoorn, P., Bollen, M., & Beeres, R. (2013). Dual loyalties in military medical care—Between ethics and effectiveness. In H. Amersfoort, R. Moelker, J. Soeters, & D. Verweij (Eds.), *Moral responsibility and military effectiveness* (pp. 79–96). Retrieved from http://philpapers.org/archive/OLSDLI

Owen, R. P., & Wanzer, L. (2014). Compassion fatigue in military healthcare teams. *Archives of Psychiatric Nursing, 28*(1), 2–9.

Redman, B. K., & Fry, S. T. (2000). Nurses' ethical conflicts: What is really known about them? *Nursing Ethics, 7*(4), 360–366.

Repine, T. B., Lisagor, P., & Cohen, D. J. (2005). The dynamics and ethics of triage: Rationing care in hard times. *Military Medicine, 170*, 505–509.

Ritchie, E. C., & Mott, R. (2002). Caring for civilians during peace keeping missions: Priorities and decisions. *Military Medicine, 167*(Suppl 3), 14–16.

Rivers, F. M., Gordon, S., Speraw, S., & Reese, S. (2013). US Army nurses' reintegration and homecoming experiences after Iraq and Afghanistan. *Military Medicine, 178*(2), 166–173.

Ross, M. C., Smith, K. K., Smith, A., Ryan, R., Webb, L., & Humphreys, S. (2008). Analysis of after-action reporting by deployed nurses. *Military Medicine, 173* (2), 210–216.

Rushton, P., Scott, J. E., & Callister, L. C. (2008). "It's what we are here for": Nurses caring for military personnel during the Persian Gulf Wars. *Nursing Outlook, 56*, 179–186.

Scannell-Desch, E., & Doherty, M. E. (2010). Experiences of U.S. military nurses in the Iraq and Afghanistan wars, 2003-2009. *Journal of Nursing Scholarship, 42*(1), 3–12.

Singh, J. A. (2007). Treating war detainees and terror suspects: Legal and ethical responsibilities of military physicians. *Military Medicine, 172*(15), 15–21.

Sundin-Huard, D., & Fahy, K. (1999). Moral distress, advocacy, and burnout: Theorizing the relationships. *International Journal of Nursing Practice, 5*, 8–13.

Thompson, S., & Mastel-Smith, B. (2012). Caring as a standard of nursing when deployed military nurses provide services to enemy insurgents. *International Journal for Human Caring, 16*(4), 22–26.

Tschudin, V. (2010). Nursing ethics: The last decade. *Nursing Ethics, 17*(1), 127–131.

Ulrich, C., Taylor, C., Soeken, K., O'Donnell, P., & Farrar, A. (2010). Everyday ethics: Ethical issues and stress in nursing practice. *Journal of Advanced Nursing, 66*(11), 2510–2519.

Zangaro, G. A., & Kelley, P. A. (2010). Job satisfaction and retention of military nurses: A review of the literature. *Annual Review of Nursing Research, 28*, 19–41.

CHAPTER 13

The Promise and Potential Perils of Big Data for Advancing Symptom Management Research in Populations at Risk for Health Disparities

Suzanne Bakken and Nancy Reame

ABSTRACT

Symptom management research is a core area of nursing science and one of the priorities for the National Institute of Nursing Research, which specifically focuses on understanding the biological and behavioral aspects of symptoms such as pain and fatigue, with the goal of developing new knowledge and new strategies for improving patient health and quality of life. The types and volume of data related to the symptom experience, symptom management strategies, and outcomes are increasingly accessible for research. Traditional data streams are now complemented by consumer-generated (i.e., quantified self) and "omic" data streams. Thus, the data available for symptom science can be considered big data. The purposes of this chapter are to (a) briefly summarize the current drivers for the use of big data in research; (b) describe the promise of big data and associated data science methods for advancing symptom management research;

http://dx.doi.org/10.1891/0739-6686.34.247

(c) explicate the potential perils of big data and data science from the perspective of the ethical principles of autonomy, beneficence, and justice; and (d) illustrate strategies for balancing the promise and the perils of big data through a case study of a community at high risk for health disparities. Big data and associated data science methods offer the promise of multidimensional data sources and new methods to address significant research gaps in symptom management. If nurse scientists wish to apply big data and data science methods to advance symptom management research and promote health equity, they must carefully consider both the promise and perils.

INTRODUCTION

Symptom management research is a core area of nursing science and one of the priorities for the National Institute of Nursing Research, which specifically focuses on understanding the biological and behavioral aspects of symptoms such as pain and fatigue, with the goal of developing new knowledge and new strategies for improving patient health and quality of life (National Institute of Nursing Research, 2015). The types and volume of data related to the symptom experience, symptom management strategies, and outcomes are increasingly accessible for research. Traditional data streams are now complemented by consumer-generated (i.e., quantified self) and "omic" data streams (Figure 13.1) (Dodd et al., 2001; Swan, 2013). Thus, the data available for symptom science can be considered big data. Nurse scientists have integrated genomics into their programs of research in symptom management (Cashion et al., 2013; Merriman et al., 2014; Reddy et al., 2014), but less research has focused on the other big data sources such as social media to capture the symptom experience and symptom management strategies (Yoon, Elhadad, & Bakken, 2013). Authors are increasingly noting the vital role of quantified self (phenome) and environmental (envirome) big data for research as well as personalized medicine (Dudley, Listgarten, Stegle, Brenner, & Parts, 2015; Hansen, Miron-Shatz, Lau, & Paton, 2014; Swan, 2013).

Big data are typically conceptualized in terms of volume, variety, and velocity (e.g., sensor or streaming data) and more recently, veracity, which refers to the level of uncertainty associated with the collection of data sources (IBM, 2015). These multiple attributes of big data reflect an additional complexity beyond that of simple volume (e.g., Medicare claims data). Some authors also consider a fifth "V" in data science attributes—value, an attribute that points to the necessity of the rigorous methods of data science to extract knowledge from data so that it is of value (Marr, 2015). The National Consortium for Data Science has emphasized value in its definition of data science as "the systematic study of the

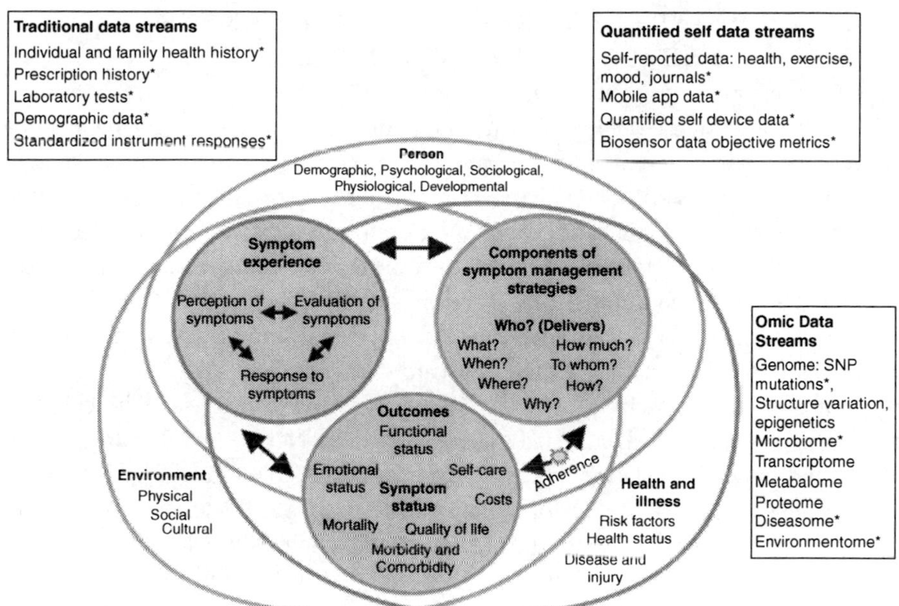

FIGURE 13.1 Data streams for symptom management research.
Note. SNP = single nucleotide polymorphism.
*consumer available, Swan (2013).

organization and use of digital data in order to accelerate discovery, improve critical decision-making processes, and enable a data-driven economy" (Ahalt et al., 2014, p. iii). Data science draws upon theories and techniques from multiple fields such as mathematics, statistics, and information technology and includes methods such as probability models, machine learning, statistical learning, computer programming, pattern recognition and learning, visualization, predictive analytics, uncertainty modeling, data warehousing, and high-performance computing (Wikipedia, 2015).

The purposes of this chapter are to (a) briefly summarize the current drivers for the use of big data in research; (b) describe the promise of big data and associated data science methods for advancing symptom management research; (c) explicate the potential perils of big data and data science from the perspective of the ethical principles of autonomy, beneficence, and justice; and (d) illustrate strategies for balancing the promise and the perils of big data through a case study of a community at high risk for health disparities.

WHAT ARE THE CURRENT DRIVERS FOR THE USE OF BIG DATA IN RESEARCH?

There are several important drivers for the use of big data in research that are relevant to advancing the science of symptom management. First, electronic health-related data have increased in volume and variety. Consumer-generated data from mobile apps, wearables, medical devices, and sensors along with multiple sources of environmental and "omic" data complement traditional electronic sources of research data such as surveys, clinical data warehouses, and transaction data. Second, the number of research networks has expanded. For example, the development of the National Patient-Centered Clinical Research Network by the Patient-Centered Outcomes Research Institute (PCORI) has increased the availability of data from a variety of data sources through its Clinical Data Research Networks and Patient-Powered Research Networks (PCORI, 2015). Also, the Clinical Translational Science Award Accrual to Clinical Trials Network was launched recently to develop a nationwide network of sites that share electronic health record data (National Center for Advancing Translational Sciences, 2015). Third, initiatives related to precision medicine and biobanking are growing, including the recent launch of President Obama's Precision Medicine Initiative (Collins & Varmus, 2015). Fourth, through the Big Data to Knowledge initiative (National Institutes of Health [NIH], 2015), the NIH has acknowledged the role of big data to advance scientific knowledge and launched a set of funding opportunities designed to develop resources and increase the competency of the biomedical workforce in data science in three core areas: computer science, biostatistics, and biomedical science.

WHAT IS THE PROMISE OF BIG DATA FOR ADVANCING SYMPTOM SCIENCE IN POPULATIONS AT RISK FOR HEALTH DISPARITIES?

In terms of the promise of big data for advancing symptom science in populations at risk for health disparities, research studies suggest that there are differences—which have been attributed to race and ethnicity—in symptom experiences, symptom management strategies, and symptom outcomes. In terms of the symptom experience, illustrative studies report

- Higher rates of pain among multiracial individuals with lung and colorectal cancer (Martinez, Snyder, Malin, & Dy, 2014)
- Increased severity of pain in Black patients with lung and colorectal cancer (Martinez et al., 2014)
- Lower rates of 14 physical symptoms among Asian Americans (Bauer, Chen, & Alegria, 2012)

- Decreased depression symptom severity among African Americans exposed to trauma (Ghafoori, Barragan, Tohidian, & Palinkas, 2012)
- Risk for moderate lower urinary tract symptoms higher in Hispanic and Black men and lower in Asian men (Van Den Eeden et al., 2012)
- Black women younger than 50 years more likely to report frequent and intense prodromal symptoms of myocardial infarction (McSweeney et al., 2010)

Studies have also reported racial differences in symptom strategies. For example, there are lower rates of recognition of late-life depression and treatment in Blacks (Pickett, Greenberg, Bazelais, & Bruce, 2014). In terms of differences in symptom outcomes, one example is that the time to reach functional decline in multiple sclerosis is shorter in Black Caribbeans than British Whites (Koffman et al., 2013).

A few recent studies are briefly described to support the potential of a variety of big data sources working in parallel to increase the understanding of the symptom experience. In a study that examined genes, environment, and depression symptoms in adolescents, female 5-HTTLPR genotype carriers had a marginally significant protective effect for depressive symptoms and no significant influences of environment (Uddin et al., 2011). In contrast, males residing in neighborhoods with relatively poor building conditions had higher depressive symptoms but no differences related to genotype. There were no significant gene–environment interactions.

Important distinctions between genotype and phenotype symptom expression, especially in underserved minorities, can be elucidated with big data approaches. One area of special interest for symptom research relates to racial/ethnic differences in drug pharmacokinetics, as clearance rates are known to affect treatment efficacy as well as risk for adverse effects. For example, in a study of the drug olanzapine, used in the treatment of acute psychosis, genotype rather than race, as previously documented, was a significant predictor of clearance rate (Bigos et al., 2011). At standard antipsychotic doses, 50% of individuals with the high-clearance genotype have trough blood levels below the therapeutic range and more African Americans carry the allele. After accounting for CYP3A43 genotype, race was no longer a significant predictor of olanzapine clearance.

Through remote monitoring using a smart inhaler, Van Sickle et al. (Van Sickle, Magzamen, Truelove, & Morrison, 2013) combined data about the use of inhaled, short-acting bronchodilators and location and presented these data to 30 asthma patients electronically. This resulted in improved asthma control and a decline in day-to-day asthma symptoms. Participants' reports suggest that the mechanisms for this improvement included increased awareness and understanding of asthma patterns, level of control, bronchodilator use (timing, location) and triggers, and improved preventive practices.

Studies such as these provide examples of how the use of big data can contribute to advancing the science of symptom management. However, the use of big data and data science methods for these purposes is in its infancy, and nurse scientists have much to offer regarding defining important questions, applying relevant theories, contributing to the design of new data science methods, and considering the ethical, legal, and social implications (Brennan & Bakken, 2015).

WHAT ARE THE POTENTIAL PERILS OF BIG DATA AND DATA SCIENCE FROM THE PERSPECTIVE OF THE ETHICAL PRINCIPLES OF AUTONOMY, BENEFICENCE, AND JUSTICE?

There exist a number of potential perils of big data related to advancing symptom management research in populations at risk for health disparities, most of which are also relevant to big data research beyond symptom science. These are briefly summarized in the following paragraphs using the three principles for the ethical conduct of research subjects as articulated in the historic Belmont Report: respect for persons (i.e., autonomy), beneficence, and justice (The National Commission for the Protection of Human Subjects of Biomedical and Behavioral Research, 1979).

The principle of respect for persons includes two separate moral requirements: the requirement to acknowledge autonomy and the requirement to protect those with diminished autonomy (The National Commission for the Protection of Human Subjects of Biomedical and Behavioral Research, 1979). The primary mechanism for protection of autonomy is informed consent that includes adequate information—understandable in lay terms—to make an informed decision about participation (Reame, 2013). Some big data sources have explicit opt-in or opt-out consent processes, and the use of protected health information for research has ethical and regulatory oversight from institutional review boards and the Health Insurance Accountability and Portability Act. However, users of social network sites and other quantified self technologies may not fully comprehend in what ways their data can be used and who may access them. Terms of service are usually lengthy and use of data for research or commercial purposes may not be highlighted. Consequently, although an individual may technically consent by clicking "I agree," the consent does not meet typical research criteria. Kahn and colleagues (Kahn, Vayena, & Mastroianni, 2014) recommend that "approaches to informed consent must be reconceived for research in the social-computing environment, taking advantage of the technologies available and developing creative solutions that will empower users who participate in research, yield better results, and foster greater trust" (p. 13678).

Beneficence involves optimizing benefits while minimizing risks. Methodological rigor is an ethical requirement, not just a scientific one, to ensure that scarce resources are used wisely and decisions are not made based on unsound findings. This requirement remains critical in big data, although the methods vary from traditional research designs (Vayena, Salathe, Madoff, & Brownstein, 2015). Thus, poor methodological rigor is a potential peril for big data research. For example, rigor is needed in terms of selection of appropriate data streams; understanding data provenance; data extraction techniques; calibration and recalibration of algorithms designed or selected for application to the data sources; handling of confounders and biases; and approaches for pattern recognition, uncertainty modeling, predictive analytics, and so forth. Other important perils relate to risks associated with loss of confidentiality and commodification of patient-/consumer-generated data. One way these risks occur is through prosumption, a process by which digital content is both produced and consumed by individuals as websites are accessed, mobile health applications are used, messages are posted and responded to on social network sites, and tweeters are followed. Vayena et al. (2015) delineate the importance of context of use and differentiating between public health (e.g., digital disease detection for outbreaks) and commercial purposes. In the "digital patient opinion economy" (Lupton, 2013), commercial use may vary along a continuum from activities such as postmarket surveillance for drugs and medical devices to tailored advertisements for products or services. So although individuals may benefit from their prosumption activities, they do not typically reap financial benefits from commodification of their data.

The principle of justice gives rise to moral requirements that there be fair procedures and equitable outcomes in the selection of research participants. In regard to big data, the investigator is typically using existing data sources that may result in biases against underrepresented groups. For example, Latinos are less likely than Whites or Blacks to use an app for health tracking (Fox & Duggan, 2013). Differences in those represented in clinical and quantified self data sources could result in a limited understanding of the range of symptom experiences and a lack of cultural context. Similarly, racial and ethnic minorities are less likely to participate in biobanks (Dang et al., 2014; Shaibi, Coletta, Vital, & Mandarino, 2013), thus hindering discoveries based on "omic" data sources that may be of particular relevance to race or ethnicity.

BALANCING THE PROMISE AND PERILS: THE WASHINGTON HEIGHTS INWOOD INFORMATICS INFRASTRUCTURE FOR COMPARATIVE EFFECTIVENESS RESEARCH PROJECT

The Washington Heights Inwood Informatics Infrastructure for Comparative Effectiveness Research (WICER) project is used as a case study to illustrate balancing the promise and the perils associated with big data. The overall goals of WICER were to understand the health of the Washington Heights Inwood (WaHI) community in order to improve it and to build an informatics infrastructure for comparative effectiveness research. Funded as part of the Agency for Healthcare Research and Quality's PROSPECT portfolio, WICER included creating a research data warehouse comprising data from multiple clinical sources (e.g., inpatient, outpatient, home care) about WaHI residents, building tools that supported exploration of the research data warehouse and conduct of comparative effectiveness research, and a large community survey of almost 6,000 residents (Sittig et al., 2012; Wilcox, Fort, & Bakken, 2014). For the last, bilingual community health workers gathered data about social determinants of health, symptoms (e.g., depression, fatigue, anxiety), health behaviors (e.g., medication adherence, physical activity), patient-reported outcomes (e.g., quality of life), and selected physical measures (i.e., blood pressures, body mass index; Lee, Boden-Albala, Larson, Wilcox, & Bakken, 2014) to complement the clinical data about WaHI residents in the research data warehouse. A subsample of several thousand participants was also asked to provide saliva and dried blood spot samples for biomarker (e.g., oxytocin), DNA, and exome analyses (Bakken, Suero-Tejeda, Yoon, Weng, & Reame, 2015). In terms of environment, geocoded food environment data are being integrated with survey data to enable analyses about the role of environment and behaviors on selected health outcomes, and the WICER survey and research data warehouse has been compared in terms of content with other behavioral surveys according to the County Health Rankings Framework (Yoon, Wilcox, & Bakken, 2013). Given these data sources, the WICER data meet the big data attributes of volume and variety, but not necessarily veracity and velocity. However, we continue to augment our data sources. In regard to the last attribute, we have applied data mining and other data science methods to examine one type of quantified self data, tweets related to physical activity, but have not limited the tweets to those within WaHI (Yoon, Elhadad, & Bakken, 2013). Despite these caveats, the WICER project offers some useful insights related to balancing the promise and perils of big data in patients at risk for health disparities.

The major research promise of WICER is the rich characterization of the WaHI community based on the variety of data. This was considered particularly important, given that the primarily Latino immigrant community experienced significant levels of health disparities and that Latinos are often underrepresented in research (Glickman et al., 2008; Gwadz et al., 2010) and historically have low levels of participation in biobanks (Dang et al., 2014; Shaibi et al., 2013).

The key mechanism for acknowledgment of autonomy was a detailed consent form that was administered by a bilingual community health worker in the participant's language of choice (English or Spanish) during the community survey. Potential participants not only consented to the survey but also explicated their willingness for each of the following: (a) contact for potential participation in other research studies by Columbia investigators; (b) linkage of community survey data with other electronic clinical data (e.g., research data warehouse); (c) use of biospecimens by the WICER team for biomarker and genetic studies related to heart disease and stroke; (d) use of biospecimens by WICER for research in general; (e) use of biospecimens linked to WICER data by investigators outside the WICER team; and (f) long-term storage and use of biospecimens for health-related research (Bakken et al., 2015). Using this "stepped" approach, participants maintained autonomy over the use of their data. Consistent with other literature (Dash et al., 2014), WICER participants were more willing to share their data for specific reasons and with researchers they knew. In a sample of 2,290 WICER survey respondents, consent rates for biospecimens were highest for use by the WICER team for studies related to heart disease and stroke (58%) and lowest for long-term storage and use for health-related research by investigators outside the WICER team (53.2%; Bakken et al., 2015).

In regard to beneficence, because WICER was noninterventional, the potential risks associated with participation related to a loss of confidentiality and these risks were minimized by data storage on secure systems including tablet computers (Wilcox, Gallagher, Boden-Albala, & Bakken, 2012), as well as institutional regulations (e.g., institutional review board approval) and policies (e.g., data use agreement). At the same time, there were multiple strategies in place aimed at optimizing potential benefits from the perspective of various WaHI stakeholders. First, data were collected using reliable and valid measures including Patient-Reported Outcomes Measurement Information System (PROMIS) scales for depression, anxiety, fatigue, social role performance, and health-related quality of life (Bevans, Ross, & Cella, 2014; Cella et al., 2010). Second, taking advantage of the WICER's informatics infrastructure and the nature of the data and biospecimens collected, our dissemination plan included data sharing with researchers beyond the WICER study team. Third, aggregated community survey data were shared with WaHI community-based organizations and health-care organizations to inform program development and community outreach (Bakken, Suero-Tejeda, Bigger, Wilcox, & Boden-Albala, 2014).

Fourth, the WICER team conducted 20 participatory design sessions, primarily in Spanish, with a subsample of community survey participants to design and iteratively refine infographics for returning participants' data to them in a manner suitable for various levels of health literacy (Arcia et al., 2013; Arcia et al., 2015). It is hoped that such approaches can lay the foundation for greater community engagement and ultimately serve as cues to action for health behavior change. Sample infographics for PROMIS anxiety score and depression are shown in Figure 13.2. To further optimize the benefits of the project, resources were designed for sharing. These included the system that was developed to create the infographics (the Electronic Tailored Infographics for Community Education, Engagement, and Empowerment system; Velez, Bales, Arcia, & Bakken, 2014), the style guide (Arcia & Bakken, 2015) that provided the programming specifications for matching the type of data to infographic design, and infographic designs.

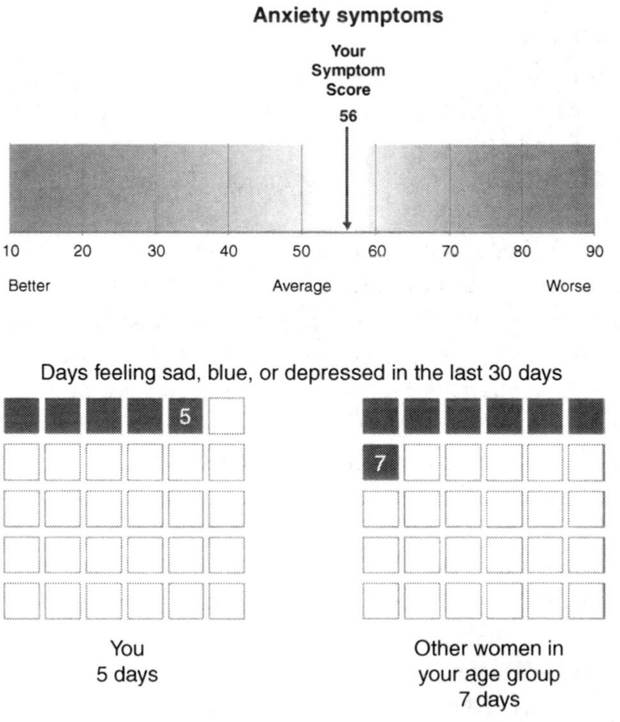

FIGURE 13.2 Example infographics for Patient-Reported Outcomes Measurement Information System anxiety score and Centers for Disease Control and Prevention 30-day depression score.

To support fair procedures and equitable outcomes in the selection of research participants (i.e., justice), WICER was explicitly designed to have multiple recruitment strategies (Lee et al., 2014). First, participants were recruited primarily from nonclinical settings including a community center and households. Second, the household sample started as a probability sample to recruit participants to reflect the demographics of WaHI. This was subsequently augmented by snowball sampling to take advantage of the connections among the community members. Although the final sample had more Latinos and more females than the community demographics as a whole, given the underrepresentation of Latinos in research and the high risk for health disparities of Latinos, this was considered to be justified. The enriched population of Latino participants ultimately shaped the infographic presentations of health data and allowed for the return of individual health information in a culturally competent manner to better promote behavior change.

CONCLUSION

Symptom management is a key area of research for nurse scientists. Big data and associated data science methods offer the promise of multidimensional data sources and new methods to address significant research gaps. The potential perils resulting from research using big data may be more problematic for those at high risk for health disparities. If nurse scientists wish to apply big data and data science methods to advance symptom management research and promote health equity, they must carefully consider the promise and perils.

ACKNOWLEDGMENTS

Manuscript preparation was supported by the Agency for Healthcare Research and Quality (R01HS022961) and the National Center for Advancing Translational Sciences (UL1TR000040).

REFERENCES

Ahalt, S., Bizon, C., Evans, J., Erlich, Y., Ginsberg, G., Krishnamurthy, A., et al. (2014). *Data to discovery: Genomes to health.* A white paper from the National Consortium for Data Science. RENCI, University of North Carolina at Chapel Hill. Text. http://dx.doi.org/10.7921/G03X84K4

Arcia, A., & Bakken, S. (2015). Style Guide: An interdisciplinary communication tool to support the process of generating tailored infographics from electronic health data using EnTICE3. *eGEMs (Generating Evidence & Methods to Improve Patient Outcomes), 3*(1), 1120.

Arcia, A., Bales, M. E., Brown, W., 3rd., Co, M. C., Jr., Gilmore, M., Lee, Y. J., et al. (2013). Method for the development of data visualizations for community members with varying levels of health literacy. *AMIA Annual Symposium Proceedings, 2013*, 51–60.

Arcia, A., Suero-Tejeda, N., Bales, M. E., Merrill, J. A., Yoon, S., Woollen, J., et al. (2015). Sometimes more is more: Iterative participatory design of infographics for engagement of community members with varying levels of health literacy. *Journal of the American Medical Informatics Association*. http://dx.doi.org/10.1093/jamia/ocv079

Bakken, S., Suero-Tejeda, N., Bigger, J. T., Wilcox, A., & Boden-Albala, B. (2014). Weaving a strong trust fabric through community-engaged research: Lessons from the WICER Project about digital infrastructure for the Learning Health System. *AMIA Joint Summits Translational Science Proceedings, eCollection 2014*, p. 126.

Bakken, S., Suero-Tejeda, N., Yoon, S., Weng, C., & Reame, N. (2015). Sociodemographic factors and health literacy are related to consent for collection, use, and storage, of biospecimens in a Latino community sample. *AMIA Joint Summits Translational Science Proceedings, eCollection 2015*, p. 241.

Bauer, A. M., Chen, C. N., & Alegria, M. (2012). Associations of physical symptoms with perceived need for and use of mental health services among Latino and Asian Americans. *Social Science in Medicine, 75*(6), 1128–1133. http://dx.doi.org/10.1016/j.socscimed.2012.05.004

Bevans, M., Ross, A., & Cella, D. (2014). Patient-Reported Outcomes Measurement Information System (PROMIS): Efficient, standardized tools to measure self-reported health and quality of life. *Nursing Outlook, 62*(5), 339–345. http://dx.doi.org/10.1016/j.outlook.2014.05.009

Bigos, K. L., Bies, R. R., Pollock, B. G., Lowy, J. J., Zhang, F., & Weinberger, D. R. (2011). Genetic variation in CYP3A43 explains racial difference in olanzapine clearance. *Molecular Psychiatry, 16*(6), 620–625. http://dx.doi.org/10.1038/mp.2011.38

Brennan, P. F., & Bakken, S. (2015). Nursing needs big data and big data needs nursing. *Journal of Nursing Scholarship, 47*(5), 477–484. http://dx.doi.org/10.1111/jnu.12159

Cashion, A., Stanfill, A., Thomas, F., Xu, L., Sutter, T., Eason, J., et al. (2013). Expression levels of obesity-related genes are associated with weight change in kidney transplant recipients. *PLoS One, 8*(3), e59962. http://dx.doi.org/10.1371/journal.pone.0059962

Cella, D., Riley, W., Stone, A., Rothrock, N., Reeve, B., Yount, S., et al. (2010). The Patient-Reported Outcomes Measurement Information System (PROMIS) developed and tested its first wave of adult self-reported health outcome item banks: 2005–2008. *Journal of Clinical Epidemiology, 63*(11), 1179–1194. http://dx.doi.org/10.1016/j.jclinepi.2010.04.011

Collins, F. S., & Varmus, H. (2015). A new initiative on precision medicine. *New England Journal of Medicine, 372*(9), 793–795. http://dx.doi.org/10.1056/nejmp1500523

Dang, J. H., Rodriguez, E. M., Luque, J. S., Erwin, D. O., Meade, C. D., & Chen, M. S., Jr. (2014). Engaging diverse populations about biospecimen donation for cancer research. *Journal of Community Genetics, 5*(4), 313–327. http://dx.doi.org/10.1007/s12687-014-0186-0

Dash, C., Wallington, S. F., Muthra, S., Dodson, E., Mandelblatt, J., & Adams-Campbell, L. L. (2014). Disparities in knowledge and willingness to donate research biospecimens: A mixed-methods study in an underserved urban community. *Journal of Community Genetics, 5*(4), 329–336. http://dx.doi.org/10.1007/s12687-014-0187-z

Dodd, M., Janson, S., Facione, N., Faucett, J., Froelicher, E. S., Humphreys, J., et al. (2001). Advancing the science of symptom management. *Journal of Advance Nursing, 33*(5), 668–676.

Dudley, J. T., Listgarten, J., Stegle, O., Brenner, S. E., & Parts, L. (2015). Personalized medicine: From genotypes, molecular phenotypes and the quantified self, towards improved medicine. *Pacific Symposium in Biocomputing, 20*, 342–346.

Fox, S., & Duggan, M. (2013). Tracking for health. *Pew Research Center's Internet & American Life Project*. Retrieved from http://www.pewinternet.org/2013/01/28/tracking-for-health/

Ghafoori, B., Barragan, B., Tohidian, N., & Palinkas, L. (2012). Racial and ethnic differences in symptom severity of PTSD, GAD, and depression in trauma-exposed, urban, treatment-seeking adults. *Journal of Traumatic Stress, 25*(1), 106–110. http://dx.doi.org/10.1002/jts.21663

Glickman, S. W., Anstrom, K. J., Lin, L., Chandra, A., Laskowitz, D. T., Woods, C. W., et al. (2008). Challenges in enrollment of minority, pediatric, and geriatric patients in emergency and acute care clinical research. *Annals of Emergency Medicine, 51*(6), 775–780.e3. http://dx.doi.org/10.1016/j.annemergmed.2007.11.002

Gwadz, M. V., Colon, P., Ritchie, A. S., Leonard, N. R., Cleland, C. M., Riedel, M., et al. (2010). Increasing and supporting the participation of persons of color living with HIV/AIDS in AIDS clinical trials. *Current HIV/AIDS Report, 7*(4), 194–200. http://dx.doi.org/10.1007/s11904-010-0055-3

Hansen, M. M., Miron-Shatz, T., Lau, A. Y., & Paton, C. (2014). Big data in science and healthcare: A review of recent literature and perspectives. Contribution of the IMIA Social Media Working Group. *Yearbook of Medical Informatics, 9*(1), 21–26. http://dx.doi.org/10.15265/iy-2014-0004

IBM. (2015). *IBM big data & analytics hub*. Retrieved from http://www.ibmbigdatahub.com/infographic/four-vs-big-data

Kahn, J. P., Vayena, E., & Mastroianni, A. C. (2014). Opinion: Learning as we go: Lessons from the publication of Facebook's social-computing research. *Proceedings of the National Academy of Sciences U S A, 111*(38), 13677–13679. http://dx.doi.org/10.1073/pnas.1416405111

Koffman, J., Gao, W., Goddard, C., Burman, R., Jackson, D., Shaw, P., et al. (2013). Progression, symptoms and psychosocial concerns among those severely affected by multiple sclerosis: A mixed-methods cross-sectional study of Black Caribbean and White British people. *PLoS One, 8*(10), e75431. http://dx.doi.org/10.1371/journal.pone.0075431

Lee, Y. J., Boden-Albala, B., Larson, E., Wilcox, A., & Bakken, S. (2014). Online health information seeking behaviors of Hispanics in New York City: A community-based cross-sectional study. *Journal of Medical Internet Research, 16*(7), e176. http://dx.doi.org/10.2196/jmir.3499

Lupton, D. (2013). *The commodification of patient opinion: The digital patient experience economy in the age of big data*. Sydney, Australila: Sydney Health & Society Group.

Marr, B. (2015). *Big Data: The 5 Vs*. Retrieved February, 2015 from http://www.slideshare.net/BernardMarr/140228-big-data-volume-velocity-variety-varacity-value

Martinez, K. A., Snyder, C. F., Malin, J. L., & Dy, S. M. (2014). Is race/ethnicity related to the presence or severity of pain in colorectal and lung cancer? *Journal of Pain and Symptom Management, 48*(6), 1050–1059. http://dx.doi.org/10.1016/j.jpainsymman.2014.02.005

McSweeney, J. C., O'Sullivan, P., Cleves, M. A., Lefler, L. L., Cody, M., Moser, D. K., et al. (2010). Racial differences in women's prodromal and acute symptoms of myocardial infarction. *American Journal of Critical Care, 19*(1), 63–73. http://dx.doi.org/10.4037/ajcc2010372

Merriman, J. D., Aouizerat, B. E., Cataldo, J. K., Dunn, L. B., Kober, K., Langford, D. J., et al. (2014). Associations between catecholaminergic, GABAergic, and serotonergic genes and self-reported attentional function in oncology patients and their family caregivers. *European Journal of Oncology Nursing*. http://dx.doi.org/10.1016/j.ejon.2014.11.004

The National Commission for the Protection of Human Subjects of Biomedical and Behavioral Research. (1979). *The belmont report: Ethical principles and guidelines for the protection of human subjects of research*. Bethesda, MD: The Commission.

National Center for Advancing Translational Sciences. (2015). *Accural to clinical trials network*. Retrieved February 28, 2015, from http://www.ncats.nih.gov/news-and-events/features/ctsa-act.html

National Institutes of Health. (2015). *NIH Big Data to Knowledge (BD2K)*. Retrieved February 28, 2015, from http://bd2k.nih.gov/index.html#sthash.8SsjsH39.dpbs

National Institute of Nursing Research. (2015). *Spotlight on symptom management*. Retrieved February 28, 2015 from https://www.ninr.nih.gov/researchandfunding/symptommanagement#.VPM-DvnF8QE

Patient-Centered Outcomes Research Institute. (2015). *PCORnet: The national patient-centered clinical research network*. Retrieved February 28, 2015, from http://www.pcornet.org/

Pickett, Y. R., Greenberg, R. L., Bazelais, K. N., & Bruce, M. L. (2014). Depression treatment disparities among older minority home healthcare patients. *American Journal of Geriatric Psychiatry, 22*(5), 519–522. http://dx.doi.org/10.1016/j.jagp.2013.01.078

Reame, N. (2013). Research ethics. In A. Peirce & J. Smith (Eds.), *Ethical and legal issues for doctoral nursing students* (pp. 33–78). Lancaster, PA: Destech.

Reddy, S. Y., Rasmussen, N. A., Fourie, N. H., Berger, R. S., Martino, A. C., Gill, J., et al. (2014). Sleep quality, BDNF genotype and gene expression in individuals with chronic abdominal pain. *BioMed Central Medical Genomics, 7*(1), 61. http://dx.doi.org/10.1186/s12920-014-0061-1

Shaibi, G. Q., Coletta, D. K., Vital, V., & Mandarino, L. J. (2013). The design and conduct of a community-based registry and biorepository: A focus on cardiometabolic health in Latinos. *Clinical and Translational Science, 6*(6), 429–434. http://dx.doi.org/10.1111/cts.12114

Sittig, D. F., Hazlehurst, B. L., Brown, J., Murphy, S., Rosenman, M., Tarczy-Hornoch, P., et al. (2012). A survey of informatics platforms that enable distributed comparative effectiveness research using multi-institutional heterogenous clinical data. *Medical Care, 50*(Suppl), S49–S59. http://dx.doi.org/10.1097/mlr.0b013e318259c02b

Swan, M. (2013). The quantified self: Fundamental disruption in big data science and biological discovery. *Big Data, 1*(2), 85–99. http://dx.doi.org/10.1089/big.2012.0002

Uddin, M., Koenen, K. C., Aiello, A. E., Wildman, D. E., de los Santos, R., & Galea, S. (2011). Epigenetic and inflammatory marker profiles associated with depression in a community-based epidemiologic sample. *Psychology Medicine, 41*(5), 997–1007. http://dx.doi.org/10.1017/s0033291710001674

Van Den Eeden, S. K., Shan, J., Jacobsen, S. J., Aaronsen, D., Haque, R., Quinn, V. P., et al. (2012). Evaluating racial/ethnic disparities in lower urinary tract symptoms in men. *Journal of Urology, 187*(1), 185–189. http://dx.doi.org/10.1016/j.juro.2011.09.043

Van Sickle, D., Magzamen, S., Truelove, S., & Morrison, T. (2013). Remote monitoring of inhaled bronchodilator use and weekly feedback about asthma management: An open-group, short-term pilot study of the impact on asthma control. *PLoS One, 8*(2), e55335. http://dx.doi.org/10.1371/journal.pone.0055335

Vayena, E., Salathe, M., Madoff, L. C., & Brownstein, J. S. (2015). Ethical challenges of big data in public health. *PLoS Computational Biolology, 11*(2), e1003904. http://dx.doi.org/10.1371/journal.pcbi.1003904

Velez, M., Bales., M. E., Arcia, A., & Bakken, S. (2014). Electronic Tailored Infographics for Community Engagement, Education, and Empowerment (EnTICE3). *AMIA Joint Summits Translational Science Proceedings, eCollection 2014*, p. 206.

Wikipedia. (2015). *Data science*. Retrieved February 28, 2015 from http://en.wikipedia.org/wiki/Data_science

Wilcox, A., Fort, D., & Bakken, S. (2014). Creating a next-generation research informatics infrastructure: WICER lessons for data integration. *AMIA Joint Summits Translational Science Proceedings, eCollection 2014*, p. 167.

Wilcox, A. B., Gallagher, K. D., Boden-Albala, B., & Bakken, S. R. (2012). Research data collection methods: From paper to tablet computers. *Medical Care, 50*(Suppl), S68–S73. http://dx.doi.org/10.1097/mlr.0b013e318259c1e7

Yoon, S., Elhadad, N., & Bakken, S. (2013). A practical approach for content mining of Tweets. *American Journal of Preventive Medicine, 45*(1), 122–129. http://dx.doi.org/10.1016/j.amepre.2013.02.025

Yoon, S., Wilcox, A., & Bakken, S. (2013). Comparisons among health behavior surveys: Implications for the design of informatics infrastructures that support comparative effectiveness research. *eGEMs (Generating Evidence & Methods to improve patient outcomes), 1*(1), Article 9. http://dx.doi.org/10.13063/2327-9214.1021

Index

NOTE: Page references followed by *f* and *t* denote figures and tables, respectively.

SERIES EDITOR

Christine E. Kasper, PhD, RN, FAAN, FACSM
Department of Veterans Affairs
Office of Nursing Services, Washington, DC
and
Professor, Daniel K. Inouye Graduate School of Nursing
Uniformed Services University of the Health Sciences,
Bethesda, MD

VOLUME EDITOR

Yvette Perry Conley, PhD
Professor of Nursing and Human Genetics
University of Pittsburgh
Pittsburgh, PA

ANNUAL REVIEW OF NURSING RESEARCH

VOLUME 33, 2015

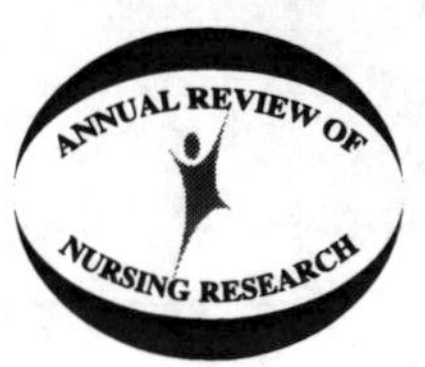

Annual Review of Nursing Research

Traumatic Brain Injury

VOLUME 33, 2015

Series Editor

CHRISTINE E. KASPER, PhD, RN, FAAN, FACSM

Volume Editor

YVETTE PERRY CONLEY, PhD

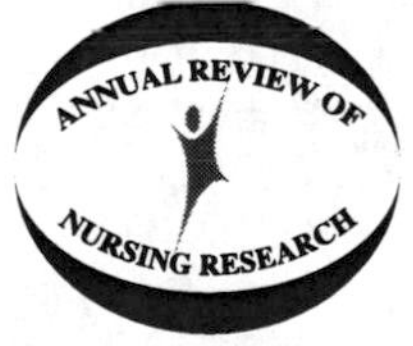

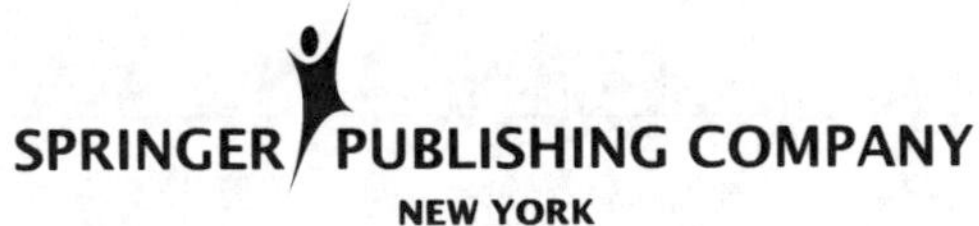

Springer Publishing Company, LLC
11 West 42nd Street
New York, NY 10036
www.springerpub.com

Acquisitions Editor: Joseph Morita
Composition: Exeter Premedia Services Private Ltd

ISBN: 978-0-8261-7162-7
E-book ISBN: 978-0-8261-2922-2
ISSN: 0739-6686
Online ISSN: 1944-4028

15 16 17/ 5 4 3 2 1

Printed in the United States of America by Gasch Printing

Contents

About the Volume Editor

Yvette P. Conley, PhD, is Professor of Nursing and Human Genetics at the University of Pittsburgh. Dr. Conley received her MS in Genetic Counseling and her PhD in Human Genetics, and she has spent her entire faculty career dedicated to the education and training of the next generation of nurse scientists. Her research uses genomic and epigenomic approaches to understand symptom development and patient outcomes after neurological insult, including traumatic brain injury. She is faculty for the Summer Genetics Institute sponsored by the National Institute of Nursing Research and director of an institutional training grant (T32) titled "Targeted Research and Academic Training for Nurses in Genomics" (T32NR009759) also sponsored by the National Institute of Nursing Research; this educates and trains nurses at the predoctoral and postdoctoral levels to incorporate genomics into their research trajectories. She serves on the editorial boards of *Biological Research for Nursing* and *Heart & Lung: The Journal of Acute and Critical Care*. She has served on many study sections of the National Institutes of Health and Department of Defense, including as a standing member of the Nursing and Related Clinical Sciences Study Section. She is a long-time and active member of the American Society of Human Genetics, the Council for the Advancement of Nursing Science, and the International Society of Nurses in Genetics.

Contributors

Sheila Alexander, PhD, RN
Associate Professor
School of Nursing
University of Pittsburgh
Pittsburgh, PA

Malcolm I. Anderson, RN, PhD
Faculty of Nursing & Health
Avondale College of Higher Education
Sydney, Australia

Taura Barr, PhD, RN
Assistant Professor
School of Nursing
West Virginia University
Morgantown, WV

Tristin Baxter, AAS
Research Assistant
Madigan Army Medical Center
Tacoma, WA

Ellen Bennett, PhD
Assistant Professor
Department of Neurology
Duke University School of Medicine
Durham, NC

Suzanna Boyce Berndt, BA, MPA
Clinical Research Coordinator
Duke University School of Nursing
Durham, NC

Patricia A. Blissitt, PhD, RN, CCRN, CNRN, CCNS, CCM, ACNS-BC
Assistant Professor
School of Nursing
University of Washington
Seattle, WA

Teresita L. Briones, PhD, RN
Associate Professor
College of Nursing
Wayne State University
Detroit, MI

Maysaa Daher, BPsych
Brain Injury Rehabilitation Research Group
Ingham Institute of Applied Medical Research
Sydney, Australia

Julia K. Eads, BA
Undergraduate Student
Duke University
Durham, NC

Jessica Gill, PhD, RN
Lasker Clinical Research Scholar
National Institute of Nursing Research Division of Intramural Research
National Institutes of Health
Bethesda, MD

Pedro Guardado, BS
Postbaccalaureate Fellow
National Institute of Nursing Research Division of Intramural Research
National Institutes of Health
Bethesda, MD

Christine E. Kasper, PhD, RN, FAAN, FACSM
Department of Veterans Affairs
Office of Nursing Services
Washington, DC
Uniformed Services University of the Health Sciences
Daniel K. Inouye Graduate School of Nursing
Bethesda, MD

Catherine Kirkness, PhD, RN
Associate Professor
School of Nursing
University of Washington
Seattle, WA

Whitney Livingston, BA
Postbaccalaureate Fellow
National Institute of Nursing Research Division of Intramural Research
National Institutes of Health
Bethesda, MD

Lucinda Matheson, RN, BN, GCNEd
Faculty of Nursing & Health
Avondale College of Higher Education
Sydney, Australia

Pamela H. Mitchell, PhD, RN, FAAN, FAHA
Professor
School of Nursing
University of Washington
Seattle, WA

Vincent Mysliwiec, MD, FCCP
Department of Pulmonary, Critical Care and Sleep Medicine
Madigan Army Medical Center
Tacoma, WA

Ava M. Puccio, PhD, RN
Assistant Professor
Department of Neurological Surgery
University of Pittsburgh
Pittsburgh, PA

Karin Reuter-Rice, PhD, CPNP-AC, FCCM
Assistant Professor
Duke University School of Nursing
Durham, NC

Frederick P. Rivara, MD, MPH
Professor
Department of Pediatrics
University or Washington
Seattle, WA

Grahame K. Simpson, PhD
Liverpool Brain Injury Rehabilitation Unit
Liverpool Hospital
Rehabilitation Studies Unit
Sydney School of Medicine
University of Sydney
Brain Injury Rehabilitation Research Group
Ingham Institute of Applied Medical Research
New South Wales, Australia

Hilaire J. Thompson, PhD, RN, CNRN, ACNP-BC, FAAN
Associate Professor
School of Nursing
University of Washington
Seattle, WA

Monica S. Vavilala, MD
Professor
Departments of Pediatrics and Anesthesiology & Pain Medicine
University of Washington
Seattle, WA

Preface

Traumatic brain injury (TBI), in its many forms, has been prominent in the national and international media as it involves injury due to global military conflict as well as the often-tragic outcomes following years of repeated sports-related concussions. This 33rd volume of the *Annual Review of Nursing Research* series delves into the continually expanding area of TBI research. TBI has long been recognized as the result of accident, vehicular crashes, gunshot, blunt force trauma, and explosion; however, only recently has TBI been linked to long-term cognitive disability, neuropsychiatric symptoms, chronic traumatic encephalopathy, Alzheimer's disease, and neurodegeneration following mild and repeated concussive events. Persistent impairment in neurophysiological function, learning, and memory following TBI significantly affect an individual's quality of life and activities of daily living, core areas of clinical nursing concern.

The research topics for the chapters were carefully chosen and compiled into this review of nursing research by Dr. Yvette Conley, Professor of Nursing and Human Genetics and Vice Chair for Research at the University of Pittsburgh School of Nursing, who has served with distinction as the volume editor. She has long excelled as one of the leaders in the study of TBI, focusing on mitochondrial genetics during recovery from neuroinflammation. As series editor, it is my hope that these topically based chapters will be used not only by those conducting research studies but also as texts and supplements to nursing curricula for both the undergraduate and graduate students.

This volume is composed of eight chapters. These begin with Hilaire J. Thompson and coauthors reviewing how common data elements among federal agencies are advancing the study of TBI in Chapter 1. In Chapter 2, Christine E. Kasper reviews TBI research in military populations. In Chapter 3, Teresita L. Briones reviews the various animal models used in TBI research, while Ava M. Puccio and Sheila Alexander provide an *in-depth review* on the role of genomic, transcriptomic, and epigenomic approaches in TBI research in Chapter 4.

The issue continues with Pamela H. Mitchell and coauthors reviewing the research in cerebral perfusion pressure and intracranial pressure changes following TBI in Chapter 5. In Chapter 6, Karin Reuter-Rice and coauthors review the research in TBI in pediatric populations. In Chapter 7, Malcom I. Anderson and colleagues provide a systematic review of the relationship between coping and psychological adjustment in family caregivers of individuals who have suffered a TBI. Jessica Gill and colleagues discuss the changes in sleep and the occurrence of posttraumatic stress disorder following TBI in Chapter 8.

Nursing science has played a significant role in the development of basic, applied, and clinical research in TBI over the past 20 years. These advances in the scientific understanding of TBI have been greatly facilitated by the support and funding of these studies by the National Institute of Nursing Research, the National Institutes of Health, the Department of Veterans Affairs, the Department of Defense, as well as a number of individual foundations. Fortunately, a large number of doctoral and postdoctoral students have been trained over these past two decades to expand and develop the science presented here as independent scientists. As with the progress and development of all nursing research, it is hoped that the result will be the alleviation of human suffering and the restoration of quality of life.

Christine E. Kasper, PhD, RN, FAAN, FACSM
Series Editor

ANNUAL REVIEW OF NURSING RESEARCH

VOLUME 33, 2015

CHAPTER 1

Common Data Elements and Federal Interagency Traumatic Brain Injury Research Informatics System for TBI Research

Hilaire J. Thompson, Monica S. Vavilala, and Frederick P. Rivara

ABSTRACT

Despite increased attention to traumatic brain injury (TBI), there remains no specific treatment and available interventions focus rather on the prevention of secondary injury. One of the reasons posited for the lack of a successful therapy is the amalgamation of various types of injuries under the same severity category in clinical trials. Informatics approaches have been suggested as a means to develop an improved classification system for TBI. As a result of federal interagency efforts, common data elements (CDEs) for TBI have now been developed. Further, the Federal Interagency Traumatic Brain Injury Research Informatics System (FITBIR) has been created and is now available for TBI researchers to both add and retrieve data. This chapter will discuss the goals, development, and evolution of the CDEs and FITBIR and discuss how these tools can be used to support TBI research. A specific exemplar using the CDEs and lessons learned from working with the CDEs and FITBIR are included to aid future researchers.

http://dx.doi.org/10.1891/0739-6686.33.1

INTRODUCTION

Previously termed a *silent epidemic* (Centers for Disease Control, 2001), there has been increased attention to the problem of traumatic brain injury (TBI) in recent years primarily due to increased interest in sports-related concussion and combat-related TBI. This is evidenced by an increase in the number of PubMed citations on TBI (more than doubling from 1,844 in 2000 to 4,299 in 2013). Despite this increased emphasis in the biomedical and nursing literature, there remains no specific treatment for TBI and interventions continue to focus on the prevention of secondary injury. In response to this identified problem, the National Institute of Neurological Disorders and Stroke (NINDS), together with National Institute on Disability and Rehabilitation Research (NIDRR), the Defense and Veterans Brain Injury Center, and the Brain Injury Association of America, sponsored a workshop in October 2007 examining barriers to TBI clinical trial effectiveness, specifically the current classification system of TBI severity based solely on the Glasgow Coma Scale score. As a result of this workshop's recommendations, an effort ensued to develop the common data elements (CDEs) for TBI and the Federal Interagency Traumatic Brain Injury Research Informatics System (FITBIR). This chapter discusses the goals, development, and evolution of the CDEs and FITBIR and how these tools can be used to support TBI research. A specific exemplar using the CDEs and lessons learned from working with the CDEs and FITBIR are included to aid future researchers.

Recommendations from the October 2007 Workshop for the Classification of TBI for Targeted Therapies specifically identified that (a) a set of CDEs should be developed and instituted in collaboration with the NINDS CDEs initiative and (b) a new databank should be launched in order to allow for data sharing and analysis (Saatman et al., 2008). The development of a new databank was desired as much of the current evidence base for the treatment of severe TBI came from the analysis of a similar resource, the U.S. Traumatic Coma Data Bank (TCDB). However, the TCDB data was gathered in the 1980s and focused solely on severe TBI, so it was viewed as outdated and too limited in scope. The development of the new database was recommended to characterize injury patterns across the life span and across injury severities and to improve injury classification, diagnosis, and treatment (Saatman et al., 2008).

DEVELOPMENT OF THE CDEs FOR TBI

The overarching purpose of the NINDS CDE Project (www.commondataelements.ninds.nih.gov) is to standardize data acquisition so that it is collected similarly across studies for the same constructs and to foster the movement of data into actionable information by enabling comparison across studies (National

Insitute of Neurologic Disorders and Stroke, 2014). In response to the 2007 workshop recommendations, the Interagency Common Data Elements Project for TBI was launched in 2008 and the first set of recommendations for CDEs for TBI in adults was published (Version 1 [V1]) in 2010. CDEs V1 included various domains for data collection including demographics and clinical assessment, trial protocols, outcome, neuroimaging, and biomarkers (Haacke et al., 2010; Maas et al., 2010, 2011; Manley et al., 2010). The primary emphasis of V1 was the coding of data. Each data element identified in CDEs V1 had three levels of coding—basic, intermediate, and advanced—to allow for crosswalking of data from multiple studies when collapsed to the "basic" level if measured at different levels of specificity (Maas et al., 2011). Data elements were further classified as "core," "supplemental," or "emerging." Data elements regarded as "core" were recommended to be collected for all clinical studies of TBI. This first version of the CDEs was subsequently followed by the publication of the pediatric CDEs for TBI (Adelson et al., 2012; Berger, Beers, Papa, & Bell, 2012; Miller, Odenkirchen, Duhaime, & Hicks, 2012).

Following the publication of the adult and pediatric CDEs for TBI V1, it was recognized that some modification and revision was necessary. There were several limitations with V1, including the realization that more than half of the 480 CDEs were classified as "core" and many of these were highly specific to population or setting and not broadly applicable (Hicks et al., 2013). Further, the first version lacked recommendations for mild TBI and was viewed as more focused on the acute phase following TBI. New workgroups, organized around the type of study (epidemiologic, acute hospitalized, rehabilitation for moderate-severe, and mild TBI/concussion), were then formed in 2012 to revisit the TBI CDEs. The specific procedures followed by the workgroups are detailed by Hicks and colleagues (2013). An emphasis of the workgroups was to clearly distinguish "core" elements from others in order to make data collection of the CDEs across multiple studies more feasible. This resulted in the reduction of core elements from 242 to 16. Those CDEs recommended data collection specific to the type of study questions (e.g., acute hospitalized or epidemiology). Data elements considered necessary to these study types were categorized as "basic" and all others as "supplemental" (replacing "emerging" category from V1). Significantly, draft CDEs were subject to external review prior to finalization and were endorsed by the American Association of Neurological Surgeons and the American Congress of Rehabilitation Medicine. The resulting Version 2 of the TBI CDEs is publically available at www.commondataelements.ninds.nih.gov/TBI.aspx#tab=Data_Standards. One excellent feature of the CDE website is that case report forms for the CDEs including questionnaires and instruments can be directly accessed from the website. Tests, tools, and questionnaires included in the CDEs are provided with a brief description and references supporting validity and reliability. For those instruments or tools that are copyrighted or trademarked, information is provided on how to obtain permission to use the resource.

EXEMPLAR OF CDE USE IN TBI RESEARCH

To date, two studies have published their experiences with implementing the V1 TBI CDEs in a prospective (Yue et al., 2013) and a retrospective (Stead et al., 2013) study, respectively. We recently consulted the TBI CDEs in the development of the Impact of Aging on the Immune Response to Injury (AIm:TBI) study protocol. The design is a prospective cohort study, which follows subjects to 6 months post injury or from enrollment for age- and gender-matched controls. The goal of the AIm:TBI study is to test a model of impairment and disability following mild TBI in adults in which aging modulates the immune response following TBI. The model is based on the Institute of Medicine's Disability Framework (Pope & Tarlov, 1991) and examines measures in four domains, injury, impairment, functional limitation, and health-related quality of life, as well as transitional factors, which modify the individual response across all domains (see Figure 1.1).

In study design, we referenced recommendations from the TBI CDEs to help tailor this study. This included reviewing core elements as well as relevant basic elements from the mild TBI, epidemiologic, and biospecimen and biomarker elements for their fit with our proposed model (Figure 1.1; Table 1.1). We also examined the CDEs for their specific applicability and validity with older adult populations.

We were able to easily use CDEs in place of elements used in the pilot study to allow for the improved harmonization of the present study with that of other researchers. For example, for our construct of "Impairment" (Figure 1.1), we exchanged the head injury symptom checklist (HISC) used in the pilot study with the CDE Rivermead Postconcussion Symptom Questionnaire (RPQ). To enrich the assessment in some areas, we chose to add supplemental measures (e.g., social support; Short Form [SF]-36) to the study protocol.

We implemented the study protocol using the CDEs; data collection is ongoing. Subjects are able to complete visits within a 60- to 90-minute timeframe including all outcome measures and do not report the testing to be burdensome. The AIm:TBI study presently maintains >90% retention to 6 months, with more than 225 of 300 planned subjects recruited. Thus, researchers interested in using the CDEs should be able to balance the quality and quantity of data collected with subject burden.

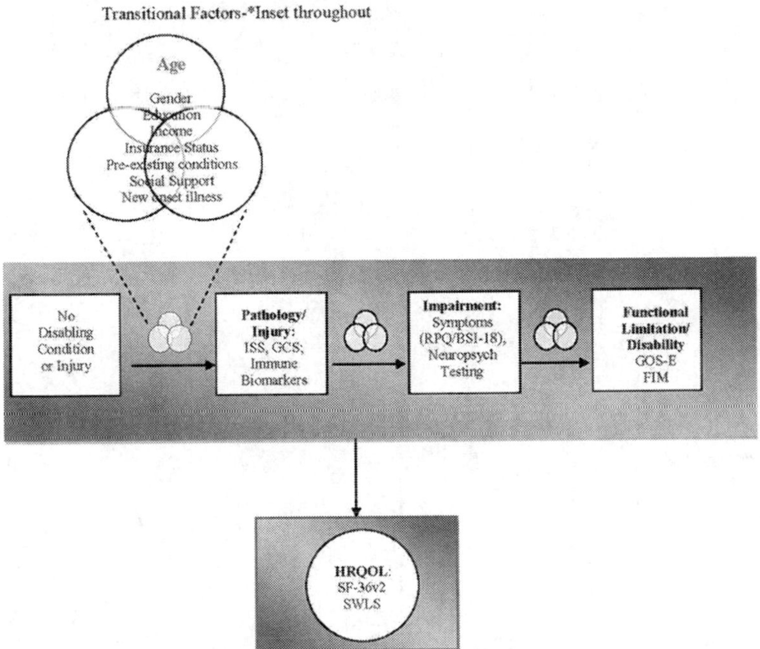

FIGURE 1.1 Conceptual model tested in the AIm:TBI study with associated common data elements.

Note. ISS = Injury Severity Score; GCS = Glasgow Coma Scale; RPQ = Rivermead Post-concussion questionnaire; BSI-18 = Brief Symptom Inventory-18; GOS-E = Glasgow Outcome Scale-Extended; FIM = Functional Independence Measure; SF-36 = MOS Short Form-36; SWLS = Satisfaction with Life Scale.

The implementation of the CDEs into the study protocol required some additional staff training. For example, research staff were trained and validated by a licensed neuropsychologist to administer the recommended basic CDE neuropsychological tests. This training was able to be completed within the planned 3-month startup period. The neuropsychologist also performs ongoing review of a subset of the subject testing. Investigators planning to use neuropsychological testing should include these costs in planned study budgets.

In planning for the use of the Brief Symptom Inventory-18 (BSI-18), a mental health protocol was developed, should subjects endorse anxiety, depressive symptoms, or suicidal ideation. In the initial 2 years of the study, we have had approximately 20% of subjects enrolled endorse suicidal ideation within the prior week and have needed to implement the mental health protocol for further evaluation and referral. The prevalence of suicidal ideation in this sample of individuals in the acute/subacute period following mild TBI

TABLE 1.1

Mapping of AIm:TBI Study Domains and Measures to Common Data Elements

Domain	Measure	Common Data Elements	Core, Basic, or Supplemental[a]
Transitional factors	Age	Birth date (age calculated from date of birth)	Core
	Insurance status	Type of insurance	Supplemental
	Gender	Gender	Core
	Race/ethnicity	U.S. racial category; ethnicity	Core
	Education	Education level	Core
	Income	Employment status; income range	Core; supplemental
	Preexisting conditions	Medical history conditions coded by SNOMED	Core
	Social support	MOS Social Support Survey	Supplemental
Pathology: injury	Injury	GCS: motor, eye, verbal, total score	Core
		Loss of consciousness indicator	Basic
		Posttraumatic amnesia indicator	Basic
		Abbreviated Injury Scale region and scores	Basic
		Injury mechanism E-code	Core
		Findings from head imaging if any	Core

Impairment: symptoms	Symptom presence and burden	Rivermead Postconcussion Symptom Questionnaire (RPQ)	Basic
		Brief Symptom Inventory-18 (BSI-18)	Basic
	Neuropsychological impairment	Rey Auditory Verbal Learning Test (RAVLT)	Basic
		Trail Making Test (TMT)	Basic
		Processing Speed Index from Wechsler Adult Intelligence Scale	Basic
Functional limitation/ disability	Functional change/ postinjury disability	Functional Independence Measure	Basic (motor and cognitive subscales only) all others supplemental
		Glasgow Outcome Scale-Extended (GOS-E)	Core
Quality of life	Health-related quality of life	MOS Short Form-36	Supplemental
		Satisfaction with Life Scale (SWLS)	Basic

Note. AIm:TBI = Impact of Aging on the Immune Response to Injury; E-code = External cause of injury code; GCS = Glasgow Coma Scale; MOS = Medical Outcomes Study; SNOMED = Systematized Nomenclature of Medicine.

[a]The study questions of the AIm:TBI study fit both the epidemiologic and mild TBI/concussion research categories; data elements noted as basic may be for only one or both of the categories listed.

is similar to that reported in a prior study of chronic mild TBI with a mean length since injury of 5 years (Tsaousides, Cantor, & Gordon, 2011). Based on the prevalence, we strengthened our mental health protocol by having a psychiatrist specializing in the care of injured patients available for evaluation as needed. Research staff were also provided with the opportunity for additional specialized training to address suicidal ideation. Researchers planning to use the BSI-18 in similar samples should plan to have similar protocols and referral resources available.

FITBIR: CONSIDERATIONS FOR RESEARCHERS

FITBIR (https://fitbir.nih.gov/) was launched in mid-2012. It takes a "big data" approach, and its stated purpose is "to help accelerate TBI research by creating an infrastructure that integrates heterogeneous data sets allowing access to much more quality research data than an investigator would be able to collect independently" (FITBIR, 2014). FITBIR implements the data dictionary developed from the TBI CDEs. Investigators planning to submit applications for the funding of TBI research to the National Institutes of Health (NIH) or other federal sources like the Department of Defense should carefully read funding announcements to determine if they are required to submit to FITBIR and include this information in the data-sharing plan of the grant application.

An application approval process is in place in order for investigators to contribute data to or access data from FITBIR. In setting up their study databases, investigators need to carefully review the data dictionary in order to upload data meeting FITBIR quality standards. One of the challenges with the current data dictionary is that many FITBIR elements are coded alphanumerically rather than numerically. This can become a challenge if the use of a single data set for both FITBIR upload and data analysis is desired. The conversion of the study dataset from one format to the other may be required, necessitating additional human resources with informatics expertise for data management. It is critical that investigators have the necessary resources, both human and financial, to support data management associated with meeting FITBIR data-sharing requirements. FITBIR provides a cost model and project estimation tool for researchers to assist in estimating the necessary resources (FITBIR, 2014). Technical support is available to researchers through weekly FITBIR users' conference calls and individual project consultations.

For investigators with approved projects, data are submitted quarterly to FITBIR. Investigators identify which data are considered experimental (i.e., testing study hypotheses). Core and basic CDEs used for experimental purposes are made available to other researchers contributing data to FITBIR 6 months following the end of the study funding period and 12 months for all other researchers

(FITBIR, 2014). This is an important deadline for researchers to consider when planning for the dissemination of project findings.

In order to allow researchers to share data regarding individual subjects without disclosing personally identifiable information (PII), researchers create global unique identifiers (GUIDs) using a local tool. Pseudo-GUIDs are available for submitting data from retrospective studies when the data required to create one is not available. The generated GUID is a random number that does not contain any PII. The specific information required to create a GUID includes full name at birth; date of birth including month, day, and year; city and country of birth; and sex at birth. Therefore, investigators who will be submitting data to FITBIR from prospective studies need to include these items in their data collection plans. Additional tools available from FITBIR are the Protocol & Form Research Management System, which allows for the creation of case report forms linked to the FITBIR data dictionary, and the Medical Image Processing, Analysis, and Visualization, which is used for imaging data.

CONCLUSIONS

Integrating the CDEs for studies of TBI is feasible and does not add substantively to subject or researcher burden. In many cases, the recommended basic CDEs for each category may overlap, and it is up to the individual researcher to determine which is best for the planned study and sample. Newer computer-adapted tests such as the Patient Reported Outcomes Measurement Information System (PROMIS) measures and the NIH toolbox for neurological function hold some promise to address this gap, but require validation in TBI patients prior to widespread adoption. Depending on the CDEs selected for use, some additional staff training and validation may be needed prior to implementing the study protocol and may have implications for the study budget.

Building on the foundation of the TBI CDEs, FITBIR holds promise for accelerating TBI research by leveraging data from multiple studies. Investigators contributing data should consult the FITBIR/CDE data dictionary carefully in planning for database and case report form setup in order to minimize the post-processing of study data. It is also critical that researchers have adequate data management and informatics support on the study team. FITBIR should be an invaluable resource in the future for secondary data analysis as there are clear quality standards for the studies accepted to contribute data. Presently data available for analysis in FITBIR are limited as the project was recently launched. However, it should eventually allow for the examination of research questions that cannot presently be answered through a single study or through existing databases.

ACKNOWLEDGMENTS

This work was supported, in part, by a grant from the NIH/National Institute of Neurologic Diseases and Stroke R01NS077913. Its contents are solely the responsibility of the authors and do not necessarily represent the official view of the granting agency.

REFERENCES

Adelson, P. D., Pineda, J., Bell, M. J., Abend, N. S., Berger, R. P., Giza, C. C., et al. (2012). Common data elements for pediatric traumatic brain injury: Recommendations from the working group on demographics and clinical assessment. *Journal of Neurotrauma, 29*(4), 639–653. http://dx.doi.org/10.1089/neu.2011.1952

Berger, R. P., Beers, S. R., Papa, L., & Bell, M. (2012). Common data elements for pediatric traumatic brain injury: Recommendations from the biospecimens and biomarkers workgroup. *Journal of Neurotrauma, 29*(4), 672–677. http://dx.doi.org/10.1089/neu.2011.1861

Centers for Disease Control and Prevention (CDC). (2001). *Traumatic Brain Injury in the United States: A report to Congress*. Atlanta, GA: CDC.

Federal Interagency Traumatic Brain Injury Research Informatics System (FITBIR). (2014). *FAQs*. Retrieved August 29, 2014 from https://fitbir.nih.gov/jsp/about/faqs.jsp

Haacke, E. M., Duhaime, A. C., Gean, A. D., Riedy, G., Wintermark, M., Mukherjee, P., et al. (2010). Common data elements in radiologic imaging of traumatic brain injury. *Journal of Magnetic Resonance Imaging, 32*(3), 516–543. http://dx.doi.org/10.1002/jmri.22259

Hicks, R., Giacino, J., Harrison-Felix, C., Manley, G., Valadka, A., & Wilde, E. A. (2013). Progress in developing common data elements for traumatic brain injury research: Version two—The end of the beginning. *Journal of Neurotrauma, 30*(22), 1852–1861. http://dx.doi.org/10.1089/neu.2013.2938

Maas, A. I., Harrison-Felix, C. L., Menon, D., Adelson, P. D., Balkin, T., Bullock, R., et al. (2011). Standardizing data collection in traumatic brain injury. *Journal of Neurotrauma, 28*(2), 177–187. http://dx.doi.org/10.1089/neu.2010.1617

Maas, A. I., Harrison-Felix, C. L., Menon, D., Adelson, P. D., Balkin, T., Bullock, R., et al. (2010). Common data elements for traumatic brain injury: Recommendations from the interagency working group on demographics and clinical assessment. *Archives of Physical Medicine and Rehabilitation, 91*(11), 1641–1649.

Manley, G. T., Diaz-Arrastia, R., Brophy, M., Engel, D., Goodman, C., Gwinn, K., et al. (2010). Common data elements for traumatic brain injury: Recommendations from the biospecimens and biomarkers working group. *Archives of Physical Medicine and Rehabilitation, 91*(11), 1667–1672.

Miller, A. C., Odenkirchen, J., Duhaime, A. C., & Hicks, R. (2012). Common data elements for research on traumatic brain injury: Pediatric considerations. *Journal of Neurotrauma, 29*(4), 634–638. http://dx.doi.org/10.1089/neu.2011.1932

National Institute of Neurologic Disorders and Stroke (NINDS). (2014). *NINDS Common Data Elements*. Retrieved August 29, 2014 from http://www.commondataelements.ninds.nih.gov/#page=Default

Pope, A. M., & Tarlov, A. R. (Eds.). (1991). *Disability in America: A National Agenda for prevention*. Washington, DC: National Academies Press.

Saatman, K. E., Duhaime, A. C., Bullock, R., Maas, A. I., Valadka, A., & Manley, G. T. (2008). Classification of traumatic brain injury for targeted therapies. *Journal of Neurotrauma, 25*(7), 719–738. http://dx.doi.org/10.1089/neu.2008.0586

Stead, L. G., Bodhit, A. N., Patel, P. S., Daneshvar, Y., Peters, K. R., Mazzuoccolo, A., et al. (2013). TBI surveillance using the common data elements for traumatic brain injury: A population study. *International Journal of Emergency Medicine, 6*(1), 5. http://dx.doi.org/10.1186/1865-1380-6-5

Tsaousides, T., Cantor, J. B., & Gordon, W. A. (2011). Suicidal ideation following traumatic brain injury: Prevalence rates and correlates in adults living in the community. *Journal of Head Trauma Rehabilitation, 26*(4), 265–275. http://dx.doi.org/10.1097/HTR.0b013e3182225271

Yue, J. K., Vassar, M. J., Lingsma, H. F., Cooper, S. R., Okonkwo, D. O., Valadka, A. B., et al. (2013). Transforming research and clinical knowledge in traumatic brain injury pilot: Multicenter implementation of the common data elements for traumatic brain injury. *Journal of Neurotrauma, 30*(22), 1831–1844. http://dx.doi.org/10.1089/neu.2013.2970

CHAPTER 2

Traumatic Brain Injury Research in Military Populations

Christine E. Kasper

ABSTRACT

Traumatic brain injury (TBI) in all of its forms—blast, concussive, and penetrating—has been an unfortunate sequela of warfare since ancient times. The continued evolution of military munitions and armor on the battlefield, as well as the insurgent use of improvised explosive devices, has led to blast-related TBI whose long-term effects on behavior and cognition are not yet known. Advances in medical care have greatly increased survival from these types of injuries. Therefore, an understanding of the potential health effects of TBI is essential. This review focuses on specific aspects of military-related TBI. There exists a large body of literature reporting the environmental conditions, forces, and staging of injury. Many of these studies are focused on the neuropathology of TBI, due to blast overpressure waves, and the emergence of large numbers of mild blast-related TBI cases.

A Marine died after exposure to a shot that did not result in any noted external injury.

—*A Case of Death from the Wind of a Shot* (McTaran, 1812)

http://dx.doi.org/10.1891/0739-6686.33.13

INTRODUCTION

Traumatic brain injury (TBI) has been an unfortunate byproduct of warfare since early human history; however, until the recent effective use of rapid evacuation to forward military hospitals, those with TBI usually died of their injury. Personal protective equipment, that is, body armor, has effectively prevented life-threatening wounds to the abdomen and thorax, leaving TBI, due to concussive blasts, a survivable injury. This review examines the history and current research in the context of combat and the military.

ANCIENT WARFARE AND HEAD TRAUMA

The earliest wars, circa 4000 BCE in Egypt and Mesopotamia, used stone tools and weapons. Within 500 years, the Bronze Age emerged, bringing new weapons, the wheel, chariot, armor, helmet, composite bow, and penetrating axe (Gabriel & Metz, 1992). At this time, warfare remained relatively rare and ritualistic, and combat deaths were limited. While stone tools permitted killing one's enemy by blunt force and penetrating wounds, the arrival of organized aggression during the Bronze Age enabled warfare on a large scale. During the period of 4000–2000 BCE, the world's first armies emerged in Sumer and Egypt, and death and destruction were achieved on a modern scale (Gabriel & Metz, 1992). The first appearance of defensive protective equipment, the helmet, is seen on the commemorative Stele of Vultures, erected by Eannatum of Lagash following the defeat of the State of Umma in 2525 BCE. These early helmets were made of copper with a leather cap or lining. Early body armor also emerged at the same time in response to the use of the highly lethal sickle-sword, bronze socket-axe, and the pointed penetrating axe, which remained in use for the next 2000 years (Gabriel & Metz, 1992).

Large battles during ancient times often resulted in significant casualties and few long-term survivors due to lack of battlefield medicine or immunizations and the poor general health of the troops. In later antiquity, it is chronicled that Roman losses during the Battle of Cannae, Second Punic War 216 BCE, thus: "45,500 foot soldiers and 2,700 horsemen were slain in almost equal proportion of citizens and allies"; Hannibal lost "about 8,000 of his bravest men" (Livy, 1965).

Ancient warfare was intentionally deadly and little effort was made to provide organized medical care for their soldiers. Battlefield care for head wounds, while attempted, was largely ineffective (Gabriel & Metz, 1992; Iserson & Moskop, 2007). Few could have survived the severe TBIs that were inflicted by those weapons. Recent analysis of the newly recovered remains of Richard III reveals in great detail the trauma that axe and sword can inflict on a human skull (Appleby et al., 2015).

THE U.S. CIVIL WAR

During the U.S. Civil War, 1861–1865 CE, the weapons of choice were the cannon, bayonet, and rifles using slow-velocity, soft lead, conoidal bullets (Adams, 1952). These soft slow-moving bullets flattened during impact and were exceptionally damaging to soft tissue and bone, creating large wounds, exposed to infection (Weiss, 2001). Neither protective body armor nor helmets were worn by either army in this conflict. In all, approximately 620,000 men died during this war. Most of the injuries were to the limbs, 71%, followed by 18% torso wounds, and only 11% were to the head, neck, or face (Adams, 1952; Livermore, 1957). Reports from the medical literature of the time do not yet use the terminology of traumatic brain injury; few with direct wounds to the head survived. Relatively few injuries were incurred by cannonballs, 359 wounds out of a reported total of 144,000 (Adams, 1952; Livermore, 1957). The shells, case projectiles, and canisters shot from field artillery were deadly and scattered "shrapnel" on the field of battle (Cole, 2002). As those injured by these shells did not usually survive, it is difficult to determine whether they were of sufficient explosive power to create the explosive blast wave necessary to cause serious TBI.

WORLD WAR I

The clinical phenomena now attributed to battlefield TBI first appeared during World War I (WWI): concussion, amnesia, tremor, tinnitus, headaches, and sensitivity to noise; the battlefield physicians of WWI were confounded by the large numbers of soldiers reporting these symptoms. This cluster of symptoms was first reported in the journal *Lancet* in 1915 (Meyers, 1915). By 1916, approximately 40% of reported casualties described this cluster of symptoms and the disorder came to be known as "shell shock" (Mcleod, 2004). Initially, it was unclear whether to attribute this symptom cluster to physical or psychiatric causes, as not all of the soldiers manifesting these symptoms had been exposed to active explosive shelling (Mott, 1916b; Shephard, 2000). Early reports attributed causality to carbon monoxide poisoning and concussive shell explosion or regarded the illness as a result of compressive forces to the brain (Jones, Fear, & Wessely, 2007; Jones, Thomas, & Ironside, 2007).

Given the wide range of symptoms, it was difficult to attribute these solely to organic origin. Thus, the first clinical research studies of what we now know as military-related TBI and posttraumatic stress disorder (PTSD) were conducted in an attempt to lessen the losses of soldiers reporting these symptoms in active battle. The concept of concussive damage to the brain without the presence of penetration of the skull was first described by Fredrick Mott (Mott, 1916b), while early advances in the understanding of the neurological damage from penetrating head wounds were achieved by the British neurologists Gordon Holmes, Percy Sargent, and Harvey Cushing (Holmes & Lister, 1916; McDonald, 2007). The first modern metal helmets were introduced in 1916 in an effort to protect the cranium from the explosions and shrapnel in the hope of reducing the incidence of TBI and shell shock (Lanska, 2009). Unfortunately, these helmets were shallow and did not provide sufficient cranial protection to the base of the head, which exposed the soldier to potential occipital and cerebellar injuries (Dean, 1927). While all of the armies engaged in WWI wore helmets, none wore any form of protective body armor to protect the torso from injury.

As previously discussed, a portion of the soldiers suffering from shell shock had not been exposed to explosions. Research conducted by the British consulting psychiatrist Myers during 1915–1916 resulted in his hypothesis that the explanation for symptoms in this group was psychological and "emotional" shock (Jones et al., 2003; Jones & Wessely, 2003). Unfortunately, the idea that these symptom clusters were largely "emotional" rather than neurologic became the favored prevailing military medical concept, as it permitted the commanding officers to limit the medical losses of soldiers from the front lines and return them to duty after a few days of rest (Jones et al., 2007). One can speculate that the very rapid redeployment of "shell-shocked" soldiers only increased their PTSD, assuming that they survived the trenches. Thus, a soldier presenting with memory loss, dizziness, changes in vision, or fatigue without visible injury was considered a shell shock or "mental case," and 10% of all British casualties were so classified (Jones et al., 2007). Excluding wounds, one-third of all discharges from the British Army by 1918, or 32,000 soldiers, were for shell shock (Salmon, 1917). It became clear by 1917 that many of these shell shock cases had no explosive exposure and efforts were made to restrict the diagnosis, and those invalided were given the preliminary label of "not yet diagnosed, nervous" (Jones et al., 2003). To the modern clinician, these clinical symptom clusters, in the absence of exposure to explosion, appear to be signs of PTSD.

WORLD WAR II

By the start of World War II in the late 1930s, it was clear that the ever-increasing explosive power of munitions was related to nonpenetrating concussive disorders. However, improvements in the protective steel and leather helmets characteristic of this war arose from significant casualties due to motorcycle accidents and the death of Colonel Thomas Edward Lawrence ("Lawrence of Arabia"), rather than from a desire to avoid other forms of head trauma (Maartens, Wills, & Adams, 2002). After the start of the war, Hugh Cairns, Advisor on Head Injuries to the Ministry of Health and honorary Consulting Neurosurgeon to the British Army at Home, noted that there was a marked 20% increase in fatal injuries of military motorcycle dispatch riders and their passengers (Cairns, 1941). As he had formed one of the first mobile neurosurgical units for the war, he was able to pay close attention specifically to the cases of head trauma. Cairns found that most of the deaths in fatal motorcycle accidents due to TBI "might have been avoided if adequate protection for the head had been worn" (Cairns, 1941). He was able to compare his observations of the fatalities to those who survived wearing crash helmets. In a few of these cases, significant damage to the helmets had been sustained and the rider suffered only mild TBI. The modern helmet was constructed from his instructions to construct helmets with a solid outer shell and web slings to support and secure the helmet, with a gap between them to contain energy-absorbing material (Cairns, 1941). By 1941, there was an abrupt decline in military motorcycle injuries to single digits, once the British Army required the use of these helmets. The use of these helmets also spread to the Royal Air Force in 1942 (Cairns, 1946).

The research of Cairns was pivotal in spreading the use of a new and more protective design of the helmet throughout the military; however, his legacy was to consist of continued research into the physics of concussive forces to the head and its association with measurable brain and skull injury, which was the start of serious clinical research into the causes and prevention of TBI (Lanska, 2009). The contemporaries of Cairns were British neurologists Derek Denny-Brown and Ritchie Russell, both majors in the Royal Army Medical Corps, who developed the first clinically relevant animal model of TBI (Denny-Brown & Russell, 1941). This model created closed head injury on an animal with a pendulum-attached hammer. Unlike other TBI models of the time, the head of the animal was unrestrained. They found that concussion occurred if the head was allowed to move and did not occur if the head was restrained during impact. This work demonstrated the fundamental association of sudden head acceleration in the causation of concussion, and created a distinction between the now classic acceleration/deceleration concussion and concussions due to compression or crush injuries (Lanska, 2009). Denny-Brown and Russell's research eventually lead them to propose neuronal injury, increased intracranial pressure, respiratory dysfunction, vascular mechanisms, and the release of toxic chemicals as the actual causes of concussion. While an important advance in research at that time, their model was based on the idea that the brain "sloshed" around in the skull (Denny-Brown & Russell, 1941). Further studies using a macaque monkey wearing a small metal helmet found that cushioned helmets were necessary to slow acceleration of concussive events (Denny-Brown & Russell, 1941).

The theoretical role of acceleration was further clarified by the work of Holbourn in 1943 who proposed two main causes of closed head injuries: deformation of the skull without fracture resulting in localized and minor damage and "sudden rotation of the head," which is causal to the contrecoup injury, intracranial hemorrhage, and concussion (Holbourn, 1943). He effectively separated the concepts of "compression" and "acceleration" concussion and introduced rotational shear injury with a mechanical model constructed from gelatin within a paraffin wax skull (Holbourn, 1943, 1945). Pudenz and Sheldon in 1946 and Ommaya and colleagues later experimentally confirmed Holbourn's theoretical predictions (Ommaya, Goldsmith, & Thibault, 2002; Ommaya, Grubb, & Naumann, 1971; Pudenz & Shelden, 1946).

THE VIETNAM WAR

There were 58,000 U.S. combat fatalities during the Vietnam War and 40% of these were due to head and neck trauma (Caveness, 1979). This war was the first to use rapid air evacuation using the helicopter to military combat hospitals located at the front. Rapid air evacuation dramatically increased overall survival rate from combat casualties in Vietnam. Unfortunately, soldiers did not have protective body armor, only the helmet, which had not significantly changed its protective characteristics since World War II. The M1 helmet was used from World War II through the Korean War and Vietnam War and was made of a steel shell with an inner lining. This helmet provided limited protection of the temporal area, was oddly balanced, and could not be worn while using communication devices (Thama, Tanb, & Leea, 2008). While effective at providing ballistic protection from 15 g, 0.45-caliber rounds moving at a velocity of 244 m/s, it was unfortunately not often worn in the heat of the jungles of Vietnam (Thama et al., 2008).

Early treatment by mobile military hospitals was successful in decreasing mortality in the wounded from 30% in World War II to 24% in Vietnam (Gawande, 2004; Rish, Dillon, & Weiss, 1983). In relation to head trauma during the Vietnam War, 12%–14% of all combat injuries involved brain injury. Another 2%–4% of lethal injuries to the thorax and abdomen also had brain injury (Okie, 2005). Death from brain injury among the U.S. armed forces exceeded 75% of all brain injury; few survived to reach mobile surgical hospitals (Okie, 2005; Rish et al., 1983).

TBI: IRAQ AND AFGHANISTAN

One of the earliest reports of blast injury of the central nervous system (CNS) was during WWI at the Lettsonian lectures of the Medical Society of London, and concussion was attributed to "aerial compression" (Mott, 1916a). Others at the time disputed Mott, claiming that the injuries arouse from carbon monoxide toxicity. Later, Fulton more accurately noted that "death from primary blast is a clinical entity that requires close study, because of its intimate connection with concussion" and with the syndrome's association with shell shock and psychiatry (Denny-Brown & Russell, 1941; Fulton, 1942).

Blast injuries, resulting mostly from improvised explosive devices (IEDs), vehicle-borne IEDs, and improvised rocket-assisted mortars currently represent the single largest cause of military TBI. Since 2000 and the "Global War on Terror," 307,283 soldiers and military personnel have suffered TBI, and 208,952 or 68% of these cases were blast related (Kovacs, Leonessa, & Ling, 2014; Ling, Bandak, Armonda, Grant, & Ecklund, 2009; Okie, 2005). Current statistics on TBI in the U.S. military is available at the Defense and Veterans Brain Injury Center (http://dvbic.dcoe.mil/dod-worldwide-numbers-tbi), and overall casualties are compiled by the Department of Defense's casualty website (www.defense.gov/news/casualty.pdf).

The Department of Defense (DoD) has conducted extensive research over the past decade to determine the effects of blast trauma to the body in order to improve the construction of protective body armor and helmets (Gupta & Przekwas, 2013). Improvements to protective equipment have greatly reduced the injuries to the thorax from munitions and shrapnel; however, the exposed areas of the face, brain, and extremities continue. Unfortunately, the helmet cannot completely protect against the blast wave, as large areas of the head remain exposed. Improvements to the helmet replaced the sling suspension system with foam pads to reduce the effects of the blast wave (Gupta & Przekwas, 2013).

BLASTS AND BLAST WAVES

Blast "winds" are extreme, have velocities exceeding 300 miles/hour, and are more intense than any gust of wind historically recorded on the surface of the earth (Goldstein et al., 2012). Damage to biological tissue varies significantly with multiple environmental factors in relation to the blast, such as, distance from the explosion, angle of the head, and whether personal protective equipment was worn (Moore et al., 2008). A blast is defined as "an explosion in the atmosphere and refers to the release of energy in such a period of time and within such a volume as to be small enough for the creation of a pressure wave of finite amplitude spreading from the source of the explosion, the energy radiated can be nuclear, chemical, electrical or pressure energy" (Strehlow & Baker, 1976).

An explosion converts chemical energy to kinetic energy, propelling a shock wave, acoustic energy, electromagnetic field energy, and shrapnel away from the source and colliding with the brain and biological tissues at a great velocity (Moore et al., 2008). The blast wave can be magnified eightfold depending on the structural environment of the explosion, as in a walled courtyard

(Cullis, 2001; Kambouchev, Radovitzky, & Noels, 2007). Such reflective blast waves can produce significantly more tissue damage than an open field blast (Bauman et al., 2009; Cullis, 2001; Magnuson, Leonessa, & Ling, 2012).

BLAST INJURIES

A blast injury is classified in four groups: primary blast injury due to the shockwave; secondary due to propelled debris and shrapnel, which causes penetrating or blunt trauma; tertiary injuries due to tissue and skeletal translocations from blast load and impact on rigid objects; and quaternary injury, which includes all other associated injuries such as burns or toxic exposure to metals. Detailed discussions of the clinical phenomena and research associated with each of these conditions have been extensively discussed in the military medical literature (Champion, Holcomb, & Young, 2009; DePalma, Burris, Champion, & Hodgson, 2005; Elsayed & Atkins, 2008; Kalinich & Kasper, 2014; Mac Donald et al., 2011; Stuhmiller et al., 1999).

Body armor and other protective equipment on the battlefield in combination with the extraordinary performance of medical first responders and military healthcare providers have saved soldiers' lives from previously lethal injuries (Okie, 2005). Unlike previous wars, the use of individual body armor systems reduces the incidence of fatal wounds to the thorax and abdomen following exposure to explosion and increases survival from attack, albeit with the comorbidity of blast TBI (bTBI; Hoge et al., 2008; Ling & Ecklund, 2011). Mild bTBI is the most prevalent of all forms of bTBI (see Table 2.1). The very large numbers of neurotrauma victims who suffer from blast injuries display varying degrees of memory impairment, anxiety, and so forth, preventing them from normal activities of daily living and from returning to active duty. Most mild TBI (mTBI) cases show cognitive deficits immediately following the blast injury and few, ~5%, report brief loss of consciousness (Hoge et al., 2008; Ling et al., 2009). Most mild bTBI cases recover; however, many continue to report symptoms long after injury and are strongly associated with depression, chronic dizziness, fatigue, headaches, subtle cognitive impairment, PTSD, and other physical health problems in the first 3 to 4 months after returning from deployment (Elder & Cristian, 2009; Heltemes, Holbrook, Macgregor, & Galarneau, 2012; Hoge et al., 2008). The sequela of bTBI can be temporary or chronic. Posttraumatic epilepsy (PTE) may also develop in 10%–25% of closed head TBI cases and in 50% of those with a penetrating head injury (Kovacs et al., 2014). The risk for developing PTE is correlated to the severity of TBI.

Moderate-to-severe bTBI occurs when the explosive blast causes gross structural brain damage. Cases present with altered mental status ranging from

TABLE 2.1
Department of Defense Classification of Traumatic Brain Injury

TBI	Casualties 2000–2014	Classification Definition
Concussion/ mild	253,350	A confused or disoriented state, which lasts less than 24 hours; loss of consciousness for up to 30 minutes; memory loss lasting less than 24 hours; and structural brain imaging (MRI or CT scan) yielding normal results.
Moderate	25,370	A confused or disoriented state, which lasts more than 24 hours; loss of consciousness for more than 30 minutes, but less than 24 hours; memory loss lasting greater than 24 hours, but less than 7 days; and structural brain imaging yielding normal or abnormal results.
Severe	3,088	A confused or disoriented state, which lasts more than 24 hours; loss of consciousness for more than 24 hours; memory loss for more than 7 days; and structural brain imaging yielding normal or abnormal results.
Penetrating	4,538	A head injury in which the dura mater, the outer layer of the meninges, is penetrated. Penetrating injuries can be caused by high-velocity projectiles or objects of lower velocity such as knives, or bone fragments from a skull fracture that are driven into the brain.
Not classifiable	20,937	

Note. From Fischer (2014).

confusion to lethargy to coma (Magnuson et al., 2012). Intracranial hemorrhage, skull fracture, cerebral edema, and parenchymal contusions appear clearly abnormal with neuroimaging (Davenport, Lim, Armstrong, & Sponheim, 2012). Cerebral vasospasm occurs in 50% of severe bTBI, and unlike concussive TBI, can present up to 30 days after the blast injury (Oertel et al., 2005).

The sudden change in ambient pressure of the body, secondary to the blast, causes injury primarily to organs that contain air, such as the lungs, or composed of tissues with varying specific weight, such as the ears and intestines (Elsayed, 1997; Guy, Glover, & Cripps, 2000; Mayorga, 1997). However, increasing evidence shows that even peripheral blast trauma without direct injury to the head causes secondary alterations in the brain (Cernak, Wang, Jiang, Bian, & Savic, 2001a; Trudeau et al., 1998). This can result from multiple factors, including kinetic energy transfer of blast overpressure/wave to the brain. Indirect bTBIs are the most frequent and challenging types because they are frequently without any external injuries. Individuals exposed to blast waves have been reported to suffer from both acute and chronic complex neuropsychiatric symptoms (Cernak, Savic, Lazarov, Joksimovic, & Markovic, 1999; Cernak et al., 2001a; Guy et al., 2000; Mayorga, 1997; Sylvia, Drake, & Wester, 2001; Trudeau et al., 1998).

The emotional and cognitive abnormalities implicate damage to various subcompartments of the hippocampus. The ventral hippocampus, along with the prefrontal cortex and amygdala, is involved in mediating anxiety-related functions. The dorsal part of the hippocampus is predominantly involved in mediating spatial learning and memory (Bannerman et al., 2004; McEwen, 2002). Pathologies affecting these brain regions and/or their afferent and efferent connections can be responsible for the observed emotional and cognitive impairments.

One of the most frequently occurring symptoms reported in bTBI patients is memory impairment. The limited numbers of studies using the rodent model of the injury have also demonstrated significant memory deficit and have identified some structural changes probably mediated by increased nitric oxide levels (Cernak et al., 2001a; Cernak, Wang, Jiang, Bian, & Savic, 2001b). These changes include neuronal swelling, altered dendritic morphology, glial reaction, and massive microglia invasion (Cernak et al., 1996; Elsayed, 1997; Guy et al., 2000; Kaur, Singh, Lim, Ng, & Ling, 1997; Kaur, Singh, Lim, Ng, Yap, et al., 1997; Mayorga, 1997; Saljo, Bao, Haglid, & Hansson, 2000).

PATHOLOGY OF BLAST-RELATED BRAIN INJURY

Blast-related TBI causes the loss of axons and neurons, leading to disrupted neuronal functions (Nortje & Menon, 2004). A cascade of humeral and cellular responses follows damage to the CNS parenchyma. Humeral components include the release of chemokines, cytokines, and other intercellular signaling molecules both from injured resident cells and from the cells that invade the damaged site (Landis, 1994). These soluble molecules are involved in coordinating the complex cellular response to injury including glia response and increased stem cell proliferation and de novo neurogenesis. The primary astroglia that participate in the early cellular response after TBI are called reactive astroglia because they appear hypertrophic with stellar-shaped morphology and elevated levels of glial fibrillary acidic protein, the astroglia-specific intermediate filament. Probably one of the most significant responses to TBI is the increased division of stem and progenitor cells in the adult hippocampus (Norton, 1999; Yoshimura et al., 2003).

CHRONIC TRAUMATIC ENCEPHALOPATHY

Research and clinical reports of bTBI often report the phenomena of injury as if it is a singular event; for some this may be accurate. Unfortunately, combat personnel are often chronically exposed to bTBI when using explosives during training, while deployed for offensive operations, as well as when attacked with IEDs or other explosive devices. The clinical presentation of chronic mild bTBI is similar to chronic traumatic encephalopathy (CTE), a tau protein–associated disorder that has been previously linked to neurodegenerative pathology in athletes who have experienced multiple chronic concussive TBI (McKee et al., 2009; McKee et al., 2010; Omalu et al., 2005). Presenting symptoms include executive dysfunction, affective lability, memory loss, cognitive deficit, and dementia.

In a recent and seminal work, Goldstein and colleagues (Goldstein et al., 2012) demonstrated that the neuropathology of CTE in athletes was similar to the CTE found in military personnel exposed to chronic bTBI and was differentiated from age-related dementia. Post-mortem brains from blast/concussion Veterans, athletes with multiple concussion injuries, and brains from control subjects were compared. Tau pathology with axon dystrophy and degeneration, with clusters of activated microglia were found in the Veterans brains. These signs of neuropathology were also found in a previously reported case of CTE as well as in the athlete subject group. None of the pathologic signs of CTE were found in the control group. This suggested that bTBI and CTE might have similar physiologic mechanisms and biomechanical causes. To verify the apparent relationship between bTBI and CTE, Goldstein developed a mouse model of blast neurotrauma where the mice were exposed to a single experimental air blast scaled to the intensity of common IED explosions. The mice were monitored by high-speed video, and it was found that the blast caused rapid acceleration–deceleration oscillatory movements of the head for 8 minutes (Goldstein et al., 2012). These rodent brains were sampled 2 weeks following the experimental blast and signs of neuroinflammation in the cortex, hippocampus, cerebellum, brainstem, and corticospinal tract were present. There was also evidence of phosphorylated tau neuropathology in the superficial cortical layers and hippocampus, along with a number of other signs of neuropathology. Functional changes in the brain were also compared to mice in which the head was immobile during the blast wave, preventing oscillation. Mice in the experimental blast group also demonstrated learning and memory deficits in behavioral tasks related to hippocampal function, while the immobilized group did not have these deficits. In summary, it was found that a single blast exposure was sufficient to cause brain pathology and memory impairment. This finding replicates the findings of Kovesdi and colleagues, conducted in an F344 rat model (Kovesdi et al., 2011).

The findings of Goldstein and colleagues are important, as the neuropathology found following bTBI were indistinguishable from the changes seen in sport-related CTE. This indicates that the underlying pathologic processes of CTE and bTBI are similar and that bTBI research could be examined in a sport concussive model.

Given the large numbers of veterans and current military exposed to chronic bTBI over multiple deployments since the start of the Operation Iraqi Freedom/Operation Enduring Freedom operations in Iraq and Afghanistan, it seems prudent that close clinical monitoring of the mental status and behavior of all blast-exposed military and veterans is warranted as well as of those reporting concussion from sport- or vehicle-associated trauma.

INTERVENTION POST-BTBI

To date, pharmacologic therapies for the treatment of bTBI in humans have yet to show efficacy. However, a few studies of bTBI in rodent models have shown the efficacy of selected drugs and behavioral measures to decrease anxiety and diminish gliosis and secondary damage to the brain. Enriched environments—group housing in large cages with toys—for rats exposed to a single mild bTBI appear to play a role in the recovery of memory functions but not in anxiety. Also, behavioral stimulation using enriched environments decreased IL-6 and IFNγ in the ventral hippocampus (Kovesdi et al., 2011). As a class of drugs, anti-inflammatory agents are being extensively studied. One of the first used acute minocycline administration to mitigate the symptoms of mild blast-induced traumatic brain injury, likely by reducing inflammation secondary to the injury (Kovesdi et al., 2012).

The TriService Nursing Research Program (TSNRP) is a unique program funding and supporting rigorous scientific research in the field of military nursing with a goal to advance military nursing science and optimize the health of military members and their families (Institute of Medicine Committee on Military Nursing Research, 1996). In the past 8 years, TSNRP has funded a number of military nurse scientists to study various aspects of TBI. Many of these studies are currently underway and a few have begun to present and publish their findings (TriService Nursing Research Program, 2014).

CONCLUSIONS

Research related to military-associated TBI continues to be a focus of significant importance both to the Department of Defense and to the Department of Veterans Affairs whose hospitals and clinical sites are charged with the immediate and long-term care of those recovering from these often-devastating injuries. Early care and effective transport of the injured has recently emerged as an area with extensive clinical nursing involvement (De Jong et al., 2008; Nagra, 2011). The Joint Theater Trauma System has been developed as a formal system of trauma care to improve the health-care outcomes for combat casualties in the current wars in Iraq and Afghanistan. As each injury and TBI is entered into this comprehensive database, it is hoped that it will provide the evidence for practice as well as form a basis to indicate where the future research in military-related TBI should focus. Unfortunately, as wars continue to emerge globally, the incidence of TBI will continue. It is hoped that improvements in care will promote effective intervention and recovery for the military and the veteran.

REFERENCES

Adams, G. W. (1952). *Doctors in blue; the medical history of the Union Army in the Civil War*. New York, NY: Henry Schuman.

Appleby, J., Rutty, G. N., Hainsworth, S. V., Woosnam-Savage, R. C., Morgan, B., Brough, A., et al. (2015). Perimortem trauma in King Richard III: a skeletal analysis. *The Lancet, 385*(9964), 253–259.

Bannerman, D. M., Rawlins, J. N., McHugh, S. B., Deacon, R. M., Yee, B. K., Bast, T., et al. (2004). Regional dissociations within the hippocampus—memory and anxiety. *Neuroscience & Biobehavioral Reviews*, *28*(3), 273–283. http://dx.doi.org/10.1016/j.neubiorev.2004.03.004

Bauman, R. A., Ling, G., Tong, L., Januszkiewicz, A., Agoston, D., Delanerolle, N., et al. (2009). An introductory characterization of a combat-casualty-care relevant swine model of closed head injury resulting from exposure to explosive blast. *Journal of Neurotrauma*, *26*(6), 841–860.

Cairns, H. S. (1941). Head injuries in motorcyclists: The importance of the crash helmet. *British Medical Journal*, 2(4213), 465–483.

Cairns, H. S. (1946). Crash helmets. *British Medical Journal*, *2*, 322–324.

Caveness, W. F. (1979). Incidence of craniocerebral trauma in the United States in 1976 with trend from 1970 to 1975. *Advances in Neurological*, 22, 1–3.

Cernak, I., Savic, J., Malicevic, Z., Zunic, G., Radosevic, P., Ivanovic, I., et al. (1996). Involvement of the central nervous system in the general response to pulmonary blast injury. *Journal of Trauma*, *40*(3 Suppl), S100–S104.

Cernak, I., Savic, V. J., Lazarov, A., Joksimovic, M., & Markovic, S. (1999). Neuroendocrine responses following graded traumatic brain injury in male adults. *Brain Injury*, *13*(12), 1005–1015.

Cernak, I., Wang, Z., Jiang, J., Bian, X., & Savic, J. (2001a). Cognitive deficits following blast injury-induced neurotrauma: possible involvement of nitric oxide. *Brain Injury*, *15*(7), 593–612.

Cernak, I., Wang, Z., Jiang, J., Bian, X., & Savic, J. (2001b). Ultrastructural and functional characteristics of blast injury-induced neurotrauma. *Journal of Trauma*, *50*(4), 695–706.

Champion, H. R., Holcomb, J. B., & Young, L. A. (2009). Injuries from explosions: Physics, biophysics, pathology, and required research focus. *Journal of Trauma-Injury, Infection, and Critical Care*, *66*(5), 1468–1477.

Cole, P. M. (2002). *Civil War artiliary at Gettsburg*. New York, NY: Da Capo Press.

Cullis, I. (2001). Blast waves and how they interact with structures. *Journal of the Royal Army Medical Corps*, *147*(1), 16–26.

Davenport, N. D., Lim, K. O., Armstrong, M. T., & Sponheim, S. R. (2012). Diffuse and spatially variable white matter disruptions are associated with blast-related mild traumatic brain injury. *NeuroImage*, *59*(3), 2017–2024. http://dx.doi.org/10.1016/j.neuroimage.2011.10.050

De Jong, M. J., Martin, K. D., Huddleston, M., Spott, M. A., McCoy, J., Black, J. A., et al. (2008). Performance improvement on the battlefield. *Journal of Trauma Nursing*, *15*(4), 174–180. http://dx.doi.org/10.1097/01.JTN.0000343322.70334.12

Dean, B. (1927). Helmets and body armor- the medical viewpoint. In M. Ireland (Ed.), *The Medical Department of the United States Army in the World War* (Vol. 9, pp. 1–8). Washington, DC: Government Printing Office.

Denny-Brown, D., & Russell, W. (1941). Experimental cerebral concusion. *Brain*, *64*, 93–164.

DePalma, R. G., Burris, D. G., Champion, H. R., & Hodgson, M. J. (2005). Blast injuries. *New England Journal of Medicine*, *352*(13), 1335–1342.

Elder, G. A., & Cristian, A. (2009). Blast-related mild traumatic brain injury: Mechanisms of injury and impact on clinical care. *The Mount Sinai Journal of Medicine, New York*, *76*(2), 111–118. http://dx.doi.org/10.1002/msj.20098

Elsayed, N., & Atkins, J. (2008). *Explosion and blast-related injuries*. Burlington, MA: Elsevier Inc.

Elsayed, N. M. (1997). Toxicology of blast overpressure. *Toxicology*, *121*(1), 1–15.

Fischer, H. (2014). A Guide to U.S. Military Casualty Statistics: Peration New Dawn, Operation Iraqi Freedom, and Operation Enduring Freedom CRS Report for Congress. Washington, DC : Congressional Research Service.

Fulton, J. (1942). Blast and concussion in the present war. *New England Journal of Medicine*, *226*, 1–8.

Gabriel, R. A., & Metz, K. S. (1992). A short history of war: The evolution of warfare and weapons. *Professional Readings in Military Strategy, No. 5*. Retrieved October 1, 2014 from http://www.au.af.mil/au/awc/awcgate/gabrmetz/gabr0000.htm

Gawande, A. (2004). Casualties of war—military care for the wounded from Iraq and Afghanistan. *The New England Journal of Medicine*, *351*(24), 2471–2475. http://dx.doi.org/10.1056/NEJMp048317

Goldstein, L. E., Fisher, A. M., Tagge, C. A., Zhang, X. L., Velisek, L., Sullivan, J. A., et al. (2012). Chronic traumatic encephalopathy in blast-exposed military veterans and a blast neurotrauma mouse model. *Science Translation Medicine*, *4*(134), 134ra160. http://dx.doi.org/10.1126/scitranslmed.3003716

Gupta, R. K., & Przekwas, A. (2013). Mathematical models of blast-induced TBI: Current status, challenges, and prospects. *Frontiers in Neurology*, *4*, 59. http://dx.doi.org/10.3389/fneur.2013.00059

Guy, R. J., Glover, M. A., & Cripps, N. P. (2000). Primary blast injury: Pathophysiology and implications for treatment. Part III: Injury to the central nervous system and the limbs. *Journal of the Royal Naval Medical Service*, *86*(1), 27–31.

Heltemes, K. J., Holbrook, T. L., Macgregor, A. J., & Galarneau, M. R. (2012). Blast-related mild traumatic brain injury is associated with a decline in self-rated health amongst US military personnel. *Injury*, *43*(12), 1990–1995. http://dx.doi.org/10.1016/j.injury.2011.07.021

Hoge, C. W., McGurk, D., Thomas, J. L., Cox, A. L., Engel, C. C., & Castro, C. A. (2008). Mild traumatic brain injury in U.S. Soldiers returning from Iraq. *The New England Journal of Medicine*, *358*(5), 453–463. http://dx.doi.org/10.1056/NEJMoa072972

Holbourn, A. (1943). Mechanics of head injury. *Lancet*, *242*, 438–441.

Holbourn, A. (1945). The mechanics of brain injuries. *British Medical Bulletin*, *3*, 147–149.

Holmes, G., & Lister, W. (1916). Disturbances of vision from cerebral lesions, with special reference to the cortical representation of the macula. *Brain*, *39*, 34–73.

Institute of Medicine Committee on Military Nursing Research. (1996). *The program for research in military nursing: Progress and future direction*. Washington, DC: Institute of Medicine.

Iserson, K. V., & Moskop, J. C. (2007). Triage in medicine, part I: Concept, history, and types. *Annals of Emergency Medicine*, *49*(3), 275–281. http://dx.doi.org/10.1016/j.annemergmed.2006.05.019

Jones, E., Fear, N. T., & Wessely, S. (2007). Shell shock and mild traumatic brain injury: A historical review. *American Journal of Psychiatry*, *164*(11), 1641–1645. http://dx.doi.org/10.1176/appi.ajp.2007.07071180

Jones, E., Thomas, A., & Ironside, S. (2007). Shell shock: An outcome study of a First World War 'PIE' unit. *Psychological Medicine*, *37*(2), 215–223. http://dx.doi.org/10.1017/S0033291706009329

Jones, E., Vermaas, R. H., McCartney, H., Beech, C., Palmer, I., Hyams, K., et al. (2003). Flashbacks and post-traumatic stress disorder: The genesis of a 20th-century diagnosis. *British Journal of Psychiatry*, *182*, 158–163.

Jones, E., & Wessely, S. (2003). "Forward psychiatry" in the military: Its origins and effectiveness. *Journal of Traumatic Stress*, *16*(4), 411–419. http://dx.doi.org/10.1023/A:1024426321072

Kalinich, J. F., & Kasper, C. E. (2014). Do metals that translocate to the brain exacerbate traumatic brain injury? *Medical Hypotheses*, *82*(5), 558–562. http://dx.doi.org/10.1016/j.mehy.2014.02.011

Kambouchev, N., Radovitzky, R., & Noels, L. (2007). Fluid–structure interaction effects in the dynamic response of free-standing plates to uniform shock loading. *Journal of Applied Mechanics*, *74*(5), 1042–1045.

Kaur, C., Singh, J., Lim, M. K., Ng, B. L., & Ling, E. A. (1997). Macrophages/microglia as 'sensors' of injury in the pineal gland of rats following a non-penetrative blast. *Neuroscience Research*, *27*(4), 317–322.

Kaur, C., Singh, J., Lim, M. K., Ng, B. L., Yap, E. P., & Ling, E. A. (1997). Ultrastructural changes of macroglial cells in the rat brain following an exposure to a non-penetrative blast. *Annals of the Academy of Medicine, Singapore*, *26*(1), 27–29.

Kovacs, S. K., Leonessa, F., & Ling, G. S. (2014). Blast TBI models, neuropathology, and implications for seizure risk. *Frontiers in Neurology*, *5*, 47. http://dx.doi.org/10.3389/fneur.2014.00047

Kovesdi, E., Gyorgy, A. B., Kwon, S. K., Wingo, D. L., Kamnaksh, A., Long, J. B., et al. (2011). The effect of enriched environment on the outcome of traumatic brain injury; a behavioral, proteomics, and histological study. *Frontiers in Neuroscience*, *5*, 42. http://dx.doi.org/10.3389/fnins.2011.00042

Kovesdi, E., Kamnaksh, A., Wingo, D., Ahmed, F., Grunberg, N. E., Long, J. B., et al. (2012). Acute minocycline treatment mitigates the symptoms of mild blast-induced traumatic brain injury. *Frontiers in Neurology*, *3*, 111. http://dx.doi.org/10.3389/fneur.2012.00111

Landis, D. M. (1994). The early reactions of non-neuronal cells to brain injury. *Annual Review of Neuroscience*, *17*(1), 133–151.

Lanska, D. J. (2009). Historical perspective: Neurological advances from studies of war injuries and illnesses. *Annals of Neurology*, *66*(4), 444–459. http://dx.doi.org/10.1002/ana.21822

Ling, G., Bandak, F., Armonda, R., Grant, G., & Ecklund, J. (2009). Explosive blast neurotrauma. *Journal of Neurotrauma*, *26*(6), 815–825. http://dx.doi.org/10.1089/neu.2007.0484

Ling, G. S., & Ecklund, J. M. (2011). Traumatic brain injury in modern war. *Current Opinion in Anaesthesiology*, *24*(2), 124–130. http://dx.doi.org/10.1097/ACO.0b013e32834458da

Livermore, T. L. (1957). *Numbers & losses in the Civil War in America, 1861-65*. Bloomington, IN: Indiana University Press.

Livy. (1965). *The war with Hannibal; books XXI-XXX of The History of Rome from its foundation* (Vol. 22). Baltimore, MD: Penguin Books.

Maartens, N. F., Wills, A. D., & Adams, C. B. (2002). Lawrence of Arabia, Sir Hugh Cairns, and the origin of motorcycle helmets. *Neurosurgery*, *50*(1), 176–179; discussion 179–180.

Mac Donald, C. L., Johnson, A. M., Cooper, D., Nelson, E. C., Werner, N. J., Shimony, J. S., et al. (2011). Detection of blast-related traumatic brain injury in US military personnel. *New England Journal of Medicine*, *364*(22), 2091–2100.

Magnuson, J., Leonessa, F., & Ling, G. S. (2012). Neuropathology of explosive blast traumatic brain injury. *Current Neurology and Neuroscience Reports*, *12*(5), 570–579. http://dx.doi.org/10.1007/s11910-012-0303-6

Mayorga, M. A. (1997). The pathology of primary blast overpressure injury. *Toxicology*, *121*(1), 17–28. http://dx.doi.org/S0300483X97036524

McDonald, I. (2007). Gordon Holmes Lecture: Gordon Holmes and the neurological heritage. *Brain*, *130*(Pt 1), 288–298. http://dx.doi.org/10.1093/brain/awl335

McEwen, B. S. (2002). Sex, stress and the hippocampus: Allostasis, allostatic load and the aging process. *Neurobiology of Aging*, *23*(5), 921–939.

McKee, A. C., Cantu, R. C., Nowinski, C. J., Hedley-Whyte, E. T., Gavett, B. E., Budson, A. E., et al. (2009). Chronic traumatic encephalopathy in athletes: Progressive tauopathy following repetitive head injury. *Journal of Neuropathology and Experimental Neurology*, *68*(7), 709.

McKee, A. C., Gavett, B. E., Stern, R. A., Nowinski, C. J., Cantu, R. C., Kowall, N. W., et al. (2010). TDP-43 proteinopathy and motor neuron disease in chronic traumatic encephalopathy. *Journal of Neuropathology and Experimental Neurology*, *69*(9), 918.

Mcleod, A. D. (2004). Shell shock, Gordon Holmes and the Great War. *Journal of the Royal Society of Medicine*, *97*(2), 86–89.

Meyers, S. (1915). A contribution to the study of Shell Shock. *Lancet*, *1*, 316–320.

Moore, D. F., Radovitzky, R. A., Shupenko, L., Klinoff, A., Jaffee, M. S., & Rosen, J. M. (2008). Blast physics and central nervous system injury. *Future Neurology*, *3*(3), 243–250.

Mott, F. (1916a). The effects of high explosives on the central nervous system. *Lancet*, *1*, 332–353.

Mott, F. (1916b). Special discussion on shell shock without visible signs of injury. *Proceedings of the Royal Society of Medicine*, *9*, i–xxiv.

Nagra, M. (2011). Optimizing wartime en route nursing care in Operation Iraqi Freedom. *US Army Medical Department Journal*, Oct/Dec, 51–58.

Nortje, J., & Menon, D. K. (2004). Traumatic brain injury: Physiology, mechanisms, and outcome. *Current Opinion in Neurology*, *17*(6), 711–718.

Norton, W. T. (1999). Cell reactions following acute brain injury: A review. *Neurochemical Research*, *24*(2), 213–218.

Oertel, M., Boscardin, W. J., Obrist, W. D., Glenn, T. C., McArthur, D. L., Gravori, T., et al. (2005). Posttraumatic vasospasm: The epidemiology, severity, and time course of an underestimated phenomenon: A prospective study performed in 299 patients. *Journal of Neurosurgery*, *103*(5), 812–824. http://dx.doi.org/10.3171/jns.2005.103.5.0812

Okie, S. (2005). Traumatic brain injury in the war zone. *The New England Journal of Medicine*, *352*(20), 2043–2047. http://dx.doi.org/10.1056/NEJMp058102

Omalu, B. I., DeKosky, S. T., Minster, R. L., Kamboh, M. I., Hamilton, R. L., & Wecht, C. H. (2005). Chronic traumatic encephalopathy in a National Football League player. *Neurosurgery*, *57*(1), 128–134.

Ommaya, A. K., Goldsmith, W., & Thibault, L. (2002). Biomechanics and neuropathology of adult and paediatric head injury. *British Journal of Neurosurgery*, *16*(3), 220–242.

Ommaya, A. K., Grubb, R. L., Jr., & Naumann, R. A. (1971). Coup and contre-coup injury: Observations on the mechanics of visible brain injuries in the rhesus monkey. *Journal of Neurosurgery*, *35*(5), 503–516. http://dx.doi.org/10.3171/jns.1971.35.5.0503

Pudenz, R. H., & Shelden, C. H. (1946). The lucite calvarium; a method for direct observation of the brain; cranial trauma and brain movement. *Journal of Neurosurgery*, *3*(6), 487–505.

Rish, B. L., Dillon, J. D., & Weiss, G. H. (1983). Mortality following penetrating craniocerebral injuries. An analysis of the deaths in the Vietnam Head Injury Registry population. *Journal of Neurosurgery*, *59*(5), 775–780. http://dx.doi.org/10.3171/jns.1983.59.5.0775

Saljo, A., Bao, F., Haglid, K. G., & Hansson, H. A. (2000). Blast exposure causes redistribution of phosphorylated neurofilament subunits in neurons of the adult rat brain. *Journal of Neurotrauma*, *17*(8), 719–726.

Salmon, T. (1917). The care and treatment of mental diseases and war neuroses ("shell shock") in the British army. *Mental Hygiene*, *1*, 309–347.

Shephard, B. A. (2000). *A war of nerves: Soldiers and psychiatrists 1914-1994*. London: Jonathan Cape.

Strehlow, R. A., & Baker, W. E. (1976). The characterization and evaluation of accidental explosions. *Progress in Energy and Combustion Science*, 2(1), 27–60.

Stuhmiller, J. H., Masiello, P. J., Ho, K. H., Mayorga, M. A., Lawless, N., & Argyros, G. (1999). Biomechanical modeling of injury from blast overpressure. Paper presented at the Proceedings of the Specialists' Meeting of the RTO Human Factors and Medicine Panel, Wright-Patterson Air Force Base, OH.

Sylvia, F. R., Drake, A. I., & Wester, D. C. (2001). Transient vestibular balance dysfunction after primary blast injury. *Military Medicine*, *166*(10), 918–920.

Thama, C., Tanh, V., & Leea, H. (2008). Ballistic impact of a KEVLAR® helmet: Experiment and simulations. *International Journal of Impact Engineering*, *35*(5), 304–318. http://dx.doi.org/10.1016/j.ijimpeng.2007.03.008

TriService Nursing Research Program. (2014). *Funded Studies*. Retrieved September 15, 2014 from http://www.usuhs.mil/tsnrp/FundedStudies/funded.php

Trudeau, D. L., Anderson, J., Hansen, L. M., Shagalov, D. N., Schmoller, J., Nugent, S., et al. (1998). Findings of mild traumatic brain injury in combat veterans with PTSD and a history of blast concussion. *The Journal of Neuropsychiatry and Clinical Neurosciences*, *10*(3), 308–313.

Weiss, E. D. (2001). The second sacrifice: Costly advances in medicine and surgery during the Civil War. *The Yale Journal of Biology and Medicine*, *74*(3), 169–177.

Yoshimura, S., Teramoto, T., Whalen, M. J., Irizarry, M. C., Takagi, Y., Qiu, J., et al. (2003). FGF-2 regulates neurogenesis and degeneration in the dentate gyrus after traumatic brain injury in mice. *The Journal of Clinical Investigation*, *112*(8), 1202–1210.

CHAPTER 3

Animal Models of Traumatic Brain Injury

Is There an Optimal Model That Parallels Human Brain Injury?

Teresita L. Briones

ABSTRACT

Traumatic brain injury (TBI) is the leading cause of mortality and morbidity in the younger population worldwide. Survivors of TBI often experience long-term disability in the form of cognitive, sensorimotor, and affective impairments. Despite the high prevalence in, and cost of TBI to, both individuals and society, some of its underlying pathophysiology is not completely understood. Animal models have been developed over the past few decades to closely replicate the different facets of TBI in humans to better understand the underlying pathophysiology and behavioral impairments and assess potential therapies that can promote neuroprotection. However, no effective treatment for TBI has been established to date in the clinical setting, despite promising results generated in preclinical studies in the use of neuroprotective strategies. The failure to translate results from preclinical studies to the clinical setting underscores a compelling need to revisit the current state of knowledge in the use of animal models in TBI.

http://dx.doi.org/10.1891/0739-6686.33.31

INTRODUCTION

Traumatic brain injury (TBI), broadly defined, encompasses any damage to the brain resulting from any external mechanical force that can cause rapid acceleration or deceleration, blast waves, crush, and impact or penetration by a projectile. TBI results in altered brain function leading to temporary or permanent impairment of cognitive, physical, and psychosocial functions and is the major cause of death and disability for people under the age of 45 years (Langlois, Rutland-Brown, & Wald, 2006). TBI is often referred to as a *silent epidemic* because of the fact that it ranks as the leading cause of mortality and disability in the young population worldwide (Langlois, Marr, Mitchko, & Johnson, 2005). Reports show that someone in the United States suffers a TBI every 18.5 seconds (Faul, Xu, & Wald, 2010). Indeed, worldwide, 10 million deaths and/or hospitalizations annually are directly attributable to TBI (Masel & DeWitt, 2010); in the United states alone, the Centers for Disease Control and Prevention estimates that during 2002–2006, approximately 1.7 million Americans per year (new cases) suffered from TBI (Faul, Xu, & Wald, 2010). This estimate is higher than the incidence of Alzheimer's disease, Parkinson's disease, and multiple sclerosis combined, and greater than the incidence of individuals diagnosed with brain, breast, colon, lung, and prostate cancer combined (Corrigan, Selassie, & Orman, 2010). What is most alarming is that this estimate does not include data from military personnel, where the signature injury of those who served in the Iraq and/or Afghanistan wars is TBI related. It is estimated that nearly 60% of all casualties among soldiers admitted to Walter Reed National Military Medical Center suffer from TBI (Ling & Ecklund, 2011). Furthermore, the Department of Defense Medical Surveillance System estimates that the number of personnel who experienced some degree of TBI between the years 2000 and 2013 was 266,810 (AFHS Center, 2013).

The purpose of this review is to succinctly summarize the current knowledge on preclinical reports in modeling the pathogenesis and the common rehabilitation strategies related to TBI and to demonstrate how data generated from these animal studies are clinically relevant. In doing this review, the PubMed and Scopus databases were searched using keywords such as *TBI* and *animal models*, which initially yielded 675 articles and none were published in nursing journals. The search was limited to the last 20 years because the use of animal models in the field of TBI research continues to evolve. More focused searches using keywords *adults*, *cognitive impairment*, and *nonpharmacologic therapy* returned less than 300 results, the majority of which are articles on mild TBI. The inclusion criteria used in this review comprised studies that: (a) were original data-based papers; (b) used established measures of morphological and behavioral outcomes of TBI; (c) were studies in rats and mice only; and (d) were studies that included shams as comparison control groups. Additionally, studies on TBI models using young animals were excluded. These filtering strategies resulted in the exclusion of more than half of the articles generated for the review.

Are Animal Models of TBI Clinically Relevant?

Most pathophysiological and neurobehavioral consequences of TBI may be reproduced using an animal model even if it is not possible to mimic the entire complexity of TBI effects. In determining whether the use of animal models of TBI is clinically relevant, it is important to focus the discussion in terms of its validity and reliability. Questions on the face and construct validity and predictive validity and reliability of using an animal model that need to be addressed are (a) *face validity*, which refers to the phenomenological similarity in the behavior being examined between the animals used to model the condition and humans. Because it is unrealistic to expect exactly similar behaviors in rodents and humans, the aim is to search for relevant equivalents in the behavior based upon the brain regions assumed to be involved; (b) *construct validity*, which refers to the similarity in underlying mechanisms even though the precise expression of behaviors may be different in animals and humans; and (c) *predictive validity and reliability*, which, respectively, refer to (i) the predictive value that observations made in animals will be similar or equivalent to the human condition, and (ii) to the similarity in the accuracy with which both the experimental and the clinical observations are made. When studying behavioral consequences of TBI using animal models, at the minimum, issues of predictive validity and reliability should be met.

MODELING TBI USING ANIMALS

Animal models of TBI have always been an important element in the study of how the central nervous system (CNS) responds to injury. The ultimate goal in using animal models is to reproduce in the laboratory setting the clinically relevant and standardized patterns of brain injury that closely reflect the morphological, biochemical, molecular, and behavioral changes seen following TBI. Several animal models of TBI have been developed since the 1980s using a variety of species including cats, dogs, and nonhuman primates. But in the 1990s, the use of rodents dominated the research in the field of TBI, and to date, it is the most widely used approach in preclinical studies. Several issues contributed to the preponderance of rodent models such as ethical issues in the use of nonhuman primates as well as the need to establish complex surgical facilities to accommodate their postsurgery needs; cost and availability involved in using larger animals; and the simplicity of carrying out the procedures required in using rodent models. At present, several types of animal models of TBI exist that use rodents, and the advantages and disadvantages of each model are discussed in the following text.

Fluid Percussion Injury Model

The fluid percussion injury (FPI) model is among the most commonly used models in studying TBI and there are several types available, but generally, head injury is inflicted following a craniotomy using a weighted pendulum positioned at a desired height that strikes the piston of a reservoir of fluid creating a fluid wave that impacts against the intact dura. The craniotomy is created using the skull coordinates, and a fluid wave is generated either centrally around the midline between the bregma and lambda or laterally over the parietal bone between the bregma and lambda (McIntosh, Noble, Andrews, & Faden, 1987; McIntosh et al., 1989). The FPI injury model produces a brief displacement and deformation of brain tissue, and the severity of injury depends on the strength of the fluid wave (McIntosh et al., 1989).

The FPI model of TBI produces a combination of focal cortical contusion and diffuse subcortical neuronal injury including injury in the hippocampus and thalamus. The FPI model also causes blood–brain barrier (BBB) disruption, intracranial hemorrhage, brain swelling, and sometimes cavity formation. The damage produced by the FPI model occurs within minutes of the impact with progressive loss of neurons, but the damage does not markedly expand into the contralateral brain regions (Hicks, Soares, Smith, & McIntosh, 1996). Conversely, the progressive neuronal degeneration that occurs beneath the contused cortex can continue to expand up to 1 year after injury owing to ongoing cell death (Bramlett & Dietrich, 2002). Over days to months after injury, the progressive degenerative cascade can persist in selectively vulnerable brain areas in the ipsilateral regions such as the hippocampus, thalamus, medial septum, striatum, and amygdala (Hicks et al., 1996, Liu et al., 2010).

Strengths and Weaknesses

The FPI models replicate the common pathophysiological features seen in human TBI (Thompson et al., 2005). Another advantage of the FPI is that it is highly reproducible, and the investigator can regulate the severity of TBI. However, since this model does not produce skull fracture and results mainly in focal injury, it cannot replicate moderate-to-severe TBI in humans where skull fractures and contusions across multiple brain regions are present (Hardman & Manoukian, 2002). The two FPI models are midline where the injury is induced at the center of the sagittal suture and lateral where the injury is induced approximately 3.5 mm left or right of the sagittal suture (McIntosh et al., 1987; McIntosh et al.,

1989). The midline FPI was the first developed model, which was then modified and subsequently adapted for use in rats to produce the lateral FPI; the lateral FPI model is the most widely used (Thompson et al., 2005) for studying TBI pathophysiology and pharmacology. The site of craniotomy is crucial in determining the extent and location of tissue injury produced by the FPI model (Vink, Mullins, Temple, Bao, & Faden, 2001). Lateral FPI primarily results in unilateral cortical damage, and involvement of the contralateral cortex and brain stem is rare, whereas midline FPI causes bilateral cortical alterations associated with direct axial movement of the lower brain stem causing apnea (Dixon et al., 1987); this injury is the reason that there is a higher mortality rate associated with midline FPI compared to other models.

Controlled Cortical Impact Injury Model

In the controlled cortical impact (CCI) injury model, a craniotomy is performed between the bregma and lambda, and a pneumatic or electromagnetic impact device is used to drive a rigid impactor to deliver mechanical force onto the exposed, intact dura, causing a deformity in the underlying cortex. The controlled impact is delivered to the intact dura through a unilateral craniotomy between the bregma and lambda, which causes deformation of the underlying cortex (Dixon, Clifton, Lighthall, Yaghmai, & Hayes, 1991). The CCI model is considered to induce focal injury, but in some instances, diffuse damage can occur. The damage induced by the CCI model occurs proximal to the mechanical impact and induces injury to both cortical and subcortical structures (Dixon et al., 1991).

The injury created by the CCI model mimics the cortical tissue loss, acute subdural hematoma, axonal injury, concussion, contusion, BBB dysfunction, and even coma (Lighthall, 1988; Marmarou et al., 1994) seen in human TBI. A comprehensive neuropathological evaluation of the CCI TBI model revealed that ventricular enlargement is also seen following CCI (Dixon et al., 1987). The damage induced by CCI can persist up to 1 year after injury, and the accompanying neurological deficit may be associated with brain atrophy (Lighthall, 1988; Dixon et al., 1991; Pierce, Smith, Trojanowski, & McIntosh, 1998) and progressive decline in cerebral blood flow (Kochanek et al., 2002).

Strengths and Weaknesses

The advantage of CCI over other TBI models is that the time, velocity, and depth of impact can be controlled, making it more useful in studying the biomechanical changes that occur following TBI (Dixon et al., 1991). An additional advantage of the CCI injury compared with other models is the lack of rebound injury because the impact delivered by the device is gravity driven (Lighthall, 1988).

The severity of CCI-induced injury increases proportionally with the degree of impact delivered and the resulting cortical deformity; thus, this model is ideal for experimental purposes in studying the consequences of mild, moderate, and severe TBI (Goodman, Cherian, Bryan, & Robertson, 1994; Saatman, Feeko, Pape, & Raghupathi, 2006). The CCI model also has low mortality rate compared to most TBI models (Dixon et al., 1991). The disadvantage is similar to that of the FPI model in that only unilateral damage is produced, with rare involvement of the contralateral cortex. Furthermore, the need for a craniotomy could be a disadvantage in using this TBI model.

Weight-Drop TBI Model

In weight-drop models, a free-falling guided weight is dropped onto the skull, which can be exposed either with or without craniotomy (Morales et al., 2005). The severity of injury induced by these models can be regulated by adjusting the weight mass and the height from which it falls. There are three commonly used weight-drop models: *Feeney's model* where the weight is delivered to the intact dura through a craniotomy, which produces cortical contusion (Feeney, Boyeson, Linn, Murray, & Dail, 1981) and *Shohami's model*, which mimics a closed head injury where the weight-drop impact is delivered without craniotomy to one side of an unprotected skull (Chen, Constantini, Trembovler, Weinstock, & Shohami, 1996) while the head is placed on a hard surface. This closed head injury model can cause focal blunt trauma to the unprotected skull (Flierl et al., 2009) and breakdown of the BBB resulting from the impact. *Marmarou's* (Marmarou et al., 1994) is another weight-drop head injury model that produces an impact acceleration injury, which mimics the diffuse axonal injury seen in human TBI, typically caused by falls or motor vehicle accidents (Johnson, Stewart, & Smith, 2013). Of all the weight-drop models, Marmarou's is the most commonly used in experimental studies. In this model, an anesthetized rat is strapped on a foam block with the skull exposed through a midline incision between the lambda and bregma. The use of the foam enables the dorsal/ventral acceleration of the unrestrained head. A stainless steel disc is mounted with glue to the skull to prevent fracture when the weight is dropped. Trauma is induced using a device consisting of a brass weight that is set to fall freely from a desired height through a Plexiglas tube, and dropping the brass weight onto the stainless steel disc distributes the energy diffusely over the brain, causing widespread axonal damage, while maintaining an intact cranium.

More recently, a modification of Marmarou's model has been developed to reproduce the frontal impact commonly encountered in motor vehicle and sports accidents (Kilbourne et al., 2009). This new TBI model is known as the Maryland model where the impact force is applied to the anterior part of the cranium and produces TBI by causing anterior–posterior plus sagittal rotational acceleration of the brain inside the intact cranium (Kilbourne et al., 2009). The Maryland model is also a closed head injury type that produces diffuse damage via the coup-contrecoup action.

The damage produced by Feeney's model includes cortical contusion that progresses to intracerebral hemorrhage during the first few hours of injury (Dail, Feeney, Murray, Linn, & Boyeson, 1981; Feeney et al., 1981). Meanwhile, both the Shohami and Marmarou models are characterized by widespread and bilateral damage of neurons, axons, dendrites, and microvasculature as well as extensive diffuse axonal injury, particularly in the corpus callosum, internal capsule, optic tracts, cerebral and cerebellar peduncles, and the long tracts in the brain stem (Foda & Marmarou, 1994; Albert-Weissenberger, Varrallyay, Raslan, Kleinschnitz, & Sirén, 2012); however, the presence of skull fracture is only seen in the Shohami model (Chen et al., 1996). The Maryland model on the other hand can cause concussion but not contusion, and skull fracture is also absent but cortical petechial hemorrhages and diffuse axonal injury are common.

Strengths and Weaknesses

The weight-drop injury models, specifically the Marmarou, mimics closed head injury with accompanying concussion and contusion, a common type of TBI in humans. Moreover, it is inexpensive, easy to perform, and capable of producing graded diffuse axonal injury. A major disadvantage of the weight-drop models is the relatively high variability in injury severity that is produced. Furthermore, mortality is higher in weight-drop models compared to CCI because respiratory depression is common due to brain stem injury (Foda & Marmarou, 1994; Marmarou et al., 1994). In addition, the Maryland model needs further characterization, and more studies are needed to establish its reproducibility.

Penetrating Ballistic-Like Brain Injury Model

The penetrating ballistic-like brain injury (PBBI) is a model of focal brain injury, even though in some instances, it can also result in diffuse damage. The PBBI model mimics the damage caused by gunshot wounds to the brain. The injury produced by this model results from the transmission of projectiles with high energy accompanied by a shock wave that then creates a temporary cavity in the brain that is larger than the size of the projectile itself (Williams et al., 2005). Specifically, the injury is created by inserting a probe with an inflatable balloon at the tip into the desired location in the brain followed by fast inflation of the balloon to mimic the cavity produced by a penetrating bullet. The injury severity caused by the PBBI model is directly related to the anatomical path of the projectile and the degree of energy transfer (Williams et al., 2006, Williams, Ling, & Tortella, 2006).

The PBBI model mimics the ballistic effect in brain trauma. Several pathophysiological characteristics of PBBI are similar to those reported in other brain trauma models, including the presence of hemispheric swelling, increased intracranial pressure, and white matter injury as well as neuroinflammation in brain regions remote from the core lesion (Williams et al., 2006). Aside from the white matter, marked gray matter damage and increased blood–brain permeability as well as seizures are also seen in PBBI. Even though PBBI is considered to be a model of focal brain injury, it can result in intracerebral hemorrhage and degeneration of neurons and fiber tracts remote from the core lesion (Williams et al., 2006; Williams et al., 2006).

Strengths and Weaknesses

The PBBI rat model is helpful in characterizing the immediate and subacute (up to 7 days) changes in intracranial pressure seen after brain trauma (Wei, Lu, Yang, Tortella, 2010). The model also captures several unique temporal aspects of a ballistic brain injury and may be a highly relevant model of moderate-to-severe brain trauma for mechanistic studies. However, compared to other TBI models, PBBI causes extensive intracerebral hemorrhage on the primary lesion site owing to the penetrating nature of the injury and the temporary cavity that it forms to truly model gunshot wound injuries to the brain. However, its primary disadvantage concerns the expertise required of the investigator performing the procedure. Furthermore, this TBI model is associated with a high mortality rate because of the complete loss of brain tissue created by the ballistic impact.

Blast Injury Model

With the increasing incidence of TBI among military personnel involved in modern warfare, it became necessary to develop another TBI model because the existing ones could not mimic the blast-induced mild TBI increasingly reported. According to a Rand Corporation study, it is estimated that approximately 19% of the returning service personnel had mild TBI in 2008 alone, and many of them did not have external injuries (Warden, 2006; Cernak & Noble-Haeussein, 2010). Many of the mild TBI cases reported among service personnel are associated with exposure to blast waves caused by improvised explosive devices (Warden, 2006; Benzinger, 2009). To elucidate the effects of primary blast waves on the CNS, animal models of blast TBI have been established, mainly in rodents (Long et al., 2009; Cheng 2010) and swine (Bauman et al., 2009; de Lanerolle et al., 2011). In this model, a long compression-driven metal tube that is closed on one end is used to deliver blast waves. An air pressure wave or an explosion is used to deliver over or underpressure waves beginning at the closed end of the tube, while the animal wearing a Kevlar vest to protect the thoracic cavity is placed at the open end of the tube to receive the shock wave affecting the whole body as well as the head (Risling & Davidsson, 2012). The Kevlar vest encases the thorax and part of the abdomen so that mortality associated with the systemic effects of the blast wave, specifically hypotension and lung injury or hemorrhage (DeWitt & Prough, 2009), is greatly reduced.

Injury induced by blast is interestingly different from other forms of TBI. Blast injury is characterized by diffuse cerebral brain edema, intracranial hemorrhage, and delayed vasospasm (de Lanerolle et al., 2011). Diffuse axonal injury is the most prominent feature during the initial 2 weeks following blast exposure in rats with body shielding (Cernak et al., 2011). Other common damages induced by the blast injury model include neuronal degeneration, reactive gliosis, and neuroinflammation (de Lanerolle et al., 2011).

Strengths and Weaknesses

The blast-induced model developed in rats mimics the real morphological damage seen in the personnel who sustained TBI from the military conflicts in Iraq and Afghanistan. This model is superior to other animal models of TBI in mimicking the injury seen in the battlefield because it does not involve direct impact to create the injury but still results in the unique pathological features seen in blast-induced mild TBI. For example, a pathological feature seen in blast injury that is not common in most TBI models is chronic traumatic encephalopathy (CTE), a condition characterized by the presence of neurofibrillary tangles as a result of hyperphosphorylated tau associated with progressive neurodegeneration (Goldstein et al., 2012; Magnuson, Leonessa, & Ling, 2012). Current blast TBI models focus mainly on reproducing the morphological injury due to blast waves; however, they do not replicate the posttraumatic seizures, a common consequence of blast-induced mild TBI seen in humans. Therefore, finding an ideal and reliable experimental blast induced TBI model that can produce equivalent symptomatic characteristics of the injury seen in human is still in progress.

Repetitive Brain Injury Model

With increasing recognition that repeated mild TBI commonly observed in athletes (soccer, football, boxing, ice hockey, etc.) may have cumulative adverse effects on cognitive function, several studies have attempted to reproduce the clinical consequences of repetitive mild TBI. Several models have been developed using versions of the weight drop, modified versions of the CCI or FPI, and momentum exchange methods in lightly anesthetized animals where injury is induced at repeated intervals, up to four times, to produce mild concussive insults (reviewed in Weber, 2007). Results from studies on repetitive mild TBI show that motor function is impaired and that axonal pathology is increased if the second injury and subsequent injuries occur within a 3- to 5-day period of the first trauma, but no skull fracture and increase in BBB permeability are seen (Laurer et al., 2001; Longhi et al., 2005). Additionally, animals exposed to five head impacts (1 per day for 5 days) show delays in recovery of the righting reflex (recovery of consciousness) by comparison to controls, and a transient decrement in balance and coordination is also evident after repeated injury (Allen, Gerami, & Esser, 2000; Angoa-Perez et al., 2014). Further, rats that receive repeated mild TBI show greater cognitive impairment evidenced by poor performance in the Barnes maze when compared to controls (DeFord et al., 2002; Creeley, Wozniak, Bayly, Olney, & Lewis, 2004). Repeated mild impacts also show persistent gliosis and CTE-like increase in phosphorylated tau levels at 30 days after the last impact (Kane et al., 2012).

Strengths and Weaknesses

The animal models of sports-related mild TBI have been very effective in characterizing the molecular and cellular bases of repetitive injury, thus providing us a beginning foundation in understanding this unique phenomenon. However, current reports are somewhat inconsistent in their findings that in comparison to single injuries, multiple insults worsen (Laurer et al., 2001; Longhi et al., 2005), make little difference (Creeley et al., 2004), or actually improve outcome (DeRoss et al., 2002). These conflicting findings are most likely due to the variable times used to deliver the repeated injury and the different animal age groups used (from adolescent to adults). Furthermore, the greatest shortcoming of the existing models on repeated mild TBI is that they do not replicate the head movements, both the rotational and angular acceleration that are common in sports-related injury (Guskiewicz & Mihalik, 2011).

PATHOPHYSIOLOGICAL CONSEQUENCES IN ANIMAL MODELS OF TBI

Common to all animal models are two of the main pathological hallmarks of TBI seen in humans: neuronal cell death and white matter damage; and both of them can occur as a result of primary as well as secondary injury. The primary injury induced by TBI causes rapid deformation of brain tissue with destruction of brain parenchyma and blood vessels resulting in contusion, intracerebral hemorrhage, and damage to cell membranes with the immediate release of intracellular contents (McIntosh, 1994; Rink et al., 1995). The initial injury that occurs at the moment of trauma cannot be treated, only prevented. By contrast, the secondary injury induced by TBI can occur from minutes to days or months after the initial trauma. Animal models of TBI greatly aid our current understanding of the secondary injuries seen following trauma as well as the progressive nature of the neuronal and glial damage after injury. A detailed overview of all aspects of the secondary injury cascade seen in human TBI is beyond the scope of this review. However, the key pathophysiological features seen in the different animal models that mimic the human condition are highlighted in the following text and in Table 3.1.

Studies on animal models of TBI show that there is a massive disturbance of the cellular ion homeostasis initiated by the excessive release of the excitatory amino acid neurotransmitters glutamate and aspartate, with the subsequent activation of glutamate receptors leading to excitotoxicity during the immediate period following the primary injury. The release of glutamate results in the cellular influx of Na^+ and Ca^{2+} and efflux of K^+ (Faden, Demediuk, Panter, & Vink, 1989; Katayama, Becker, Tamura, & Hovda, 1990; Nilsson, Hillered, Olsson, Sheardown, & Hansen, 1993), which are regarded as vital events that lead to mitochondrial damage, an increase in free radical production, changes in gene expression, and activation of calcium dependent proteases including caspases, calpains, and phospholipases. This cascade of events eventually results in extensive cytoskeletal damage (Kupina, Detloff, Bobrowski, Snyder, & Hall, 2003; Stiefel, Tomita, & Marmarou, 2005) and marked mitochondrial perturbation (Lifshitz, Sullivan, Hovda, Wieloch, & McIntosh, 2004; Mazzeo, Beat, Singh, & Bullock, 2009).

An increase in glucose utilization has also been reported in animal models of TBI (Giri, Krishnappa, Bryan, Robertson, & Watson, 2000). The high demand for glucose and increase in local cerebral metabolic rate of glucose occurs at a time of reduced regional cerebral blood flow (Nilsson, Hillered, Pontén, & Ungerstedt, 1990; Marklund, Sihver, Långström, Bergström, & Hillered, 2002) and causes the uncoupling of blood flow–cerebral metabolism that is deleterious to the injured brain post-TBI (Chen et al., 2004). Disruption in the balance between cerebral blood flow and cerebral metabolism leads to the overproduction of reactive oxygen species or free radicals due to the perturbation of the mitochondrial respiratory chain, increased free iron production as a result of the breakdown of extravasated hemoglobin, oxidation of catecholamines, breakdown of membrane phospholipids and NADPH (the reduced form of nicotinamide adenine dinucleotide phosphate), and activation of nitric oxide synthase (Lewen, Matz, & Chan, 2000; Lewen et al., 2001; Stiefel et al., 2005). All of these events increase the production of free radicals and challenges and exhaust both the intra and extracellular antioxidant defense systems (Shohami, Beit-Yannai, Horowitz, & Kohe, 1997; Hall, Vaishnav, & Mustafa, 2010) leading to oxidative stress. The emerging consensus from studies in animal models show that oxidative stress is currently the major contributor to the secondary injuries seen following TBI, which can then lead to further damage by inducing lipid peroxidation, protein oxidation, and deoxyribonucleic acid (DNA) damage (Lewen et al., 2000).

TABLE 3.1

Key Pathological Features Seen in Human TBI That Are Replicated in TBI Animal Models

TBI Model	Injury Type	Species	Key Pathological Features					Replicates Human Condition	Reference
			Concussion	Contusion	TAI	Hemorrhage	Skull Fracture		
FPI	Focal/ diffuse	Rat, mouse	√	√	√	—	Occasional	+	McIntosh et al. (1987) Hicks et al. (1996) Bramlett and Dietrich (2002) Liu et al. (2010) Thompson et al. (2005) Hardman and Manoukian (2002) McIntosh et al. (1989) Vink et al. (2001) Dixon et al. (1987)
CCI	Mainly focal	Rat, mouse, swine	√	√	√	—	—	++	Dixon et al. (1991) Dixon et al. (1987) Lighthall (1988) Marmarou et al. (1994) Pierce et al. (1998) Kochanek et al. (2002) Goodman et al. (1994) Saatman et al. (2006)
Weight drop: Marmarou	Mainly diffuse	Rat, mouse	√	√	√	—	—	+	Marmarou et al. (1994) Johnson et al. (2013) Foda and Marmarou (1994) Albert-Weissenberger et al. (2012)

Weight drop: Feeney	Mainly focal	Rat, mouse	√	√	√	—	—	+	Feeney et al. (1981) Dail et al. (1981)
Weight drop: Shohami	Mainly focal	Rat, mouse	√	√	√	—	—	+	Chen et al. (1996) Flierl et al. (2009)
PBBI	Mainly focal	Cat, rat	√	√	√	√	Occasional	+/-	Williams et al. (2005) Williams et al. (2006) Wei et al. (2010)
Blast	Mainly diffuse	Rat, mouse, swine	√	√	√	ND	√	-	Long et al. (2009) Cheng (2010) Bauman et al. (2009) de Lanerolle et al. (2011) Risling and Davidsson (2012) DeWitt and Pough (2009) Cernak et al. (2011)
Repetitive	Mainly diffuse	Rat, mouse, swine	√	√	√	ND	occasional		Laurer et al. (2001) Longhi et al. (2005) Allen et al. (2000) Angoa-Perez et al. (2014) DeFord et al. (2002) Creeley et al. (2004) Kane et al. (2012)

Note. CCI = controlled cortical impact; FPI = fluid percussion injury; ND = not determined; PBBI = penetrating ballistic-like brain injury; TBI = traumatic brain injury; TAI = traumatic axonal injury; + = replicates the human condition to some degree; – = does not replicate the human condition; +/– = not consistently observed in animal models; √ = closely parallels the human condition.

Animal models of TBI also induce a robust immune activation including an acute neuroinflammatory response with breakdown of the BBB, edema formation, proliferation of peripheral immune cells, activation of resident microglia and astrocytes, and release of cytokines (Habgood et al., 2007; Ziebell & Morganti-Kossman, 2010). An upregulation of several cytokines, both proinflammatory and anti-inflammatory, have also been reported such as tumor necrosis factor (TNF) and the interleukin (IL) family of peptides (Kelly, Lifshitz, & Povlishock, 2007; Lenzlinger, Morganti-Kossman, Laurer, & McIntosh, 2001; Lu et al., 2009). More important, the infiltrating leukocytes secreting myeloperoxidase is also an important source for the generation of free radicals through the increased production of hypochlorous acid (Lewen et al., 2000). Both human and animal studies demonstrate that neuroinflammation can persist up to years after injury (Schwab, Beschorner, Meyermann, Gözalan, & Schluesener, 2002; Ziebell & Morganti-Kossman, 2010). The TBI-induced inflammatory process is believed to be a double-edged sword in that it can have both destructive and beneficial effects (Lenzlinger et al., 2001; Morganti-Kossman, Rancan, Stahel, & Kossmann, 2002; Morganti-Kossmann, Satgunaseelan, Bye, & Kossmann, 2007). A major participant in the neuroinflammatory process is microglia since these cells are among the first to display very early activation following injury and are capable of contributing to neuronal damage by expressing potentially harmful molecules, such as IL-1β, TNF-α, and reactive oxygen species (Morganti-Kossmann et al., 2007). However, microglia can also provide protective effects after injury and participate in restoring damaged tissues (repair function) by engulfing neutrophils, and through the release of growth factors and anti-inflammatory cytokines such as IL-4 and IL-10 (Lenzlinger et al., 2001; Morganti-Kossman et al., 2002; Lalancette-Hebert, Gowing, Simard, Weng, & Kriz, 2007).

Neuronal injury in brain regions such as the cerebral cortex, hippocampus, thalamus, and in rare instances, parts of the brain stem is well documented in the first few hours after both human and animal models of TBI. However, neuronal injury can also occur as part of secondary injury likely influenced by the role of neuronal gap junctions during glutamate-mediated excitotoxicity (Stoica & Faden, 2010; Sun et al., 2013). The neuronal injury seen as part of primary trauma presents characteristics of necrotic cell death (Mustafa & Alshboul, 2013). In contrast, it is believed that the neuronal cell death in secondary injury presents characteristics of apoptotic cell death (Belousov & Fontes, 2013). Initiation of apoptotic cell death occurs following mitochondrial damage when an opening of the mitochondrial permeability transition pore causes the release and activation of proapoptotic factors including soluble cytochrome c, apoptosis inducing factor, and caspases (Lifshitz et al., 2004; Mazzeo et al., 2009). Regardless of whether necrosis or apoptosis is the cause of TBI-induced neuronal cell death, damage may be observed not just at the site of injury but also in areas remote from the site of impact, especially in vulnerable regions of the brain such as the hippocampus, the region involved in memory processing (Saatman et al., 2006).

Although neuronal cell death has received the most attention in the field of TBI research, axonal injury is also common after trauma as demonstrated both in clinical and in animal studies (reviewed in Kou & Vandevord, 2014). Traumatic axonal injury is often referred to as diffuse axonal injury and is believed to be a dominant contributor to the neurological deficits observed following TBI. Axonal injury is observed across all TBI subtypes (mild, moderate, and severe), and acute disconnection of axons at the time of impact is observed primarily in severe TBI. Studies show that the degree of axonal injury usually determines mortality rate at the time of injury (Johnson et al., 2013; Wang & Ma, 2010). Stretching and shearing of axons seen in TBI can also occur in areas remote to the site of impact usually due to intra-axonal cytoskeleton damage that eventually leads to axonal disconnection (Büki & Povlishock, 2006).

More recently, two biochemical processes have been identified as chronic consequences of TBI: the *formation of amyloid plaques* and *tau pathology*, and both of these biochemical processes are key contributors to neurodegeneration (Chauhan, 2014; McKee, Daneshvar, Alvarez, & Stein, 2014). Reports on the presence of neurofibrillary tangles in neocortical areas in boxers diagnosed with CTE exist since the early 1970s, and subsequent studies have since confirmed the findings of extensive neurofibrillary tangle pathology in postmortem studies (reviewed in Kokjohn et al., 2013). Neurofibrillary tangles are threadlike aggregates of hyperphosphorylated tau protein (Iqbal & Grundke-Iqbal, 2006). Tau is a normal axonal protein that binds to microtubules via its microtubule-binding domains and promotes microtubule assembly and stability (Grundke-Iqbal, Iqbal, & Wisniewski, 1986). In TBI, the hyperphosphorylation of the tau protein reduces its ability to bind to microtubules (Figure 3.1), which causes the disassembly of microtubules resulting in impaired axonal transport and eventually leading to compromised neuronal and synaptic function via the increased aggregation of tau and formation of neurofibrillary tangles (Mandelkow & Mandelkow, 2012). Animal studies of repetitive TBI and blast injuries show that tau accumulation intra-axonally and its hyperphosphorylation are associated with repeated brain trauma evidenced by increased tau immunoreactivity in the perinuclear cytoplasm and in neurites (Abisambra & Scheff, 2014; Goldstein et al., 2012; Mouzon et al., 2014). Other models of TBI also show that tau and neurofilament proteins accumulate in damaged axons (Blennow, Hardy, & Zetterberg, 2012; Hawkins et al., 2013). Consistent in all these studies is the demonstrated correlation between tau hyperphosphorylation and injury severity (Abisambra & Scheff, 2014; Hawkins et al., 2013).

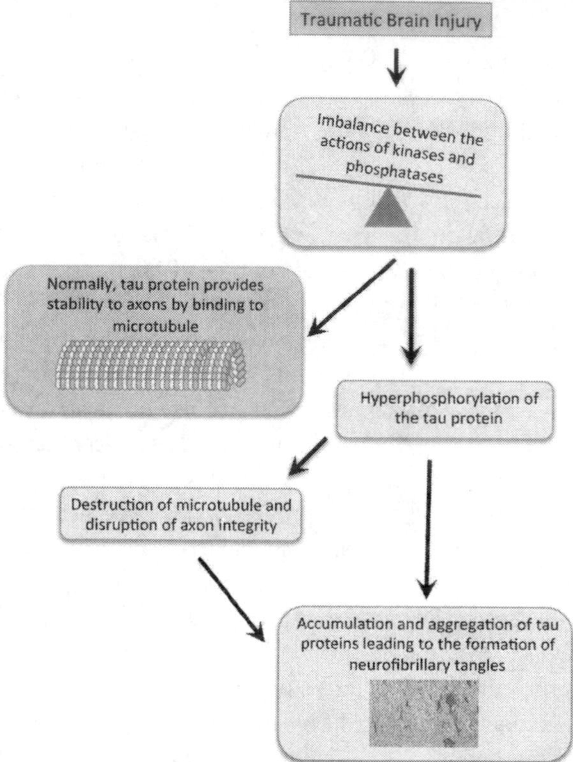

FIGURE 3.1 Pathway to tau pathology in CTE. The schematic diagram shows that TBI affects the normal function of the tau protein via the actions of kinases and phosphatases. Phosphorylation of the tau protein is regulated by the actions of kinases and phosphatases, and when an imbalance on the functioning of these two enzymes happens following TBI, it leads to increased phosphorylation (hyperphosphorylation) of the tau protein. Hyperphosphorylation disrupts the ability of the tau protein to bind to microtubules, creating instability in axon structure. Hyperphosphorylation of the tau protein also leads to its accumulation. Tau aggregation together with the disruption of axon integrity can result in the formation of neurofibrillary tangles, which is a common feature in CTE and other neurodegenerative disorders such as Alzheimer's disease.

The other biochemical process that is a major contributor to neurodegeneration in TBI is the accumulation of beta amyloid, a key component of plaques in Alzheimer's disease (Blennow et al., 2012; Smith, Johnson, & Stewart, 2013). Clinical studies show that amyloid plaques are present in boxers after repeated head injury and also in victims of automobile accidents (Kokjohn et al., 2013; Malkki, 2014). Studies of fresh surgically excised brain tissue samples also provided further support that acute severe brain trauma can result in the accumulation of amyloid plaques (Ikonomovic et al., 2004). Amyloid beta (Aβ) is generated from the beta amyloid precursor protein (βAPP) by the concerted action of β-secretase and γ-secretase (Figure 3.2). Generally, βAPP is involved in the regulation of neuronal growth and survival (Mattson, 1997; Selkoe, 1991). Under physiologic conditions, βAPP undergoes normal processing where it is cleaved in the middle of the β-amyloidogenic sequence by the α-secretase enzyme, resulting in the generation of the secreted form of βAPP (Popa-Wagner, Schröder, Walker, Kessler, & Futrell, 1998; Selkoe 1991). Under pathologic conditions, alternative processing of βAPP is carried out by the concerted efforts of the β-secretase amyloid cleaving enzyme (BACE) and the γ-secretase enzyme, resulting in the production of the carboxyl-terminal portion of βAPP and the liberation as well as the accumulation of Aβ oligomers, which can be neurotoxic (Cleary et al., 2005; Popa-Wagner et al., 1998; Wen, Onyewuchi, Yang, Liu, & Simpkins, 2004). Furthermore, the carboxyl-terminal fragment of βAPP is shown to destabilize calcium homeostasis and render neuronal cells vulnerable to glutamate-induced excitotoxicity (Kim et al., 1998). Studies on rotational acceleration models of TBI show an accumulation of βAPP and diffuse amyloid plaques within damaged axons throughout the white matter (Li, Li, Feng, & Gu, 2010; Tran, Sanchez, Esparza, & Brody, 2011). The accumulation of βAPP, together with increased expression of BACE-1 and presenilin enzymes, is seen in the terminal bulbs of disconnected axons and in some cortical neurons (Stone et al., 2004). Studies show that the intensity of amyloid plaque deposition in TBI is comparable to that found in Alzheimer's disease cases (Blennow et al., 2012; Chauhan, 2014).

BEHAVIORAL CONSEQUENCES OF TBI IN ANIMAL MODELS

TBI results in a multitude of deficits following injury and the long-term neurological consequences include impairments in sensation and perception, motor control, cognition, and affective behaviors such as depression and anxiety. These neurological impairments are due to the primary and secondary events that are triggered following TBI and can persist for months to years after injury even in mild TBI. Basic and preclinical animal research attempts to model aspects of the neurological impairments associated with TBI pathology seen in humans using different injury paradigms and measuring different types of neurological outcomes. Behavioral assessments in animal models of TBI can be divided into three major categories: (a) sensorimotor; (b) cognitive; and (c) affective, such as neuropsychiatric symptoms as shown in Table 3.2, while the different tests are described in the following text.

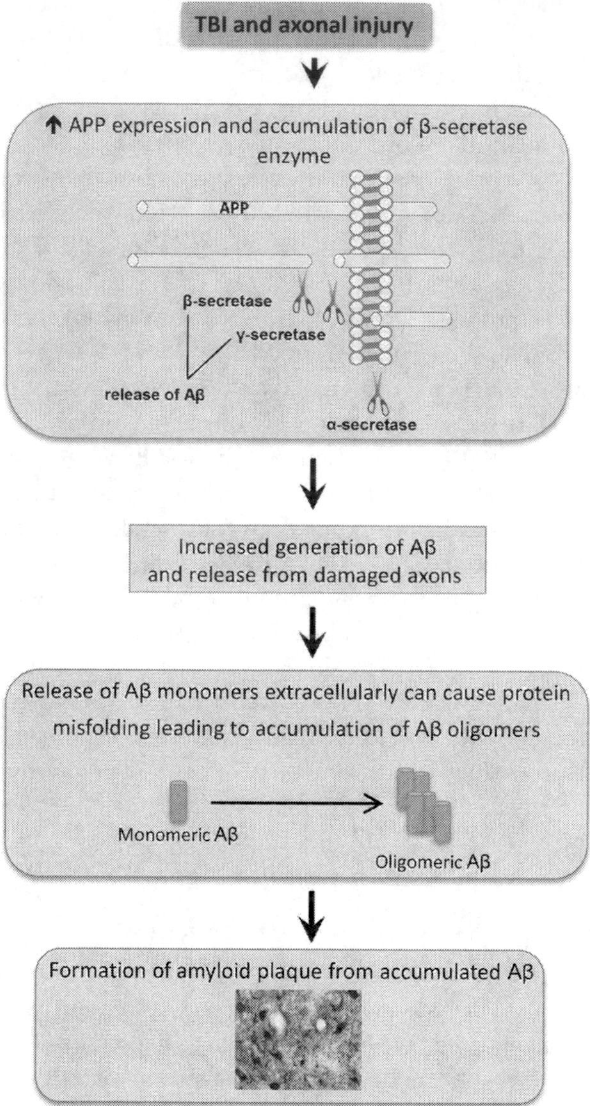

FIGURE 3.2 Pathway to amyloid beta (Aβ) pathology. The schematic diagram shows that the amyloid precursor protein is processed via the alternative pathway following traumatic brain injury (TBI). Although the α-secretase enzyme normally cleaves the amyloid precursor protein, following TBI, it is cleaved by the concerted actions of the β-secretase and γ-secretase enzymes. Increased expression of the precursor protein following TBI, together with processing via the alternative pathway, leads to more extracellular release of Aβ. Increased Aβ leads to accumulation, eventually resulting in the formation of amyloid plaques, which can initiate CTE and other neurodegenerative disorders such as Alzheimer's disease.

TABLE 3.2
Types of Behavioral Tests Employed in the Different TBI Models

	Type of Behavioral Measure				
Injury Model	Sensorimotor	Cognitive	Affective	Species	Reference
FPI	Balance beam/beam walking Rotarod Cylinder test	Barnes maze	–	Rat, mouse	Hallam et al. (2004) Bramlett, Dietrich, and Green (1999) Piot-Grojean, Wahl, Goobno, and Stutzmann (2001) Carballosa, Blaya, Alonso, Bramlett, and Hentall (2013) Maegele et al. (2005) Maegele et al. (2014)
CCI	Balance beam/beam walking Cylinder test Rotarod	Morris water maze Barnes maze Nonmatching-to-sample task Spontaneous object recognition	Elevated plus maze Open field	Rat, mouse	Singleton, Yan, Fellows-Mayle, and Dixon (2010) Fox and Faden (1998) Shaw et al. (2013) Dixon et al. (1999) Dapul et al. (2013) Monaco et al. (2013) Tajiri, Kellogg, Shimizu, Arendash, and Borlongan (2013) Jacqmain, Nudi, Fluharty, and Smith (2014) Gu et al. (2014) Liu et al. (2014) Briones and Woods (2013) Moritz, Geeck, Underly, Searles, and Smith (2014) Darwish, Mahmood, Schallert, Chopp, and Therrien (2014)

(*Continued*)

TABLE 3.2

Types of Behavioral Tests Employed in the Different TBI Models (Continued)

	Type of Behavioral Measure				
Injury Model	Sensorimotor	Cognitive	Affective	Species	Reference
PBBI	Rotarod		–		Shear et al. (2010)
Blast	Rotarod	Morris water maze	Elevated plus maze Open field test		Kovesdi et al. (2012) Budde et al. (2013)
Repetitive	Rotarod Balance beam/ beam walking	Barnes maze Morris water maze	–		Mouzon et al. (2014) Kane et al. (2012) DeFord et al. (2002) Creeley et al. (2004) DeRoss et al. (2002)

Note. CCI = controlled cortical impact; FPI = fluid percussion injury; PBBI = penetrating ballistic-like brain injury; TBI = traumatic brain injury; – = not assessed.

Balance Beam

The balance beam is a test for sensorimotor and vestibular functions and involves the use of an elevated narrow beam, which the animal balances on, and the latency for the animal to fall off the beam is recorded (typically a maximum latency of 60 seconds is provided). A round or narrower beam can be used to increase the difficulty of the task. The brain regions involved in carrying out this sensorimotor function are the motor cortex (Singleton et al., 2010) and possibly cerebellum (Colombel, Lalonde, & Caston, 2002; Lekic et al., 2011). Studies show deficits in balance beam performance in the TBI rats following CCI and FPI compared to their uninjured counterparts, and this behavioral impairment can be present up to 1 month after injury (Fox & Faden, 1998; Fox, Fan, Levasseur, & Faden, 1998; Hallam et al., 2004; Liu et al., 2013; Shaw et al., 2013).

A permutation of the balance beam test is beam walking, which is a test for fine motor coordination in rodents and uses a negative reinforcement paradigm. In this test, animals must escape from ambient light and/or high-decibel white noise by crossing an elevated narrow beam and entering a dark goal box on the other end of the beam. The time that it takes an animal to cross the beam and the number of foot slips it makes while crossing are recorded. The scoring ranges from 1 to 7, with 1 indicating the inability to traverse the beam and to place the affected limb on the horizontal surface and 7 indicating that the animal is able to traverse the beam normally with no more than two foot slips. The brain regions thought to be involved in performing these motor functions are the motor cortex, sensory cortex, thalamus, brain stem, and cerebellum (Barth, Jones, & Schallert, 1990; Colombel et al., 2002; Lekic et al., 2011). Deficits in beam walking performance are reported in the CCI and FPI models and may be present up to 1 month after trauma (Bramlett et al., 1999; Dixon et al., 1999; Piot-Grosjean et al., 2001; Singleton et al., 2010).

Cylinder Test

The cylinder test is used to assess asymmetries in forelimb function. In this test, an animal is placed in a cylinder and the number of times it places its contralateral, ipsilateral, or both paws on the wall of the cylinder during rearing are counted. Injured animals often do not use their contralateral limbs (injured site) to balance themselves while rearing along the walls of the cylinder (Woodlee et al., 2005). Brain structures suggested to be involved in the cylinder test are the midbrain median raphe and dorsal raphe nuclei (Carballosa et al., 2013). Experimental studies on TBI using the CCI and lateral FPI models demonstrate that the use of the contralateral limb to maintain posture during the cylinder test is significantly less in injured animals when compared to the sham-operated group (Carballosa et al., 2013; Dapul et al., 2013; Lekic et al., 2011).

Rotarod

The rotarod task is a sensitive measure for integrated motor abilities that requires animals to maintain balance on a rotating rod (Hamm et al., 1994). The amount of time spent balanced on the rotarod before falling off or gripping the rod itself and spinning around once is measured. Increased slips and falls while performing the rotarod test may be due to tissue loss in the cortex, striatum, and corticostriatal connections (Fujimoto et al., 2004). Deficits in rotarod performance are reported in animals subjected to the CCI, weight-drop, FPI, and penetrating ballistic-like injury models of TBI in comparison to those that received sham surgery (Shear et al., 2010; Maegele et al., 2014; Monaco et al., 2013; Mouzon et al., 2014).

Morris Water Maze

The Morris water maze task is primarily a cognitive test to assess spatial learning and memory where animals are placed into a large tank filled with tepid water to find a platform hidden below the surface of the water. Distal cues in the testing room are used to locate the platform (Briones & Therrien, 2000; Morris, 1984). The animals are tested individually and placed into different starting positions of the tank (north, south, west, or east). Spatial learning involves encoding information about the environment to facilitate navigation through space. Animals are given several trials a day for several days to facilitate learning (first few days) and recall (last days of testing) of the encoded information. Performance in the Morris water maze requires an intact hippocampus. Specific deficits in water maze performance have been reported in animals with damage to the hippocampus, striatum, basal forebrain, cerebellum, prefrontal cortex, insular cortex, and entorhinal and perirhinal cortices (Briones & Therrien, 2000; D'Hooge & De Deyn, 2001). The Morris water maze is the most common task used to assess cognitive impairment in several models of TBI (Budde et al., 2013; Gu et al., 2014; Jacqmain et al., 2014; Liu et al., 2014; Tajiri, Kellogg et al. 2013). Outcome measures to determine performance in the water include swim latency, the path taken to reach the platform, and swimming speed.

Barnes Water Maze

The Barnes maze is also a cognitive test of spatial learning and memory in rodents and is dependent on an intact hippocampus (Barnes 1979). In this test, animals are placed on a circular board elevated several feet from the ground, with holes lining the entire perimeter of the board. The holes allow the animals to look through the ground below, except for one hole that contains a dark, escape compartment. Animals are trained over several days to learn the location of this compartment, and during testing, the latency to find the compartment is used as a measure of spatial learning. To assess for working memory, the location of the hole with the escape compartment is moved during each test trial. Reports show that rats subjected to the CCI, FPI, weight-drop, and repetitive TBI models have longer latency in locating the escape compartment compared to the uninjured group during the spatial learning and working memory trials in the Barnes maze (Kovesdi et al., 2012; Maegele et al., 2005, Maegele et al., 2014; Moritz et al., 2014).

Nonmatching-to-Sample Tasks

The nonmatching-to-sample task (NMTS) consists of a series of paired sample and test trials and is designed to assess learning and memory function that is not dependent on an intact hippocampus. This cognitive task is not commonly used in TBI and used mostly in aging (Dumitriu et al., 2010) and other neurodegenerative studies where damage to the prefrontal cortex and entorhinal and perirhinal cortices are evident (Blanchet et al., 2000). In a recent study in our laboratory, we showed impaired performance of adults rats in the NMTS task following CCI (Briones & Woods, 2013). For the NMTS task, either a black or a white cylinder is suspended directly above the submerged platform in the water maze at the beginning of each sample trial. In subsequent test trials, both cylinders are present, but the cylinder not present during the preceding sample trial is suspended over the platform and serves as a cue for the location of the goal. Thus, if on a given sample trial, the black cylinder cues the platform, then on the succeeding test trial, the white cylinder is used to cue the platform. The black and white cylinders are selected as sample stimuli for each pair of trials according to a semirandom schedule that ensures that each cylinder serves as the sample stimulus on 50% of the trials over the phase of the experiment. For each test trial, the platform is moved to a different quadrant in the water maze with the nonsample cylinder located directly above it. Based on a random schedule, the position of the submerged platform is changed after each sample and test trial to eliminate the use of spatial cues. All quadrants are used equally for locating cues in the sample and test trials and the platform is positioned randomly. Parameters recorded in the NMTS task are swim latency and errors made in locating the platform.

Spontaneous Object Recognition

The spontaneous object recognition task evaluates nonspatial hippocampal-mediated memory (Tam, Robinson, Jennings, & Bonardi, 2014). In this task, animals are allowed to explore two identical objects in a chamber for a predetermined amount of time, and then, after an intertrial interval, are placed back into the chamber with one familiar object and one novel object. The time spent with the novel and familiar objects is recorded. Animals without injury spend more time exploring the novel object in relation to the familiar object. Brain structures implicated in this task are the dentate gyrus, the hippocampus, and the perirhinal cortex (Darwish et al., 2014; Ennaceur, Neave, & Aggleton, 1996). Reports show that animals subjected to the CCI and weight-drop models of TBI have persistent deficits in the spontaneous object recognition test, compared with the uninjured rats (Darwish et al., 2014; Schreiber et al., 2014; Tsenter et al., 2008).

Elevated Plus Maze

The elevated plus maze (EPM) is a task that assesses anxiety. Anxiety disorders develop in 10%–70% of patients with mild TBI (Bhalerao et al., 2013; Vaishvai, Rao, & Fann, 2009), so it is important to determine if it can be reproduced in animal models. The elevated maze is cross-shaped, with two open arms and two closed arms. Rodents have a preference for dark places; therefore, behavior differences are assessed by the time spent in the closed arms of the maze, relative to the open arms. Animals are placed in the center of the maze facing an open arm and tracked using motion detection software. The number of entries, time spent in each arm (open vs. closed), and distance traveled are typically measured. The brain structures implicated in this task are the amygdala and hippocampus. Studies show differences in anxiety in animals subjected to the CCI, lateral FPI, weight-drop, and blast TBI models compared with uninjured controls, and this symptom can persist at 1 month after injury (Budde et al., 2013; Kovesdi et al., 2012; Moritz et al., 2014; Schreiber et al., 2014).

Sucrose Preference Test

The most common psychiatric complaint in patients with TBI is depression (Bhalerao et al., 2013; Riggio & Wong, 2009). The reported prevalence of depression varies between studies and ranges from 10% to 77% (Hart et al., 2012). Rates of depression in patients with TBI are highest in the first year after the injury is sustained, but the risk for the appearance of depression remains elevated even decades after an injury (Hart et al., 2012). The brain structures implicated in depressive symptoms are the frontal cortex, amygdala, posterior cingulate, insula, and hippocampus (Godsil, Kiss, Spedding, & Jay, 2013; Leech & Sharp, 2014; Wiebking et al., 2014). The two clinical hallmarks of a major depressive disorder are anhedonia and behavioral despair (APA, 2000). Anhedonia is a phenomenon in which there is a loss of interest in pleasure derived from typically enjoyable experiences or activities. The sweet taste of sugar is a potent motivator both in humans and in rodents (Sclafani, 2006);

so an-often employed, nonoperant method in assessing hedonic sensitivity in rodents is the measurement of preference for consuming sweetened fluids (sucrose/saccharin) over water.

For the *sucrose preference test,* rats are acclimated to a two-bottle choice of drinking water or 1% sucrose solution for a few days followed by testing days. On the day of testing, two preweighted bottles of 5% sucrose solution and tap water are presented to the animals. To prevent side preference in drinking behavior, the position of the bottle containing the liquids is changed daily during the test. Liquid consumption from each bottle is recorded and corrected by body weight to calculate sucrose solution intake, water intake, and total liquid consumption by the end of the test period. Sucrose preference is calculated using the following equation: sucrose preference (%) = sucrose intake/(sucrose intake + water intake) × 100. Some studies that explored the effects of TBI on depressive-like symptoms in rats following FPI showed no significant differences between injured rats and the sham control group in the sucrose preference test at 1, 3, and 6 months after the primary injury (Jones et al., 2008). However, other investigators report that rats subjected to CCI showed a significantly decreased preference for saccharin compared to the control sham rats at 8 days following injury (Milman et al., 2005; Moritz et al., 2014). The limited number of studies on depressive-like symptoms in rodents subjected to TBI and the contrasting findings reported to date support the notion that it is premature to assert that the phenomenon of depression can be reproduced in the animal model.

Open Field Test

The other hallmark of major depression in humans is behavioral despair, and in rodents, it is manifested as a significant decline in the animal's effort to avoid or escape aversive situations (APA, 2000). The open field test is commonly used to assess behavioral despair in animals (Paré, 1994), and in this test, the animal is placed in a black Plexiglas box for a few days for habituation training; testing is carried out once the animals are habituated to the apparatus. The box is divided into two areas: peripheral area and center area. During testing, the rats are placed in the peripheral area and allowed to freely explore for 5 minutes. Activity in the open field is recorded either by manual observation or by using a computerized videotracking system. The measures recorded include immobility time, horizontal movement (distance covered during locomotion), and number of entries in the center area. Deficits in open field behavior in TBI rodents are reported following CCI, FPI, weight–drop, and blast injuries compared with uninjured controls and can persist up to 1 month after injury (Budde et al., 2013; Jacqmain et al., 2014; Kovesdi et al., 2012, Moritz et al., 2014).

TBI REHABILITATION STRATEGIES USED IN ANIMAL MODELS

Humans and animals often show a surprisingly high degree of spontaneous behavioral recovery after TBI. This spontaneous behavioral recovery is believed to reflect the brain's ability to compensate for the injury, a phenomenon commonly known as brain plasticity. Brain plasticity involves compensatory neuroanatomical restructuring or regrowth of connections in the CNS in response to an injury or environmental change that is accompanied by improvement in behavior. Studies show that plasticity mechanisms can be enhanced by increased expression of neurotrophic factors together with modulation of the injury response (Garcia, Shah, Dixon, Wagner, & Kline, 2011). Earlier basic and preclinical TBI research had focused heavily on strategies to attenuate the early expansion of damage, but with the increased recognition of the role of brain plasticity during recovery, current TBI therapies emphasize the use of strategies that can provide neuroprotection, modulate oxidative stress and inflammation, and also enhance regeneration (Garcia et al., 2011). To date, there is no effective pharmacologic therapy for TBI, and this failure rate highlights the necessity for examining alternative strategies. The most common nonpharmacological alternative therapies examined in animal models of TBI are summarized in the following text.

Use of Exercise in TBI

Experimental data support the use of exercise as a treatment for TBI. Postinjury exercise improves performance in spatial learning and memory tasks of rats that receive FPI and weight-drop injury when compared with that of their sedentary counterparts (reviewed in Griesbach, 2011; Archer, 2012). This cognitive improvement induced by exercise after TBI is linked to the enhanced facilitation of endogenous repair mechanisms through the increased expression of plasticity-related molecules such as brain-derived neurotrophic factor (BDNF), cytochrome c oxidase, neurotrophin-3, and synapsin I within the hippocampus (Griesbach, Hovda, Gomez-Pinilla, & Sutton, 2008; Griesbach, Hovda, & Gomez-Pinilla,. 2009; Gu et al., 2014; Hicks et al., 1998; Lima et al., 2009; Koo, Lee, & Kim, 2013). In addition, exercise has neuroprotective properties through counteracting increases in the production of free radicals after TBI that leads to oxidative stress (Griesbach et al., 2008; Lima et al., 2009). The increased lipid peroxidation and protein oxidation induced by oxidative stress after TBI compromises cell signaling that can eventually lead to cell death (Shohami et al., 1997). In fact, exercise modulated neuronal cell death in the ipsilateral cortex by decreasing the levels of oxidized proteins that contain carbonyl groups following CCI in rats (Griesbach et al., 2008; Itoh et al., 2011). A recent study also showed that exercise for 6 weeks before CCI increased the survival of cerebellar neurons (Seo et al., 2010). Additionally, reports show that the neuroprotective effect of exercise may be mediated by the modulation of the inflammatory process through the reduction of cytokine production. For instance, studies indicate that exercise decreases the production of the cytokine, TNF-α, after injury (Ding et al., 2006), and elevations in TNF-α in brain injury are linked to increased neuronal death and depression (Feuerstein, Liu, & Barone, 1994).

Despite the neuroprotective effects of exercise seen in most studies, contradicting findings are reported when physical activity is implemented early during the acute period post-TBI (reviewed in Griesbach, 2011). For example, early implementation of exercise following weight-drop injury is linked to an exacerbation of postconcussive symptomatology, such as depression, anxiety, and cognitive deterioration (Jones et al., 2008). Additionally, animal studies in rats with FPI that undergo acute voluntary exercise present with more pronounced learning and memory deficits in comparison with the unexercised, injured rats (Crane, Fink, & Smith, 2012). Likewise, results of other animal studies show that early forced exercise after a unilateral sensorimotor cortex injury increases the brain lesion size and results in greater behavioral impairment (Humm, Kozlowski, James, Gotts, & Schallert, 1998; Kozlowski, James, & Schallert, 1996). In addition to worsening outcome, early exercise post-TBI appears to suppress a neuroplasticity response to brain injury that has been observed both in humans (Weiller, Chollet, Friston, Wise, & Frackowiak, 1992) and in animals (Dunn-Meynell & Levin, 1995; Kozlowski & Schallert, 1998). It is possible that compensatory and/or restorative responses that are often times observed in areas of the brain that have endured a lesser amount of harm are aggravated by the exertion induced by early exercise after brain injury, thus disrupting the compensatory reorganization that usually follow TBI to facilitate recovery (Dancause et al., 2005; Stein & Hoffman, 2003). This line of reasoning is supported by studies that demonstrate disruption in increased plasticity-related molecules such as synapsin, cAMP response element-binding protein (CREB), and Ca^{2+}/calmodulin-dependent protein kinase II (CAMKII) in rats allowed to exercise within 24 hours after TBI (Griesbach, Gomez-Pinilla, & Hovda, 2004). In contrast, increased molecular markers of plasticity are observed when voluntary exercise is delayed 2 weeks after FPI, wherein increased cortical BDNF, a key plasticity molecule, is accompanied by a significant enhancement in cognitive performance (Griesbach, Hovda, Molteni, Wu, & Gomez-Pinilla, 2004). These studies indicate not only that a delayed time window is preferable to achieve the beneficial effects of exercise after injury but also that the early use of exercise may impede recovery after TBI. It is possible that premature stimulation of the brain post-TBI through exercise imposes an increased energetic demand at a time when the brain is already metabolically compromised.

Use of Environmental Enrichment

Although it is recognized that intensive therapy and rehabilitation programs are essential for maximizing recovery and quality of life post-TBI, current available treatments are often minimally successful. Clearly, new methods of brain repair after TBI should be examined in order to enhance brain plasticity, and the most studied rehabilitation strategy post-TBI in animal models is the use of environmental enrichment (EE). There is over 50 years of evidence to suggest that exposure to an enriched or complex environment is a powerful stimulus that can alter brain cell numbers, structure, function, and chemistry as well as influence recovery from CNS injury (reviewed in van Praag, Kempermann, & Gage, 2000). The earliest report that the external environment altered behavior came in 1949 when Hebb (1949) demonstrated that rodents who received EE had better problem-solving skills in a complex task compared to the standard laboratory-caged animals. Subsequent reports show that EE in rats increased total brain weight and total DNA or ribonucleic acid (RNA) content in the brain in addition to its influence on brain neurochemistry, specifically acetylcholine expression (Rosenzweig, Love, & Bennett, 1968; Rosenzweig & Bennett, 1978).

EE consists of an enlarged living environment with increased social interaction and novel stimuli that, together, promote physical and cognitive stimulation (Figure 3.3). Results of studies in experimental models of TBI suggest that relatively brief exposure (e.g., 3 weeks) of EE can confer behavioral benefits (Cheng et al., 2012; de Witt et al., 2011). EE facilitates learning and memory as well as improves motor performance after both CCI and FPI in rats (Hamm, Temple, Pike, O'dell, & Lyeth, 1996; Held, Gordon, & Gentile, 1985;

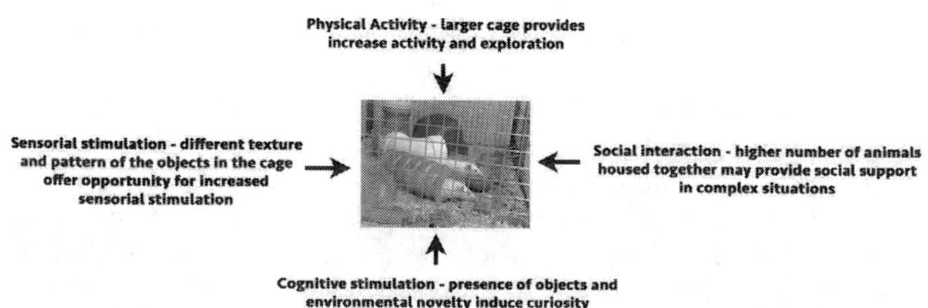

FIGURE 3.3 Enriched environment (EE) paradigm. In EE, rats are housed together in a large cage so that physical activity and social interactions are facilitated. In addition, the variety of objects in the cage and the daily changing of the objects provide multisensory stimuli and novelty.

Hoffman et al., 2008; Johnson et al., 2013; Passineau, Green, & Dietrich, 2001; Matter, Folweiler, Curatolo, & Kline, 2011; Maegele et al., 2014; Sozda et al., 2010). In addition to CCI and FP brain injury, EE has also been shown to provide benefit after blast TBI. The beneficial effects of EE on behavioral, cellular, and molecular alterations induced by blast injury, a leading cause of disability among soldiers, are associated with memory impairments and increased anxiety (Kovesdi et al., 2011). Briefly, rats were tested on the EPM and Barnes maze tests on separate days starting at 15, 44, and 66 days after blast injury induced through a compression-driven shock tube in order to provide a more longitudinal behavioral study relevant for the clinical setting. The study results show that long-term EE exposure significantly improved spatial memory compared to normal housing. The study also shows that the vascular endothelial growth factor, a signaling protein acting as a positive regulator of adult de novo hippocampal neurogenesis (Rosenstein & Krum, 2004), and tau protein expression in the hippocampus are normalized after long-term EE exposure, compared to normally housed rats. Moreover, enriched housing reduced the expression of the proinflammatory cytokine, IL-6, in the hippocampus (Kovesdi et al., 2011).

In a recent study from our laboratory (Briones & Woods, 2013), we showed that 4 weeks of continuous EE exposure significantly normalized CCI-induced cognitive impairment evidenced by decrease in mean swim latency and decreased errors made in an NMTS task conducted in a water maze. Also, in a delayed NMTS task, we showed that TBI rats displayed greater performance errors as the time delay between the sample and test trials increased, whereas EE attenuated the injury-related behavioral deficits. Furthermore, we demonstrated that EE housing is able to decrease the expression of the proinflammatory cytokines IL-1β and TNF-α, while expression of the anti-inflammatory cytokine (IL-10) increased, and this modulation of the inflammatory response is accompanied by the restoration of the TBI-induced disruption in brain energy metabolism. These findings suggest that overall, enhanced functional recovery attributed to EE housing after TBI may involve complex plasticity processes as well as modulation of the inflammatory response. As we continue to generate more data to increase our understanding of the mechanisms involved in the beneficial effects of EE, our laboratory conducted a gene microarray study and our results show that the genes associated with energy metabolism as well as plasticity mechanisms, including dendritic growth, synaptogenesis, neurogenesis, myelin synthesis, and memory, are upregulated. However, the genes associated with apoptosis, protein folding, and protein aggregation are down-regulated after EE housing. Our findings suggest that the EE experience can trigger genomic alterations in the brain that can initiate interacting signaling cascades culminating in enhanced neuronal plasticity and neuroprotection, and this line of thinking is depicted in our interactive model (Figure 3.4). Thus, it is reasonable to suggest that EE may be a rodent correlate of clinical physiotherapy for TBI rehabilitation.

Although the overwhelming consensus of all the published studies is that EE confers benefits after TBI and can therefore be considered a viable neurorehabilitation strategy, there are caveats to the EE effect. First, the effect of EE after TBI in female rats is not as clear as it is in male rats since only two reports are available to date that examined gender differences on the effects of enrichment following CCI. One study show beneficial effects of EE on improving cognitive and motor deficits (Monaco et al., 2013), while the other study shows that EE-enhanced cognitive performance is limited only to males, but no effect is seen in females (Wagner et al., 2002). The marked EE-induced behavioral differences between the two CCI studies in female animals may be a result of the inclusion of the rotarod task in one that may have provided additional rehabilitation that manifests in previously undetected cognitive improvement.

Second, even though the time frame of clinical rehabilitation may be varied, it is certainly shorter than the continuous nature of EE housing in the laboratory. The difference between the relatively short duration of daily clinical rehabilitation after TBI and the continuous nature of experimental EE emphasizes a disparity between the experimental model and the clinical environment that it attempts to replicate. It is possible that a certain threshold of EE is necessary to elicit the beneficial effects during neurobehavioral recovery to determine its translational potential to human beings who suffer from TBI. Third, it is not clear whether the benefits of early EE exposure are similar between humans and animals. That is, the benefits of early EE exposure seen in the animal models of TBI may be disadvantageous to humans just like the use of physical activity during the acute period following injury. To address these issues, future studies should focus on the importance of timing, such as when is the earliest or latest time that EE can be initiated to promote optimal outcomes and what is the least amount of EE that is capable of conferring benefits.

SUMMARY

Animal models have been extremely useful in elucidating the morphological, biochemical, and molecular changes that occur following TBI, and to some extent, these models also help in increasing our understanding of the behavioral impairments following injury. Impairments in cognitive functioning, such as attention, processing speed, and memory, have frequently been cited as significant contributors to disability following head injury both in humans and in animals,

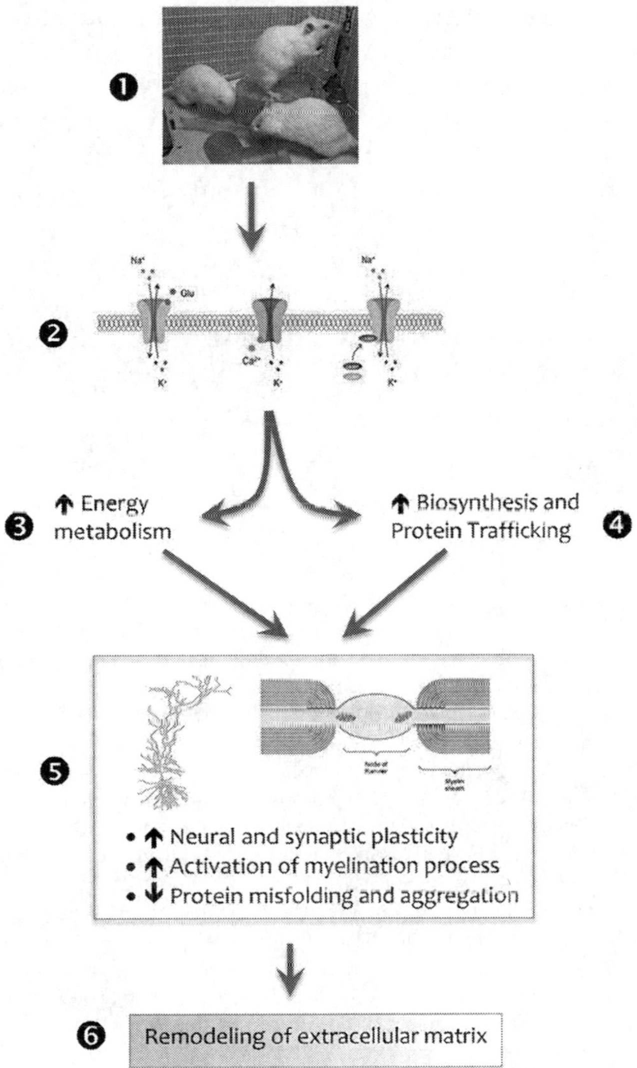

FIGURE 3.4 Integrative model of EE effects on brain plasticity and neuroprotection. ❶Exposure to EE promotes ❷signaling through neurotransmitter-activated channels, Ca^{2+}-regulated channels, or G-protein–mediated channels leading to heightened activity-dependent signaling, which then ❸boosts brain energy metabolism and ❹promotes biosynthesis and protein trafficking. Consequently, ❺neuronal and synaptic plasticity is enhanced and myelination process is activated; and together with decreased protein misfolding and aggregation, these steps culminate in the ❻remodeling of the extracellular matrix. All these interacting processes then lead to increased brain plasticity and protection from neuronal injury.

and these impairments affect the normal functioning ability of the individual. Given that current clinical therapies for TBI are ineffective, studies investigating nonpharmacologic approaches must be evaluated. The potential benefits of exercise and enriched environmental exposure is proven in animal studies, and even though it is obvious that studies of TBI in rodents cannot directly be compared to those in humans, clinically designed protocols for the implementation of exercise and EE exposure should be examined.

ACKNOWLEDGMENT

This work was supported in part by the Wayne State University Faville Endowment Funds.

REFERENCES

Abisambra, J. F., & Scheff, S. (2014). Brain injury in the context of tauopathies. *Journal of Alzheimers Disease & Parkinsonism, 40*(3), 495–518.

AFHS Center. (2013). *DoD TBI statistics 2000-2013*. Washington, DC: Department of Defense.

Albert-Weissenberger, C., Várrallyay, C., Raslan, F., Kleinschnitz, C., & Sirén, A. L. (2012). An experimental protocol for mimicking pathomechanisms of traumatic brain injury in mice. *Experimental & Translational Stroke Medicine, 4*, 1.

Allen, G. V., Gerami, D., & Esser, M. J. (2000). Conditioning effects of repetitive mild neurotrauma on motor function in an animal model of focal brain injury. *Neuroscience, 99*, 93–105.

American Psychiatric Association. (2000). *Diagnostic and statistical manual of mental disorders* (4th ed., text rev.). Washington, DC: American Psychiatric Association.

Angoa-Perez, M., Kane, M. J., Briggs, D. I., Herrera-Mundo, N., Viano, D. C., & Kuhn, D. M. (2014). Animal models of sports-related head injury: Bridging the gap between pre-clinical research and clinical reality. *Journal of Neurochemistry, 129*(6), 916–931.

Archer, T. (2012). Influence of physical exercise on traumatic brain injury deficits: Scaffolding effect. *Neurotoxicity Research, 21*(4), 418–434.

Barnes, C. A. (1979). Memory deficits associated with senescence: A neurophysiological and behavioral study in the rat. *Journal of Comparative and Physiological Psychology, 93*(1), 74–104.

Barth, T. M., Jones, T. A., & Schallert, T. (1990). Functional subdivisions of the rat somatic sensorimotor cortex. *Behavioural Brain Research, 39*(1), 73–95.

Bauman, R. A., Ling, G. S. F., Tong, L., Januszkiewicz, A., Agoston, D., Delanerolle, N., et al. (2009). An introductory characterization of a combat-casualty-care relevant swine model of closed head injury resulting from exposure to explosive blast. *Journal of Neurotrauma, 26*, 841–860.

Belousov, A. B., & Fontes, J. D. (2013). Neuronal gap junctions: Making and breaking connections during development and injury. *Trends in Neurosciences, 36*(4), 227–236.

Benzinger, T. L. (2009). Blast-related brain injuty: Imaging for clinical and research applications: Report of the 2008 St. Louis worshop. *Journal of Neurotrauma, 26*, 2233–2243.

Bhalerao, S. U., Geurtjens, C., Thomas, G. R., Kitamura, C. R., Zhou, C., & Marlborough, M. (2013). Understanding the neuropsychiatric consequences associated with significant traumatic brain injury. *Brain Injury, 27*, 767–774.

Blanchet, S., Marie, R. M., Dauvillier, F., Landeau, B., Benali, K., Eustache, F., et al. (2000). Cognitive processes involved in delayed non-matching-to-sample performance in Parkinson's disease. *European Journal of Neurology, 7*(5), 473–483.

Blennow, K., Hardy, J., & Zetterberg, H. (2012). The neuropathology and neurobiology of traumatic brain injury. *Neuron, 76*, 886–899.

Bramlett, H. M., & Dietrich, W. D. (2002). Quantitative structural changes in white and gray matter 1 year following traumatic brain injury in rats. *Acta Neuropathologica, 103*(6), 607–614.

Bramlett, H. M., Dietrich, W. D., & Green, E. J. (1999). Secondary hypoxia following moderate fluid percussion brain injury in rats exacerbates sensorimotor and cognitive deficits. *Journal of Neurotrauma, 16*(11), 1035–1047.

Briones, T. L., & Therrien, B. A. (2000). Behavioral effects of transient cerebral ischemia. *Biological Research for Nursing, 1*(4), 276–287.

Briones, T. L., & Woods, J. (2013). Decreased neuroinflammation and increased brain energy homeostasis following environmental enrichment after mild traumatic brain injury is associated with improvement in cognitive function. *Acta Neuropathologica Communications, 1*(1), 57.

Budde, M. D., Shah, A., McCrea, M., Cullinan, W. E., Pintar, F. A., & Stemper, B. D. (2013). Primary blast traumatic brain injury in the rat: Relating diffusion tensor imaging and behavior. *Frontiers in Neurology, 4*, 154.

Büki, A., & Povlishock, J. T. (2006). All roads lead to disconnection? - traumatic axonal injury revisited. *Acta Neurochirurgica, 148*(2), 181–194.

Carballosa, G. M. M., Blaya, M. O., Alonso, O. F., Bramlett, H. M., & Hentall, I. D. (2013). Midbrain raphe stimulation improves behavioral and anatomical recovery from fluid-percussion injury. *Journal of Neurotrauma, 30*(2), 119–130.

Cernak, I., & Noble-Haeussein, L. J. (2010). Traumatic brain injury: An overview of pathobiology with emphasis on military population. *Journal of Cerebral Blood Flow & Metabolism, 30*, 255–266.

Cernak, I., Merkle, A. C., Koliatsos, V. E., Bilik, J. M., Luong, Q. T., Mahota, T. M., et al. (2011). The pathobiology of blast injuries and blast-induced neurotrauma as identified using a new experimental model of injury in mice. *Neurobiology of Disease, 41*(2), 538–551.

Chauhan, N. B. (2014). Chronic neurodegenerative consequences of traumatic brain injury. *Restorative Neurology and Neuroscience, 32*, 337–365.

Chen, S. F., Richards, H. K., Smielewski, P., Johnstrm, P., Salvador, R., Pickard, J. D., et al. (2004). Relationship between flow-metabolism uncoupling and evolving axonal injury after experimental traumatic brain injury. *Journal of Cerebral Blood Flow & Metabolism, 24*, 1025–1036.

Chen, Y., Constantini, S., Trembovler, V., Weinstock, M., & Shohami, E. (1996). An experimental model of closed head injury in mice: Pathophysiology, histopathology, and cognitive deficits. *Journal of Neurotrauma, 13*(10), 557–568.

Cheng, J. P. (2010). Development of a rat model for studying blast-induced traumatic brain injury. *Journal of the Neurological Sciences, 294*(1–2), 23–28.

Cheng, J. P., Shaw, K. E., Monaco, C. M., Hoffman, A. N., Sozda, C. N., Olsen, A. S., et al. (2012). A relatively brief exposure to environmental enrichment after experimental traumatic brain injury confers long-term cognitive benefits. *Journal of Neurotrauma, 29*(17), 2684–2688.

Cleary, J. P., Walsh, D. M., Hofmeister, J. J., Shankar, G. M., Kuskowski, M. A., Selkoe, D. J., et al. (2005). Natural oligomers of the amyloid-beta protein specifically disrupts cognitive function. *Nature Neuroscience, 8*(1), 79–84.

Colombel, C., Lalonde, R., & Caston, J. (2002). The effects of unilateral removal of the cerebellar hemispheres on motor functions and weight gain in rats. *Brain Research, 950*(1–2), 231–238.

Corrigan, J. D., Selassie, A. W., & Orman, J .A. (2010). The epidemiology of traumatic brain injury. *Journal of Head Trauma Rehabilitation*, *25*, 72–80.

Crane, A. T., Fink, K. D., & Smith, J. S. (2012). The effects of acute voluntary wheel running on recovery of function following medial frontal cortical contusions in rats. *Restorative Neurology and Neuroscience*, *30*, 325–333.

Creeley, C. E., Wozniak, D. F., Bayly, P. V., Olney, J. W., & Lewis, L. M. (2004). Multiple episodes of mild traumatic brain injury result in impaired cognitive performance in mice. *Academic Emergency Medicine*, *11*, 809–819.

Dail, W. G., Fenney, D. M., Murray, H. M., Linn, R. T., & Boyeson, M. G. (1981). Responses to cortical injury II: Widespread depression of the activity of an enzyme in cortex remote from a focal injury. *Brain Research*, *211*(1), 79–89.

Dancause, N., Barbay, S., Frost, S. B., Plautz, E. J., Chen, D., Zoubina, E. V., et al. (2005). Extensive cortical rewiring after brain injury. *Journal of Neuroscience*, *25*, 10167–10179.

Dapul, H. R., Park, J., Zhang, J., Lee, C., DanEshmand, A., Lok, J., et al. (2013). Concussive injury before or after controlled cortical impact exacerbates histopathology and functional outcome in a mixed traumatic brain injury model in mice. *Journal of Neurotrauma*, *30*, 382–391.

Darwish, H., Mahmood, A., Schallert, T., Chopp, M., & Therrien, B. (2014). Simvastatin and environmental enrichment effect on recognition and temporal order memory after mild-to-moderate traumatic brain injury. *Brain Injury*, *28*, 211–226.

de Lanerolle, N. C., Bandak, F., Kang, D., Li, A. Y., Du, F., Swauger, P., Parks, S., et al. (2011). Characteristics of an explosive blast-induced brain injury in an experimental model. *Journal of Neuropathology and Experimental Neurology*, *70*(11), 1046–1057.

de Witt, B. W., Ehrenberg, K. M., McAloon, R. L., Panos, A. H., Shaw, K. E., Raghavan, P. V., et al. (2011). Abbreviated environmental enrichment enhances neurobehavioral recovery comparably to continuous exposure after traumatic brain injury. *Neurorehabilitation and Neural Repair*, *25*(4), 343–350.

DeFord, S. M., Wilson, M. S., Rice, A. C., Clausen, T., Rice, L. K., Barabnova, A., et al. (2002). Repeated mild brain injuries result in cognitive impairment in B6C3F1 mice. *Journal of Neurotrauma*, *19*(4), 427–438.

DeRoss, A. L., Adams, J. E., Vane, D. W., Russell, S. J., Terella, A. M., & Wald, S. L. (2002). Multiple head injuries in rats: Effects on behavior. *Journal of Trauma*, *52*, 708–714.

DeWitt, D. S., & Prough, D. S. (2009). Blast-induced brain injury and posttraumatic hypotension and hypoxemia. *Journal of Neurotrauma*, *26*, 877–887.

D'Hooge, R., & De Deyn, P. P. (2001). Applications of the Morris water maze in the study of learning and memory. *Brain Research Reviews*, *36*(1), 60–90.

Ding, Y. H., Mrizek, M., Lai, Q., Wu, Y., Reyes, R., Li, J., et al. (2006). Exercise preconditioning reduces brain damage and inhibits TNF-alpha receptor expression after hypoxia/reoxygenation: An in vivo and in vitro study. *Current Neurovascular Research*, *3*(4), 263–271.

Dixon, C. E., Clifton, G. L., Lighthall, J. W., Yaghmai, A. A., & Hayes, R. L. (1991). A controlled cortical impact model of traumatic brain injury in the rat. *Journal of Neuroscience Methods*, *39*(3), 253–262.

Dixon, C. E., Kraus, M. F., Kline, A. E., Ma, X., Yan, H. Q., Griffith, R. G., et al. (1999). Amantadine improves water maze performance without affecting motor behavior following traumatic brain injury in rats. *Restorative Neurology and Neuroscience*, *14*(4), 285–294.

Dixon, C. E., Lyeth, B. G., Povlishock, J. T., Findling, R. L., Hamm, R. J., Marmarou, A., et al. (1987). A fluid percussion model of experimental brain injury in the rat. *Journal of Neurosurgery*, *67*, 110–119.

Dumitriu, D., Hao, J., Hara, Y., Kaufmann, J., Janssen, W. G., Lou, W., et al. (2010). Selective changes in thin spine density and morphology in monkey prefrontal cortex correlate with aging-related cognitive impairment. *Journal of Neuroscience*, *30*(22), 7507–7515.

Dunn-Meynell, A. A., & Levin, B. E. (1995). Lateralized effect of unilateral somatosensory cortex contusion on behavior and cortical reorganization. *Brain Research*, *675*, 143–156.

Ennaceur, A., Neave, N., & Aggleton, J. P. (1996). Neurotoxic lesions of the perirhinal cortex do not mimic the behavioural effects of fornix transection in the rat. *Behavioural Brain Research*, *80*, 9–25.

Faden, A. I., Demediuk, P., Panter, S., & Vink, R. (1989). The role of excitatory amino acids and NMDA receptors in traumatic brain injury. *Science*, *244*(4906), 798–800.

Faul, M. D., Xu, L., & Wald, M. M. (2010). *Traumatic brain injury in the United States: Emergency department visits, hospitalizations and deaths 2002–2006*. Atlanta, GA: Centers for Disease Control and Prevention, National Center for Injury Prevention and Control.

Feeney, D. M., Boyeson, M. G., Linn, R. T., Murray, H. M., & Dail, W. G. (1981). Responses to cortical injury I: Methodology and local effects of contusions in the rat. *Brain Research*, *211*(1), 67–77.

Feuerstein, G. Z., Liu, T., & Barone, F. C. (1994). Cytokines, inflammation, and brain injury: Role of tumor necrosis factor-alpha. *Cerebrovascular Brain Metabolic Reviews*, *6*, 341–360.

Flierl, M. A., Stahel, P. F., Beauchamp, K. M., Morgan, S. J., Smith, W. R., & Shohami, E. (2009). Mouse closed head injury model induced by a weight-drop device. *Nature Protocols*, *4*, 1328–1337.

Foda, M. A., & Marmarou, A. (1994). A new model of diffuse brain injury in rats Part II: Morphological characterizations. *Journal of Neurosurgery*, *80*, 301–313.

Fox, G. B., & Faden, A. I. (1998). Traumatic brain injury causes delayed motor and cognitive impairment in a mutant mouse strain known to exhibit delayed Wallerian degeneration. *Journal of Neuroscience Research*, *53*, 718–727.

Fox, G. B., Fan, L., Levasseur, R. A., & Faden, A. I. (1998). Sustained sensory/motor and cognitive deficits with neuronal apoptosis following controlled cortical impact brain injury in the mouse. *Journal of Neurotrauma*, *5*, 599–614.

Fujimoto, S. T., Longhi, L., Saatman, K. E., Conte, V., Stocchetti, N., & McIntosh, T. K. (2004). Motor and cognitive function evaluation following experimental traumatic brain injury. *Neuroscience and Biobehavioral Reviews*, *28*, 365–378.

Garcia, A. N., Shah, M. A., Dixon, C. E., Wagner, A. K., & Kline, A. E. (2011). Biologic and plastic effects of experimental traumatic brain injury treatment paradigms and their relevance to clinical rehabilitation. *PM&R*, *3*(6 Suppl 1), S18–S27.

Giri, B. K., Krishnappa, I. K., Bryan, R. M., Robertson, C., & Watson, J. (2000). Regional cerebral blood flow after cortical impact injury complicated by a secondary insult in rats. *Stroke, 31*, 961–967.

Godsil, B. P., Kiss, J. P., Spedding, M., & Jay, T. M. (2013). The hippocampal-prefrontal pathway: The weak link in psychiatric disorders? *European Neuropsychopharmacology*, *23*, 1165–1181.

Goldstein, L. E., Fisher, A. M., Tagge, C. A., Zhang, X. L., Velisek, L., Sullivan, J. A., et al. (2012). Chronic traumatic encephalopathy in blast-exposed military veterans and a blast neurotrauma mouse model. *Science Translational Medicine*, *4*, 134–160.

Goodman, J. C., Cherian, L., Bryan, R. M., & Robertson, C. S. (1994). Lateral cortical impact injury in rats: Pathologic effects of varying cortical compression and impact velocity. *Journal of Neurotrauma*, *11*(5), 587–597.

Griesbach, G. S. (2011). Exercise after traumatic brain injury: Is it a double-edged sword? *PM&R*, *3*(6 Suppl 1), S64–S72.

Griesbach, G. S., Gomez-Pinilla, F., & Hovda, D. A. (2004). The upregulation of plasticity-related proteins following TBI is disrupted with acute voluntary exercise. *Brain Research, 1016*(2), 154–162.

Griesbach, G. S., Hovda, D. A., & Gomez-Pinilla, F. (2009). Exercise-induced improvement in cognitive performance after traumatic brain injury in rats is dependent on BDNF activation. *Brain Research, 1288*, 105–115.

Griesbach, G. S., Hovda, D. A., Gomez-Pinilla, F., & Sutton, R. L. (2008). Voluntary exercise or amphetamine treatment, but not the combination, increases hippocampal BDNF and synapsin I following cortical contusion in rats. *Neuroscience, 154*, 530–540.

Griesbach, G. S., Hovda, D. A., Molteni, R., Wu, A., & Gomez-Pinilla, F. (2004). Voluntary exercise following traumatic brain injury: Brain-derived neurotrophic factor upregulation and recovery of function. *Neuroscience, 125*(1), 129–139.

Grundke-Iqbal, I., Iqbal, K., & Wisniewski, H. M. (1986). Microtubule-associated protein tau. A component of Alzheimer paired helical filaments. *Journal of Biological Chemistry, 261*, 6084–6089.

Gu, Y. L., Zhang, L., Ma, N., Ye, L., Wang, D., & Gao, X. (2014). Cognitive improvement of mice induced by exercise prior to traumatic brain injury is associated with cytochrome c oxidase. *Neuroscience Letters, 570*, 86–91.

Guskiewicz, K. M., & Mihalik, J. P. (2011). Biomechanics of sport concussion: Quest for the elusive injury threshold. *Exercise and Sport Sciences Reviews, 39*(1), 4–11.

Habgood, M. D., Bye, N., Dziegielewska, K. M., Ek, C. J., Lane, M. A., Potter, A., et al. (2007). Changes in blood-brain barrier permeability to large and small molecules following traumatic brain injury in mice. *European Journal of Neuroscience, 25*(1), 231–238.

Hall, E. D., Vaishnav, R. A., & Mustafa, A. G. (2010). Antioxidant therapies for traumatic brain injury. *Neurotherapeutics, 7*(1), 51–61.

Hallam, T. M., Floyd, C. L., Folkerts, M. M., Lee, L. L., Gong, Q.-Z., Lyeth, B. G., et al. (2004). Comparison of behavioral deficits and acute neuronal degeneration in rat lateral fluid percussion and weight-drop brain injury models. *Journal of Neurotrauma, 21*, 521–539.

Hamm, R. J., Pike, B. R., O'dell, D. M., Lyeth, B. G., & Jenkins, L. W. (1994). The rotarod test: An evaluation of its effectiveness in assessing motor deficits following traumatic brain injury. *Journal of Neurotrauma, 11*(2), 187–196.

Hamm, R. J., Temple, M. D., Pike, B. R., O'dell, D. M., & Lyeth, B. G. (1996). Exposure to environmental complexity promotes recovery of cognitive function after traumatic brain injury. *Journal of Neurotrauma, 13*(1), 41–47.

Hardman, J. M., & Manoukian, A. (2002). Pathology of head trauma. *Neuroimaging Clinics of North America, 12*, 175–187.

Hart, T., Hoffman, J. M., Pretz, C., Kennedy, R., Clark, A. N., & Brenner, L. A. (2012). A longitudinal study of major and minor depression following traumatic brain injury. *Archieves of Physical Medicine and Rehabilitation, 93*(8), 1343–1349.

Hawkins, B. E., Krishnamurthy, S., Castillo-Carranza, D. L., Sengupta, U., Prough, D. S., Jackson, G. R., et al. (2013). Rapid accumulation of endogenous tau oligomers in a rat model of traumatic brain injury: Possible link between traumatic brain injury and sporadic tauopathies. *Journal of Biological Chemistry, 288*(23), 17042–17050.

Hebb, D. O. (1949). *The organization of behavior*. New York, NY: Wiley.

Held, J. M., Gordon, J., & Gentile, A. M. (1985). Environmental influences on locomotor recovery following cortical lesions in rats. *Behavioral Neuroscience, 99*(4), 678–690.

Hicks, R. R., Boggs, A., Leider, D., Kraemer, P., Brown, R., Scheff, S. W., et al. (1998). Effects of exercise following lateral fluid percussion brain injury in rats. *Restorative Neurology and Neuroscience, 12*, 41–47.

Hicks, R., Soares, H., Smith, D., & McIntosh, T. (1996). Temporal and spatial characterization of neuronal injury following lateral fluid-percussion brain injury in the rat. *Acta Neuropathologica*, *91*(3), 236–246.

Hoffman, A. N., Malena, R. R., Westergom, B. P., Luthra, P., Cheng, J. P., Aslam, H. A., et al. (2008). Environmental enrichment-mediated functional improvement after experimental traumatic brain injury is contingent on task-specific neurobehavioral experience. *Neuroscience Letters*, *431*(3), 226–230.

Humm, J. L., Kozlowski, D. A., James, D. C., Gotts, J. E., & Schallert, T. (1998). Use-dependent exacerbation of brain damage occurs during an early post-lesion vulnerable period. *Brain Research*, *783*(2), 286–292.

Ikonomovic, M. D., Uryu, K., Abrahamson, E. E., Ciallella, J. R., Trojanowski, J. Q., Lee, V., et al. (2004). Alzheimer's pathology in human temporal cortex surgically excised after severe brain injury. *Experimental Neurology*, *190*(1), 192–203.

Iqbal, K., & Grundke-Iqbal, I. (2006). Discoveries of tau, abnormally hyperphosphorylated tau and others of neurofibrillary degeneration: A personal historical perspective. *Journal of Alzheimers Disease*, *9*(3 Suppl), 219–242.

Itoh, T., Imano, M., Nishida, S., Tsubaki, M., Hashimoto, S., Ito, A., & Satou, T. (2011). Exercise inhibits neuronal apoptosis and improves cerebral function following rat traumatic brain injury. *Journal of Neural Transmission*, *118*(9), 1263–1272.

Jacqmain, J., Nudi, E. T., Fluharty, S., & Smith, J. S. (2014). Pre and post-injury environmental enrichment effects functional recovery following medial frontal cortical contusion injury in rats. *Behavioural Brain Research*, *275*, 201–211. http://dx.doi.org/10.1016/j.bbr.2014.08.056

Johnson, E. M., Traver, K. L., Hoffman, S. W., Harrison, C. R., & Herman, J. P. (2013). Environmental enrichment protects against functional deficits caused by traumatic brain injury. *Frontiers in Behavioral Neuroscience*, *7*. http://dx.doi.org/10.3389/fnbeh.2013.00044

Johnson, V. E., Stewart, W., & Smith, D. H. (2013). Axonal pathology in traumatic brain injury. *Experimental Neurology*, *246*, 35–43.

Jones, N. C., Cardamone, L., Williams, J. P., Salzberg, M. R., Myers, D., & O'Brien, T. J. (2008). Experimental traumatic brain injury induces pervasive hyperanxious phenotype in rats. *Journal of Neurotrauma*, *25*(11), 1367–1374.

Kane, M. J., Angoa-Pérez, M., Briggs, D. I., Viano, D. C., Kreipke, C. W., & Kuhn, D. M. (2012). A mouse model of human repetitive mild traumatic brain injury. *Journal of Neuroscience Methods*, *203*(1), 41–49.

Katayama, Y., Becker, D. P., Tamura, T., & Hovda, D. A. (1990). Massive increases in extracellular potassium and the indiscriminate release of glutamate following concussive brain injury. *Journal of Neurosurgery*, *73*(6), 889–900.

Kelly, B. J., Lifshitz, J., & Povlishock, J. T. (2007). Neuroinflammatory responses after experimental diffuse traumatic brain injury. *Journal of Neuropathology and Experimental Neurology*, *66*(11), 989–1001.

Kilbourne, M., Kuehn, R., Tosun, C., Caridi, J., Keledjian, K., Bochicchio, G., et al. (2009). Novel model of frontal impact closed head injury in the rat. *Journal of Neurotrauma*, *26*(12), 2233–2243.

Kim, H.-S., Lee, S. H., Kim, S. S, Kim, Y. K., Jeong, S. J., Ma, J., et al. (1998). Post-ischemic changes in the expression of Alzheimer's APP isoforms in rat cerebral cortex. *Neuroreport*, *9*(3), 533–537.

Kochanek, P. M., Hendrich, K. S., Dixon, C. E., Schiding, J. K., Williams, D. S., & Ho, C. (2002). Cerebral blood flow at one year after controlled cortical impact in rats: Assessment by magnetic resonance imaging. *Journal of Neurotrauma*, *19*(9), 1029–1037.

Kokjohn, T. A., Maarouf, C. L., Daugs, I. D., Hunter, J. M., Whiteside, C. M., Malek-Ahmadi, M., et al. (2013). Neurochemical profile of dementia pugilistica. *Journal of Neurotrauma*, *30*(11), 981–997.

Koo, H. M., Lee, S. M., & Kim, M. H. (2013). Spontaneous wheel running exercise induces brain recovery via neurotrophin-3 expression following experimental traumatic brain injury in rats. *Journal of Physical Therapy Science*, *25*(9), 1103–1107.

Kou, Z., & Vandevord, P. J. (2014). Traumatic white matter injury and glial activation: From basic science to clinics. *Glia*, *62*(11), 1831–1855. http://dx.doi.org/10.1002/glia.22690

Kovesdi, E., Gyorgy, A. B., Kwon, S. C., Wingo, D. L., Kamnaksh, A., Long, J. B., et al. (2011). The effect of enriched environment on the outcome of traumatic brain injury: A behavioral, proteomics, and histological study. *Frontiers in Neuroscience*, *15*, 42.

Kovesdi, E., Kamnaksh, A., Wingo, D., Ahmed, F., Grunberg, N. E., Long, J. B., et al. (2012). Acute minocycline treatment mitigates the symptoms of mild blast-induced traumatic brain injury. *Frontiers in Neurology*, 3, 111.

Kozlowski, D. A., & Schallert, T. (1998). Relationship between dendritic pruning and behavioral recovery following sensorimotor cortex lesions. *Behavioural Brain Research*, *97*(1–2), 89–98.

Kozlowski, D. A., James, D. C., & Schallert, T. (1996). Use-dependent exaggeration of neuronal injury after unilateral sensorimotor cortex lesions. *Journal of Neuroscience*, *16*, 4776–4786.

Kupina, N. C., Detloff, M. R., Bobrowski, W. F., Snyder, B. J., & Hall, E. D. (2003). Cytoskeletal protein degradation and neurodegeneration evolves differently in males and females following experimental head injury. *Experimental Neurology*, *180*(1), 55–73.

Lalancette-Hebert, M., Gowing, G., Simard, A., Weng, Y. C., & Kriz, J. (2007). Selective ablation of proliferating microglial cells exacerbates ischemic injury in the brain. *Journal of Neuroscience*, *27*(10), 2596–2605.

Langlois, J. A., Marr, A., Mitchko, J., & Johnson, R. L. (2005). Tracking the silent epidemic and educating the public: CDC's traumatic brain injury-associated activities under the TBI Act of 1996 and the Children's Health Act of 2000. *Journal of Head Trauma Rehabilitation*, *20*(3), 196–204.

Langlois, J. A., Rutland-Brown, W., & Wald, M. M. (2006). The epidemiology and impact of traumatic brain injury: A brief overview. *Journal of Head Trauma Rehabilitation*, *21*(5), 375–378.

Laurer, H. L., Bareyre, F. M., Lee, M. Y. C., Trojanowski, J. Q., Longhi, L., Hoover, R., et al. (2001). Mild head injury increasing the brain's vulnerability to a second concussive impact. *Journal of Neurosurgery*, *95*(5), 859–870.

Leech, R., & Sharp, D. J. (2014). The role of the posterior cingulate cortex in cognition and disease. *Brain*, *137*(Pt 1), 12–32.

Lekic, T., Rolland, W., Hartman, R., Kamper, J., Suzuki, H., Tang, J., et al. (2011). Characterization of the brain injury, neurobehavioral profiles, and histopathology in a rat model of cerebellar hemorrhage. *Experimental Neurology*, *227*(1), 96–103.

Lenzlinger, P. M., Morganti-Kossmann, M., Laurer, H. L., & McIntosh, T. K. (2001). The duality of the inflammatory response to TBI. *Molecular Neurobiology*, *24*(1–3), 169–181.

Lewen, A., Fujimura, M., Sugawara, T., Matz, P., Copin, J., & Chan, P. H. (2001). Oxidative stress-dependent release of mitochondrial cytochrome c after traumatic brain injury. *Journal of Cereb Blood Flow and Metabolism*, *21*, 914–920.

Lewen, A., Matz, P., & Chan, P. H. (2000). Free radical pathway in CNS injury. *Journal of Neurotrauma*, *17*(10), 871–890.

Li, X. Y., Li, J., Feng, D. F., & Gu, L. (2010). Diffuse axonal injury induced by simultaneous moderate linear and angular head accelerations in rats. *Neuroscience*, *169*(1), 357–369.

Lifshitz, J., Sullivan, P. G., Hovda, D. A., Wieloch, T., & McIntosh, T. K. (2004). Mitochondrial damage and dysfunction in traumatic brain injury. *Mitochondrion*, *4*, 705–713.

Lighthall, J. W. (1988). Controlled cortical impact: A new experimental brain injury model. *Journal of Neurotrauma*, *4*, 1–15.

Lima, F. D., Oliveira, M. S., Furian, A. F., Souza, M. A., Rambo, L. M., Ribeiro, L. R., et al. (2009). Adaptation to oxidative challenge induced by chronic physical exercise prevents Na+, K+-ATPase activity inhibition after traumatic brain injury. *Brain Research*, *1279*, 147–155.

Ling, G. S., & Ecklund, J. M. (2011). Traumatic brain injury in modern war. *Current Opinion in Anaesthesiology*, *24*(2), 124–130.

Liu, N. K., Zhang, Y.-P., O'Connor, J., Gianaris, A., Oakes, E., Lu, Q.-B., et al. (2013). A bilateral head injury that shows graded brain damage and behavioral deficits in adult mice. *Brain Research*, *1499*, 121–128.

Liu, N. K., Zhang, Y.-P., Zou, J., Verhovshek, T., Chen, C., Lu, Q.-B, et al. (2014). A semicircular controlled cortical impact produces long-term motor and cognitive dysfunction that correlates well with damage to both the sensorimotor cortex and hippocampus. *Brain Research*, *1576*, 18–26.

Liu, Y. R., Cardamone, L., Hogan, R. E., Gregoire, M.-C., Williams, J. P., Hicks, R. J., et al. (2010). Progressive metabolic and structural cerebral perturbations after traumatic brain injury: An in vivo imaging study in the rat. *Journal of Nuclear Medicine*, *51*(11), 1788–1795

Long, J. B., Bentley, T. L., Wessner, K. A., Cerone, C., Sweeney, S., & Bauman, R. A. (2009). Blast overpressure in rats: Recreating a battlefield injury in the laboratory. *Journal of Neurotrauma*, *26*(6), 827–840.

Longhi, L., Saatman, K. E., Fujimoto, S., Raghupathi, R., Meaney, D. F., Davis, J., et al. (2005). Temporal window of vulnerability to repetitive experimental concussive brain injury. *Neurosurgery*, *56*(2), 364–374.

Lu, J., Goh, S. J., Tng, P. Y., Deng, Y. Y., Ling, E. A., & Moochhala, S. (2009). Systemic inflammatory response following acute traumatic brain injury. *Frontiers in Bioscience*, *14*, 3795–3813.

Maegele, M., Braun, M., Wafaisade, A., Schäfer, N., Lippert-Gruener, M., Kreipke, C., et al. (2014). Long-term effects of enriched environment on neurofunctional outcome and CNS lesion volume after traumatic brain injury in rats. *Physiological Research*. PMID: 25194132

Maegele, M., Lippert-Gruener, M., Ester-Bode, T., Garbe, J., Bouillon, B., Neugebauer, E., et al. (2005). Multimodal early onset stimulation combined with enriched environment is associated with reduced CNS lesion volume and enhanced reversal of neuromotor dysfunction after traumatic brain injury. *European Journal of Neuroscience*, *21*(9), 2406–2418.

Magnuson, J., Leonessa, F., & Ling, G. S. F. (2012). Neuropathology of explosive blast traumatic brain injury. *Current Neurology and Neuroscience Reports*, *12*(5), 570–579.

Malkki, H. (2014). Traumatic brain injury: PET imaging detects amyloid deposits after TBI. *Nature Reviews Neurology*, *10*(1), 3. http://dx.doi.org/10.1038/nrneurol.2013.250

Mandelkow, E. M., & Mandelkow, E. (2012). Biochemistry and cell biology of tau protein in neurofibrillary degeneration. *Cold Spring Harbor Perspectives in Medicine*, *2*(7), a006247.

Marklund, N., Sihver, S., Långström, B., Bergström, M., & Hillered, L. (2002). Effect of traumatic brain injury and nitrone radical scavengers on relative changes in regional cerebral blood flow and glucose uptake in rats. *Journal of Neurotrauma*, *19*(10), 1139–1153.

Marmarou, A., Foda, M. A. A.-E., van den Brink, W., Campbell, J., Kita, H., & Demetriadou, K. (1994). A new model of diffuse brain injury in rats. Part I: Pathophysiology and biomechanics. *Journal of Neurosurgery*, *80*(2), 291–300.

Masel, B. E., & DeWitt, D. S. (2010). Traumatic brain injury: A disease process, not an event. *Journal of Neurotrauma*, *27*, 1529–1540.

Matter, A. M., Folweiler, K. A., Curatolo, L. M., & Kline, A. E. (2011). Temporal effects of environmental enrichment-mediated functional improvement after experimental traumatic brain injury in rats. *Neurorehabilitation and Neural Repair*, *25*(6), 558–564.

Mattson, M. P. (1997). Cellular actions of beta-amyloid precursor protein and its soluble and fibrillogenic derivatives. *Physiological Review*, *77*, 1081–1132.

Mazzeo, A. T., Beat, A., Singh, A., & Bullock, M. R. (2009). The role of mitochondrial transition pore, and its modulation, in traumatic brain injury and delayed neurodegeneration afer TBI. *Experimental Neurology*, *218*(2), 363–370.

McIntosh, T. K. (1994). Neurochemical sequela of traumatic brain injury: Therapeutic implications. *Cerebrovascular Brain Metabolic Reviews*, *6*, 109–162.

McIntosh, T. K., Noble, L., Andrews, B., & Faden, A. I. (1987). Traumatic brain injury in the rat: Characterization of a midline fluid-percussion model. *Central Nervous System Trauma*, *4*, 119–134.

McIntosh, T. K., Vink, R., Noble, L., Yamakami, I., Fernyak, S., Soares, H., et al. (1989). Traumatic brain injury in the rat: Characterization of a lateral fluid-percussion model. *Neuroscience*, *28*, 233–244.

McKee, A. C., Daneshvar, D. H., Alvarez, V. E., & Stein, T. D. (2014). The neuropathology of sport. *Acta Neuropathologica*, *127*(1), 29–51.

Milman, A., Rosenberg, A., Weizman, R., & Pick, C. G. (2005). Mild traumatic brain injury induces persistent cognitive deficits and behavioral disturbances in mice. *Journal of Neurotrauma*, *22*(9), 1003–1010.

Monaco, C. M., Mattiola, V. V., Folweiler, K. A., Tay, J. K., Yelleswarapu, N. K., Curatolo, L. M., et al. (2013). Environmental enrichments promotoes robust functional and histological benefits in female rats after controlled cortical impact injury. *Experimental Neurology*, *247*, 410–418.

Morales, D. M., Marklund, N., Lebold, D., Thompson, H. J., Pitkanen, A., Maxwell, W. L., et al. (2005). Experimental models of traumatic brain injury: Do we really need to build a better mousetrap? *Neuroscience*, *136*(4), 971–989.

Morganti-Kossman, M. C., Rancan, M., Stahel, P. F., & Kossmann, T. (2002). Inflammatory response in acute traumatic brain injury: A double-edged sword. *Current Opinion in Critical Care*, *8*(2), 101–105.

Morganti-Kossmann, M. C., Satgunaseelan, L., Bye, N., & Kossmann, T. (2007). Modulation of immune response by head injury. *Injury*, *38*(12), 1392–1400.

Moritz, K. E., Geeck, K., Underly, R. G., Searles, M., & Smith, J. S. (2014). Post-operative environmental enrichment improves spatial and motor deficits but may not ameliorate anxiety- or depression-like symptoms in rats following traumatic brain injury. *Restorative Neurology and Neuroscience*, *32*(5), 701–716.

Morris, R. G. (1984). Developments of a water-maze procedure for studying spatial learning in the rat. *Journal of Neuroscience Methods*, *11*(1), 47–60.

Mouzon, B. C., Bachmeier, C., Ferro, A., Ojo, J.-O., Crynen, G., Acker, C. M., et al. (2014). Chronic neuropathological and neurobehavioral changes in a repetitive mild traumatic brain injury model. *Annals of Neurology*, *75*(2), 241–254.

Mustafa, A. G., & Alshboul, O. A. (2013). Pathophysiology of traumatic brain injury. *Neurosciences*, *18*, 222–234.

Nilsson, P., Hillered, L., Olsson, Y., Sheardown, M. J., & Hansen, A. J. (1993). Regional changes in interstitial K+ and Ca2+ levels following cortical compression contusion trauma in rats. *Journal of Cerebral Blood Flow and Metabolism*, *13*(2), 183–192.

Nilsson, P., Hillered, L., Pontén, U., & Ungerstedt, U. (1990). Changes in cortical extracellular levels of energy-related metabolites and amino acids following concussive brain injury in rats. *Journal of Cerebral Blood Flow and Metabolism*, *10*(5), 631–637.

Paré, W. P. (1994). Open field, learned helplessness, conditioned defensive burying, and forced-swim tests in WKY rats. *Physiology and Behavior*, *55*(3), 433–439.

Passineau, M. J., Green, E. J., & Dietrich, W. D. (2001). Therapeutic effects of environmental enrichment on cognitive function and tissue integrity following severe traumatic brain injury in rats. *Experimental Neurology*, *168*(2), 373–384.

Pierce, J. E., Smith, D. H., Trojanowski, J. Q., & McIntosh, T. K. (1998). Enduring cognitive, neurobehavioral and histopathological changes persist for up to one year following severe experimental brain injury in rats. *Neuroscience*, *87*(2), 359–369.

Piot-Grosjean, O., Wahl, F., Gobbo, O., & Stutzmann, J.-M. (2001). Assessment of sensorimotor and cognitive deficits induced by a moderate traumatic injury in the right parietal cortex of the rat. *Neurobiology of Disease*, *8*(6), 1082–1093.

Popa-Wagner, A., Schroder, E., Walker, L. C., Kessler, C., & Futrell, N. (1998). Beta-amyloid precursor protein and beta-amyloid peptide immunoreactivity in the rat brain after middle cerebral artery occlusion. *Stroke*, *29*, 2196–2202.

Riggio, S., & Wong, M. (2009). Neurobehavioral sequelae of traumatic brain injury. *Mount Sinai Journal of Medicine*, *76*(2), 163–172.

Rink, A., Fung, K. M., Trojanowski, J. Q., Lee, V. M., Neugebauer, E., & McIntosh, T. K. (1995). Evidence of apoptotic cell death after experimental traumatic brain injury in the rat. *American Journal of Pathology*, *147*(6), 1575–1583.

Risling, M., & Davidsson, J. (2012). Experimental animal models for studies on the mechanisms of blast-induced neurotrauma. *Frontiers in Neurology*, *3*, 30.

Rosenstein, J. M., & Krum, J. M. (2004). New roles for VEGF in nervous tissue - beyond blood vessels. *Experimental Neurology*, *87*, 246–253.

Rosenzweig, M. R., & Bennett, E. L. (1978). Experimental influences on brain anatomy and brain chemistry in rodents. In G. Gottlieb (Eds.), *Studies on the development of behavior and the nervous system* (Vol. 4, pp. 429–532). New York, NY: Academic Press.

Rosenzweig, M. R., Love, W., & Bennett, E. L. (1968). Effects of a few hours a day of enriched experience on brain chemistry and brain weights. *Physiology and Behavior*, *3*(6), 819–825.

Saatman, K. E., Feeko, K. J., Pape, R. L., & Raghupathi, R. (2006). Differential behavioral and histopathological responses to graded cortical impact injury in mice. *Journal of Neurotrauma*, *23*(8), 1241–1253.

Schreiber, S., Lin, R., Haim, L., Baratz-Goldstien, R., Rubovitch, V., Vaisman, N., et al. (2014). Enriched environment improves the cognitive effects from traumatic brain injury in mice. *Behavioural Brain Research*, *271*, 59–64.

Schwab, J. M., Beschorner, R., Meyermann, R., Gözalan, F., & Schluesener, H. J. (2002). Persistent accumulation of cyclooxygenase-1-expressing microglial cells and macrophages and transient upregulation by endothelium in human brain injury. *Journal of Neurosurgery*, *96*(5), 892–899.

Sclafani, A. (2006). Sucrose motivation in sweet “sensitive” (C57BL/6J) and subsensitive (129P3/J) mice measured by progressive ratio licking. *Physiology and Behavior*, *87*, 734–744.

Selkoe, D. J. (1991). The molecular pathology of Alzheimer's disease. *Neuron*, *6*, 487–498.

Seo, T. B., Kim, B.-K., Ko, I.-G., Kim, D.-H., Shin, M.-S, Kim, C.-J., et al. (2010). Effect of treadmill exercise on Purkinje cell loss and astrocytic reaction in the cerebellum after traumatic brain injury. *Neuroscience Letters*, *481*(3), 178–182.

Shaw, K. E., Bondi, C. O., Light, S. H., Massimino, L. A., McAloon, R. L., et al. (2013). Donepezil is ineffective in promoting motor and cognitive benefits after controlled cortical impact injury in male rats. *Journal of Neurotrauma*, *30*(7), 557–564.

Shear, D. A., Lu, X. M., Bombard, M. C., Pedersen, R. P., Chen, Z., Davis, A., et al. (2010). Longitudinal characterization of motor and cognitive deficits in a model of penetrating ballistic-like brain injury. *Journal of Neurotrauma*, *27*, 1911–1923.

Shohami, E., Beit-Yannai, E., Horowitz, M., & Kohe, R. (1997). Oxidative stress in closed-head injury: Brain antioxidant capacity as an indicator of functional outcome. *Journal of Cerebral Blood Flow and Metabolism*, *17*, 1007–1019.

Singleton, R. H., Yan, H. Q., Fellows-Mayle, W., & Dixon, C. E. (2010). Resveratrol attenuates behavioral impairments and reduces cortical and hippocampal loss in a rat controlled cortical impact model of traumatic brain injury. *Journal of Neurotrauma*, *27*, 1091–1099.

Smith, D. H., Johnson, V. E., & Stewart, W. (2013). Chronic neuropathologies of single and repetitive TBI: Substrates of dementia? *Nature Reviews Neurology*, *9*, 211–221.

Sozda, C. N., Hoffman, A. N., Olsen, A. S., Cheng, J. P., Zafonte, R. D., & Kline, A. E. (2010). Empirical comparison of typical and atpical environmental enrichment paradigms on functional and histological putcome after experimental traumatic brain injury. *Journal of Neurotrauma*, *27*, 1047–1057.

Stein, D. G., & Hoffman, S. W. (2003). Concepts of CNS plasticity in the context of brain damage and repair. *Journal of Head Trauma Rehabilitation*, *18*(4), 317–341.

Stiefel, M. F., Tomita, Y., & Marmarou, A. (2005). Secondary ischemia impairing the restoration of ion homeostasis following traumatic brain injury. *Journal of Neurosurgery*, *103*(4), 707–714.

Stoica, B. A., & Faden, A. I. (2010). Cell death mechanisms and modulation in traumatic brain injury. *Neurotherapeutics*, *7*, 3–12.

Stone, J. R., Okonkwo, D. O., Dialo, A. O., Rubin, D. G., Mutlu, L. K., Povlishock, J. T., et al. (2004). Impaired axonal transport and altered axolemmal permeability occur in distinct populations of damaged axons following traumatic brain injury. *Experimental Neurology*, *190*(1), 59–69.

Sun, D., McGinn, M., Hankins, J. E., Mays, K. M., Rolfe, A., & Colello, R. J. (2013). Aging- and injury-related differential apoptotic response in the dentate gyrus of the hippocampus in rats following brain trauma. *Frontiers in Aging Neuroscience*, *5*.

Tajiri, N., Kellogg, S. L., Shimizu, T., Arendash, G. W., & Borlongan, C. V. (2013). Traumatic brain injury precipitates cognitive impairment and extracellular Aβ aggregation in Alzheimer's disease transgenic mice. *PLoS One*, *8*(11), e78851.

Tam, S. K., Robinson, J., Jennings, D. J., & Bonardi, C. (2014). Dissociations in the effect of delay on object recognition: Evidence for an associative model of recognition memory. *Journal of Experimental Psychology: Animal Learning and Cognition*, *40*(1), 106–115.

Thompson, H. J., Lifshitz, J., Marklund, N., Grady, M. S., Graham, D. I., Hovda, D. A., et al. (2005). Lateral fluid percussion brain injury: A 15-year review and evaluation. *Journal of Neurotrauma*, *22*(1), 42–75.

Tran, H. T., Sanchez, L., Esparza, T. J., & Brody, D. L. (2011). Distinct temporal and anatomical distributions of amyloid-β and tau abnormalities following controlled cortical impact in transgenic mice. *PLoS One*, *6*, e25475.

Tsenter, J., Beni-Adani, L., Assaf, Y., Alexandrovich, A. G., Trembovler, V., & Shohami, E. (2008). Dynamic changes in the recovery after traumatic brain injury in mice: Effect of injury severity on T2-weighted MRI abnormalities, and motor and cognitive functions. *Journal of Neurotrauma*, *25*(4), 324–333.

Vaishvai, S., Rao, V., & Fann, J. R. (2009). Neuropsychiatric problems after traumatic brain injury: Unraveling the silent epidemic. *Psychosomatics*, *50*(3), 198–205.

van Praag, H., Kempermann, G., & Gage, F. H. (2000). Neural consequences of environmental enrichment. *Nature Reviews Neuroscience*, *1*(3), 191–198.

Vink, R., Mullins, P. G. M., Temple, M. D., Bao, W., & Faden, A. I. (2001). Small shifts in craniotomy position in the lateral fluid percussion injury model are associated with differential lesion development. *Journal of Neurotrauma*, *18*(8), 839–847.

Wagner, A. K., Kline, A. E., Sokoloski, J., Zafonte, R. D., Capulong, E., & Dixon, C. E. (2002). Intervention with environmental enrichment after experimental brain trauma enhances cognitive recovery in male but not female rats. *Neuroscience Letters, 334*(3), 165–168.

Wang, H. C., & Ma, Y. B. (2010). Experimental models of traumatic axonal injury. *Journal of Clinical Neuroscience, 17*(2), 157–162.

Warden, D. (2006). Military TBI during the Iraq and Afghanistan wars. *Journal of Head Trauma Rehabilitation, 21*, 398–402.

Weber, J. T. (2007). Experimental models of repetitive brain injuries. *Progress in Brain Research, 161*, 253–261.

Wei, G., Lu, X. M., Yang, X., & Tortella, F. C. (2010). Intracranial pressure following penetrating ballistic-like brain injury in rats. *Journal of Neurotrauma, 27*, 1635–1641.

Weiller, C., Chollet, F., Friston, K. J., Wise, R. J. S., & Frackowiak, R. S. J. (1992). Functional reorganization of the brain in recovery from striatocapsular infarction in man. *Annals of Neurology, 31*(5), 463–472.

Wen, Y., Onyewuchi, O., Yang, S., Liu, R., & Simpkins, J. W. (2004). Increased β-secretase activity and expression in rats following transient cerebral ischemia. *Brain Research, 1009*, 1–8.

Wiebking, C., Duncan, N. W., Tiret, B., Hayes, D. J., Marjanňska, M., Doyon, J., et al. (2014). GABA in the insula - a predictor of the neural response to interoceptive awareness. *Neuroimage, 86*, 10–18.

Williams, A. J., Hartings, J. A., May Lu, X.-C., Rolli, M. L., Dave, J. R., & Tortella, F. C. (2005). Characterization of a new rat model of penetrating ballistic brain injury. *Journal of Neurotrauma, 22*(2), 313–331.

Williams, A. J., Hartings, J. A., May Lu, X.-C., Rolli, M. L., Dave, J. R., & Tortella, F. C. (2006). Penetrating ballistic-like brain injury in the rat: Differential time courses of hemorrhage, cell death, inflammation, and remote degeneration. *Journal of Neurotrauma, 23*(12), 1828–1846.

Williams, A. J., Ling, G. S. F., & Tortella, F. C. (2006). Severity level and injury track determine outcome following a penetrating ballistic-like brain injury in the rat. *Neuroscience Letters, 408*(3), 183–188.

Woodlee, M. T., Asseogarcia, A., Zhao, X., Liu, S., Jones, T., & Schallert, T. (2005). Testing forelimb placing 'across the midline' reveals distinct, lesion-dependent patterns of recovery in rats. *Experimental Neurology, 191*(2), 310–317.

Ziebell, J. M., & Morganti-Kossman, M. C. (2010). Involvement of pro- and anti-inflammatory cytokines and chemokines in the pathophysiology of TBI. *Neurotherapeutics, 7*, 22–30.

CHAPTER 4

Genomics, Transcriptomics, and Epigenomics in Traumatic Brain Injury Research

Ava M. Puccio and Sheila Alexander

ABSTRACT

The long-term effects and significant impact of the full spectrum of traumatic brain injury (TBI) has received increased attention in recent years. Despite increased research efforts, there has been little movement toward improving outcomes for the survivors of TBI. TBI is a heterogeneous condition with a complex biological response, and significant variability in human recovery contributes to the difficulty in identifying therapeutics that improve outcomes. Personalized medicine, identifying the best course of treatment for a given individual based on individual characteristics, has great potential to improve recovery for TBI survivors. The advances in medical genetics and genomics over the past 20 years have increased our understanding of many biological processes. A substantial amount of research has focused on the genomic, transcriptomic, and epigenomic profiles in many health and disease states, including recovery from TBI. The focus of this review chapter is to describe the current state of the science in genomic, transcriptomic, and epigenomic research in the TBI population. There have been some advancements toward understanding the genomic, transcriptomic, and epigenomic processes in humans, but much of this work remains at the preclinical stage. This current evidence does improve our understanding of

http://dx.doi.org/10.1891/0739-6686.33.75

TBI recovery, but also serves as an excellent platform upon which to build further study toward improved outcomes for this population.

INTRODUCTION

Traumatic brain injury (TBI) is a major problem in the United States and worldwide, contributing significantly to mortality and disability of people of all ages, having a bimodal distribution with a high incidence in the young population related to motor vehicle accidents and a high incidence in the elderly due to falls. In 2010, 2.5 million people suffered TBI in the United States alone. The long-term negative effects of TBI are especially detrimental in the younger age strata due to severe disabilities, which may lead to many years of less-than-optimal function. Despite the poor outcome profile of people suffering TBI, and an intense focus on identifying effective therapeutics, progress toward improved outcomes has been slow. This is due to many issues including the heterogeneity of resultant injuries and multifactorial responses to TBI treatment. In addition, the unique morphology of the central nervous system (CNS), which includes multiple cell types, a distinct set of cells (neurons) with minimal repair reserves, and little to no regenerative capacity, all contribute to the difficulty to attribute "one treatment to fit all." The lack of effect of over 32 clinical trials in the TBI population may be due to this heterogeneous inherent nature of the population, lending support for identifying genetic influences on treatment and recovery following a TBI.

Recent advances in genetic and genomic technologies have led to significant advancements in our understanding of many multifactorial diseases and hold promise for increasing our understanding of the response to and recovery from TBI and for the development of therapeutics aimed at modifying pathway responses to improve outcomes. Once thought to be immune to genetic and genomic influence, recovery from acute traumatic injury has increasingly been found to be influenced by individual biologic variation.

The purpose of this review is to summarize the literature on genomics, transcriptomics, and epigenomics in TBI with special emphasis on research efforts in the adult TBI population. Literature on the single-gene effects on recovery from TBI were considered beyond the scope of this review and therefore not included except in relation to the interaction approaches.

GENOMIC APPROACHES

What Is Genomics?

Genomics is the study of summative effects of genetic variance across a genome. It includes the study of variations across the genome, interactions of genes, and gene–environment interactions. An understanding of the impact of multiple/all genes on an outcome of interest and of how genes interact with one another and with environmental factors to modify biological functioning advances the knowledge base of a given health or disease state and also provides insight into possible pathways for intervention development.

Genome Studies

The human genome contains over 20,000 genes (National Human Genome Research Institute, 2011). While changes in deoxyribonucleic acid (DNA) sequence for a gene, known as genetics, is extremely informative for single-gene disorders and some multifactorial disorders, the complex biologic human system relies on interactions among multiple genes, their gene products, and environmental factors. Genomics is one approach to tackle the challenges of studying biological variability leading to recovery in a complex system such as the human brain. The genome-wide association study (GWAS) is an approach that studies variations in the DNA sequence across the entire genome of groups of individuals from a population of interest, comparing them to a similar control group (Strawbridge et al., 2011).

The GWAS approach generates many points of potential genetic variability in people with the outcome variable of interest. Commercially available platforms for GWAS studies include the evaluation of 200,000 to over 2 million polymorphisms (Spencer, Su, Donnelly, & Marchini, 2009) and can focus on the entire genome or just the coding regions (Corvin, Craddock, & Sullivan, 2010). While this is often considered a strength of the GWAS approach as it informs about the multiple pathways involved, it may also be considered a weakness as the multiple statistical analyses performed, in combination with the small effect size of individual variants, require very large sample sizes to yield meaningful results (Clarke & Thirlaway, 2011; Hunter et al., 2007; McCarthy & Hirschhorn, 2008; Pearson & Manolio, 2008; Zondervan et al., 2007). The potential for false-positive findings is significant, and replication studies, using similar sample sizes, are necessary to confirm findings (Chanock, 2007; Hunter et al., 2007). With such a large number of data points to be compared across groups, a sample size of at least 2,000 per group (cases and controls; Corvin et al., 2010) is most likely to yield meaningful results, yet it is difficult to recruit this number of TBI subjects, given the frequency of the injury and barriers to multisite, multiyear research studies.

A well-designed GWAS study needs to have a very well-defined phenotype to be informative (Clarke et al., 2011; Corvin, et al., 2010; McCarthy et al., 2008). Groups to be compared need to be similar in all aspects except the outcome of interest, and this can be especially challenging in studies of TBI.

The heterogeneous nature of TBI—with a heterogeneous population and multiple types of injury culminating in a classification of TBI—confounds results of research (Hicks et al., 2013). There is questionable relevance for a GWAS that compares all subjects with TBI, given the variable pathophysiologic events occurring during mild, moderate, and severe TBI, and also after injury, owing to different degrees (mild, moderate, severe) and types of brain injuries (CT morphology, ischemia, infarction, etc.). Numerous potential covariates, such as sex, age, and type of injury, must be controlled for in the selection of inclusion criteria of the control group or controlled for in the analysis, adding to the complexity in the statistical approach required.

Cost is also a prohibitive factor for GWAS studies. The cost for the recruitment of a sample size needed for a GWAS study in a TBI population is exorbitant. The cost of sequencing the entire genome or the single nucleotide polymorphisms (SNPs) covering the genome is also significant, making this type of research difficult. However and is anticipated to continue to decline, increasing the feasibility of this type of research. Additionally, research in other areas focused on minimizing cost while maintaining adequate power to yield clinically meaningful results is ongoing (Muller, Pahl, & Schafer, 2007; Stanhope & Skol, 2012).

Gene–Gene Interactions

Gene–gene interactions may be studied by extracting genetic variability data from a GWAS or by sequencing or genotyping two or more genes. The premise of this research is that the effect of variation within two genes of interest is greater than the effect of either gene alone (Cordell, 2009). The genes of interest are ideally related with biologically interactive gene products but may be associational, exploring the effects of multiple genetic variants on a health or disease state. With well-selected genes identified, gene–gene interaction studies are hypothesis driven. Whether the genes have products functioning in the same biologic pathway or represent functional variability in different pathways, and promote a single outcome or have opposite effects, they have the potential to generate significant data supporting the understanding of biological interactions within the context of the phenotype under investigation (Sanjuan & Elena, 2006).

The phenotype remains an important concept for gene–gene interaction studies. Having a well-defined phenotype of interest, with an appropriate control sample for comparison, allows for a thorough investigation of the effect of a genetic/genomic variation on the outcome. Potential covariates may be explored in the statistical analysis but must be identified a priori so that appropriate data is collected. Covariates are very important for gene–gene interaction studies; the effects may only be seen in one "type" of subject (males or females) and the effects may be lost in a study of the general population without considering these sources of variability.

The focus of gene–gene interaction studies is narrower than a GWAS and as such requires a smaller sample size. The power analysis to identify an ideal sample size must consider the number of genes to be studied, allele frequencies, effect sizes of each of the genetic variants, and potential covariates (Gauderman, 2002). Given the complexity of the human brain, this approach is well suited to the study of TBI where there are multiple gene products in multiple pathways with small, individual effects that culminate in a larger scenario of recovery.

Gene–Environment Interactions

Gene–environment interaction studies explore the effects of one or more genes and one or more environmental sources of potential variation in an outcome (Aschard et al., 2012). The study of gene–environment interaction is a challenging approach. The nature of the design and the inherent flaws in collecting environmental data make it difficult to carry out (Aschard et al., 2012). Environmental exposures typically occur over a lifetime, and there is significant potential for recall bias (Aschard et al., 2012). Some conditions may only present in subjects who have a given genetic background and a given environmental exposure. Prospective cohort designs can often adequately answer questions related to gene–environment interaction; however, these require long-term follow-up and are generally costly. Selection of the genetic variant(s) should also be carefully considered for this type of research. The GWAS approach allows for decrease in the bias related to genetic risk factors, but requires very large sample sizes. The candidate gene approach may introduce bias or lead to a lack of significant findings even when there is a significant relationship for multiple reasons. Population stratification, the different allele frequencies for populations from different genetic backgrounds, may impact results such that it is difficult to determine if the causes of effects are truly due to genetic variants or to ethnic differences, such as diet (Aschard et al., 2012; Keller, 2014). Confounders, or potential confounders, add additional complexity to gene–environment research, and selection and statistical control need to be carefully planned in the design phase of research (Keller, 2014). More recent work has suggested that the use of principal component methods aids in correction of population stratification (Bhattacharjee et al., 2010). Sample size is also a consideration for gene–environment interaction studies. Studies must be adequately powered to explore the effects of the genetic and environmental effects, interactive effects, and the impact of covariates including their potential interaction with genetic and environmental effects and/or the outcome variable of interest (Aschard et al., 2012; Bookman et al., 2011).

What Is the Research That Has Been Done in TBI Using Genomic Approaches

While the gene–gene interaction is an important concept for the exploration of more than one gene within a single pathway or in multiple pathways after TBI, there are few published studies using this approach. This science has developed to the point where studies of human gene–gene interaction are beginning to be explored. One study explored the association of SNPs in the glutamic acid decarboxylase (GAD) genes, GAD1 and GAD2, and the risk of seizures after human TBI (Darrah et al., 2013). In an independent analysis, only the GAD1 SNPs were significantly associated with seizures, and two SNPs in the GAD1 gene heightened that risk of seizure development in the 6 months following TBI (Darrah et al., 2013). In another study exploring the role of serotonin pathway genes and the response to citalopram for depressive symptoms after human TBI, SNPs in two of six genes were found to exhibit interactive effects predicting greater treatment response, while one SNP predicted adverse events (Lanctot et al., 2010). Table 4.1 provides an overview of studies using the approaches outline in this chapter and gene–gene interaction studies in particular.

To date, there has been minimal research exploring gene–environment interactions in TBI. The strong evidence for a role of apolipoprotein E genotype and TBI having combined effects resulting in dementia later in life suggests that TBI may be an environmental insult interacting with genotypes to promote poor cognitive function (Jellinger, 2004; Koponen et al., 2004; Tang et al., 1996). While this work does not explore the effects of gene–environment interactions on TBI, it does show that a gene–environment approach with TBI as an environmental insult contributes to pathology and cognitive dysfunction later in life. Table 4.1 provides an overview of studies using the approaches outlined in this chapter and a gene–environment interaction study in particular.

Where Can We Go From Here?

As with any type of research, there are strengths and weaknesses of genomic approaches to research. The large amount of data generated often results in more questions than answers, and additional study is warranted to inform mechanistic research that can truly identify a source for potential therapeutic intervention. Genomic approaches are well suited to TBI research where the human response is more complex than the animal response. To date, there has been no study utilizing the GWAS approach in brain-injured humans or animals. There have been studies in other populations hallmarked by brain dysfunction and complex response

TABLE 4.1

Example Studies Using Genomic, Transcriptomic, and Epigenomic Approaches in Traumatic Brain Injury

Approach/Reference	Sample	Independent Variable	Dependent Variable	Results
DNA Polymorphism Approaches				
GWAS: No TBI Studies Completed				
Gene–Gene Interaction				
Darrah et al. (2013)	257 White adults with severe TBI (GCS ≤ 8)	GAD1 and GAD2 functional and/or tagging SNPs: 6 SNPs. 17 haplotypes	Seizures at: 1 week post-TBI 1 week to 6 months post-TBI >6 months post-TBI 6-month GOS	SNPs associated with seizures at <1 week: GAD1 rs3828725 (TT and CT genotypes). No haplotypes conferred increased risk. SNPs associated with seizures 1 week to 6 months: rs3791878 (GG genotype) rs769391(AA genotype). These genotypes conferred increased seizure risk both alone and in combination. There were no significant associations with seizure development >6 months or with 6-month outcome.

(Continued)

TABLE 4.1

Example Studies Using Genomic, Transcriptomic, and Epigenomic Approaches in Traumatic Brain Injury (Continued)

Approach/Reference	Sample	Independent Variable	Dependent Variable	Results
Lanctot et al. (2010)	90 adults with depression after mild-to-moderate TBI	Serotonergic system genes: 5HTTLPR, 5HTT rs25531, 5HT1A C1019G, 5HT2A T102C, MTHFR C677T, BDNF val66met, TPH2 G703T	Response to citalopram	MTHFR C677T and BDNF SNPs were associated with greater treatment response.
			Adverse events with citalopram use	5HTTLPR was associated with increased adverse event development.
McAllister et al. (2008)	93 adults, 1 month post-TBI 54 adults	DRD2 TAQ1 A AND SNPs in NCAM, ANKK1, and DRD2	Memory and attention tests, including the CVLT recognition task and the CPT	The TAQ1 A (rs 1800497) T allele was associated with poorer performance on CVLT recognition in both TBI subjects and control sample and CPT performance in the TBI subjects only.
				In a haploblock of 3 SNPs in ANKK1 (rs11604671, rs4938016, and rs1800497 [TAQ1A]), specifically genotype G-C-C, performance associated with CVLT was stronger than for rs1800497 alone.

Gene–Environment Interaction				
Koponen et al. (2004)	60 subjects with previous TBI of any severity based on length of loss of consciousness/ coma and subsequent referral for neuropsychological evaluation.	APOE genotype APOE ε4 allele positive/negative status	*DSM-IV* Axis I and Axis II disorders: Major depression, Anxiety disorder, Alcohol abuse or dependence, Psychotic disorders, Definite dementia, Definite + subclinical dementia, Definite SCID-II personality disorders, Definite + subthreshold SCID-II personality disorders, Definite organic personality syndrome, Definite + subclinical organic personality syndrome	In individuals with a previous history of TBI, carrying at least one APOE ε4 allele increases the risk of definite and subclinical dementia compared to subjects without the APOE ε4 allele.

(*Continued*)

TABLE 4.1

Example Studies Using Genomic, Transcriptomic, and Epigenomic Approaches in Traumatic Brain Injury (Continued)

Approach/Reference	Sample	Independent Variable	Dependent Variable	Results
		Transcriptomic Approaches		
Laird et al. (2013)	26 severe TBI patients and 9 controls' (CSF) protein levels; human and rodent tissue culture gene expression	TBI (human), TBI (mouse, CCI), or control	HMGB1 protein levels, TLR4 (microglia) and AQP4 (astrocytes) expression	There was an increase in HMGB1 in human CSF (high ICP) and increase in IL-6, TLR4, and AQP4.
Verrier et al. (2012)	Severe TBI patients' (CSF) protein levels; mouse microdialysate tissue culture gene expression	TBI (human), TBI (mouse, CCI) or control	2',3' cAMP, 3'5' cAMP, 2' AMP, 3'AMP, 5' AMP, and adenosine	TBI activates the brain 2',2'-cAMP-adenosine pathway (murine model). TBI human CSF 2',3'-cAMP significantly increased within 12 hours of injury, correlating with 2'AMP, 3'AMP, adenosine and inosine.
Liu et al. (2013)	19 severe TBI and 3 meningioma patients (brain tissue)	TBI/meningioma human brain tissue	Ferritin expression	There was a marked increase of ferritin following acute TBI (≤12 hours) and elevated > 48 hours after TBI.

Zhao et al. (2013)	TBI and control human patients	Peripheral blood mononuclear cells	Olfactory receptor biomarkers	Activation of OR11H1 and OR4M1 segregated TBI and control cases with 90% accuracy, 83% sensitivity, and 100% specificity. Downregulation correlated with severity of brain injury and TBI-specific symptoms.
Epigenomic Approaches				
Histone Acetylation and Methylation (Animal Models)				
Gao et al. (2006)	Male Sprague-Dawley rat pups (postnatal Day 17)	TBI (CCI) or sham	At 6, 24, and 72 hours after injury: CA1 and CA3 neuronal loss (H&E) CA1 and CA3 histone H3 acetylation and methylation (IHC)	There was no significant neuronal loss. No significant histone H3 acetylation or methylation in CA1 was seen at any time point. There was decreased histone H3 acetylation in CA3 at 6 and 24 hours after injury. There was decreased histone H3 methylation in CA3 at 6, 24, and 72 hours after injury.

(*Continued*)

TABLE 4.1

Example Studies Using Genomic, Transcriptomic, and Epigenomic Approaches in Traumatic Brain Injury (Continued)

Approach/Reference	Sample	Independent Variable	Dependent Variable	Results
Dash et al. (2010)	Adult male Sprague-Dawley rats	TBI (CCI) or sham and The HDAC inhibitor VPA or vehicle at 30 minutes or 3 hours after injury, then daily for 5 days or SAHA or vehicle at 30 minutes after injury, then daily for 5 days	Hippocampal GSK3 and ERK pathway (gene expression) and histone acetylation (IR) at 45 minutes after VPA administration BBB permeability at 48 hours after TBI (Evans Blue extravasation) Motor function (beam balance and paw placement) on Days 1–3 after TBI Cognitive function (MWM) on Days 14–21 after TBI	VPA increases hippocampal H3 and H4 acetylation and decreases GSK3 pathway activation in a dose–response manner. There were VPA effects on ERK pathway activation. VPA reduced BBB permeability in the ipsilateral hemisphere. VPA had no effects on beam balance but improved paw placement at any time point. VPA-treated animals also had a reduction in posttrauma weight loss, potentially confounding these effects. Higher dose (400 mg/kg vs. 100 mg/kg) VPA improved MWM functioning after TBI. The delayed VPA administration (3 hours) led to improved motor but not cognitive function after TBI.

				The more selective (Class I and Class II) HDAC inhibitor SAHA increased H3 and H4 acetylation but not GSK3 pathway activation or motor or cognitive function after TBI.
Dash, Orsi, and Moore (2009)	Adult male C57 mice	TBI (CCI) or sham AND SAHA or vehicle at 30 minutes after injury (acetylation studies) or on Day 7 (or 14) and daily for 4 weeks	Hippocampal histone acetylation 30 minutes after drug administration (IR, western blot)	SAHA increased hippocampal H3 and H4 acetylation.
			Cognitive function: spatial learning and memory (MWM; with and without training)	SAHA did not lead to any changes in baseline cognitive function, but TBI animals with MWM training had improved function over time, normalizing to sham level.
			Fear conditioning (with training): memory	SAHA AND training improved memory function as measured by fear conditioning.

(Continued)

TABLE 4.1

Example Studies Using Genomic, Transcriptomic, and Epigenomic Approaches in Traumatic Brain Injury (Continued)

Approach/Reference	Sample	Independent Variable	Dependent Variable	Results
Zhang et al. (2008)	Adult male Sprague-Dawley rats	TBI (LFP) or sham AND DMA-PB administered in 4 doses or vehicle immediately after TBI	Hippocampal histone acetylation colocalization (OX-42 for microglia; Fluoro Jade B for degenerating neurons) 24 hours after injury	DMA-PB decreased CA2 and CA3 acetylation in a dose–response manner. DMA-PB (all doses) decreased CA2 and CA3 phagocytic microglia. DMA-PB showed trends toward decreasing the number of degenerating neurons.
Yu et al. (2013)	Adult male C57BL/6 mice	TBI (CCI) or sham AND Subeffective doses of lithium, VPA, or combination or vehicle 15 minutes post-TBI and daily for up to 21 days	Lesion volume (H&E staining) Acetylhistone H3, phospho-GSK-3β, β-catenin (western blot) BBB (immunoglobulin G extravasation) Neurodegeneration (Fluoro-Jade B) Motor function (beam walk test)	Combined dosing with lithium and VPA decreased lesion volume, BBB disruption, and neurodegeneration while increasing H3 acetylation 3 days after injury AND improved motor function 21 days after injury. Either of the drugs individually did not achieve significant results in any outcome measure.

Cao, Liang, Gao, Zhao, and Liang (2013)	Adult male rats	TBI (via LFP) or sham AND MS-275 (Class I HDAC) at 15 or 40 mg/kg, 30 minutes after TBI, then daily	Spatial learning and memory (MWM) Days 10–14 post-TBI Degenerating hippocampal CA2-3 neurons (Fluro-Jade B) at 24 hours post-TBI Hippocampal CA2-3 neuronal survival (cresyl violet) at 14 days post-TBI	MS-275 improved spatial learning and memory. Higher dose of MS-275 (45 mg/kg) decreased hippocampal neuronal degeneration. Trends suggest that MS-275 may improve hippocampal neuronal survival at 14 days after TBI.
Wang et al. (2013)	Adult male C57B/6 J mice	TBI (CCI) or sham AND Scriptaid (0, 1.5, 3.5, or 5.5 mg/kg) at 30 minutes or (3.5mg/kg) 12 hours after TBI Additional study included administration of LY294002 or vehicle 1 hour before TBI	24-hour deacetylase activity (western blot) Lesion volume Hippocampal CA3 neuron survival (stereologic cell count; MAP2 IHC) and dendrite analysis Motor functioning (foot faults, wire-hanging test, cylinder test) and cognitive functioning (MWM) 35 days after TBI	Scriptaid decreased lesion volume and improved H3 acetylation, hippocampal CA3 and pericontusional neuronal survival and processes, and motor and cognitive functioning in a dose–response manner. Additional testing found that Scriptaid induced effects partially by modulating AKT signaling that improves neuronal survival.

(*Continued*)

TABLE 4.1

Example Studies Using Genomic, Transcriptomic, and Epigenomic Approaches in Traumatic Brain Injury (Continued)

Approach/Reference	Sample	Independent Variable	Dependent Variable	Results
		DNA Methylation		
Lundberg et al. (2009)	Adult male Sprague-Dawley rats	TBI (WD) or sham surgery or sham no surgery	At 1, 4, 7, and 14 days post-TBI:	
			Dnmt enzymes (IHC)	The astrocytes at or near the point of injury stained Dnmt positive in cytoplasm, with highest expression at earlier time points and minimal expression by 14 days. More distant astrocytes did not show such staining.
			Cell type and location (NeuN staining for neurons: GFAP staining for astrocytes; nestin staining for CNS progenitor cells)	BrdU-treated astrocytes did not stain positive, suggesting that these cells are not actively dividing.
			Cell division (BrdU)	Neurons and microglia did not have Dnmt cytoplasmic expression but did have nucleic Dnmt expression in noninjured brains and the contralateral side to the injury.

Zhang, Zhang, Fauser, and Schluesener (2007)	Adult male rats	TBI (WD) or sham and Dexamethasone (1mg/kg) or vehicle every other day through 24, 48, or 96 hours after TBI.	Spatiotemporal global methylation status (anti-5-methycytosine: IHC) at 6, 12, 18, 24, 48, and 96 hours after TBI. Microglia/macrophage (ED1 and EMAP-II IHC) and B cell (OX22 IHC), astrocytes (GFAP), and oligodendrocytes (MBP).	Global methylation was similar in sham animals and contralateral side in TBI animals. In TBI animals, the ipsilateral cortex showed decreased global methylation starting at 24 hours (nonsignificant) and continuing at the 48- and 96-hour (significant) time points. Most cells exhibiting hypomethylation were microglia/macrophages. No other cell type showed significant variable methylation. Dexamethasone suppresses these effects at 48 hours after injury only.

(*Continued*)

TABLE 4.1

Example Studies Using Genomic, Transcriptomic, and Epigenomic Approaches in Traumatic Brain Injury (Continued)

Approach/Reference	Sample	Independent Variable	Dependent Variable	Results
		miRNA		
Patz et al. (2013)	26 CSF samples collected from 11 adults with TBI	TBI presence	miRNA (and other microparticle) presence in the CSF	81 distinct miRNAs were present, 23 of which confirm upregulation after TBI as identified in rat studies.
	26 samples from 17 adults without TBI			Many miRNAs were present in control and TBI CSF.
				miR-451 was only found in TBI samples.
Redell, Moore, Ward, Hergenroeder, and Dash (2010)	Plasma samples from: 10 severe TBI subjects and 10 age-, gender-, and race-matched healthy controls	Presence of severe TBI	Presence of plasma miRNA	52 miRNA had altered plasma levels in severe TBI: 33 decreased, 19 increased.
		Presence of mild TBI		8 miRNAs were detected only in the plasma of severe TBI subjects; miR-16, miR-92a, and miR-765 were good markers of severe TBI.
	11 mild TBI subjects (GCS > 12; negative head computed tomography scan)			

miR-16 and miR-92a were elevated in the mild TBI cases (compared to healthy controls). There was fair diagnostic potential with either miRNA, but no diagnostic value added by combining the two.

Note. 5HTT = 5-hydroxyltryptamine (serotonin) transporter gene; 5HTTLPR = 5-hydroxytryptamine (serotonin) transporter gene–linked polymorphic region; AKT = protein kinase B; ANKK1 = ankyrin repeat and kinase domain containing 1; APOE = apolipoprotein E; AQP4 = aquaporin 4; BBB = blood–brain barrier; BDNF = brain-derived neurotrophic factor; CA = Cornu Ammonis area, cAMP = cyclic adenosine monophosphate; CCI = closed cortical impact model; CNS = central nervous system; CPT = Gordon Continuous Performance Test; CSF = cerebrospinal fluid; CVLT = California Verbal Learning Test; DMA-PB = 4-dimethylamino-N-[5-(2-mercaptoacetylamino)pentyl]benzamide; DNA = deoxyribonucleic acid; DNMT = DNA methyltransferase; DRD2 = dopamine receptor D2 gene; *DSM-IV* = *Diagnostic and Statistical Manual* (4th ed.); EMAP II = endothelial monocyte-activating polypeptide-II; ERK = extracellular signal-related kinase; GAD = glutamate decarboxylase; GCS = Glasgow Coma Scale; GOS = Glasgow Outcome Scale; GFAP = glial fibrillary acidic protein; GSK = glycogen synthase kinase; GWAS = genome-wide association study; H&E = hematoxylin and eosin; H3 = histone 3; H4 = histone 4; HDAC = histone deacetylase; HMGB1 = high-mobility group box 1; IHC = immunohistochemistry; IR = immunoreactivity; LFP = lateral fluid percussion model; MAP-2 = microtubule-associated protein 2; MBP = myelin basic protein; miRNA = micro-ribonucleic acid; MTHFR = methylenetetrahydrofolate reductase gene; MWM = Morris water maze; NCAM = neural cell adhesion molecule; OR11H1 and OR4M1 = olfactory receptors; SAHA = suberoylanilide hydroxamic acid; SCID = Structured Clinical Interview for DSM; SNP = single nucleotide polymorphism; TBI = traumatic brain injury; TLR4 = toll-like receptor 4; TPH2 = tryptophan hydroxylase 2 gene; VPA = sodium valproate; WD = weight drop model.

involving multiple biologic pathways including ischemic stroke (Gretarsdottir et al., 2002); however, results have not been replicated (International Stroke Genetics Consortium, Wellcome Trust Case-Control Consortium 2., 2010; Ikram et al., 2009). The potential causes of this difficulty in replicating studies may be due to inherent differences in study population, ancestry, survival bias, or heterogeneity among participants. Due to the heterogeneous nature of brain injuries and the population suffering TBI, future research needs to be carried out using genomic approaches. It will be important to standardize phenotype data collection, use standard data elements, and create biobanks to allow for multicenter research studies combining samples to adequately power genomic approaches. As sample and data banks become more common, sample size issues may become less of an issue for investigators willing to share samples and data and collecting common data elements as outlined in the National Institute of Neurological Disorders and Stroke common data elements for TBI subjects (Glozak & Seto, 2007). The Federal Interagency Traumatic Brain Injury Research informatics system database (http://fitbir.nih.gov/) initiatives are a start to these efforts with a National Institutes of Health mandate in TBI research to enter data into this database for future cumulative analyses.

TRANSCRIPTOMIC APPROACHES

What Is Transcriptomics?

Transcriptomics is the study of the total set of ribonucleic acid (RNA) transcripts from a given sample. This approach, when focusing on messenger RNA (mRNA) is often referred to as a gene expression study. At a given moment in time and in different cell types, different genes are silenced or transcribed ("turned on or off") at variable rates depending upon the cellular needs at the time. Results of this type of work inform us of genes and biological pathways that are active, or inactive, in response to a particular biological event. Transcription research may focus on one gene's transcription product or the transcription products of multiple genes with a single or multiple pathways. Genes work in a network of interactions, and the usage of pathway analyses interprets the data by identifying connections among biological processes, pathways, and networks (Khatri, Sirota, & Butte, 2012; Rezola et al., 2014).

What Is the Research That Has Been Done in TBI Using Transcriptomic Approaches?

The transcriptomic approach in the TBI population (as in any injury or disease process) is useful in understanding the molecular changes that occur and therefore may inform targets for treatment effects (Luo et al., 2007; Zhang, Xuan, de los Reyes, Clarke, & Ressom, 2008). Defining the underpinnings of gene regulation in primary and secondary cellular injuries, the disease process of TBI, and the heterogeneous hereditary components will potentially assist in the understanding of both the acute and the long-term outcome differences. Computational methods for analyzing gene expression results are key to identifying differences and interpreting results (Merrick & Bruno, 2004; Phan, Quo, & Wang, 2006)

The majority of research exploring gene expression in TBI has been performed in experimental animal research and/or cell culture research. The resultant target protein products are those, which may be involved in secondary injury or recovery processes following a TBI. Many of these secondary injury pathways are related to inflammation, oxidative stress, and excitatory amino acid activations. In addition, the recovery process may be adaptive to include microglia activation, assisting in the resolution of injury in the brain, or maladaptive, involving tau protein and senile plaques, which may ultimately place the individual at an increased risk for neurodegenerative disorders (i.e., Alzheimer's and Parkinson's disease). Combination research studies demonstrating protein release in human subjects correlating with gene expression in animals or human cell cultures provide evidence toward a common genetic link to a particular protein. For example, Laird and colleagues demonstrated that cerebral edema, as measured by elevated intracranial pressure in severe TBI patients, was associated with the high-mobility group box protein1 (HMGB1; Laird et al., 2014). In addition, it was reported that HMGB1 was activated by the microglial toll-like receptor 4 (TLR4) and subsequent expression of the astrocyte water channel, aquaporin 4 (AQP4), promoting cerebral edema. Genetic or pharmacological inhibition of the TLR4 receptor decreased the edema, allowing a potential therapeutic window or treatment modality. A study by Verrier and colleagues examined the metabolites that are released in a mouse controlled cortical impact TBI model via microdialysate collection and showed that the 2', 3' cAMP-adenosine pathway was activated. In correlation, the same metabolites were examined in the cerebrospinal fluid (CSF) of severe TBI patients and were significantly increased in the initial 12 hours following injury (Verrier et al., 2012).

Brain tissue obtained from craniotomies following a severe TBI or brain tumor removal has also provided gene expression data in this population. A study performed by Liu and colleagues examined 19 contused brain samples 3 hours to 17 days following a TBI and resulting in a significant increase of ferritin, which may contribute to the secondary injury cascade following a TBI (Liu et al., 2013).

Peripheral blood mononuclear cells (PBMCs) may provide a measurable correlate to brain alterations following a TBI. PBMC samples from TBI subjects were examined by Zhao and colleagues for olfactory receptor (OR) activation (Zhao et al., 2013). Downregulation of OR11H1 and OR4M1 resulted in decreased abnormal tau phosphorylation, which could result in decreased TBI-induced tauopathy. Table 4.1 includes more detailed information on select significant work exploring the effects of TBI using a transcriptomic approach.

Where Can We Go From Here?

Once basic gene expression targets are identified, potential translational therapies could be trialed. Reprogramming of the differentiated human somatic cells into a pluripotent state theoretically would allow the creation of patient- and disease-specific stem cells (Takahashi et al., 2007; Yamanaka, 2007). Also, transporting a cell "back to a primitive state," such as a neonatal gene expression, could offer potential therapy mechanisms for outcome improvement. A study performed by Cummins and Gentene examined the effect of a hyperbaric treatment on the expression of matrix metalloproteinase 9 (MMP-9), which is involved as a potential contributory factor associated with cerebral ischemia. Although only examined in one patient who acted as her own control, hyperbaric oxygen treatment mitigated MMP-9 expression following trauma (Cummins & Gentene, 2010). Additional gene expression studies examining treatment effects need to be performed to provide mechanistic, molecular evidence of a beneficial effect.

EPIGENOMIC APPROACHES

What Is Epigenomics?

Individual cells have various genes that are active or inactive depending upon the extracellular environment and the cellular needs. The epigenetic research approach focuses on the exploration of nonsequence variation (e.g., histone modification, methylation, and miRNA [micro-RNA]) modifying gene transcription, translation, and RNA stability of a given gene/gene product (Paoloni-Giacobino, 2011; Petronis, 2010; Shirodkar & Marsden, 2011). Epigenomics is the study of the combined effects of one or more of these mechanisms across the genome and its impact on the outcome of interest (Petronis, 2010). Epigenomic changes can be passed to daughter cells but are also modifiable (Paoloni-Giacobino, 2011; Petronis, 2010). These changes are different for different tissue types and cellular environments and are subject to further modification by additional factors such as maternal behavior, exercise, diet, and aging (Paoloni-Giacobino, 2011; Petronis, 2010). One particularly challenging aspect of this line of research lies in the significant sources of modification to epigenomic processes over the course of an individual life span (Paoloni-Giacobino, 2011). Epigenomics classically includes three main areas of study: histone modification, DNA methylation, and small RNA/miRNA function. The International Human Epigenome Consortium (IHEC; www.ihec-epigenomes.org) is an excellent resource for scientists, making available a series of data sets of reference epigenomes.

Histone Modification and Methylation

Histone modification has a bearing on the extent and severity (tightness) of the DNA coiling around the histone protein that assist in packaging the DNA (Zentner & Henikoff, 2013). DNA transcription machinery cannot access DNA that is tightly wound around the histone. During times of need, chemical modifications to the histone occur that loosen the DNA and make it available for transcription and translation. Quantification of these changes can tell us which areas of the genome, or more specifically which genes, are active or silenced. This research informs our knowledge of individual genes and pathways that are activated or deactivated at a given point in time relative to the outcome of interest.

Acetylation is specific to the histones anchoring the DNA to form nucleosomes. Acetylation allows the histone to release the DNA, permitting unwinding (Zentner & Henikoff, 2013). For DNA in tightly coiled regions, acetylation of the histone, and lysine acetylation in particular, or other mechanisms of histone modification are required for DNA transcription as it must be released from the histone and unwound before transcription can occur (Zentner & Henikoff, 2013). Histones are modified by other processes including, but not limited to, methylation, phosphorylation, adenosine diphosphate (ADP) ribosylation, and glycosylation (Zentner & Henikoff, 2013). Enzymes with histone acetyltransferase (HAT) activity, such as the general control non-derepressible t-related N-acetyltransferases (GNAT), monocytic leukemia zinc finger protein Ybf2/Sas3, Sas2, and Tat interacting protein 60 (MYST), p300/CBP, and others, promote histone acetylation (Yang & Seto, 2007). Enzymes with histone deactylase (HDAC) activity, such as HDAC1, HDAC2, HDAC3, HDAC11, and others, remove acetyl groups from the histone (Yang & Seto, 2007). Histone acetylation is modified by exercise, diet, immune activity, and possibly smoking and stress (Yang & Seto, 2007). Alterations in acetylation have been implicated in inflammatory disorders including asthma (Kuo et al., 2014), chronic obstructive pulmonary disease (Mroz, Noparlik, Chyczewska, Braszko, & Holownia, 2007), cancer (Cohen, Poreba, Kamieniarz, & Schneider, 2011; Glozak & Seto, 2007), cardiac hypertrophy (Wang et al., 2014), schizophrenia (Tang, Dean, & Thomas, 2011), and Huntington's disease (Lee, Hwang, Kim, Kowall, & Ryu, 2013). Histone acetylation occurs in regions where genes are to be activated (Yang & Seto, 2007).

Studies of histone acetylation are generally focused on a DNA region of interest, and as such, this type of work is primarily hypothesis-driven research.

Methylation involves attaching methyl groups to the DNA backbone. Methylation prevents DNA transcription machinery from accessing the DNA and halts transcription (Bergman & Cedar, 2013; Zentner & Henikoff, 2013). Highly methylated regions have little to no activity, while regions without methylation may be transcribed or are regulated through some other mechanism. Studies of methylation tell us which areas of the genome may not be actively transcribed and therefore have a biological role in the outcome of interest. It is important to note that there are other mechanisms involved in the regulation of DNA relaxation, histone binding, and transcription (Zentner & Henikoff, 2013). Knowledge of the areas that have variable methylation (up or down) is particularly informative in determining what genes are involved in a specific outcome (Bergman & Cedar, 2013). There are likely different genes being turned on or off in multiple pathways after TBI, some that promote cellular survival and some promoting appropriate cell death, and individuals with good outcomes likely have a distinct epigenetic pattern(s) reflecting this phenomenon.

Methylation quantification may be performed for the entire genome, or for individual genes alone, or a panel of genes within one or more identified pathways. Quantification of methylation of the entire genome may be hypothesis generating, while methylation quantification of one or more genes within a pathway is a hypothesis-driven approach. Both approaches are relevant depending upon the question being answered. Methylation has been implicated in cancer (Baylin, Herman, Graff, Vertino, & Issa, 1998; Chen, Pettersson, Beard, Jackson-Grusby, & Jaenisch, 1998; Jones & Baylin, 2002; Nakayama et al., 2004), atherosclerosis (Castro et al., 2003; Dong, Yoon, & Goldschmidt-Clermont, 2002), and aging (Gonzalo et al., 2010; Horvath, 2013). Both histone acetylation and DNA demethylation must occur before transcription can occur. Given that response to TBI driven by cellular response to damage impacting both mechanisms, they are likely to modify outcome.

Acetylation status contributes to DNA binding to histones, while methylation quantification contributes to gene transcription activity, or the lack thereof, in a given physiologic state. As such, markers of these processes facilitate understanding of the pathophysiology of the outcome measure and may identify a target for therapeutic intervention. Selection of the phenotype remains important for acetylation and methylation research as it is still important to compare groups that are similar on all but the variable of interest. Covariates are many, must be identified a priori, and incorporated in the inclusion criteria for adequate study. Specifically, epigenetic mechanisms are influenced by prenatal and sensitivity and 100% specificity (Redell, Moore, Ward, Hergenroeder, & Dash, 2010). It should be noted that the miRNA profile found in human serum versus CSF is different (Burgos et al., 2013). This work also found that miR-16 and miR-92A has diagnostic value in mild TBI (GCS > 12) up to 24 hours after injury. While the sample size was small in this work (n = approximately 10 per group), it shows the significant promise of the use of miRNA as a diagnostic tool.

miRNA has also been used as a tool to determine the mechanism of action in studies of therapeutic interventions in TBI. In a fluid percussion rat model of TBI with follow-up treatment with therapeutic hypothermia (33°C for 4 hours), there was considerable difference in miRNA expression in the cerebral cortex between groups. There were 47 miRNAs with differential expression (15 higher, 31 lower) in the TBI group at 7 hours and 16 miRNAs had variable expression (7 higher, 9 lower) in the TBI group at 24 hours. They found that seven miRNAs had higher nd five miRNAs had lower expression in the TBI-therapeutic hypothermia group ompared to the TBI-normothermic group at 7 hours after injury. Of interest, niR-9, miR-290, miR-451, and miR-874, which have previously been identified s influential in neurodevelopment and/or after TBI, were upregulated in the ther- peutic hypothermia TBI group (Truettner, Alonso, Bramlett, & Dietrich, 2011).

In a study of veterans with or without mild TBI (n = 9 TI and 9 non-TBI) ploring variable serum small noncoding RNAs, a panel of 18 small RNA iomark- s (4 miRNAs, 13 snoRNAs and 1 small scaRNA) were downregulated in subjects th mild TI (Pasinetti et al., 2012). Further analysis suggested that a panel includ- g three snoRNA biomarkers were sufficient for the differentiation of mild TBI m non-TBI subjects (Pasinetti et al., 2012). While this work had a very small nple size and needs further replication in better-powered studies of the mild TBI pulation, it makes an interesting contribution to the literature, showing the pos- lity of a blood biomarker for mild TBI and provides a platform for future work.

ere Can We Go From Here?

enomic approaches hold great promise for the studies of TBI. To date, the rity of research has occurred in animal models of TBI. Future research ld focus on human tissues to generate results that are more applicable and a er understanding of this complex recovery process.

The work in HDAC inhibitors needs to be expanded, particularly in human cations. As work in animal models including therapeutics after TBI con- s to identify the mechanism of action, translation to human populations nes feasible. Clinical trials exploring the effects of valproate and other inhibitors should focus on safety as well as efficacy. The use of HDAC tors with previous Food and Drug Administration approval will expedite rk while new agents continue to be developed and tested in both human

lifelong behaviors and exposures including genetic variants, diet, alcohol intake, cigarette smoking, exercise, endocrine function/dysfunction, heavy metals, and infectious agents (Foley et al., 2009; Paoloni-Giacobino, 2011). The temporal and physiologic nature of variable acetylation and methylation status makes time and tissue important considerations. Acetylation and methylation status changes over time and depends upon the local environment. The tissue used for this type of research needs to reflect the cellular environment and insults that drive changes in that specific tissue type (Foley et al., 2009; Paoloni-Giacobino, 2011). Samples must be collected at an appropriate time point to answer the research question, and repeated sampling may be beneficial to show changes over time contributing to the outcome. Hypoxia-inducible factor 1 (HIF1) is an excellent example of how epigenetic changes are modified by cellular environment changes over time. In states of normal oxygen, HIF1 is modified by the HIF prolyl hydrolases and quickly degraded. In hypoxic conditions when HIF prolyl hydrolases are inhibited by the lack of oxygen, HIF1 is stabilized and acts to upregulate the expression of genes involved in cellular survival during low-oxygen states (Smith, Robbins, & Ratcliffe, 2008). The epigenetic study of HIF1 effects requires the sampling of a specific tissue where hypoxia is prevalent and at the specific time when this biologic activity can be captured. Studies using whole blood may not be informative for TBI research as they speak to events occurring in the entire body rather than CNS specific effects. While less informative, this sample is often more easily available and may still be used to inform other work or identify points of potential intervention. The sample size required is again impacted by the number of acetylation and methylation points to be analyzed, the number of time points where samples are available, and the effect size of the changes.

RNA: microRNAs, Small Nucleolar RNAs, and Long Noncoding RNAs

More recent research has identified noncoding regions that are vital for the regulatory control of genes and gene products. miRNAs are short, noncoding RNAs that are important for transcription and posttranscriptional gene expression regulation (Esteller, 2011; Pasinetti, Ho, Dooley, Abbi, & Lange, 2012). miRNAs attach to messenger RNA (mRNA) to prevent translation into protein or initiate its degradation. In this way, miRNAs alter protein production and modify gene expression and the brain's biological response to TBI. A single miRNA has multiple mRNA targets and thus may impact the expression of multiple genes, contributing to the complex biological response. Small noncoding RNAs belong to a category including both miRNAs and small nucleolar RNAs (snoRNAs). Small noncoding RNAs are capable of modifying epigenetic mechanisms through effects on transcription and posttranscription gene expression regulation (Esteller 2011; Pasinetti et al., 2012). snoRNAs modify ribosomal RNA to exert effects on gene expression.

What Is the Research That Has Been Done in TBI Using Epigenomic Approaches?

Much of the work exploring epigenomic/epigenetic mechanisms in TBI has been done in preclinical animal and cell models. Given the dearth of literature in the human realm, we present the current state of the science of TBI research in epigenetics/epigenomics in animal models when human studies are not available. Table 4.1 includes more detailed information on this work, exploring the epigenetics/epigenomics work in TBI. In a study of rat TBI, Gao and colleagues found that histone H3 acetylation and methylation in the hippocampal region decreased at multiple time points up to 24 and 72 hours after injury, suggesting that histone H3 is active in the early response to TBI (Gao et al., 2006).

HDAC inhibitors have shown some neuroprotective effects in many human neurodegenerative diseases (Hahnen et al., 2008) and in animal models of TBI. Administration of the HDAC inhibitor valproate improved blood–brain barrier (BBB) permeability, decreased contusion volume, and improved functional outcome (Dash et al., 2009; Dash et al., 2010). Specific mechanisms of HDAC inhibitors, and valproate in particular, have suggested that these effects may be driven by HDAC moderation of inflammation (Dash, Orsi, & Moore, 2009; Dash et al., 2010) or, through work using the HDAC inhibitor ITF2357 in a mouse model of TBI, by glial apoptosis and microglia function (Zhang et al., 2008). These findings have been replicated with other HDAC inhibitors (Cao et al., 2013; Wang et al., 2013). Follow-up work found that HDAC inhibitors increase the expression of nerve growth factors and neurotrophic factors while decreasing apoptotic factors (Lu et al., 2013). Additional work has found that these effects of valproate were enhanced when administered in combination with lithium (a glycogen synthase kinase 3 inhibitor; Yu et al., 2013).

One study found global hypomethylation near the site of injury driven by activated microglia/macrophages in the first 24–48 hours after weight drop model TBI in a rat model (Zhang, Zhang, Fauser, & Schluesener, 2007). This effect was inhibited after 48 hours by the administration of dexamethasone. An additional study found that DNA-methyltransferase (Dnmt1) enzymes are upregulated in reactive astrocytes near the injury early after TBI and decreased by 14 days (Lundberg et al., 2009).

Significant changes in miRNA have been found to occur after TBI. miR-21 increases in the hippocampus for 3 days after closed cortical impact in a model of rat TBI. miR-21 theoretically modifies the expression of 99 potential target genes

involved in enzyme-linked receptor signaling, transcriptional regulation developmental processes (Redell, Zhao, & Dash, 2011). Another study that 35 miRNAs were upregulated and 50 were downregulated in the campus after closed cortical injury in a rat model of TBI (Redell, Liu, & 2009). Targets of these miRNAs include signal transduction, transcriptic liferation, and differentiation of proteins (Redell et al., 2009). Addition using the closed cortical impact model in rats found the modified expre miRNAs (upregulation of miR-124, miR-135a, and miR-153; downre of miR-222) with targets in the apoptotic cascade, aerobic respiration, tein folding 1 day after induced injury, while the modified expressio miRNAs (upregulation of miR-124 and miR-153; downregulation of and miR-135b) with targets in cytoskeletal organization and intrace ficking was noted 7 days after induced injury (Hu et al., 2012). also been explored in the cerebral cortex after fluid percussion inj This work generated a larger number of miRNAs with variable expre were upregulated at least twofold and 5–23 were downregulated at depending upon the time point) at 6, 24, 48, and 72 hours afte Li, Chen, Yang, & Zhang, 2009). This work highlights the tempor miRNAs as part of the temporal response to TBI and the initiatic pathways in the response pattern.

In humans, 81 miRNAs have been identified in micropart cerebrospinal fluid (CSF). Fourteen miRNAs were identified in t ing miR-451 present only in those patients with severe TBI (Glas [GCS] < 9) and miR-9 present only in the healthy controls (Pa While this work includes a small number of subjects with CSF dom time points and for convenience only, it highlights the pote markers to inform further work exploring the pathways involv TBI and the use of miRNA.

There has also been significant work exploring the use as biomarkers of TBI for specific use as diagnostic markers. and particularly mild TBI, can be difficult due to the wide v as well as the need for imaging to identify lesions. Animals fied variable expression of miR-let-71, with target proteins ubiquitin C-terminal hydrolase-1, as early as 3 hours afte (Balakathiresan et al., 2012; Hu et al., 2012) and upregulati 132 and miR-183, with target proteins in the cholinergic a naling pathway, 6 hours after repeat blast injury (Valiyav human plasma of the 52 miRNAs noted to have variable TBI (compared to healthy controls), miR-16, miR-92A, a nostic ability with a combination of the three generati

and animal models. The development of other histone modifiers should also continue, developing therapeutics to alter these processes and testing their safety and efficacy in animal models and then in human clinical trials. This work should especially focus on targeted methylation and acetylation of specific genes relevant to TBI and the biologic pathways activated, or deactivated, after TBI. Similar work needs to be carried out for miRNA. The use of small RNA and miRNA as biomarkers has the potential to increase prognostic capability, and perhaps diagnostic capability, particularly for mild and complicated mild or moderate TBI (Paoloni-Giacobino, 2011; Pasinetti et al., 2012). As we learn more from the preclinical work, the modifiers of specific miRNA relevant to pathways activated or deactivated after TBI inform the community about the pathobiologic reaction to TBI. This also identifies areas to intervene to improve the outcome from TBI. Blocking the effects of miRNA to modify one pathway that promotes worse outcome or enhancing effects of miRNA to modify another pathway promoting better outcome may enhance outcomes. The complex nature of the response to TBI with multiple biologic pathway activation or deactivation makes this translation difficult, but research is essential to identify proper targets for intervention. In the era of personalized medicine, there will likely be distinct profiles identifying different needs for different patients.

CONCLUSIONS

The "Omics" revolution has generated data contributing to our understanding of many health and disease states including TBI. There are clearly genomic, transcriptomic, and epigenomic mechanisms contributing to the brain response to injury. The knowledge generated from this line of research has increased our understanding of this response and identified potential targets for intervention. Understanding common mechanisms of recovery from TBI as well as individual differences in biologic responses contributes to the development of a paradigm shift in clinical care that promotes individualized care to maximize outcomes. The future holds great promise for the survivors of TBI. As knowledge increases, more therapeutics will be developed and distinct populations likely to receive benefit from a single therapeutic will be identified. This will facilitate individualized genomic- and epigenomic-based care, specific to the individual's biologic needs, to maximize outcomes.

REFERENCES

Aschard, H., Lutz, S., Maus, B., Duell, E. J., Fingerlin, T. E., Chatterjee, N., et al. (2012). Challenges and opportunities in genome-wide environmental interaction (GWEI) studies. *Human Genetics, 131*(10), 1591–1613. http://dx.doi.org/10.1007/s00439-012-1192-0

Balakathiresan, N., homia, M., Chandran, R., Chavko, M., McCarron, R. M., & Maheshwari, R. K. (2012). MicroRNA let-7i is a promising serum biomarker for blast-induced traumatic rain injury. *Journal of Neurotrauma, 29*(7), 1379–1387.

Baylin, S. B., Herman, J. G., Graff, J. R., Vertino, P. M., & Issa, J. P. (1998). Alterations in DNA methylation: A fundamental aspect of neoplasia. *Advances in Cancer Research, 72*, 141–196.

Bergman, Y., & Cedar, H. (2013). DNA methylation dynamics in health and disease. *Nature Structural & Molecular Biology, 20*(3), 274–281. http://dx.doi.org/10.1038/nsmb.2518

Bhattacharjee, S., Wang, Z., Ciampa, J., Kraft, P., Chanock, S., Yu, K., et al. (2010). Using principal components of genetic variation for robust and powerful detection of gene-gene interactions in case-control and case-only studies. *The American Journal of Human Genetics, 86*(3), 331–342. http://dx.doi.org/10.1016/j.ajhg.2010.01.026

Bookman, E. B., McAllister, K., Gillanders, E., Wanke, K., Balshaw, D., Rutter, J., et al. (2011). Gene-environment interplay in common complex diseases: Forging an integrative model-recommendations from an NIH workshop. *Genetic Epidemiology, 35*(4), 217–225. http://dx.doi.org/10.1002/gepi.20571

Burgos, K. L., Javaherian, A., Bomprezzi, R., Ghaffari, L., Rhodes, S., Courtright, A., et al. (2013). Identification of extracellular miRNA in human cerebrospinal fluid by next-generation sequencing. *Ribonucleic Acid, 19*(5), 712–722. http://dx.doi.org/10.1261/rna.036863.112

Cao, P., Liang, Y., Gao, X., Zhao, M. G., & Liang, G. B. (2013). Administration of MS-275 improves cognitive performance and reduces cell death following traumatic brain injury in rats. *CNS Neuroscience & Therapeutics, 19*(5), 337–345.

Castro, R., Rivera, I., Struys, E. A., Jansen, E. E., Ravasco, P., Camilo, M. E., et al. (2003). Increased homocysteine and S-adenosylhomocysteine concentrations and DNA hypomethylation in vascular disease. *Clinical Chemistry, 49*(8), 1292–1296.

Chanock, S. J., Manolio, T., Boehnke, M., Boerwinkle, E., Hunter, D. J., Thomas, G., et al. (2007). Replicating genotype–phenotype associations. *Nature, 447*(7145), 655–660. http://dx.doi.org/10.1038/447655a

Chen, R. Z., Pettersson, U., Beard, C., Jackson-Grusby, L., & Jaenisch, R. (1998). DNA hypomethylation leads to elevated mutation rates. *Nature, 395*(6697), 89–93. http://dx.doi.org/10.1038/25779

Clarke, A., & Thirlaway, K. (2011). Genetic counselling for personalised medicine. *Human Genetics, 130*(1), 27–31. http://dx.doi.org/10.1007/s00439-011-0988-7

Clarke, G. M., Anderson, C. A., Pettersson, F. H., Cardon, L. R., Morris, A. P., & Zondervan, K. T. (2011). Basic statistical analysis in genetic case-control studies. *Nature Protocols, 6*(2), 121–133. http://dx.doi.org/10.1038/nprot.2010.182

Cohen, I., Poreba, E., Kamieniarz, K., & Schneider, R. (2011). Histone modifiers in cancer: Friends or foes? *Genes Cancer, 2*(6), 631–647. http://dx.doi.org/10.1177/1947601911417176

Cordell, H. J. (2009). Detecting gene-gene interactions that underlie human diseases. *Nature Reviews Genetics, 10*(6), 392–404. http://dx.doi.org/10.1038/nrg2579

Corvin, A., Craddock, N., & Sullivan, P. F. (2010). Genome-wide association studies: A primer. *Psychological Medicine, 40*(7), 1063–1077. http://dx.doi.org/10.1017/S0033291709991723

Cummins, F. J., Jr., & Gentene, L. J. (2010). Hyperbaric oxygen effect on MMP-9 after a vascular insult. *Journal of Cardiovascular Translational Research, 3*(6), 683–687. http://dx.doi.org/10.1007/s12265-010-9221-7

Darrah, S. D., Miller, M. A., Ren, D., Hoh, N. Z., Scanlon, J. M., Conley, Y. P., et al. (2013). Genetic variability in glutamic acid decarboxylase genes: associations with post-traumatic seizures after severe TBI. *Epilepsy Research, 103*(2–3), 180–194. http://dx.doi.org/10.1016/j.eplepsyres.2012.07.006

Dash, P. K., Orsi, S. A., & Moore, A. N. (2009). Histone deactylase inihbition combined with behavioral therapy enhances learning and memory following traumatic brain injury. *Neuroscience, 163*(1), 1–8.

Dash, P. K., Orsi, S. A., Zhang, M., Grill, R. J., Pati, S., Zhao, J., et al. (2010). Valproate administered after traumatic brain injury provides neuroprotection and improves cognitive function in rats. *PLoS ONE, 5*(6), e11383.

Dong, C., Yoon, W., & Goldschmidt-Clermont, P. J. (2002). DNA methylation and atherosclerosis. *Journal of Nutrition, 132*(8 Suppl), 2406S–2409S.

Esteller, M. (2011). Non-coding RNAs in human disease. *Nature Reviews Genetics, 12*(12), 861–874. http://dx.doi.org/10.1038/nrg3074

Foley, D. L., Craig, J. M., Morley, R., Olsson, C. A., Dwyer, T., Smith, K., et al. (2009). Prospects for epigenetic epidemiology. *American Journal of Epidemiology, 169*(4), 389–400. http://dx.doi.org/10.1093/aje/kwn380

Gao, W. M., Chadha, M. S., Kline, A. E., Clark, R. S., Kochanek, P. M., Dixon, C. E., et al. (2006). Immunohistochemical analysis of histone H3 acetylation and methylation—evidence for altered epigenetic signaling following traumatic brain injury in immature rats. *Brain Research, 1070*(1), 31–34. http://dx.doi.org/S0006-8993(05)01608-2

Gauderman, W. J. (2002). Sample size requirements for association studies of gene-gene interaction. *American Journal of Epidemiology, 155*(5), 478–484.

Glozak, M. A., & Seto, E. (2007). Histone deacetylases and cancer. *Oncogene, 26*(37), 5420–5432. http://dx.doi.org/1210610

Gonzalo, V., Lozano, J. J., Munoz, J., Balaguer, F., Pellise, M., Rodriguez de Miguel, C., et al. (2010). Aberrant gene promoter methylation associated with sporadic multiple colorectal cancer. *PLoS One, 5*(1), e8777. http://dx.doi.org/10.1371/journal.pone.0008777

Gretarsdottir, S., Sveinbjornsdottir, S., Jonsson, H. H., Jakobsson, F., Einarsdottir, E., Agnarsson, U., et al. (2002). Localization of a susceptibility gene for common forms of stroke to 5q12. *The American Journal of Human Genetics, 70*(3), 593–603. http://dx.doi.org/S0002-9297(07)60263-8

Hahnen, E., Hauke, J., Trankle, C., Eyupoglu, I. Y., Wirth, B., & Blumcke, I. (2008). Histone deacetylase inhibitors: Possible implications for neurodegenerative disorders. *Expert Opinion on Investigational Drugs, 17*(2), 169–184. http://dx.doi.org/10.1517/13543784.17.2.169

Hicks, R., Giacino, J., Harrison-Felix, C., Manley, G., Valadka, A., & Wilde, E. A. (2013). Progress in developing common data elements for traumatic brain injury research: Version two—the end of the beginning. *Journal of Neurotrauma, 30*(22), 1852–1861. http://dx.doi.org/10.1089/neu.2013.2930

Horvath, S. (2013). DNA methylation age of human tissues and cell types. *Genome Biology, 14*(10), R115. http://dx.doi.org/gb-2013-14-10-r115

Hu, Z., Yu, D., Almeida-Suhett, C., Tu, K., Marini, A. M., Eiden, L., et al. (2012). Expression of miRNAs and their cooperative regulation of the pathophysiology in traumatic brain injury. *PLoS One, 7*(6), e39357. http://dx.doi.org/10.1371/journal.pone.0039357

Hunter, D. J., Kraft, P., Jacobs, K. B., Cox, D. G., Yeager, M., Hankinson, S. E., et al. (2007). A genome-wide association study identifies alleles in FGFR2 associated with risk of sporadic postmenopausal breast cancer. *Nature Genetics, 39*(7), 870–874. http://dx.doi.org/ng2075

Ikram, M. A., Sudha, S., Joshua, C. B., Myriam, F., Anita, L. D., Yurii S. A., et al. (2009). Genomewide association studies of stroke. *The New England Journal of Medicine, 360*(17):1718–1728. Epub 2009 Apr 15. http://dx.doi.org/10.1056/NEJMoa0900094

International Stroke Genetics Consortium. (2015). Recommendations from the International Stroke Genetics Consortium, part 1: Standardized phenotypic data collection. *Stroke, 46*(1), 279–284. Epub 2014 Dec 9. http://dx.doi.org/10.1161/STROKEAHA

Jellinger, K. A. (2004). Head injury and dementia. *Current Opinion in Neurology, 17*(6), 719–723. http://dx.doi.org/00019052-200412000-00012

Jones, P. A., & Baylin, S. B. (2002). The fundamental role of epigenetic events in cancer. *Nature Reviews Genetics, 3*(6), 415–428. http://dx.doi.org/10.1038/nrg816

Keller, M. C. (2014). Gene x environment interaction studies have not properly controlled for potential confounders: The problem and the (simple) solution. *Biological Psychiatry, 75*(1), 18–24. http://dx.doi.org/10.1016/j.biopsych.2013.09.006

Khatri, P., Sirota, M., & Butte, A. J. (2012). Ten years of pathway analysis: Current approaches and outstanding challenges. *PLoS Computational Biology, 8*(2), e1002375. http://dx.doi.org/10.1371/journal.pcbi.1002375

Koponen, S., Taiminen, T., Kairisto, V., Portin, R., Isoniemi, H., Hinkka, S., et al. (2004). APOE-epsilon4 predicts dementia but not other psychiatric disorders after traumatic brain injury. *Neurology, 63*(4), 749–750. http://dx.doi.org/63/4/749

Kuo, C. H., Hsieh, C. C., Lee, M. S., Chang, K. T., Kuo, H. F., & Hung, C. H. (2014). Epigenetic regulation in allergic diseases and related studies. *Asia Pacific Allergy, 4*(1), 14–18. http://dx.doi.org/10.5415/apallergy.2014.4.1.14

Laird, M. D., Shields, J. S., Sukumari-Ramesh, S., Kimbler, D. E., Fessler, R. D., Shakir, B., et al. (2014). High mobility group box protein-1 promotes cerebral edema after traumatic brain injury via activation of toll-like receptor 4. *Glia, 62*(1), 26–38. http://dx.doi.org/10.1002/glia.22581

Lanctot, K. L., Rapoport, M. J., Chan, F., Rajaram, R. D., Strauss, J., Sicard, T., et al. (2010). Genetic predictors of response to treatment with citalopram in depression secondary to traumatic brain injury. *Brain Injury, 24*(7–8), 959–969. http://dx.doi.org/10.3109/02699051003789229

Lee, J., Hwang, Y. J., Kim, K. Y., Kowall, N. W., & Ryu, H. (2013). Epigenetic mechanisms of neurodegeneration in Huntington's disease. *Neurotherapeutics, 10*(4), 664–676. http://dx.doi.org/10.1007/s13311-013-0206-5

Lei, P., Li, Y., Chen, X., Yang, S., & Zhang, J. (2009). Microarray based analysis of microRNA expression in rat cerebral cortex after traumatic brain injury. *Brain Research, 1284*, 191–201. http://dx.doi.org/10.1016/j.brainres.2009.05.074

Liu, H. D., Li, W., Chen, Z. R., Zhou, M. L., Zhuang, Z., Zhang, D. D., et al. (2013). Increased expression of ferritin in cerebral cortex after human traumatic brain injury. *Neurological Sciences, 34*(7), 1173–1180. http://dx.doi.org/10.1007/s10072-012-1214-7

Lu, J., Frerich, J. M., Turtzo, L. C., Li, S., Chiang, J., Yang, C., et al. (2013). Histone deacetylase inhibitors are neuroprotective and preserve NGF-mediated cell survival following traumatic brain injury. *Proceedings of the National Academy of Sciences of the United States of America, 110*(26), 10747–10752. http://dx.doi.org/10.1073/pnas.1308950110

Lundberg, J., Karimi, M., von Gertten, C., Holmin, S., Ekstrom, T. J., & Sandberg-Nordqvist, A. C. (2009). Traumatic brain injury induces relocalization of DNA-methyltransferase 1. *Neuroscience Letters, 457*(1), 8–11. http://dx.doi.org/10.1016/j.neulet.2009.03.105

Luo, F., Yang, Y., Zhong, J., Gao, H., Khan, L., Thompson, D. K., et al. (2007). Constructing gene co-expression networks and predicting functions of unknown genes by random matrix theory. *BMC Bioinformatics, 8*, 299. http://dx.doi.org/1471-2105-8-299

McAllister, T. W., Flashman, L. A., Harker Rhodes, C., Tyler, A. L., Moore, J. H., Saykin, A. J., et al. (2008). Single nucleotide polymorhispsm in ANKK1 and the dopamine D2 receptor gene after cognitive outcome shortly after traumatic brain injury: a replication and extension study. *Brain Injury. 22*(9); 705–714.

McCarthy, M. I., & Hirschhorn, J. N. (2008). Genome-wide association studies: Potential next steps on a genetic journey. *Human Molecular Genetics, 17*(R2), R156–R165. http://dx.doi.org/10.1093/hmg/ddn289

McCarthy, M. I., Abecasis, G. R., Cardon, L. R., Goldstein, D. B., Little, J., Ioannidis, J. P., et al. (2008). Genome-wide association studies for complex traits: Consensus, uncertainty and challenges. *Nature Reviews Genetics, 9*(5), 356–369. http://dx.doi.org/10.1038/nrg2344

Merrick, B. A., & Bruno, M. E. (2004). Genomic and proteomic profiling for biomarkers and signature profiles of toxicity. *Current Opinion in Molecular Therapeutics, 6*(6), 600–607.

Mroz, R. M., Noparlik, J., Chyczewska, E., Braszko, J. J., & Holownia, A. (2007). Molecular basis of chronic inflammation in lung diseases: New therapeutic approach. *Journal of Physiology and Pharmacology, 58 Suppl 5*(Pt 2), 453–460.

Muller, H. H., Pahl, R., & Schafer, H. (2007). Including sampling and phenotyping costs into the optimization of two stage designs for genomewide association studies. *Genetics Epidemiology, 31*(8), 844–852. http://dx.doi.org/10.1002/gepi.20245

Nakayama, M., Gonzalgo, M. L., Yegnasubramanian, S., Lin, X., De Marzo, A. M., & Nelson, W. G. (2004). GSTP1 CpG island hypermethylation as a molecular biomarker for prostate cancer. *Journal of Cellular Biochemistry, 91*(3), 540–552. http://dx.doi.org/10.1002/jcb.10740

National Human Genome Research Institute. (2011). *An overview of the human genome project*. Retrieved July 07, 2011 from http://www.genome.gov/12011238

Paoloni-Giacobino, A. (2011). Post genomic decade—the epigenome and exposome challenges. *Swiss Medical Weekly, 141*, w13321. http://dx.doi.org/10.4414/smw.2011.13321

Pasinetti, G. M., Ho, L., Dooley, C., Abbi, B., & Lange, G. (2012). Select non-coding RNA in blood components provide novel clinically accessible biological surrogates for improved identification of traumatic brain injury in OEF/OIF Veterans. *American Journal of Neuro-degenerative Diseases, 1*(1), 88–98.

Patz, S., Trattnig, C., Grunbacher, G., Ebner, B., Gully, C., Novak, A., et al. (2013). More than cell dust: Microparticles isolated from cerebrospinal fluid of brain injured patients are messengers carrying mRNAs, miRNAs, and proteins. *Journal of Neurotrauma, 30*(14), 1232–1242. http://dx.doi.org/10.1089/neu.2012.2596

Pearson, T. A., & Manolio, T. A. (2008). How to interpret a genome wide association study. *The Journal of the American Medical Association, 299*(11), 1335–1344. http://dx.doi.org/10.1001/jama.299.11.1335

Petronis, A. (2010). Epigenetics as a unifying principle in the aetiology of complex traits and diseases. *Nature, 465*(7299), 721–727. http://dx.doi.org/10.1038/nature09230

Phan, J. H., Quo, C. F., & Wang, M. D. (2006). Functional genomics and proteomics in the clinical neurosciences: Data mining and bioinformatics. *Progress in Brain Research, 158*, 83–108. http://dx.doi.org/S0079-6123(06)58004-5

Redell, J. B., Liu, Y., & Dash, P. K. (2009). Traumatic brain injury alters expression of hippocampal microRNAs: Potential regulators of multiple pathophysiological processes. *Journal of Neuroscience Research, 87*(6), 1435–1448. http://dx.doi.org/10.1002/jnr.21945

Redell, J. B., Moore, A. N., Ward, N. H., III, Hergenroeder, G. W., & Dash, P. K. (2010). Human traumatic brain injury alters plasma microRNA levels. *Journal of Neurotrauma, 27*(12), 2147–2156. http://dx.doi.org/10.1089/neu.2010.1481

Redell, J. B., Zhao, J., & Dash, P. K. (2011). Altered expression of miRNA-21 and its targets in the hippocampus after traumatic brain injury. *Journal of Neuroscience Research, 89*(2), 212–221. http://dx.doi.org/10.1002/jnr.22539

Rezola, A., Pey, J., Tobalina, L., Rubio, A., Beasley, J. E., & Planes, F. J. (2014). Advances in network-based metabolic pathway analysis and gene expression data integration. *Briefings in Bioinformatics*. Epub ahead of print. http://dx.doi.org/bbu009

Sanjuan, R., & Elena, S. F. (2006). Epistasis correlates to genomic complexity. *Proceedings of the National Academy of Sciences of the United States of America, 103*(39), 14402–14405. http://dx.doi.org/0604543103

Shirodkar, A. V., & Marsden, P. A. (2011). Epigenetics in cardiovascular disease. *Current Opinion in Cardiology, 26*(3), 209–215. http://dx.doi.org/10.1097/HCO.0b013e328345986e

Smith, T. G., Robbins, P. A., & Ratcliffe, P. J. (2008). The human side of hypoxia-inducible factor. *British Journal of Haematology, 141*(3), 325–334. http://dx.doi.org/10.1111/j.1365-2141.2008.07029.x

Spencer, C. C., Su, Z., Donnelly, P., & Marchini, J. (2009). Designing genome-wide association studies: Sample size, power, imputation, and the choice of genotyping chip. *PLoS Genetics, 5*(5), e1000477. http://dx.doi.org/10.1371/journal.pgen.1000477

Stanhope, S. A., & Skol, A. D. (2012). Improved minimum cost and maximum power two stage genome-wide association study designs. *PLoS One, 7*(9), e42367. http://dx.doi.org/10.1371/journal.pone.0042367

Strawbridge, R. J., Dupuis, J., Prokopenko, I., Barker, A., Ahlqvist, E., Rybin, D., et al. (2011). Genome-wide association identifies nine common variants associated with fasting proinsulin levels and provides new insights into the pathophysiology of type 2 diabetes. *Diabetes, 60*(10), 2624–2634. http://dx.doi.org/10.2337/db11-0415

Takahashi, K., Tanabe, K., Ohnuki, M., Narita, M., Ichisaka, T., Tomoda, K., et al. (2007). Induction of pluripotent stem cells from adult human fibroblasts by defined factors. *Cell, 131*(5), 861–872. http://dx.doi.org/S0092-8674(07)01471-7

Tang, B., Dean, B., & Thomas, E. A. (2011). Disease- and age-related changes in histone acetylation at gene promoters in psychiatric disorders. *Translational Psychiatry, 1*, e64. http://dx.doi.org/10.1038/tp.2011.61

Tang, M. X., Maestre, G., Tsai, W. Y., Liu, X. H., Feng, L., Chung, W. Y., et al. (1996). Effect of age, ethnicity, and head injury on the association between APOE genotypes and Alzheimer's disease. *Annals of the New York Academy of Sciences, 802*, 6–15.

Truettner, J. S., Alonso, O. F., Bramlett, H. M., & Dietrich, W. D. (2011). Therapeutic hypothermia alters microRNA responses to traumatic brain injury in rats. *Journal of Cerebral Blood Flow and Metabolism, 31*(9), 1897–1907. http://dx.doi.org/10.1038/jcbfm.2011.33

Valiyaveettil, M., Alamneh, Y. A., Miller, S. A., Hammamieh, R., Arun, P., Wang, Y., et al. (2013). Modulation of cholinergic pathways and inflammatory mediators in blast-induced traumatic brain injury. *Chemico-Biological Interactions, 203*(1), 371–375. http://dx.doi.org/10.1016/j.cbi.2012.10.022

Verrier, J. D., Jackson, T. C., Bansal, R., Kochanek, P. M., Puccio, A. M., Okonkwo, D. O., et al. (2012). The brain in vivo expresses the 2',3'-cAMP-adenosine pathway. *Journal of Neurochemistry, 122*(1), 115–125. http://dx.doi.org/10.1111/j.1471-4159.2012.07705.x

Wang, G., Jiang, X., Pu, H., Zhang, W., An, C., Hu, X., et al. (2013). Scriptaid, a novel histone deacetylase inhibitor, protects against traumatic brain injury via modulation of PTEN and AKT pathway: Scriptaid protects against TBI via AKT. *Neurotherapeutics, 10*(1), 124–142.

Wang, Y., Miao, X., Liu, Y., Li, F., Liu, Q., Sun, J., et al. (2014). Dysregulation of histone acetyltransferases and deacetylases in cardiovascular diseases. *Oxidative Medicine and Cellular Longevity, 2014*, 1–11. http://dx.doi.org/10.1155/2014/641979

Yamanaka, S. (2007). Strategies and new developments in the generation of patient-specific pluripotent stem cells. *Cell Stem Cell, 1*(1), 39–49. http://dx.doi.org/10.1016/j.stem.2007.05.012

Yang, X. J., & Seto, E. (2007). HATs and HDACs: From structure, function and regulation to novel strategies for therapy and prevention. *Oncogene, 26*(37), 5310–5318. http://dx.doi.org/1210599

Yu, F., Wang, Z., Tanaka, M., Chiu, C. T., Leeds, P., Zhang, Y., et al. (2013). Posttrauma cotreatment with lithium and valproate: Reduction of lesion volume, attenuation of blood-brain barrier disruption, and improvement in motor coordination in mice with traumatic brain injury. *Journal of Neurosurgery, 119*(3), 766–773. http://dx.doi.org/10.3171/2013.6.JNS13135

Zentner, G. E., & Henikoff, S. (2013). Regulation of nucleosome dynamics by histone modifications. *Nature Structural & Molecular Biology, 20*(3), 259–266. http://dx.doi.org/10.1038/nsmb.2470

Zhang, B., West, E. J., Van, K. C., Gurkoff, G. G., Zhou, J., Zhang, X. M., et al. (2008). HDAC inhibitor increases histone H3 acetylation and reduces microglia inflammatory response following traumatic brain injury in rats. *Brain Research, 1226*, 181–191 http://dx.doi.org/10.1016/j.brainres.2008.05.085

Zhang, Y., Xuan, J., de los Reyes, B. G., Clarke, R., & Ressom, H. W. (2008). Network motif-based identification of transcription factor-target gene relationships by integrating multi-source biological data. *BMC Bioinformatics, 9*, 203. http://dx.doi.org/10.1186/1471-2105-9-203

Zhang, Z. Y., Zhang, Z., Fauser, U., & Schluesener, H. J. (2007). Global hypomethylation defines a sub-population of reactive microglia/macrophages in experimental traumatic brain injury. *Neuroscience Letters, 429*(1), 1–6. http://dx.doi.org/S0304-3940(07)01039-7

Zhao, W., Ho, L., Varghese, M., Yemul, S., Dams-O'Connor, K., Gordon, W., et al. M. (2013). Decreased level of olfactory receptors in blood cells following traumatic brain injury and potential association with tauopathy. *Journal of Alzheimer's Disease, 34*(2), 417–429. http://dx.doi.org/10.3233/JAD-121894

Zondervan, K. T., Treloar, S. A., Lin, J., Weeks, D. E., Nyholt, D. R., Mangion, J., et al. (2007). Significant evidence of one or more susceptibility loci for endometriosis with near-Mendelian inheritance on chromosome 7p13-15. *Human Reproduction, 22*(3), 717–728. http://dx.doi.org/del446

CHAPTER 5

Cerebral Perfusion Pressure and Intracranial Pressure in Traumatic Brain Injury

Pamela H. Mitchell, Catherine Kirkness, and Patricia A. Blissitt

ABSTRACT

Nearly 300,000 children and adults are hospitalized annually with traumatic brain injury (TBI) and monitored for many vital signs, including intracranial pressure (ICP) and cerebral perfusion pressure (CPP). Nurses use these monitored values to infer the risk of secondary brain injury. The purpose of this chapter is to review nursing research on the monitoring of ICP and CPP in TBI. In this context, nursing research is defined as the research conducted by nurse investigators or research about the variables ICP and CPP that pertains to the nursing care of the TBI patient, adult or child. A modified systematic review of the literature indicated that, except for sharp head rotation and prone positioning, there are no body positions or nursing activities that uniformly or nearly uniformly result in clinically relevant ICP increase or decrease. In the smaller number of studies in which CPP is also measured, there are few changes in CPP since arterial blood pressure generally increases along with ICP. Considerable individual variation occurs in controlled studies, suggesting that clinicians need to pay close attention to the cerebrodynamic responses of each patient to any care maneuver. We recommend that future research regarding nursing care and ICP/CPP in TBI

http://dx.doi.org/10.1891/0739-6686.33.111

patients needs to have a more integrated approach, examining comprehensive care in relation to short- and long-term outcomes and incorporating multimodality monitoring. Intervention trials of care aspects within nursing control, such as the reduction of environmental noise, early mobilization, and reduction of complications of immobility, are all sorely needed.

INTRODUCTION

Traumatic brain injury (TBI) accounts for roughly 30% of the injury deaths for people of all ages in the United States, about 2.5 million emergency department visits and more than 280,000 hospitalizations annually (Coronado et al., 2011; Faul, Xu, Wald, & Coronado, 2010). From birth to age 20, in North America, Europe, Australia, and New Zealand, there are estimated to be 691 per 100,000 people seen in emergency departments, 74 per 100,000 people hospitalized, and 9 per 100,000 deaths related to TBI (Thurman, 2014). Most of those hospitalized with moderate-to-severe TBI (postresuscitation Glasgow Coma Scale score 9–12 and 3–8, respectively) are cared for in tertiary care centers with multimodal monitoring. The goal is to treat the primary injury, such as diffuse axonal injury, hemorrhage, contusion, and penetrating injury, while minimizing secondary injury due to systemic and brain hypoxia, ischemia, and edema (Chesnut et al., 2012). Increased intracranial pressure (ICP, intracranial hypertension) and reduced cerebral perfusion pressure (CPP) are factors contributing to secondary injury. Hawthorne and Piper provide an excellent recent summary of the current understanding of the pathophysiology and physics underlying craniocerebral dynamics and the measurement and treatment of intracranial hypertension (increased ICP; Hawthorne & Piper, 2014).

Medical therapy most often focuses on maintaining ICP and CPP within defined parameters thought to minimize secondary brain injury and reduce mortality (Bader & Palmer, 2000; Brain Trauma Foundation, 2003; Bratton et al., 2007a, 2007b, 2007c, 2007d; Carney, Chesnut, & Kochanek, 2003; Chesnut, 2014; Fakhry, Trask, Waller, & Watts, 2004). It is both assumed and demonstrated that mortality and functional outcomes worsen as ICP increases (Badri et al., 2012; Bratton et al., 2007a, 2007d; Kim, 2011; Treggiari, Schutz, Yanez, & Romand, 2007). The recent trial by Chesnut and colleagues of ICP monitoring in severe head injury patients showing no statistically significant difference in mortality for those managed with and without ICP monitoring challenged that assumption and sparked considerable critique and commentary (Chesnut et al., 2012).

Nurses use the monitored values of ICP and CPP to infer the risk of secondary brain injury related to increased ICP and reduced CPP (McNett, Doheny, Sedlak, & Ludwick, 2010; McNett & Olson, 2013). Evidence has shown there is little correlation of measured levels to the "classic" clinical signs of increasing ICP (Jones & Cayard, 1982; Price, Miller, & deScossa, 2000). The goal is to reduce the demand on the capacity of the brain to adapt to transient or sustained increased blood or cerebrospinal fluid (CSF) volume in the intracranial cavity. Indeed, nursing diagnoses have been developed to embrace this concept of predicting those at risk for secondary brain injury (Mitchell, 1986a; Rauch, Mitchell, & Tyler, 1990; Wall, Philips, & Howard, 1994). The purpose of this chapter is to review nursing research on ICP and CPP monitoring in TBI. In this context, nursing research is defined as the research conducted by nurse investigators or research about the variables ICP and CPP that pertains to nursing care of the TBI patient, adult or child.

MODIFIED SYSTEMATIC REVIEW

We conducted a modified systematic review of the literature from the onset of clinically practical ICP monitoring (1960) to August 2014, using the PRISMA (***P***referred ***R***eporting ***I***tems for ***S***ystematic ***R***eview and ***M***eta***A***nalyses) format (Moher, Liberati, Tetzlaff, & Altman, 2009). While we screened all full-text publications using the items on the PRISMA checklist, we only included the design and outcomes most relevant to our review on the evidence table. We did only qualitative comparisons of ICP/CPP changes for some nursing care activities since there was so much variability in monitoring methods over the time period reviewed.

Inclusion Criteria

Because this literature is indexed almost exclusively in PubMed (MEDLINE), we searched only that database with the terms *intracranial pressure* or *cerebral perfusion pressure* and *nursing* and *research*. This search yielded 148 items, of which 38 were reviews and 16 were classified as systematic reviews. Only two of the latter were truly systemic reviews (Fan, 2004; Jones, 2009).

This output was narrowed by excluding abstracts that were clearly clinical essays and those whose full text was not in English. We retained the 94 that involved either nurse researchers or research related to the nursing care of TBI patients, adults and children. We then added 53 relevant papers known to the authors or found in citation lists. We did not pursue theses, published abstracts, and other "gray" literature. We retrieved full-text papers for 147 papers, saved in an EndNote library. We created an evidence table, grouped by topic (measurement and specific nursing care activities: multiple activities, endotracheal suctioning, hygiene, pain, positioning, temperature management, and touch–verbal communication).

Measurement papers that were of general or historical interest were categorized and reviewed separately as part of the background (Goloskov & LeRoy,

1978; Guillaume & Janny, 1951; Lundberg, 1960; Lundberg, 1972; Lundberg, Troupp, & Lorin, 1965).

Exclusion Criteria

Nineteen full-text papers were dropped from further review for the following reasons: interventions not directly related to nursing care in increased ICP (Bisnaire & Robinson, 1999); full text not in English (Hugo, 1991; Weich, 1992); clinical essays that described the pathophysiology of TBI and nursing care, but were not critical reviews (e.g., Albano, Comandante, & Nolan, 2005; Johnson, 1999; Nolan, 2005; Walleck, 1992); descriptions of standardized management or interventions that did not specify the standardized nursing care (Leone et al., 2004; McKinley, Parmley, & Tonneson, 1999); studies with an inadequately described design or search strategy or that did not measure ICP (Chamberlain, 1998; Mavrocordatos, Bissonnette, & Ravussin, 2000; Patman, Jenkins, & Stiller, 2009; Price, Collins, & Gallagher, 2003; Sullivan, 2000; Walker, Eakes, & Siebelink, 1998); or studies of populations other than TBI (Blissitt, Mitchell, Newell, Woods, & Belza, 2006; Kirkness, Burr, Cain, Newell, & Mitchell, 2008; Kirkness, Burr, & Mitchell, 2009; Kirkness, Burr, Thompson, & Mitchell, 2008; Mitchell, Ozuna, & Lipe, 1981). Studies with mixed populations that included TBI were retained. Figure 5.1 shows the flow of included and excluded papers.

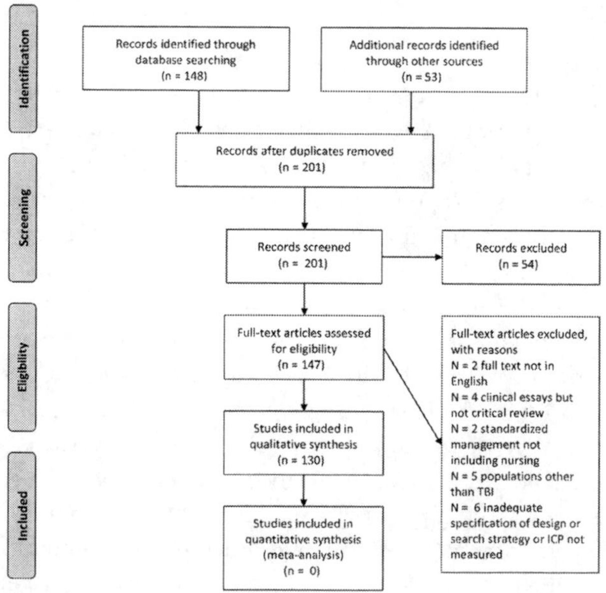

FIGURE 5.1 PRISMA 2009 flow diagram.

MEASUREMENT OF ICP AND CPP

Although Guillaume and Janny were the first to describe continuous clinical measurement of ICP (Guillaume & Janny, 1951), the modern era of feasible and safe clinical measurement stemmed from Lundberg's 1960 report of a closed system using the brain lateral ventricles for continuous and accurate measurement, compared to the snapshot of CSF fluid pressure through lumbar puncture (Lundberg, 1960). See Table 5.1 for selected studies related to measurement.

Intraventricular cannulation and external ventricular drainage remains the gold standard and the one against which subsequent methods of invasive measurement were tested. ICP is most commonly measured as the pressure of CSF in the lateral ventricles of the brain, in the parenchyma of the brain, in the subarachnoid space over the convexities of the brain, or as exerted on the dura of the brain and measured in the epidural space. CPP is the effective pressure by which the brain is perfused and is measured as the difference between arterial blood pressure (ABP) and ICP. When fluid-filled transducers are used, the values of ICP and ABP need to be referenced to standard areas. Typically, zero reference for ICP tranducers is at the head, but with a variety of reference points on the head to approximate the lateral ventricles or the foramen of Munro (Olson, Batjer, Abdulkadir, & Hall, 2014). ABP transducers are referenced to the heart purely for ABP measurement (typically the phlebostatic axis or mid-axilla). However, when the patient's head is elevated, referencing ABP to the heart can create as much as a 15-mmHg difference in the CPP value due to hydrostatic pressure differences (Rao, Klepstad, Losvik, & Solheim, 2013). Many recommend referencing both the ICP and ABP to the head in these situations (Jones, 2009). Fiberoptic sensors do not require adjustment for reference level at the head.

Two groups clearly showed that hourly hand-recorded values were, on average, closely aligned with values taken from the electronic recording, within the same intensive care unit (ICU). These findings were useful in validating the various ways that ICP and later CPP were recorded (Poca et al., 2004; Turner et al., 1988). However, the variations in reference points used and the units used to express pressures among critical care units make it difficult for accurate comparisons of ICP and CPP values among units that use different monitoring and record systems.

Electronic continuous records also form the basis for more recent attempts to identify markers of patients at risk for hyperresponsiveness (Burr, Kirkness, & Mitchell, 2008; Czosnyka et al., 2000; Fan, Kirkness, Vicini, Burr, & Mitchell, 2008, 2010; Zweifel, Dias, Smielewski, & Czosnyka, 2014). These assessments

TABLE 5.1

Selected Surveys and General Measurement

Source	Design, Including *N*	Nursing Care Studied	ICP, CPP Effects	Other Outcomes and Comments
Lundberg (1960)	134 case recordings of continuous ICP monitoring in 116 patients with brain tumors	Activities marked by bedside ink-writing potentiometer recording (strip chart recording)	Mentioned "bodily activity" and "emotional arousal" as triggers to increased ICP but did not quantitate; Figure on page 74 shows plateau wave after turning and return to baseline after VFD	Figures on pp. 74, 86, and 97 associated with activity or nursing maneuver just before showing marked increase in VFP; text on p.118 associated with figure of marked increase as patient turned right to left; p. 141: "A-waves often started when the patient was turned or turned himself in bed, when the bed was being made, on painful manipulation, when he got visitors, during preparation for operation, when he was aroused from sleep or drowsiness or when his rest was disturbed in any way....coughing and straining on defecation.."

Turner, Anderson, Ward, Young, and Marmarou (1988)	N = 5 TBI patients with concurrent computer and nurse paper recordings of ICP values; ICP measured by ventriculostomy references to external auditory meatus	Compared "end of hour" values charted by nurses with mean values sampled from the computer output. Computer ICP sampled every 5 seconds and mean calculated based on 12 values per minute. The hourly mean was based on 720 samples	Paired computer averaged and recorded values by hour, calculated difference score, which were then grouped in categories based on differences of 3 mmHg increments 84% of nurse-recorded values did not differ by more than 6 mmHg; 94% lie within 6 mmHg difference	3 mmHg is within ranges of monitor error for the monitors at that time
Jeevaratnam and Menon (1996)	N = 39 ICUs re TBI patient monitoring in the U.K.; telephone interviews with senior nursing staff	Specialized neuro ICUs in 21 of the 39 centers; general ICUs in 18 Care coordinated by anesthesiology in 25; by the neurosurgeon in 12	ICP monitoring used routinely in 19 of 39 units; invasive ABP in 36 or 39 Nursing care not discussed	

(Continued)

TABLE 5.1

Selected Surveys and General Measurement (Continued)

Source	Design, Including *N*	Nursing Care Studied	ICP, CPP Effects	Other Outcomes and Comments
Poca, Sahuquillo, Barba, Anez, and Arikan (2004)	*N* = 115 patients with hydrocephalus, ICP measured with fiberoptic extradural sensor with external computer display	ICP value displayed on monitor at the end of the hour recorded by nurse on the bedside chart, arithmetic mean calculated for this comparison The computer system sampled ICP at 1 value per second and averaged over comparable time to the nurse recordings	All nurse values fell within ± 3 mmHg and the correlation was 0.99. The Bland Altman method of comparison showed that both methods were sufficiently similar throughout the range of ICP values.	Although this study was not with TBI patients, it is relevant in terms of comparing nurse recordings and those from the monitor system, a method used in most of the nurse studies of care activities.
Jones (2009)	Systematic review papers between 2000 and 2008, search terms and methods specified	Noted lack of standard for whether to reference heart or head for CPP	None of the 57 studies reported placement of transducer reference level for CPP measurement. Concluded that Brain Trauma Foundation guidelines 2007 are not based on evidence from studies.	

Van Cleve et al. (2013)	*N* = 7,149 children with moderate-to-severe TBI in 156 U.S. hospitals over 7 continuous years	Data from National Trauma Data Bank registry, includes clinical and administrative data Used files from 2002 to 2008	27.4% had ICP monitoring; lowest rate in infants; lower rate among children in combined adult/kid centers than in adult-only ICUs	Substantial variability among hospitals, implications for whether nurses in PICU may even be able to see how activities affect ICP/CPP
Colton et al. (2014)	*N* = 117 pts with TBI, observational study with data collected from paper and electronic records	Timing and dose of ICP-directed therapy, administered when nursing records indicated ICP > 20 mmHg; drugs included hypertonic saline, mannitol, propofol or fentanyl, barbiturates	No nursing activities other than drug administration studied ICP fell after all drugs, but trended back up with propofol and fentanyl; "manually recorded data consistently overestimated treatment effectiveness. Automated data collection …more accurate…"	Statistical model applied to account for multiple sampling

Note. ABP = arterial blood pressure; CPP = cerebral perfusion pressure; ICP = intracranial pressure; ICU = intensive care unit; PICU = pediatric ICU; VFD = ventricular fluid drainage; VFP = ventricular fluid pressure.

of the comparability of various monitoring methods, such as intraventricular, subarachnoid, and epidural as well as appropriate reference levels for ICP and ABP (components of CPP) are relevant because they inform the validity of observed values in the nursing care activity papers.

It is also notable that surveys of monitoring practices throughout the world continue to show that a minority of patients with TBI have ICP, CPP, and brain oxygen levels monitored. A 1989 survey of 40 neurological units in the United Kingdom indicated that ICP monitoring occurred in nearly 79% of the units, and largely for TBI in adults. Twenty-one percent did not use ICP monitoring at all (Allan, 1989). Nearly 10 years later, 49% of 39 neurosurgical ICUs in the United Kingdom routinely monitored ICP (Jeevaratnam & Menon, 1996). This rate is similar to the 47% of adults with TBI meeting the criteria for monitoring who were actually monitored in two U.S. neurotrauma units (Talving et al., 2013). The rate is even lower in children with TBI in the United States. According to data taken from the American College of Surgeons National Trauma Databank, only about 27% of children with TBI had ICP monitoring (Van Cleve et al., 2013). In England and Wales, data from a similar time frame indicated that 47% of children with severe TBI had ICP monitoring, largely among older children (Tasker, Fleming, Young, Morris, & Parslow, 2011).

SPECIFIC ACTIVITIES OF GENERAL NURSING CARE

Studies Examining Multiple Activities (shown in Table 5.2)

Although Lundberg's classic monograph of ICP monitoring in 130 patients with brain tumors noted "bodily activity" and "emotional arousal" as triggers to increased ICP and pathologic pressure waves, the frequencies were not reported (Lundberg, 1960, pp. 74, 86, 97). The earliest observational studies specifically examining nursing care activities were reported in the late 1970s (Mitchell & Mauss, 1978; Shalit & Umansky, 1977). The earliest studies, 1977 through the 1990s, often described multiple activities, while later studies began to break apart the nursing care activities most often associated with increases in ICP. Only qualitative comparisons were possible for these papers since the different measurement techniques could result in markedly different absolute values for ICP–CPP; however, trends (increase, decrease, no change) could be compared. None of the early studies measured CPP.

However, even the earliest studies noted that no activity except for extreme neck rotation accounted for ICP increases in all the patients studied (Hobdell et al., 1989; Mitchell & Mauss, 1978; Rising, 1993; Shalit & Umansky, 1977;

TABLE 5.2
Multiple Care Activities

Source	Design, Including *N*	Nursing Care Studied	ICP, CPP Effects	Other Outcomes and Comments
Shalit and Umansky (1977)	*N* = 21 comatose patients, multiple diagnoses, intraventricular catheter or subdural sensor, reference level OK	Suction: 28 times in 7 patients	Suction: Increased with coughing when initial ICP was high (the # who increased or did not change was not qunatified)	
		Body position change: 35 times in 11 patients	Position change: Considerable increase or decrease in 7 patients; no change in 4	
		Head rotation: 60 observations in 11 patients	Head rotation: "Considerable increase" in 48 of 60 observations; most pronounced in those with initial high ICP	
		Jugular venous compression: 5 patients, 15 observations	Jugular compression: Noted with head rotation; manual compression had slower and lower increase than head rotation in 8 of 13 observations	
		Elevated HOB: 30 observations in 10 patients	10–30 mmHg decrease in 15 of 20 observations; return to flat position restored ICP to original level	

(*Continued*)

TABLE 5.2
Multiple Care Activities (Continued)

Source	Design, Including *N*	Nursing Care Studied	ICP, CPP Effects	Other Outcomes and Comments
Mitchell and Mauss (1978)	*N* = 9,TBI and other pathology, incidence of VFD as index of ICP reaching at least 15 mmHg	Turning Emotionally referenced conversation	Increase in 60%–100% of 6 patients	Magnitude of increases cannot be estimated with this method of measurement, nor can decreases be measured
		Suctioning Chewing Sleep	Consistent increase within individuals but not across individuals	
		Use of bedpan Bathing Passive range of motion Manipulation of tubes	No increase	
Bruya (1981)	*N* = 20, mixed pathology including TBI, controlled trial of planned rest periods between nursing care and no planned rest, assigned by alternate patients, observations over 70-minute period, medical care by hospital protocol, ICP measured by subarachnoid bolt	"Rest" defined as leaving patient alone between care episodes Vital sign determination Respiratory care, including suction Oral care Washing of specific body parts	Highest and mean ICP did not differ appreciably significantly between groups for any of the activities. Statistical testing not done	Method of randomization (alternate patients) could have introduced bias

Tsementzis, Harris, and Loizou (1982)	N = 39 TBI patients who had developed decerebrate rigidity, ICP, intrathoracic pressure, and BP 7–68 years, paralyzed and sedated, intraventricular catheter, pressure transducer	Suction Hygiene Injection Lights on/off Temperature taking	Group 1 (33 cases): Little or no rise in ICP or change in BP; controlled with relaxants. Suction produced transient, small rises Group 2 (6 cases): Rise of at least 20 mmHG, uncontrollable All stimuli (hygiene, injection, lights on, suction) except temperature taking led to significant increase	Change in ICP appears contingent on baseline and state of brain elastance
Snyder (1983)	9 adults, subarachnoid bolt, descriptive observation (4-hour periods with trained bedside observer and observation sheet)	Respiratory care (including suctioning)	Mean increase 12.7 mmHg, with 17/89 observations of >20 mmHg	Noted when increases were greater than monitor error. However, did not indicate if values were across all patients or mostly within a few. Many activities occurred simultaneously, thus difficult to parse out extent of increase with any single activity
		Hygiene	Did not increase	
		Positioning	Mean increase 7.9 mmHg, with 5/80 observations of >20 mmHg	
		Care of tubes	Mean increase 10.2 mmHg; in 6/118 observations, 20 mmHg or greater	
		Neuro checks	Mean increase 7.2 mmHg; in 6/135 observations, 20 mmHg or more	
		Talking about/to patient	Mean increase 8.6–9.0 mmHg; in 11/225 observations, 20 mmHg or more	

(*Continued*)

TABLE 5.2
Multiple Care Activities (Continued)

Source	Design, Including *N*	Nursing Care Studied	ICP, CPP Effects	Other Outcomes and Comments
Boortz-Marx (1985)	4 patients, TBI with GCS < 5, 365 occurrences, descriptive, 2 hours, 40 minutes of observation Subarachnoid bolt or intraventricular catheter, no mention of reference level	Health care activities Patient-initiated activities Environmental stimuli	Activities quantified as percent of observations, which could be confounded by collinearity within a given patient	In most cases, the mean increase described for any activity was within monitor error for the monitors at that time (±3 mmHg) It is also difficult to determine if the activities with increases or decreases were consistent within patients or across patients since instances of observations, and not patients, were reported
Hobdell et al. (1989)	*N* = 13 children ages 1.5–11 years, either subarachnoid bolt or intraventricular catheter, trained observers, mixed pathology including TBI	Turning Suctioning Invasive procedures Hyperventilation, conversation at bedside Cumulative effect	Mean ICP over the whole sample was increased significantly following hyperventilation but not turning, change in head position, bedside conversation, or invasive procedures	Mean values of ICP before, during, and after activity compared by *t* test; no indication if within-subject correlation taken into account

Hugo (1991)		Replicated Bruya's 1981 study with rest periods	Abstract notes; no difference in ICP for those with and without rest periods	Paper in Afrikaans (abstract in English), so details cannot be ascertained by this reader
Rising (1993)	*N* = 5, TBI case study observation, TBI, GCS 4 or more, fiberoptic catheter method, patient's RN recorded activities on an observation form		Data reported by patient as number of observations with ICP 20 mmHg or more and mean ICP before, during, and after activity	Operational definitions of each nursing care activity used. Individual's prior ICP predictive of increases
		Turning	Episodes of ICP 20 or more in 3/22, 32/53, 3/8, 9/51, and 6/25; mean increase ranged from 6 to 12 mmHG	Considerable individual variability
		Suctioning	Episodes of ICP 20 or more: 5/11; 27/45; 9/55 in the 3 patients who were suctioned; mean ICP increase ranged from 5 to 17 mmHg in the 3 who were suctioned	
		Bathing	Only 2 episodes of ICP 20 or more in 1 of the 5 patients; no episodes in the others; mean ICP increased 10 mmHg in the 1 patient, 2 or less in the others	

(*Continued*)

TABLE 5.2

Multiple Care Activities (Continued)

Source	Design, Including *N*	Nursing Care Studied	ICP, CPP Effects	Other Outcomes and Comments
Tume, Baines, and Lisboa (2011)	Observational cohort over 3 years, children in PICU *N* = 25 moderate-to-severe TBI, 2–7 years, intraparenchymal fiberoptic catheter, map and CPP via arterial line, reference level not noted	ETSMV	ETSMV: Clinical and statistical changes from baseline to maximal-presented the confidence intervals (CIs) and range of increase was greater than instrument monitor error; 95% CI for change in mean 4.14–13.2; about 75% exceeded 20 mmHg	U.K.—Northwest England care maneuvers described in detail and standardized 6-month GOS also recorded
		LR turn	LR: Clinical and statistical changes from baseline to maximal; 95% CI for change in mean 6.4–10.9	Not surprising that craniectomy prevented further increase since it created a not-closed system!
		Eye care Oral care "Washing"	No clinically significant change	Much better design and analysis than earlier studies; reasonable recommendations for practice

		After craniectomy ($N = 5$), no activity increased ICP	"To try to reduce baseline ICP to <20 mmHg before turning or suctioning, where possible; • To limit the duration of these interventions as short as possible; • To allow enough time between suctioning and turning for the children to return to their baseline ICP or at least to an ICP < 20 mmHg; • To treat aggressively an ICP > 20 mmHg that persists for more than 5 min after the intervention." (p. 82)

(*Continued*)

TABLE 5.2

Multiple Care Activities (Continued)

Source	Design, Including *N*	Nursing Care Studied	ICP, CPP Effects	Other Outcomes and Comments
Davenport-Fortune and Dunnum (1985)	*N* = 100; chart review; multiple conditions including TBI	Documentation of nursing care for patients with actual or potential for increased ICP • Nursing diagnosis of potential for change in neuro status • Complete neurologic flow sheet • MD notified when change in neuro condition • Activities such as HOB elevated 30°, bowel program, teaching to avoid straining, respiratory assessment, positioning in neutral alignment	Audit showed "significant variance in documentation" in these 4 areas Variation not quantified, ICP/CPP not reported	Not relevant for this chapter except as related to variance in documentation

Olson et al. (2013)	*N* = 28 patients and 29 nurses (paired) during a 2-hour observation; mixed pathology including TBI (21%) in ICUs in 16 hospitals in the U.S.; *N* of dyads per hospital not specified	The only multisite nursing study to date. Observers recorded on the standard case form with ICP, HR, RR, BP, temperature, and nursing activities previously reported to change ICP—any additional data were recorded free form. Analyzed in the context of ICP treatment thresholds prescribed for each patient	ICP thresholds specified at 20 cm H20 (3 patients), 20 mmHg (3 patients), no unit of measure specified (8); 11 of 28 ordered for continuous CSF drainage with intermittent monitoring; no CPP observations were reported Activities that "may" have increased ICP were turning/repositioning, tests, suction, repositioning ET tube, and repositioning c-collar Activities that "may" have decreased ICP were draining CSF, limiting stimulation, raising HOB, sedation, analgesic, anxiolytic, and ICP medication "Inconsistent" impact were facilitating visitor communication, RN talking to patient, chest percussion, and administering BP medication	Observations reported in the context of ICP value: any ICP, ICP > 15, ICP > 20, ICP > 30 Authors conclude that the fact that "interventions to reduce ICP are performed even when ICP is not elevated suggests that nurses may not rely entirely on the ICP value as a cue to initiate an intervention" (p. 191), and also that "the findings of this study fail to support the assumption of treatment similarity required for comparing the effectiveness of different ICP treatments when nursing care interventions are not included in the model." (p. 192)

(Continued)

TABLE 5.2
Multiple Care Activities (Continued)

Source	Design, Including *N*	Nursing Care Studied	ICP, CPP Effects	Other Outcomes and Comments
Reviews—Multiple Activities				
Mitchell (1986b)	Reviewed studies 1960–1980, search strategy not defined	Tables indicating increase and decrease with various activities in studies up to 1980	Only activity with consistent increase was head rotation, possibly prone positioning; some were consistent within the individual but not across individuals	Reviewed studies that are also included in this table.
Parsons and Kidd (1989)	Review of research in neurologic nursing, including factors influencing ICP in adults and children as well as prognostic indicators in TBI	Reviewed studies from 1978 to 1987, including two reviews; the studies reviewed are included in this table by individual study		
Walleck (1992)	Clinical essay that reviewed pathophysiology, current algorithm, and nursing studies		No conclusions drawn other than "nurses should be aware of the research that has been done."	Dropped from review

Chudley (1994)	Search strategy not described, included papers from 1960 to 1991		Concluded that the following may cause harmful increases in ICP: suctioning, turning, lateral rotation, extension or flexion of neck, coughing, vomiting, clusters of care, invasive procedures, and using the bedpan. Unlikely to increase ICP: hygiene care without turning, manipulation of tubes, passive limb exercise, neurologic assessment, touching, relatives' presence, and conversation with patient	
Chamberlain (1998)	Claims to be a systematic review, a guideline recommendation with strength of evidence; however, references cited are a mix of research studies, clinical essays, and textbooks; search strategy not defined	Recommendations for positioning, hyperventilation, and minimal levels based on papers used in prior reviews for this paper	Insufficient data for Class 1 and 2 standards; expert opinion for maintaining CPP > 70 mmHg is to use supine head neutral position, elevated 15°–45° first 72 hours; text recommends individualizing position based on patient response	Quality not sufficient to use in this chapter

(Continued)

TABLE 5.2

Multiple Care Activities (Continued)

Source	Design, Including *N*	Nursing Care Studied	ICP, CPP Effects	Other Outcomes and Comments
Price et al. (2003)	Review using Cochrane, CINAHL, MEDLINE, and the British Nursing Index for the care of acutely head-injured adults	Made recommendations based on existing guidelines and some selected studies	Made some statements not supported even in the studies cited. For example: "It is generally accepted that following a head injury, excessive noise, unnecessary lighting, painful procedures and an unfamiliar environment can increase ICP."	Review not used in our analysis

Note. c-collar = cervical collar; CI = confidence interval; CPP = cerebral perfusion pressure; CSF = cerebrospinal fluid; ET = endotracheal; ETSMV = endotracheal suctioning and manual ventilation; GCS = Glasgow Coma Scale; HOB = head of bed; ICP = intracranial pressure; LR = leg rolling; TBI = traumatic brain injury; VFD = ventricular fluid drainage.

Snyder, 1983). Head elevation frequently, but not always, reduced ICP (Shalit & Umansky, 1977). Further, there was a suggestion that when increases occurred, they were contingent on an already elevated ICP and reduced adaptive capacity (also called elastance or the "give" in brain tissue; Mitchell, 1986b; Mitchell & Habermann, 1999; Tsementzis, Harris, & Loizou, 1982). The early studies were characterized by small samples (9–20 patients), mixed pathologies that included, but were not limited to, TBI, and failure to account for correlated values (collinearity) in repeated measures in the same subjects (Boortz-Marx, 1985).

The only controlled trial in the early studies was Bruya's in which she alternately assigned 20 patients, mostly with TBI, whose ICP was being invasively monitored to receive 10-minute rest periods between nursing care activities or to receive the care sequentially as usually given in the unit. The mean of the highest ICP during the 70-minute trial did not differ "materially" (p. 193) between the two groups, and the increase in ICP was similar for those activities in which it increased for each group: turning, suctioning, respiratory inflation, and oral care (Bruya, 1981). The author did not provide any individual data or variance for the group data. Any adjustment for a change in position with respect to a reference point for the transducer was also not reported.

Later studies of multiple care activities in both adults and children continued to confirm that some activities such as turning, suctioning, hyperinflation, repositioning of the endotracheal tube or cervical collar could increase ICP, but did not uniformly do so. Activities that sometimes resulted in a decrease in ICP included CSF drainage, head-of-bed elevation, sedation, anxiolytics, and medications intended to reduce ICP (Olson, McNett, Lewis, Riemen, & Bautista, 2013; Tume, Baines, & Lisboa, 2011). Hygiene measures such as oral care, eye care, and bathing (exclusive of the turning involved) rarely increased ICP (Tume et al., 2011). Although these observational studies of multiple care activities could be used to determine if there was a cumulative effect of activity on ICP and CPP, none of the investigators commented on that except the Mitchell group, who noted a rising baseline with cumulative activity related to range of motion and repositioning of patients (Mitchell et al., 1981).

Specific Activities: Endotracheal Suctioning and Respiratory Care

Table 5.3 shows studies related to endotracheal suctioning and respiratory care. Endotracheal suctioning has been the most common source of increases in ICP since the earliest studies. Worries that this necessary procedure was increasing the risk for secondary brain injury in TBI patients led to a large number of studies in the 1990s. Later concern about the effects of chest compression for pulmonary physical therapy resulted in a smaller number of studies for this procedure. Increasingly sophisticated ICP and CPP measurement, study design, and

TABLE 5.3

Endotracheal Suctioning and Respiratory Care Including Chest Physiotherapy

Source	Design, Including *N*	Nursing Care Studied	ICP, CPP Effects	Other Outcomes and Comments
Campbell (1991)	Research brief; *N* = 11 with severe TBI (GCS < 8),on ventilator, "indwelling ICP monitoring device" not otherwise specified	3 hyperinflation breaths on 100% O_2 followed by 10-second suction 3 sequences with 10-minute postsuction measurement Varied hyperinflation volumes	Baseline ICP ranged from 0.18 to 11.8 mmHg. Significant ICP increases in group mean above baseline for hyperinflation and suctioning; stair-step increase with each of the 3 passes; no difference across hyperinflation volumes; return to baseline during first 3 minutes of 10-minute postsuction period. Hyperinflation at 100% O_2 did not prevent or attenuate increase in ICP with suctioning No individual values provided	Appropriate statistical treatment for repeated measures, but no reporting of variability or individual measures; so we cannot know if everyone responded the same way to suctioning
Rudy, Turner, Baun, Stone, and Brucia (1991)	*N* = 30, two-group (2 vs. 3 ETS), two-protocol (100% VT vs. 135% VT) design	2 versus 3 suctioning passes, 100% versus 135% VT, randomly assigned (randomization method not specified)	ICP, CPP, MABP, HR, and O_2 saturation Cumulative increase in MICP, MAP, and CPP with each suctioning pass, with up to 10 minutes to return to baseline	

Parsons and Shogan (1984)	N = 20 patients, TBI, ICP measured by subarachnoid bolt, referenced to the head, quasi-experimental with subject as own control	Standardized suctioning protocol, nonparticipant observer recorded mean ICP, ABP, and HR for baseline (time not specified); manual hyperventilation (20–30 seconds), ET suction 10 seconds, manual hyperventilation 20–30 seconds, suction 10 seconds, and manual hyperventilation 20–30 seconds, 1-minute recovery	Both graphs and statistical data reported as group data. Both mean ICP and mean ABP increased significantly over baseline with each suction sequence, with no significant difference between baseline and 1-minute recovery period. CPP was increased due to increase in ABP, but unchanged from baseline to recovery. The actual change in ICP for the group appears to be <2 mmHg from the graphs. Tabular data not provided	The authors conclude that suctioning is safe due to rapid recovery.
Crosby and Parsons (1992)	N = 49, all mechanically ventilated with ET tube, ICP measured with subarachnoid bolt, MABP with arterial catheter Repeated measures before and during protocol and for a 5-minute recovery period; quasi-experimental repeated measures	Data collected from electronic monitoring system; suction protocol standardized and performed by a study research nurse Procedure involved manual hyperventilation (30 seconds) followed by 15-second suction for a total of 3 suctions and 4 manual hyperventilations, and then a 5-minute recovery period	Stair-step rise in ICP, MABP, and CPP with each of the 3 manual hyperventilations, further increase with each suctioning pass; return to baseline with 5-minute rest for all variables. Both statistically significant and clinically meaningful (beyond monitor error range), but never close to dangerous levels (ICP > 20 mmHg or CPP < 50 mmHg)	Controlled for multiple measures within individuals statistically A minimum CPP of 50 mmHg was standard at the time, but has been superceded in the Brain Trauma Foundation guidelines

(*Continued*)

TABLE 5.3

Endotracheal Suctioning and Respiratory Care Including Chest Physiotherapy (Continued)

Source	Design, Including *N*	Nursing Care Studied	ICP, CPP Effects	Other Outcomes and Comments
Brucia and Rudy (1996)	*N* = 30 adults, secondary analysis of waveform data from Rudy et al. (1991) study, identified response during suction catheter insertion	Same 30 subjects as Rudy et al. (1991)—examined suction insert only—the quality of the raw data allowed this level of analysis	ICP, MABP, and CPP all increased with the insertion of catheter; statistically but not clinically significant increases in group data; HR data increased only slightly; suctioning itself only increased MICP and HR; ICP mean increase not clinically important	Careful validation of the quality of waveform data
Kerr et al. (1997)	*N* = 74 adults, repeated measures, randomized within-group design; 2 protocols with order randomized	Short-duration hyperventilation Data acquisition system from electronic monitoring Procedure baseline, 4 breaths versus 8 breaths and 4 breaths versus 30 breaths, 1-minute hyperventilation, during suction and after suction Breaths delivered via ventilator rather than manual hyperventilation	ICP, MABP, CPP, HR, and arterial O_2 saturation Short 1-minute hyperventilation reduced suction-induced increases in ICP while maintaining CPP; in discussion, noted 3 patterns of ICP change: no response, gradual rise, and dramatic rise; no compromise of CPP in any pattern; data reported as group data, so no report of the number in each pattern	Assumed that hyperventilation reduces $PaCO_2$ and thereby decreased change in ICP—in some cases, $PaCO_2$ went as low as 25 torr (mmHg), which could be problematic if sustained

Kerr et al. (1998)	Secondary analysis from data set of larger study of physiologic effects of suctioning in TBI patients N = 71, repeated measures, within-subject, between-group design Subarachnoid screw, fiberoptic catheter, intraventricular catheter	Effects of drug administration on ICP and CPP during suctioning N with no drugs = 32 Opiates only = 18 Opiates plus neuromuscular blocking = 21 Suctioning protocol: baseline, first 20-second hyperoxygenation/ hyperinflation (HH), 10-second suction, then second and third sequence, recorded after protocol at 1, 5, and 10 minutes Data extracted with digital data multimodal acquisition system	Used sophisticated regression/ survival methods to determine rate of return to baseline; likelihood ratios to determine drug effect and control for baseline ICP Significant ICP increase both statistically and clinically important with first suction pass; attenuated with opiates plus neuromuscular blocker but not with opiates alone	ICP values adjusted statistically for differences in monitoring method; supports the idea that stimulation of cough receptors is the major source of increased ICP and BP during suction

(Continued)

TABLE 5.3

Endotracheal Suctioning and Respiratory Care Including Chest Physiotherapy (Continued)

Source	Design, Including *N*	Nursing Care Studied	ICP, CPP Effects	Other Outcomes and Comments
Kerr et al. (1999)	*N* = 19 TBI adults, within-subject repeated measures ICP by external ventricular drain (closed for measurement) Jugular bulb catheter; cranial Doppler	Same suctioning protocol as 1998 paper; digital data via multimodal data acquisition system	ICP, CPP, middle cerebral artery velocity, cerebral oxygenation, jugular venous O_2, and MABP Statistically significant changes for all variables across levels of suctioning Graphs show relatively little clinically important change for ICP and CPP; jugular venous oxygenation increased and was always within adequate limits	Repeated measures statistical models
Leone et al. (2004)	Drug study—not directly relevant			Remifentanil effect similar to opiates alone in Kerr study; no attenuation of increase in any variables (Kerr et al., 1998)

Ugras and Aksoy (2012)	N = 32 adult patients who were intubated and monitored for ICP with intraventricular catheter Crossover, single-blind trial of open versus closed system suctioning, mixed pathology, only 1 TBI	Applied closed system to first 16 patients and open system to next 16; then reversed for next suctioning after ICP and CPP returned to presuction values	Appropriate reference levels used; data analyzed with repeated measures techniques Baseline values for all variables similar in both groups, but open suctioning had a significantly higher ICP value in all suction intervals and remained slightly higher after suctioning; CPP was maintained since MABP also increased; closed system returned to presuctioning baseline faster.	
Respiratory Care: Chest Physiotherapy				
Olson, Thoyre, Turner, Bennett, and Graffagnino (2007)	N = 1 single-case adult, repeated measures, TBI, intubated, and with pneumonia	Chest percussion delivered by automated bed; 10-minute sessions with 5 beats/second; ICP electronically recorded continuously; 10 minutes before and during, and 10 minutes after; used for 5 episodes of PT for analysis; no other interventions coincided	Mean values for ICP dropped significantly from before to during and after CPT (25.63 mmHg before, 23 during, 17.3 after). MAP did not change statistically or clinically	Nice N-of-1 design that is clinically applicable, although no crossover phase was done (e.g., same time interval without automated chest percussion)

(Continued)

TABLE 5.3

Endotracheal Suctioning and Respiratory Care Including Chest Physiotherapy (Continued)

Source	Design, Including *N*	Nursing Care Studied	ICP, CPP Effects	Other Outcomes and Comments
Olson, Thoyre, Bennett, Stoner, and Graffagnino (2009)	*N* = 28 adults, randomized controlled trial of CPT or not; mixed pathology with 3 TBI patients, monitored for ICP with externally drained intraventricular catheter (clamped for ICP measurement)	CPT delivered by automated bed, HOB at 30°; data collected for 10 minutes before, during, and after CPT (or for same time for control group) ICP, MAP, HR,CPP, and temperature	Analyzed and reported with repeated measures analyses; individual results reported as well ICP change was not statistically or clinically significantly different across the intervention or control time period	Concluded that chest percussion with automated bed is safe
Olson et al. (2013)	Multisite study, *N* = 30 adults enrolled in 3 hospitals (10 from each site), within-subject control, mixed pathology including TBI	Compared ICP when receiving automated CPT to baseline; each subject received 1 observed session at some point within the hour of observation; randomly assigned to receive automated CPT at 10, 20, 30, or 40 minutes after the hour (how random assignment was done, not reported)	Recorded on case report forms for the hour: BP, HR, RR, temperature, ventilator settings, ICP, CPP, brain tissue O_2 level, and bispectral index "No significant difference controlling for participants and comparing individual ICP values before and during CPT (p = .15), before and after CPT (p = .50), and during and after CPT (p = .67) or for the omnibus test of before, during, and after CPT (p = .27)."	Appropriate statistical methods for within-subject analyses and across subjects Individual values reported

Patman et al. (2009)	144 adult patients with TBI, GCS < 9, and monitored for ICP, mechanically ventilated, randomized controlled trial of CPT or not	Outcome was the incidence of VAP	Although ICP was monitored, no values of ICP or other variables were reported	Dropped from analysis
Reviews: Respiratory Care				
Wainwright and Gould (1996)	Selective review presumably from 1992 forward	Method of search and retrieval not specified	Reiterated consistent finding of increases in ICP likely related to cough; discussed effects of instilled local anesthetics as inconclusive; indicated that the use of instilled normal saline is not supported by research	Recommends survey of ET suctioning practices and use of larger samples
Tume and Jinks (2008)	21 papers; a few specifically about children with TBI and suctioning	Search strategy specified and appropriate through 2007	Papers in both adults and children; those specific to children with head injury dated and inconclusive; while suctioning and hyperventilation increased ICP and CPP, it is not clear if this is greater in children than in adults	Recommends further research specifically in children

(Continued)

TABLE 5.3

Endotracheal Suctioning and Respiratory Care Including Chest Physiotherapy (Continued)

Source	Design, Including *N*	Nursing Care Studied	ICP, CPP Effects	Other Outcomes and Comments
Pedersen, Rosendahl-Nielsen, Hjermind, and Egerod (2009)	Systematic review using an appraisal instrument; studies with ICP monitoring excluded "because ICP monitoring requires a specialized protocol"		Nothing specific to ICP/CPP	Recommendations are for suctioning in general, but are consistent with those stemming from studies of ICP and suctioning.

Note. CPP = cerebral perfusion pressure; CPT = chest physiotherapy; ET = endotracheal; ETS = endotracheal suctioning; HR = heart rate; ICP = intracranial pressure; MAP = mean arterial pressure; MABP = mean arterial blood pressure; MICP = mean intracranial pressure; $PACO_2$ = arterial carbon dioxide pressure; VAP = ventilator-associated pneumonia; VT = tidal volume.

control for multiple measurements within individuals make the results of these studies easier to compare than when suctioning was one component of multiple activities.

Parsons and colleagues found that while ICP increased during the suctioning episode, there was a rapid return to baseline at the end of the suctioning sequence (Crosby & Parsons, 1992; Parsons & Shogan, 1984; Parsons & Wilson, 1984). Rudy and colleagues established the "stair step" increase in ICP with each suctioning pass, but again a return to baseline at the end of the sequence (Rudy et al., 1991). Their data further make it clear that the insertion of the suction catheter and stimulus to cough was the key factor in increasing ICP and ABP (Brucia & Rudy, 1996). Increasingly sophisticated data capture for physiological variables and manipulation of the elements of the suctioning procedure confirmed these elements and found that changes with suctioning rapidly reversed. Only a combination of opiates and a neuromuscular blocking agent attenuated the response to suctioning (Kerr et al., 1997; Kerr et al., 1998; Kerr et al., 1999; Kerr, Weber, Sereika, Wilberger, & Marion, 2001). Most recently, Ugras and Aksoy reported a randomized trial showing that a closed suctioning system in which the patient does not need to be disconnected from mechanical ventilation allowed a significantly faster return to baseline ICP and CPP following suctioning (Ugras & Aksoy, 2012).

Despite the increasing sophistication of the measurement of physiological variables in these suctioning studies, authors continue to report results in terms of group data, with little indication of individual variability. Further, there is often a tendency to interpret statistically significant differences as clinically important. For example, a difference of 3 mmHg over multiple data points may be statistically significant, but is within the range of monitor error for the earlier monitoring systems and is of little clinical concern. More authors are using appropriate statistical techniques to correct for repeated measures or unequal observations per individual.

Olson and colleagues addressed both of these important methodological considerations in their tests of the effects of chest physiotherapy on the ICP of severely head-injured patients. They used a commercial bed that could deliver standardized chest physiotherapy through bed vibration from the posterior or lateral surface of the patient lying on the bed, first in a single patient to test safety and then in a multisite study in institutions using this same bed. Both group and individual comparisons demonstrated no statistical or clinically significant difference for ICP across the pretherapy, therapy, and posttherapy periods (Olson, Bader, Dennis, Mahanes, & Riemen, 2010; Olson et al., 2009; Olson et al., 2007).

Specific Activities: Hygiene

The earliest studies of multiple nursing care activities were somewhat equivocal with respect to whether hygiene activities such as bathing the patient, oral care, and catheter care could increase ICP (see Table 5.4). Parsons and her colleagues reported that ICP and CPP both increased significantly during each of these care procedures, but returned rapidly to baseline. The magnitude of the increases by group data was not clinically important, but there were no individual data provided to determine if these changes were problematic in any individual (Parsons et al., 1985). Szabo's review of oral care studies from 1978 to 2009 concluded that some effects attributed to oral care may have been produced by poor neck positioning (Szabo, 2011). Prendergast and colleagues conducted several careful studies regarding oral hygiene in intubated neuro critical care samples that included TBI patients. They used appropriate measurement of physiological variables and repeated measures, concluding that the mean ICP did not increase during oral care; in fact, it decreased during and after in patients with relatively high ICP (>20 mmHg; Prendergast et al., 2009; Prendergast, Jakobsson, Renvert, & Hallberg, 2012). A randomized trial of electric versus manual toothbrush had no important effect on ICP, but markedly decreased the pathologic flora of the mouth, possibly helping to prevent ventilator-associated pneumonia (VAP; Prendergast et al., 2011).

Specific Activities: Painful Procedures (see Table 5.5)

Sympathetic arousal has been assumed to be the mechanism of changes in ICP and ABP sometimes seen with presumably painful procedures, particularly in children (Arbour et al., 2014; Lundberg, 1960). For ethical reasons, few investigators have actually manipulated pain to further explore these anecdotal observations. Arbour and colleagues conducted a trial comparing ICP response to a nonnociceptive procedure (blood pressure assessment) and a nociceptive one (turning) in 45 TBI patients with varying levels of consciousness. While there were statistically significant variations in both procedures for ICP, the data were reported only by statistical *F* and *T* values, not the actual values of the physiologic variables (Arbour et al., 2014). Further, it is not clear to us that turning is uniformly painful or that manually inflating the blood pressure cuff adequately is not painful.

The study by Bellieni and colleagues of 51 healthy newborns is of more concern in generalizing care for TBI patients during painful procedures. Although their study is of healthy newborns, the fact that ICP can be measured by a sensor through the anterior fontanel makes it relevant. Peak ICP was measured during three types of blood sampling: external jugular vein, heel prick, and heel prick with sensorial saturation (providing competing sensory stimulus such as touch,

TABLE 5.4
Hygiene

Source	Design, Including *N*	Nursing Care Studied	ICP, CPP Effects	Other Outcomes and Comments
Parsons, Peard, and Page (1985)	*N* = 19 adults, severe TBI—same sample as other reports by Parsons et al. of individual activities; observation during routine care; analyzed as quasi-experimental with each patient as own control; ICP measured by subarachnoid bolt; reference levels defined	Oral care Body care (bathing) Catheter care	Group mean data: CPP never fell below 50 mmHg in any of the 3 care procedures; although ICP and CPP increases were statistically significant during each of the care procedures, they were small and not clinically important	Recorded and reported ICP and CPP; also HR and MABP at baseline, peak, and 1-minute recovery; accounted for repeated measures by analysis; individual changes not shown in tables or graphs
Prendergast, Hallberg, Jahnke, Kleiman, and Hagell (2009)	*N* = 34 intubated adult patients, mixed pathology including TBI with ICP monitors; 879 instances of oral care. ICP measured with external ventricular drainage closed every 30 minutes to record value	Oral care	ICP did not increase during or after oral care in any of the 879 instances; when ICP was >20 mmHg before oral care, it decreased during and after; showed individual plots as well as mean values	Also examined the incidence of VAP (24%) of patients enrolled 4–10 days; oral health decreased during intubation

(Continued)

TABLE 5.4
Hygiene (Continued)

Source	Design, Including *N*	Nursing Care Studied	ICP, CPP Effects	Other Outcomes and Comments
Prendergast, Hagell, and Hallberg (2011)	*N* = 47 adult patients with ICP monitor; randomized controlled trial of electric versus manual toothbrush	Oral care, specifically toothbrushing	No difference in ICP/CPP between types of toothbrush; ICP increased mean 1.7 mmHg from before to during toothbrushing and decreased 2.1 mmHg from during to after	Mean differences were statistically significant but not clinically important
Szabo (2011)	Reviewed papers from 1978 to 2009 indexed in CINAHL, MEDLINE, Cochrane, and Biosys; *N* = 4 that specifically tested or described the effect of oral care on ICP	Created tables with numerous nursing activities	Concluded that effects attributed to oral care may be confounded by neck position, arousal through stimulation of oral mucosa	

Note. CPP = cerebral perfusion pressure; ICP = intracranial pressure; HR = heart rate; MABP = mean arterial blood pressure; TBI = traumatic brain injury; VAP = ventilator-assisted pneumonia.

TABLE 5.5
Pain: Painful Procedures

Source	Design, Including N	Nursing Care Studied	ICP, CPF Effects	Other Outcomes and Comments
Arbour, Choiniere, Topolovec-Vranic, Loiselle, and Gelinas (2014)	N = 45 adults with TBI, ICP measured with unspecified method; repeated measures, within-subject design, ICP data available for 16 patients	Noninvasive blood pressure assessment (nonnociceptive),turning (considered nociceptive) Vital signs, capillary saturation, end-tidal CO_2, and ICP measured 1 minute before and 15 minutes after each of the 2 procedures conscious patients asked about level of pain with Faces Pain Thermometer	Significant fluctuations in diastolic BP, HR, capillary saturation, and ICP across the 2 procedures but similar during both; RR increased exclusively in turning; vital sign changes not exclusive to painful procedure; data reported only as group mean or with statistical f and t values; therefore no way to know if the statistically significant changes were clinically important (mean ICP change during turning is about 4 mmHg and is not clinically meaningful)	Not sure if I would agree that turning is painful compared to BP assessment; depends how high the cuff is pumped; the authors do not address this, but in fact indicate "This procedure is commonly used in the validation studies of physiologic parameters for the detection of pain in critical care" (p. 3).

(Continued)

TABLE 5.5
Pain: Painful Procedures (Continued)

Source	Design, Including *N*	Nursing Care Studied	ICP, CPP Effects	Other Outcomes and Comments
Bellieni et al. (2003)	51 healthy newborns, ICP measured by tonometer at anterior fontanel (clever use of instrument usually used to measure eye pressure)	Peak ICP measured during 3 types of blood sampling: external jugular vein, heel prick, and heel prick with sensorial sensation	Mean ICP during heel prick 26.2 mmHg versus 21 mmHg with jugular sampling; adding sensorial saturation ameliorated response with peak mean 11.75; results interpreted in the context of behavioral state; basal mean ICP of normal newborns around 5 mmHg	Although not TBI, the blood sampling is clearly painful and the ICP rise in healthy newborns is beyond the usual normal for infants, so is likely relevant to infants with TBI; variability of response depicted in graph; much wider in heel stick with sensorial stimulation

Note. BP = blood pressure; CO_2 = carbon dioxide; HR = heart rate; ICP = intracranial pressure; RR = respiratory rate; TBI = traumatic brain injury.

smell, hearing, and taste). Peak ICP was high with both jugular and heel prick sampling (21 vs. 26.2 mmHg) and much lower during heel prick with sensory saturation (11.75 mmHg), all compared to the 5 mmHg resting for normal newborns. Individual as well as group data were provided (Bellieni et al., 2003). This study also suggests a means to reduce the ICP response with competing sensory stimulation.

Specific Activities: Positioning

Positioning the patient in bed, including turning, and position of the head of the bed have been the subject of numerous studies since the early continuous ICP recordings began, as shown in Table 5.6. The studies since the 1990s have largely used appropriate statistical accounting for repeated measurements and have used computer recording of both ICP and CPP values. They have all indicated the reference levels for fluid-filled transducers, but there is no consistency in the reference level for CPP in positions where the head is elevated above the heart.

Studies of head elevation have varied the degree of head elevation (15, 30, 35, 45, and even 60°) and elevation of the whole bed (reverse Trendelenburg) versus just the backrest. The former puts less pressure on the sacrum, presumably reducing the threat of pressure ulcers, but makes it difficult to keep the patient in alignment and without slipping to the foot of the bed. Lee also studied the head down 30°, compared to 0° (Lee, 1989).

On average, ICP decreases with elevation of the head, with mean decrease ranging from less than 3 mmHg to 6 mmHg, and CPP either does not change or does not decrease to levels below 50 mmHg. However, the studies that report individual data show that as few as half the patients drop ICP, many have no change, and a few increase. Although the Brain Trauma Foundation guidelines recommend nursing the patient with head elevated 15°–30° (Rao et al., 2013), there is no strong support in the research literature for this. Lee's study in Taiwan positioning adult TBI patients with the head down 30° replicates a practice not common in the United States and indicated only a modest increase in the group mean ICP (3.5 mmHg). However, some individuals increased ICP as much as 30 mmHg over an already high baseline, while a few decreased ICP 5 mmHg or more (Lee, 1989).

Being turned in bed from supine to right or left lateral position, with or without neck flexion or rotation, appeared to be a potent stimulus to increases in ICP in the early purely observational studies. However, with the standardization of turning procedures and maintenance of neck in neutral position, this effect decreased in later studies. Mean changes in ICP and CPP were relatively small for the group data in all studies that examined turning alone (Ledwith et al., 2010; Lee, 1989; Parsons & Wilson, 1984). The changes in ICP was smallest

TABLE 5.6

Positioning and Position Change

Source	Design, Including *N*	Nursing Care Studied	ICP, CPP Effects	Other Outcomes and Comments
Lipe and Mitchell (1980)	*N* = 15, healthy adult volunteers, ICP not measured, only internal jugular vein flow			Omitted from analysis
Mitchell et al. (1981)	*N* = 20 adults, ICP measured with lateral ventricle pressure–controlled ventriculostomy (fluid drained when pressure exceeded 15 mmHg)	Mixed pathology that did not include TBI		Omitted from analysis
		Head Elevation		
Ropper, O'Rourke, and Kennedy (1982)	*N* = 19 adults, mostly TBI, ICP measured with intraventricular catheters or subarachnoid screw (4 had both), transducers referenced to head	ICP compared between flat (0°) and 60° head elevation	Data reported by individual (in graphs) and group mean; 10/19 had significantly lower mean ICP when head raised to 60°; 2/19 had lower ICP at 0°, 7/19 had no change; only 3 who had raised ICP in the supine position lowered it when raised to 60° Mean drop after raising HOB was 9 torr (mmHg), mean drop with head lowering was 7 torr	Considerably higher head elevation than most practices

Meixensberger, Baunach, Amschler, Dings, and Roosen (1997)	*N* = 22 adults, most with TBI, ICP measured with intraparenchymal fiberoptic catheter as well as brain tissue O_2	99 measurements in 22 patients, started with HOB at 30° for 10 minutes, then flat (0°) for 10–15 minutes; data analyzed by calculating difference in values when patient flat from when HOB at 30°, *t* tests and regressions used	Graphs show changes in ICP for N of observations; ICP significantly higher when flat than when head elevated (mean 20 mmHg vs. 14 mmHg), CPP significantly lower at head elevation (70 mmHg vs. 76 mmHg); no correlation of tissue O_2 with ICP and CPP values	Inadequate adjustment for repeated measures within individuals; no indication if particularly responsive individuals accounted for the clinically important changes
Mavrocordatos et al. (2000)	*N* = 15 adults scheduled for elective craniotomy, ICP measured by lumbar puncture and indwelling catheter during surgery; not specified where the transducer was referenced	Observations made 20 minutes after anesthetic induction at different operating table positions: neutral, 30° head up, 30° head down with patient's neck neutral, flexed, or extended, and with head angled 45° to the right and to the left One-way analysis of variance used with Bonferroni correction for group data	ICP increased every time the head was in a nonneutral position Statistically and clinically important increases when table in 30° Trendelenburg with the head straight or rotated right or left	Anesthetic was propofol and fentanyl, which have their own effects on ICP Bonferroni correction accounts for multiple *t* tests but not for within-individual collinearity. Sufficiently confounded by non-TBI patients and location of ICP measuring transducer to preclude use in this analysis

(*Continued*)

TABLE 5.6
Positioning and Position Change (Continued)

Source	Design, Including *N*	Nursing Care Studied	ICP, CPP Effects	Other Outcomes and Comments
Winkelman (2000)	*N* = 8 adults with TBI, crossover randomized design, intraventricular catheter or subarachnoid screw for ICP, intra-arterial catheter for ABP	Backrest position (0°, reverse Trendelenburg 30° head up, no knee gatch) randomly assigned; 65–75 minutes of baseline in the opposite position (to achieve hemodynamic equilibrium) and then placed in assigned initial position. Measurements at 5, 15, 30, and 60 minutes after position change and then placed in the other positions.	Repeated measures analysis of variance used. Individual as well as group mean data presented. Seven patients decreased ICP with head elevation, 1 did not change; all 8 increased CPP with head elevation. Mean change 4 mmHg for ICP	

Ng, Lim, and Wong (2004)	N = 38 adults with TBI, intraparenchymal sensor, arterial BP, reference level for CPP not noted	All patients started at 30° supine and then lowered to 0°; all variables measured after 15 minutes of stabilization	ICP was significantly lower at 30° than 0° of head elevation—mean change was <3 mmHg; MAP unchanged; CPP slightly higher	Paired t tests to account for within-subject effects
Turning or Repositioning Neck				
Gonzalez-Arias, Goldberg, Baumgartner, Hoopes, and Ruben (1983)	N = 10 adults, on oscillating (kinetic) bed, observational design, mixed pathology including TBI, ICP monitored with intraventricular catheter, subarachnoid screw or subdural catheter, transducer mounted on patient's head at level of insertion point of ICP catheter	Observers recorded digital readout of ICP every half hour during the bed's arc of rotation: supine to extreme left back to supine and to extreme right. Values at supine, extreme left, and right were used Total of 2,054 readings obtained in the 10 patients, ranging from a low of 158 in one patient to a high of 260 in another.	Used Pearson product-moment correlations to determine direction and degree of relationship among the 3 positions. Data are reported by individual (mean, standard deviation) Difference between any two ICP means in an individual is small (largest was 4.4 torr [mmHg].) As a group, the mean ICP was lowest in supine and highest in left lateral. The difference in means was less than 2 torr. Correlation within individuals is high (0.82–0.87 across all patients). Only patients for whom correlation was not high had initially normal ICP levels and little variation	Reported individual as well as group data and accounted for individual repeated measurement

(Continued)

TABLE 5.6

Positioning and Position Change (Continued)

Source	Design, Including *N*	Nursing Care Studied	ICP, CPP Effects	Other Outcomes and Comments
Parsons and Wilson (1984)	*N* = 18 adults, all with TBI, ICP measured with subarachnoid bolt, BP with intra-arterial catheter, both referenced to head, quasi-experimental within-subject control	Baseline measured for unspecified time prior to position change. Although continuous electronic monitoring was used, for this study, bedside observers recorded highest and lowest displayed value of each variable for each time period. One minute allowed for recovery between position change	Data graphed as group means for all variables. N varied with position change. Although ICP and CPP reported as significantly increased for all position changes with rapid return to baseline, the increase appears small on the graphs and probably not clinically significant. They report that no subject's CPP fell below 50 mmHg.	One-way analysis of variance used for analysis, which may not have adequately accounted for repeated measures.

		Position changes were standardized to (a) turn side to back with extension of lower extremities, (b) turn back to side with flexion of lower and upper extremities, (c) range of motion of upper and lower extremities, (d) head rotation to right or left, (e) elevation of HOB to 35°, (f) lowering of HOB from 35° to 0°		
Yordy and Hanigan (1985)	*N* = 13 preterm infants at high risk for secondary brain injury; ICP measured by epidural monitor on the anterior fontanel; ABP through umbilical artery	Nursing noted on strip chart recordings Suctioning Positioning Turning	Handling (a): marked increase in ICP due to pressure waves Head positioning (b): marked increase in ICP with later decrease in CPP; both returned after head repositioned	Not TBI sample, but included because one of few with infants Mortality 23%

(Continued)

TABLE 5.6
Positioning and Position Change (Continued)

Source	Design, Including *N*	Nursing Care Studied	ICP, CPP Effects	Other Outcomes and Comments
Lee (1989)	*N* = 30 adult patients with TBI, ICP measured by subarachnoid screw referenced to foramen of Munro Systematic observational design Study from China	Four positions: head at 0°, supine with head down 30°, three-fourths supine with bed flat, and three-fourths prone with bed flat, neck in neutral alignment for all, ICP measures recorded every 10 seconds for 1 minute after a 5-minute stabilization between position change Order of positions not specified	Group data compared with Student's *t* test (not specified if for paired data), individual graphs also presented Mean ICP at 0°, 20.50 +/- 1.75 (mean +/- SEM) mmHg; head down 30°, 24.15 +/- 1.75 mmHg; three-fourths supine, 28.83 +/- 2.69 mmHg; and three-fourths prone, 30.85 +/- 2.90 mmHg. Although group mean showed increase over 0°, 6 patients in head down, 4 in three-fourths supine, and 1 in three-fourths prone showed decrease in ICP Graphs also showed higher ICP levels than usually seen in U.S. samples; patients with higher baseline ICPs (20–45 mmHg) had the greatest increases (as high as 60 mmHg) However, 3 patients with baseline ICP around 20–30 mmHg decreased 5 mmHg or more.	No mention is made whether repositioning was discontinued for those patients whose ICP increased to 30 mmHg and beyond. The author did conclude that head down positioning is hazardous for TBI patients. Prone results are similar to those of Beuret at al.

Williams and Coyne (1993)	*N* = 10, some with TBI, alternating treatment design with patient as own control and recovery period between treatments, ICP measured with intraventricular catheters or subarachnoid bolts, referenced to foramen of Munro	Four nonneutral neck positions: rotation to the right and to the left, extension and flexion; sequence was assigned as patient entered, whether random or not was not specified Values from digital monitor recorded at 1-minute intervals	Mean ICP calculated for each individual for each positon Group data reported—mean ICP significantly higher for rotation to right or left than for baseline neutral (roughly 4 mmHg difference, but with about 5–6 mmHg standard deviations)	Analysis of variance for repeated measures used
Brimioulle, Moraine, Norrenberg, and Kahn (1997)	*N* = 65, ICP measured by intraventricular catheter Observation during passive range of motion or limb exercise, mixed pathology including TBI	Mixed observational design in comatose patients, passive range of motion done while supine with head 30° Patients with normal ICP had head up 45° and ICP observed during exercises involving limb movement, flexion, and extension at hip and knee and isometric contractions of hip	Some statistically significant changes in HR, ICP, and CPP with change in body position and passive range of motion in both normal and elevated ICP patients, but none was clinically important; similar results with exercise; no changes more than 3 mmHg; presumably these are group mean values, although that is not specified. A tracing is shown of 1 patient whose ICP increased to 30 mmHG with hip flexion. (p. 1687)	Appropriate referencing for transducers; both arterial pressure and ICP referenced to head; appropriate repeated measures analysis

(*Continued*)

TABLE 5.6
Positioning and Position Change (Continued)

Source	Design, Including *N*	Nursing Care Studied	ICP, CPP Effects	Other Outcomes and Comments
Beuret et al. (2002)	*N* = 51 patients requiring mechanical ventilation and with GCS 9 or less; randomized controlled trial comparing daily prone positioning for 4 hours to no prone position; ICP monitored in 23%, method not specified	Prone position Prone group for 4 hours once daily until able to sit in chair; supine group with head elevated to 20° also once daily also until able to sit in chair; no lateral positioning in either group. Primary end point was worsening lung injury score. Secondary end point was incidence of VAP.	ICP increased significantly in the prone position group Mean ICP reported for 17 periods in prone group (denominator not specified); supine mean value 11 ± 8.8, with prone ranging from 20 to 23 mmHg. Not specified if this was 1 patient or a composite, discussion noted this was in head-injured patients “There was a significant increase of ICP in PP compared to the values in SP when the head and trunk were elevated to 20°. Prone positioning had to be stopped for two patients because of increases in ICP over 30 mmHg in prone; the ICP decreased after return to the SP.” (p. 568)	VAP incidence lower but not significantly in prone group, lung worsening significantly lower

Ledwith et al. (2010)	*N* = 33, mixed pathology including TBI, quasi-experimental, within-subject control with order of 12 positons randomized, ICP, brain temperature and brain O_2 measured with triple lumen parenchymal catheter (Licox); HR, BP with 12-lead electrocardiogram and intra-arterial catheter referenced to phlebostatic axis	Turning to 12 position combinations	Group data—differences between preposition and postposition changes analyzed for each subject, apparently averaged over all patients. Group data analyzed using either paired *t* test or Wilcoxon sign rank test for paired data Mean values at baseline: ICP 10 ± 6.15 mmHg; CPP 90.88 ± 16.58 mmHg; brain O_2 37.6 ± 13.6 mmHg Both ICP and CPP increased and decreased after position changes, no mean change outside that was clinically meaningful; similar findings for brain tissue oxygenation	Appropriate tests for repeated measures, but data not reported individually. Fairly large standard deviations suggest individual variability occurred. Although the author concludes that lateral positions should be used with caution, the group data do not support that conclusion.

(*Continued*)

TABLE 5.6

Positioning and Position Change (Continued)

Source	Design, Including *N*	Nursing Care Studied	ICP, CPP Effects	Other Outcomes and Comments
		Reviews: Positioning		
Hugo (1992)	Review Also reports empirical study $N = 23$, TBI, epidural transducer	Literature search prior to 1990 Repositioning by log rolling (2 nurses)	Qualitative table In 4 studies ICP was up; in 1 study ICP was down. In 7 studies ICP was up; in 1 study ICP was down. Neck flexion or head rotation: 6 studies, ICP up Turning: 6 studies, ICP up; 2 studies, up or down ICP both increased and decreased from baseline, with most increases when turning to left lateral; no indication if these changes were consistent across patients or more within a given person	

	Reviews: Body Position		
Simmons (1997)	Risk/benefit review of published research on head positioning in adults, included TBI as well as medical causes of intracranial hypertension Search strategy and appraisal criteria not discussed	Considered ICP greater than 15 mmHg to be risky for secondary brain injury and CPP less than 70 mmHg to risk "pathological changes in autoregulation" This article analyzes research on head positioning that provides individual outcome measurements versus group means in adult patients with various conditions. "The risk/benefit method of analysis used in this review revealed that in addition to only monitoring and controlling for ICP, we must also monitor and control CPP with a greater emphasis on this particular measurement"	Concluded there is no strong research base for raising the HOB for all adult patients needing ICP management; recommended future studies show both group and individual values and that head position be individually managed by patient's own response

(*Continued*)

TABLE 5.6
Positioning and Position Change (Continued)

Source	Design, Including *N*	Nursing Care Studied	ICP, CPP Effects	Other Outcomes and Comments
Beitel (1998)	Review of 7 studies from 1983 to 1992 regarding ICP and CPP and head elevation, searched MEDLINE from 1980 to 1992	Appraisal for explicitness of research purposes, ICP and CPP measurement, whether individual as well as group means used and relevance to the clinical question	Concluded there is insufficient evidence to recommend routine head elevation at 45°. Most benefited from 30°; however, studies had various levels and all showed individual variability; CPP also varied, but most studies maintained there was adequate CPP with head elevation; suggested support for a minimal CPP of 70 mmHg	
Sullivan (2000)	Stated as a critical and synthetic review of multisystem response to positioning in TBI patients	Search strategy not defined. Strength of evidence for recommendations not defined		Not used in this review

Fan (2004)	Systematic review using keywords: *position*, *intracranial pressure*, *cerebral perfusion pressure*, and *head elevation*. Searched MEDLINE, CINAHL, PsychInfo, Health Star, and Cochrane, 1980–2003	Eleven papers reviewed that met criteria; included patients with many pathologies, including TBI	Statistically significant decrease in ICP with head elevation to 30° (6 studies), 35° (1), 45° (1), and 60° (1). CPP had no statistically significant change from flat to head up (4 studies), was increased (2 studies), and no change (1 studies) Attempted meta-analysis with effect size, but few reported it	Does not comment on whether data reported by group or individual or both

Note. ABP = arterial blood pressure; BP = blood pressure; CPP = cerebral perfusion pressure; GCS = Glasgow Coma Scale; HOB = head of bed; HR = heart rate; ICP = intracranial pressure; TBI = traumatic brain injury; VAP = ventilator-associated pneumonia.

with a study using an oscillating bed to produce slow turning, over an hour's period (Gonzalez-Arias et al., 1983). However, turning patients on mechanical ventilation to a prone position in an attempt to reduce VAP resulted in a clinically important increase in mean ICP (from 11 mmHg to 23 mmHg; Beuret et al., 2002). It is not clear in the text if this is an average over all patients or an extreme individual case. It was noted that prone positioning was stopped in two cases because of ICP increases over 30 mmHg (p. 568). Lee's study also shows large increases in ICP with three-quarters prone position, particularly in those patients with ICP baseline greater than 20 mmHg. Only 1 of 30 adults with TBI decreased ICP in this position (Lee, 1989).

Neck rotation and flexion in both adults and infants produced larger ICP increases than when the head was positioned neutrally (Parsons & Wilson, 1984; Williams & Coyne, 1993; Yordy & Hanigan, 1985).

Passive and active range of motion with the patient supine and head elevated showed no clinically or statistically significant group effects on ICP or CPP (Brimioulle et al., 1997). However, one patient did increase ICP by 30 mmHg with hip flexion as shown in an individual tracing (Brimioulle et al., 1997, p. 1687).

Specific Activities: Temperature Management

Although there are no studies of nursing management of fever in TBI patients, there are a few reports of increased ICP in patients with noninfectious hyperthermia, compared to normothermic patients (McIlvoy, 2007; Oh et al., 2012; Thompson et al., 2007; see Table 5.7). These reports suggest that any studies examining the effects of nursing care on ICP and CPP should account for the influence of hyperthermia in interpreting their results. Studies of therapeutic hypothermia were not reviewed for this chapter since this is not an independent nursing therapy.

Specific Activities: Touch and Verbal Communication

Finally, several investigators have attempted to tease out aspects of nonprocedural touch and communication with the patient by nurses and families that influence ICP and CPP (Hepworth et al., 1994; Mitchell & Habermann, 1999; Mitchell et al., 1986; Prins, 1989; see Table 5.8). Designs have improved in sophistication from pure observation to controlled trials testing familiar and unfamiliar voices (Treolar et al., 1991), content about the patient versus unrelated social content (Johnson et al., 1989; Schinner et al., 1995), or various kinds of meaningful versus ambient noise (Schinner et al., 1995). In all cases, there were minimal changes in the group mean values of ICP, but considerable individual differences. Mitchell and colleagues identified in children a contingent relationship of

TABLE 5.7
Temperature Management

Source	Design, Including *N*	Nursing Care Studied	ICP, CPP Effects	Other Outcomes and Comments
McIlvoy (2007)	*N* = 40 patients with "brain injury," mixed pathology: TBI, tumor, stroke, retrospective chart review, ICP measures with intraventricular catheter, which measured brain temperature; core with pulmonary artery catheter	Compared core (pulmonary artery catheter) and brain (intraventricular catheter) temperature and relationship of each to ICP and CPP; normothermia defined as core >36°C and hyperthermia. >38.3°C	Paired *t* tests showed hyperthemic mean brain temperature significantly higher than mean core (101.6°F vs. 101.3°F) Mean ICP in hyperthermic and normothermic states not statistically different and varied by about 1 mmHg ; individual data shown, and there was considerable variability in mean, maximal ICP, and CPP, but little variability in brain or core temperature	Not clear that these statistically significant differences are clinically meaningful
Thompson, Kirkness, and Mitchell (2007)	*N* = 108 severe TBI patients, medical record review of patients (2000–2002) in the Mitchell et al. 2002 monitoring study	Temperature data from records with contemporaneous nursing documentation of fever intervention, adherence to normothermia from Brain Trauma Foundation guidelines	85 (79%) had at least on record tympanic membrane temperature >38.5°C; only 31% of the episodes had documented nursing intervention	Contemporaneous ICP not recorded in this report, but is relevant for confounding features in current ICU treatment

(*Continued*)

TABLE 5.7

Temperature Management (Continued)

Source	Design, Including *N*	Nursing Care Studied	ICP, CPP Effects	Other Outcomes and Comments
Oh, Jeong, and Seo (2012)	*N* = 126 brain injury patients within first 72 hours of injury; record review, case control, mixed pathology: stroke, trauma, and tumor; ICP measured via intraventricular catheter	Determined ICP, GCS, and CPP in those who developed noninfectious hyperthermia (tympanic membrane temperature >38°C) and those who did not; used daily maximum and minimum for all variables	No differences found for measured ICP, CPP, and GCS on first hospital day between those who were hyperthermic for at least 1 day (*N* = 32); hyperthermic had significantly higher ICP and lower CPP on second and third days and much poorer GCS.	
McIlvoy (2007)	*N* = 40 patients with "brain injury," mixed pathology: TBI, tumor, stroke, retrospective chart review, ICP measures with intraventricular catheter which measured brain temp; core with pulmonary artery catheter	Compared core (pulmonary artery catheter) and brain (intraventricular catheter temperature and relationship of each to ICP and CPP Normothermia defined as core >36 degrees C and 38.3 degrees C	Paired t tests showed hyperthemic mean brain temp significantly higher than mean core (101.6 vs. 101.3) Mean ICP in hyperthermic and normothermic states not statistically different and varied by about 1 mmHg; individual data shown and there was considerable variability in mean, maximal ICP and CPP but little variability in brain or core temp	Not clear that these statistically significant differences are clinically meaningful

Note. CPP = cerebral perfusion pressure; GCS = Glasgow Coma Scale; ICP = intracranial pressure; TBI = traumatic brain injury.

TABLE 5.8

Touch and Verbal Communication

Source	Design, Including *N*	Nursing Care Studied	ICP, CPP Effects	Other Outcomes and Comments
Hepworth, Hendrickson, and Lopez (1994)	*N* = 24 patients with ICP monitoring (reanalysis of 1987 data [Hendrickson, 1987]), ICP measured with ventricular catheters, subarachnoid screws	ICP recorded every 15 minutes, time series model developed to assess impact of family presence and other nursing activities Time series analysis independently assessed trends in ICP	Effects presented within individual; 6 of 24 parameter estimates indicated significant reduction in ICP when family present; all significant changes were to decrease ICP Group-level effects also noted, again showing a reliable decrease in ICP with family presence	Although this paper is really about how to do a time series analysis, it was the first to apply a more sophisticated analysis to repeated measures, time series, in nursing ICP research.

(Continued)

TABLE 5.8
Touch and Verbal Communication (Continued)

Source	Design, Including *N*	Nursing Care Studied	ICP, CPP Effects	Other Outcomes and Comments
Johnson, Omery, and Nikas (1989)	*N* = 8, includes TBI, time series design with each subject as own control, ICP measured with subdural fiberoptic catheter or ventriculostomy catheter, referenced to outer canthus of eye	ICP values recorded from digital monitor readout Type 1 conversation was performed by 2 nurses and simulated change-of-shift report related to the patient, Type 2 conversation was also performed by 2 nurses and was a social conversation, unrelated to the patient; 15-minute preconversation rest period, 3-minute baseline, 3-minute conversation (order of conversation alternated sequentially), and 3-minute postbaseline values	Significant decrease in ICP in all 8 when baseline was compared to average minimum ICP when maximal, minimal, and average ICP values were calculated for each patient for each sequence of events. Data analyzed with repeated measures ANOVA and paired *t* tests. Tables are group data and individual variations reported narratively. As a group, there were no significant differences in minimum, maximum, or average ICP among baseline, Type 1 conversation, and postbaseline values. There was a statistically significant decrease during the Type 2 (social) conversation, but the actual value was only 2 mmHg. The individual graphs show marked increases and decreases in ICP during the study time period.	Individual variability in ICP was most marked in those with initially higher ICP (20–25 mmHg). The fluctuations seen on the individual graphs may well have been unrelated to the experimental condition.

Mitchell and Habermann (1999); Mitchell, Johnson, Habermann LIttle, VanInwegen-Scott, and Tyler (1986)	N = 8 children (7 months to 12 years) with mixed pathology, including TBI Reanalysis of data previously reported Observation during parent, nurse, and investigator touching/talking ICP measured by epidural fiberoptic sensor	Procedural versus nonprocedural touch and deliberative investigator touch; reanalyzed with respect to baseline stability at the time of touch or touch/talk Change in ICP of last minute prior to touch and first minute after a cluster of touch/talk. Clinical importance determined by whether change fell outside the limits of individual resting variability (95% confidence interval of pooled standard deviation for 5-minute resting sample for each child)	288 episodes of nonprocedural touch. Almost always had talking concurrent, so are reported as touch/talk; 23 episodes of investigator touch (without talking) Clinically important decreases in ICP much more likely to occur when touch/talk occurred on an unstable baseline. No clinically or statistically significant change on a stable baseline Concluded that response to touch/talk is state dependent	Individual variability accounted for in analysis by using the individual pooled standard deviations as the measure of resting variability for each child.

(*Continued*)

TABLE 5.8
Touch and Verbal Communication (Continued)

Source	Design, Including *N*	Nursing Care Studied	ICP, CPP Effects	Other Outcomes and Comments
Prins (1989)	*N* = 15 during 47 family interactions, descriptive design, ICP measured by subarachnoid bolt and intraventricular catheter, head elevated to 30°, patient supine, reference level not noted	ICP values from digital readout 5 minutes prior to family visit, every 2 minutes during 10-minute visit, and for 5 minutes after visit Quality of interaction by PFIS (4–19 range of possible scores), low scores considered more supportive	Repeated measures ANOVA used for ICP values before, during, and after visit, Pearson correlations for PFIS and ICP at all 3 times. Reported as group data. No statistically significant difference in ICP mean across the 3 time periods. Reported mean decrease from before visit to visit (9.52–8.75). Some individual data shown for those who had more than 1 visit recorded; again the changes were small and within monitor error.	Decrease reported is small and within monitor error

Treolar, Nalli, Guin, and Gary (1991)	N = 12 with TBI, experimental within-subject design, ICP measured by subarachnoid screw, referenced to external auditory canal	Tape-recorded message with familiar and unfamiliar voice, of duration 75 seconds, and taped at 60 dB level to simulate normal conversation was played from a battery-operated cassette recorder. Placement not specified Familiar voice played first: ICP recorded during last 60 seconds of a 10-minute undisturbed baseline. 5-second interval recordings of ICP for 1 minute of the recording and at 90, 120, and 180 seconds after. After a 30-minute rest period, the unfamiliar voice message was played.	Results reported as group means; baseline ICP 10.48 + 4.33, familiar voice 10.4 + 4.87, unfamiliar voice 9.64 + 4.3, minimums 1.65–2.38, maximums 15–17, presumably in mmHg; no clinically or statistically significant differences among conditions	
Weich (1992)	Afrikaans			Only abstract was available in English—dropped

(*Continued*)

TABLE 5.8
Touch and Verbal Communication (Continued)

Source	Design, Including *N*	Nursing Care Studied	ICP, CPP Effects	Other Outcomes and Comments
Schinner et al. (1995)	*N* = 15 with TBI, randomized crossover trial of the effect of 3 types of auditory stimuli on ICP and CPP ICP measured by ventricular catheter with external drain (clamped during measurement), ABP measured with intra-arterial catheter, referenced to head for CPP calculation	Data gathered electronically from bedside computer Conditions consisted of (a) noise reduction earplug with earphones placed over earplugs, (b) recording of classical piano music at 70 dB, and (c) recording of environmental ICU noise set at 70 dB Not clear if recordings were played over a Walkman with headphones over those earbuds	Analysis by ANOVA "appropriate for crossover design"—it is assumed that it accounted for repeated measures Data presented as group means and standard deviations—all 3 auditory conditions increased ICP and CPP slightly over baseline (<2 mmHg), with no clinically or statistically important difference in mean values among the 3 conditions	

Walker et al. (1998)	N = 10 comatose patients, taped message, ICP not measured	Computer generated random order to conditions ICP and CPP recorded for 5-minute baseline, 15-minute audio intervention, and 10 minutes between conditions. Measures recorded every 30 seconds by computer and averaged for "a mean"		Dropped from analysis

Note. ABP = arterial blood pressure; ANOVA = analysis of variance; CPP = cerebral perfusion pressure; ICP = intracranial pressure; ICU = intensive care unit; PFIS = Patient Family Interaction Scale; TBI = traumatic brain injury.

magnitude of ICP change with the stability of the ICP baseline. There was greater change, usually a decrease, with a more unstable baseline and often a higher ICP (Mitchell & Habermann, 1999).

CONCLUSIONS

There is now a large body of research investigating the effects of routine nursing care on ICP and, to a lesser extent, on CPP. Designs and measurement have become increasingly sophisticated, with some controlled trials and analyses that account for repeated measurement within individuals. These replications and continued studies about the effect of nursing care activities continue to show that, except for sharp head rotation and prone positioning, there are no body positions or nursing activities that uniformly or nearly uniformly result in clinically relevant ICP increase or decrease. In the smaller number of studies in which CPP is also measured, there are few changes in CPP since ABP generally increases along with ICP. Considerable individual variation occurs in controlled studies, suggesting that clinicians need to pay close attention to the cerebrodynamic responses of each patient to any care maneuver. A report by Olson and colleagues of a pilot study regarding the safety of chest physiotherapy illustrates how such an observation can be made at the bedside during everyday care (Olson et al., 2007). For the large proportion of both adults and children with TBI that surveys have shown do not have ICP monitoring, clinicians can extrapolate safe care from the studies, which show that oral hygiene, maintenance of neutral head alignment during turns, and brief suctioning result in small changes in ICP, on average, which returns quickly to baseline. The nurse and family talking with the patient, oral hygiene, bathing, and the care of catheters have rarely been shown to increase ICP or reduce CPP. Nurses need not be reluctant to engage in the care that prevents skin breakdown and pulmonary complications and improves patient hygiene and comfort for fear of causing dangerous changes in ICP or CPP.

Although the studies of nursing care maneuvers are based on the premise that we are trying to reduce intracranial adaptive demand and thus decrease the risk of secondary injury, very few have studied the impact beyond the immediate changes in ICP and CPP. Prendergast and colleagues did document a significant reduction of 2.1 cases per 1,000 ventilator days in the incidence of VAP after instituting an oral care protocol that previous research had shown did not affect adversely affect ICP (Prendergast, Kleiman, & King, 2013). Mitchell and colleagues showed that TBI patients who had an easily observed visual display of CPP relative to the recommended optimal level had significantly better odds of survival in hospital than the patients randomized to the usual bedside multivariable display (Mitchell, Burr, & Kirkness, 2002). These patients had better

Extended Glasgow Outcome Scale scores at 6 months than did those with the usual bedside display as well (Kirkness, Burr, Cain, Newell, & Mitchell, 2006). Further, those with greater ICP waveform variability, which may reflect intracranial adaptive capacity, had significantly better 6-month outcomes than those with lesser variability (Kirkness, Burr, & Mitchell, 2008).

Questions remain regarding the optimal levels for ICP and CPP in both adults and children. Chambers and Kirkham reviewed a number of studies in children, noting that survival is rare when CPP is less than 30 mmHg and that even at a level of 50 mmHg, moderate to severe disability is common. Because children have lower blood pressure than adults, they speculate that a CPP of 60 mmHg might be better tolerated in children than adults (Chambers & Kirkham, 2003). As noted earlier, Chesnut and colleagues randomized a trial of monitoring versus no monitoring in severe TBI at six sites in Bolivia and Ecuador; this showed no significant difference in mortality or functional status at 6 months in survivors (Chesnut et al., 2012). Severity of injury was tracked by the Abbreviated Injury Scale, serial CT scans, and the Glasgow Coma Scale score. Cumulative survival was slightly higher in the ICP-monitored group than in the imaging and clinical examination group, but the differences were not statistically significant. Trials to strictly manage to specific levels of ICP and CPP have suggested that the most powerful predictor of patient worsening is ICP 20 mmHg or greater with no correlation with CPP, so long as the latter is at least 60 mmHg (Dizdarevic, Hamdan, Omerhodzic, & Kominlija-Smajic, 2012; Juul, Morris, Marshall, & Marshall, 2000).

Future research regarding nursing care and ICP/CPP in TBI patients needs to have a more integrated approach, examining comprehensive care in relation to short- and long-term outcomes and incorporating multimodality monitoring (Le Roux et al., 2014). Although older adults are experiencing an increasing amount of TBI, they are rarely studied, particularly in terms of their potentially reduced resilience to traumatic insult (Thompson, McCormick, & Kagan, 2006; Thompson et al., 2008). Intervention trials of care aspects within nursing control, such as the reduction of environmental noise, early mobilization, and reduction of complications of immobility are all sorely needed.

REFERENCES

Albano, C., Comandante, L., & Nolan, S. (2005). Innovations in the management of cerebral injury. *Critical Care Nursing Quarterly, 28*(2), 135–149.

Allan, D. (1989). Intracranial pressure monitoring: A study of nursing practice. *Journal of Advanced Nursing, 14*(2), 127–131.

Arbour, C., Choiniere, M., Topolovec-Vranic, J., Loiselle, C. G., & Gélinas, C. (2014). Can fluctuations in vital signs be used for pain assessment in critically ill patients with a traumatic brain injury? *Pain Research and Treatment, 2014*, 1–11. http://dx.doi.org/10.1155/2014/175794

Bader, M. K., & Palmer, S. (2000). Keeping the brain in the zone. Applying the severe head injury guidelines to practice. *Critical Care Nursing Clinics of North America, 12*(4), 413–427.

Badri, S., Chen, J., Barber, J., Temkin, N. R., Dikmen, S. S., Chesnut, R. M., et al. (2012). Mortality and long-term functional outcome associated with intracranial pressure after traumatic brain injury. *Intensive Care Medicine, 38*(11), 1800–1809. http://dx.doi.org/10.1007/s00134-012-2655-4

Beitel, J. (1998). Positioning and intracranial hypertension: Implications of the new critical pathway for nursing practice. *Official Journal of the Canadian Association Critical Care Nurses, 9*(4), 12–16; quiz 17–18.

Bellieni, C. V., Burroni, A., Perrone, S., Cordelli, D. M., Nenci, A., Lunghi, A., et al. (2003). Intracranial pressure during procedural pain. *Biology of the Neonate, 84*(3), 202–205.

Beuret, P., Carton, M. J., Nourdine, K., Kaaki, M., Tramoni, G., & Ducreux, J. C. (2002). Prone position as prevention of lung injury in comatose patients: A prospective, randomized, controlled study. *Intensive Care Medicine, 28*(5), 564–569.

Bisnaire, D., & Robinson, L. (1999). Accuracy of leveling hemodynamic transducer systems. *Official Journal of the Canadian Association Critical Care Nurses, 10*(4), 16–19.

Blissitt, P. A., Mitchell, P. H., Newell, D. W., Woods, S. L., & Belza, B. (2006). Cerebrovascular dynamics with head-of-bed elevation in patients with mild or moderate vasospasm after aneurysmal subarachnoid hemorrhage. *American Journal of Critical Care, 15*(2), 206–216.

Boortz-Marx, R. (1985). Factors affecting intracranial pressure: A descriptive study. *Journal of Neurosurgical Nursing, 17*(2), 89–94.

Brain Trauma Foundation. (2003). *Update notice: Guidelines for the Management of Severe Head Injury: Cerebral perfusion pressure*. New York, NY: Brain Trauma Foundation.

Bratton, S. L., Chestnut, R. M., Ghajar, J., McConnell Hammond, F. F., Harris, O. A., Hartl, R., et al. (2007a). Guidelines for the management of severe traumatic brain injury. IX. Cerebral perfusion thresholds. *Journal of Neurotrauma, 24*(Suppl 1), S59–S64. http://dx.doi.org/10.1089/neu.2007.9987

Bratton, S. L., Chestnut, R. M., Ghajar, J., McConnell Hammond, F. F., Harris, O. A., Hartl, R., et al. (2007b). Guidelines for the management of severe traumatic brain injury. VI. Indications for intracranial pressure monitoring. *Journal of Neurotrauma, 24*(Suppl 1), S37–S44. http://dx.doi.org/10.1089/neu.2007.9990

Bratton, S. L., Chestnut, R. M., Ghajar, J., McConnell Hammond, F. F., Harris, O. A., Hartl, R., et al. (2007c). Guidelines for the management of severe traumatic brain injury. VII. Intracranial pressure monitoring technology. *Journal of Neurotrauma, 24*(Suppl 1), S45–S54. http://dx.doi.org/10.1089/neu.2007.9989

Bratton, S. L., Chestnut, R. M., Ghajar, J., McConnell Hammond, F. F., Harris, O. A., Hartl, R., et al. (2007d). Guidelines for the management of severe traumatic brain injury. VIII. Intracranial pressure thresholds. *Journal of Neurotrauma, 24*(Suppl 1), S55–S58. http://dx.doi.org/10.1089/neu.2007.9988

Brimioulle, S., Moraine, J. J., Norrenberg, D., & Kahn, R. J. (1997). Effects of positioning and exercise on intracranial pressure in a neurosurgical intensive care unit. *Physical Therapy, 77*(12), 1682–1689.

Brucia, J., & Rudy, E. (1996). The effect of suction catheter insertion and tracheal stimulation in adults with severe brain injury. *Heart & Lung, 25*(4), 295–303.

Bruya, M. A. (1981). Planned periods of rest in the intensive care unit: Nursing care activities and intracranial pressure. *Journal of Neurosurgical Nursing, 13*(4), 184–194.

Burr, R. L., Kirkness, C. J., & Mitchell, P. H. (2008). Detrended fluctuation analysis of intracranial pressure predicts outcome following traumatic brain injury. *IEEE Transactions on Biomedical Engineering, 55*(11), 2509–2518. http://dx.doi.org/10.1109/tbme.2008.2001286

Campbell, V. G. (1991). Effects of controlled hyperoxygenation and endotracheal suctioning on intracranial pressure in head-injured adults. *Applied Nursing Research, 4*(3), 138–140.

Carney, N. A., Chesnut, R., & Kochanek, P. M. (2003). Guidelines for the acute medical management of severe traumatic brain injury in infants, children, and adolescents. *Pediatric Critical Care Medicine, 4*(3 Suppl), S1.

Chamberlain, D. J. (1998). The critical care nurse's role in preventing secondary brain injury in severe head trauma: Achieving the balance. *Australian Critical Care, 11*(4), 123–129.

Chambers, I. R., & Kirkham, F. J. (2003). What is the optimal cerebral perfusion pressure in children suffering from traumatic coma? *Neurosurgical Focus, 15*(6), E3.

Chesnut, R. M. (2014). What is wrong with the tenets underpinning current management of severe traumatic brain injury? *Annals of the New York Academy of Sciences*. http://dx.doi.org/10.1111/nyas.12482 (July 21, epub ahead of print).

Chesnut, R. M., Temkin, N., Carney, N., Dikmen, S., Rondina, C., Videtta, W., et al. (2012). A trial of intracranial-pressure monitoring in traumatic brain injury. *The New England Journal of Medicine, 367*(26), 2471–2481. http://dx.doi.org/10.1056/NEJMoa1207363

Chudley, S. (1994). The effect of nursing activities on intracranial pressure. *British Journal of Nursing, 3*(9), 454–459.

Colton, K., Yang, S., Hu, P. F., Chen, H. H., Bonds, B., Scalea, T. M., et al. (2014). Intracranial pressure response after pharmacologic treatment of intracranial hypertension. *Journal of Trauma and Acute Care Surgery, 77*(1), 47–53. http://dx.doi.org/10.1097/ta.0000000000000270

Coronado, V. G., Xu, L., Basavaraju, S. V., McGuire, L. C., Wald, M. M., Faul, M. D., et al. (2011) Surveillance for traumatic brain injury-related deaths--United States, 1997–2007. *MMWR Surveillance Summaries, 60*(5), 1–32.

Crosby, L. J., & Parsons, L. C. (1992). Cerebrovascular response of closed head-injured patients to a standardized endotracheal tube suctioning and manual hyperventilation procedure. *The Journal of Neuroscience Nursing, 24*(1), 40–49.

Czosnyka, M., Smielewski, P., Piechnik, S., Schmidt, E. A., Seeley, H., al-Rawi, P., et al. (2000). Continuous assessment of cerebral autoregulation--clinical verification of the method in head injured patients. *Acta Neurochirurgica Supplement, 76*, 483–484.

Davenport-Fortune, P., & Dunnum, L. R. (1985). Professional nursing care of the patient with increased intracranial pressure. Planned or 'hit and miss'? *Journal of Neurosurgical Nursing, 17*(6), 367–370.

Dizdarevic, K., Hamdan, A., Omerhodzic, I., & Kominlija-Smajic, E. (2012). Modified Lund concept versus cerebral perfusion pressure-targeted therapy: A randomised controlled study in patients with secondary brain ischaemia. *Clinical Neurology and Neurosurgery, 114*(2), 142–148. http://dx.doi.org/10.1016/j.clineuro.2011.10.005

Fakhry, S. M., Trask, A. L., Waller, M. A., & Watts, D. D. (2004). Management of brain-injured patients by an evidence-based medicine protocol improves outcomes and decreases hospital charges. *The Journal of Trauma, 56*(3), 492–499; discussion 499–500.

Fan, J. Y. (2004). Effect of backrest position on intracranial pressure and cerebral perfusion pressure in individuals with brain injury: A systematic review. *The Journal of Neuroscience Nursing, 36*(5), 278–288.

Fan, J. Y., Kirkness, C., Vicini, P., Burr, R., & Mitchell, P. (2008). Intracranial pressure waveform morphology and intracranial adaptive capacity. *American Journal of Critical Care, 17*(6), 545–554.

Fan, J. Y., Kirkness, C., Vicini, P., Burr, R., & Mitchell, P. (2010). An approach to determining intracranial pressure variability capable of predicting decreased intracranial adaptive capacity in patients with traumatic brain injury. *Biological Research for Nursing, 11*(4), 317–324. http://dx.doi.org/10.1177/1099800409349164

Faul, M., Xu, L., Wald, M., & Coronado, V. (2010). *Traumatic brain injury in the United States: Emergency department visits, hospitalizations, and deaths*. Atlanta, GA: CDC, National Center for Injury Prevention and Control. Retrieved June 2, 2014 from http://www.cdc.gov/traumaticbraininjury/get_the_facts.html

Goloskov, J. W., & LeRoy, P. L. (1978). The role of the nurse in quantitative intracranial pressure determinations. *Journal of Neurosurgical Nursing, 10*(1), 17–19.

Gonzalez-Arias, S. M., Goldberg, M. L., Baumgartner, R., Hoopes, D., & Ruben, B. (1983). Analysis of the effect of kinetic therapy on intracranial pressure in comatose neurosurgical patients. *Neurosurgery, 13*(6), 654–656.

Guillaume, J., & Janny, P. (1951). Continuous intracranial manometry; importance of the method and first results. *Revue Neurologique, 84*(2), 131–142.

Hawthorne, C., & Piper, I. (2014). Monitoring of intracranial pressure in patients with traumatic brain injury. *Frontiers of Neurology, 5*, 121. http://dx.doi.org/10.3389/fneur.2014.00121

Hendrickson, S. L. (1987). Intracranial pressure changes and family presence. *The Journal of Neuroscience Nursing, 19*(1), 14–17.

Hepworth, J. T., Hendrickson, S. G., & Lopez, J. (1994). Time series analysis of physiological response during ICU visitation. *Western Journal of Nursing Research, 16*(6), 704–717.

Hobdell, E. F., Adamo, F., Caruso, J., Dihoff, R., Neveling, E., & Roncoli, M. (1989). The effect of nursing activities on the intracranial pressure of children. *Critical Care Nurse, 9*(6), 75–79.

Hugo, M. J. (1991). The effect of various nursing procedures and of rest on the intracranial pressure of the head-injured patient. *Curationis, 14*(4), 1–3.

Jeevaratnam, D. R., & Menon, D. K. (1996). Survey of intensive care of severely head injured patients in the United Kingdom. *British Medical Journal, 312*(7036), 944–947.

Johnson, L. (1999). Factors known to raise intracranial pressure and the associated implications for nursing management. *Nursing in Critical Care, 4*(3), 117–120.

Johnson, S. M., Omery, A., & Nikas, D. (1989). Effects of conversation on intracranial pressure in comatose patients. *Heart & Lung, 18*(1), 56–63.

Jones, C. C., & Cayard, C. H. (1982). Care of ICP monitoring devices: a nursing responsibility. *Journal of Neurosurgical Nursing, 14*(5), 255–261.

Jones, H. A. (2009). Arterial transducer placement and cerebral perfusion pressure monitoring: A discussion. *Nursing in Critical Care, 14*(6), 303–310. http://dx.doi.org/10.1111/j.1478-5153.2009.00352.x

Juul, N., Morris, G. F., Marshall, S. B., & Marshall, L. F. (2000). Intracranial hypertension and cerebral perfusion pressure: Influence on neurological deterioration and outcome in severe head injury. The Executive Committee of the International Selfotel Trial. *Journal of Neurosurgery, 92*(1), 1–6.

Kerr, M. E., Rudy, E. B., Weber, B. B., Stone, K. S., Turner, B. S., Orndoff, P. A., et al. (1997). Effect of short-duration hyperventilation during endotracheal suctioning on intracranial pressure in severe head-injured adults. *Nursing Research, 46*(4), 195–201.

Kerr, M. E., Sereika, S. M., Orndoff, P., Weber, B., Rudy, E. B., Marion, D., et al. (1998). Effect of neuromuscular blockers and opiates on the cerebrovascular response to endotracheal suctioning in adults with severe head injuries. *American Journal of Critical Care, 7*(3), 205–217.

Kerr, M. E., Weber, B. B., Sereika, S. M., Darby, J., Marion, D. W., & Orndoff, P. A. (1999). Effect of endotracheal suctioning on cerebral oxygenation in traumatic brain-injured patients. *Critical Care Medicine, 27*(12), 2776–2781.

Kerr, M. E., Weber, B. B., Sereika, S. M., Wilberger, J., & Marion, D. W. (2001). Dose response to cerebrospinal fluid drainage on cerebral perfusion in traumatic brain-injured adults. *Neurosurgical Focus, 11*(4), E1.

Kim, Y. J. (2011). A systematic review of factors contributing to outcomes in patients with traumatic brain injury. *Journal of Clinical Nursing, 20*(11–12), 1518–1532. http://dx.doi.org/10.1111/j.1365-2702.2010.03618.x

Kirkness, C. J., Burr, R. L., & Mitchell, P. H. (2008). Intracranial pressure variability and long-term outcome following traumatic brain injury. *Acta Neurochirurgica Supplement, 102*, 105–108.

Kirkness, C. J., Burr, R. L., & Mitchell, P. H. (2009). Intracranial and blood pressure variability and long-term outcome after aneurysmal sub-arachnoid hemorrhage. *American Journal of Critical Care, 18*(3), 241–251. http://dx.doi.org/10.4037/ajcc2009743

Kirkness, C. J., Burr, R. L., Cain, K. C., Newell, D. W., & Mitchell, P. H. (2006). Effect of continuous display of cerebral perfusion pressure on outcomes in patients with traumatic brain injury. *American Journal of Critical Care, 15*(6), 600–609; quiz 610.

Kirkness, C. J., Burr, R. L., Cain, K. C., Newell, D. W., & Mitchell, P. H. (2008). The impact of a highly visible display of cerebral perfusion pressure on outcome in individuals with cerebral aneurysms. *Heart & Lung, 37*(3), 227–237. http://dx.doi.org/10.1016/j.hrtlng.2007.05.015

Kirkness, C. J., Burr, R. L., Thompson, H. J., & Mitchell, P. H. (2008). Temperature rhythm in aneurysmal subarachnoid hemorrhage. *Neurocritical Care, 8*(3), 380–390. http://dx.doi.org/10.1007/s12028-007-9034-y

Le Roux, P., Menon, D. K., Citerio, G., Vespa, P., Bader, M. K., Brophy, G. M., et al. (2014). Consensus summary statement of the International Multidisciplinary Consensus Conference on Multimodality Monitoring in Neurocritical Care : A statement for healthcare professionals from the Neurocritical Care Society and the European Society of Intensive Care Medicine. *Intensive Care Medicine, 40*(9), 1189–1209. http://dx.doi.org/10.1007/s00134-014-3369-6

Ledwith, M. B., Bloom, S., Maloney-Wilensky, E., Coyle, B., Polomano, R. C., & Le Roux, P. D. (2010). Effect of body position on cerebral oxygenation and physiologic parameters in patients with acute neurological conditions. *The Journal of Neuroscience Nursing, 42*(5), 280–287.

Lee, S. (1989). Intracranial pressure changes during positioning of patients with severe head injury. *Heart & Lung, 18*(4), 411–414.

Leone, M., Albanese, J., Viviand, X., Garnier, F., Bourgoin, A., Barrau, K., & Martin, C. (2004). The effects of remifentanil on endotracheal suctioning-induced increases in intracranial pressure in head-injured patients. *Anesthesia and Analgesia, 99*(4), 1193–1198.

Lipe, H. P., & Mitchell, P. H. (1980). Positioning the patient with intracranial hypertension: How turning and head rotation affect the internal jugular vein. *Heart & Lung, 9*(6), 1031–1037

Lundberg, N. (1960). Continuous recording and control of ventricular fluid pressure in neurosurgical practice. *Acta Psychiatrica Scandinavica, 36*(Suppl 149), 1–193.

Lundberg, N. (1972). Monitoring of intracranial pressure. *Proceedings of the Royal Society of Medicine, 65*(1), 19–22.

Lundberg, N., Troupp, H., & Lorin, H. (1965). Continuous recording of the ventricular-fluid pressure in patients with severe acute traumatic brain injury. A preliminary report. *Journal of Neurosurgery, 22*(6), 581–590. http://dx.doi.org/10.3171/jns.1965.22.6.0581

Mavrocordatos, P., Bissonnette, B., & Ravussin, P. (2000). Effects of neck position and head elevation on intracranial pressure in anaesthetized neurosurgical patients: Preliminary results. *Journal of Neurosurgery Anesthesiol, 12*(1), 10–14.

McIlvoy, L. (2007). The impact of brain temperature and core temperature on intracranial pressure and cerebral perfusion pressure. *The Journal of Neuroscience Nursing, 39*(6), 324–331.

McKinley, B. A., Parmley, C. L., & Tonneson, A. S. (1999). Standardized management of intracranial pressure: A preliminary clinical trial. *Journal of Trauma, 46*(2), 271–279.

McNett, M. M., & Olson, D. M. (2013). Evidence to guide nursing interventions for critically ill neurologically impaired patients with ICP monitoring. *The Journal of Neuroscience Nursing, 45*(3), 120–123. http://dx.doi.org/10.1097/JNN.0b013e3182901f0a

McNett, M., Doheny, M., Sedlak, C. A., & Ludwick, R. (2010). Judgments of critical care nurses about risk for secondary brain injury. *American Journal of Critical Care, 19*(3), 250–260. http://dx.doi.org/10.4037/ajcc2009293

Meixensberger, J., Baunach, S., Amschler, J., Dings, J., & Roosen, K. (1997). Influence of body position on tissue-pO2, cerebral perfusion pressure and intracranial pressure in patients with acute brain injury. *Neurological Research, 19*(3), 249–253.

Mitchell, P. H. (1986a). Decreased adaptive capacity, intracranial: A proposal for a nursing diagnosis. *The Journal of Neuroscience Nursing, 18*(4), 170–175.

Mitchell, P. H. (1986b). Intracranial hypertension: Influence of nursing care activities. *The Nursing Clinics of North America, 21*(4), 563–576.

Mitchell, P. H., & Habermann, B. (1999). Rethinking physiologic stability: Touch and intracranial pressure. *Biological Research for Nursing, 1*(1), 12–19.

Mitchell, P. H., & Mauss, N. K. (1978). Relationship of patient-nurse activity to intracranial pressure variations: A pilot study. *Nursing Research, 27*(1), 4–10.

Mitchell, P. H., Burr, R. L., & Kirkness, C. J. (2002). Information technology and CPP management in neuro intensive care. *Acta Neurochirurgica Supplement, 81*, 163–165.

Mitchell, P. H., Johnson, F. B., Habermann LIttle, B., VanInwegen-Scott, D., & Tyler, D. (1986). Effects of touching and talking in children. In J. D. Miller, G. M. Teasdale, J. O. Rowan, S. L. Galbraith & A. D. Mendelow (Eds.), *Intracranial Pressure VI* (Vol. 6, pp. 703–704). Berlin: Springer-Verlag.

Mitchell, P. H., Ozuna, J., & Lipe, H. P. (1981). Moving the patient in bed: Effects on intracranial pressure. *Nursing Research, 30*(4), 212–218.

Moher, D., Liberati, A., Tetzlaff, J., & Altman, D. G. (2009). Preferred reporting items for systematic reviews and meta-analyses: The PRISMA statement. *PLoS Medicine, 6*(7), e1000097. http://dx.doi.org/10.1371/journal.pmed.1000097

Ng, I., Lim, J., & Wong, H. B. (2004). Effects of head posture on cerebral hemodynamics: Its influences on intracranial pressure, cerebral perfusion pressure, and cerebral oxygenation. *Neurosurgery, 54*(3), 593–597; discussion 598.

Nolan, S. (2005). Traumatic brain injury: A review. *Critical Care Nursing Quarterly, 28*(2), 188–194.

Oh, H. S., Jeong, H. S., & Seo, W. S. (2012). Non-infectious hyperthermia in acute brain injury patients: Relationships to mortality, blood pressure, intracranial pressure and cerebral perfusion pressure. *International Journal of Nursing Practice, 18*(3), 295–302. http://dx.doi.org/10.1111/j.1440-172X.2012.02039.x

Olson, D. M., Bader, M. K., Dennis, C., Mahanes, D., & Riemen, K. (2010). Multicenter pilot study: Safety of automated chest percussion in patients at risk for intracranial hypertension. *The Journal of Neuroscience Nursing, 42*(3), 119–127.

Olson, D. M., Batjer, H. H., Abdulkadir, K., & Hall, C. E. (2014). Measuring and monitoring ICP in Neurocritical Care: Results from a national practice survey. *Neurocritical Care, 20*(1), 15–20. http://dx.doi.org/10.1007/s12028-013-9847-9

Olson, D. M., Lewis, L. S., Bader, M. K., Bautista, C., Malloy, R., Riemen, K. E., et al. (2013). Significant practice pattern variations associated with intracranial pressure monitoring. *The Journal of Neuroscience Nursing, 45*(4), 186–193. http://dx.doi.org/10.1097/JNN.0b013e3182986400

Olson, D. M., McNett, M. M., Lewis, L. S., Riemen, K. E., & Bautista, C. (2013). Effects of nursing interventions on intracranial pressure. *American Journal of Critical Care, 22*(5), 431–438. http://dx.doi.org/10.4037/ajcc2013751

Olson, D. M., Thoyre, S. M., Bennett, S. N., Stoner, J. B., & Graffagnino, C. (2009). Effect of mechanical chest percussion on intracranial pressure: A pilot study. *American Journal of Critical Care, 18*(4), 330–335. http://dx.doi.org/10.4037/ajcc2009523

Olson, D. M., Thoyre, S. M., Turner, D. A., Bennett, S., & Graffagnino, C. (2007). Changes in intracranial pressure associated with chest physiotherapy. *Neurocritical Care, 6*(2), 100–103. http://dx.doi.org/10.1007/s12028-007-0015-y

Parsons, L. C., & Kidd, P. S. (1989). Neurologic nursing research. *Annual Review of Nursing Research, 7*, 3–25

Parsons, L. C., & Shogan, J. S. (1984). The effects of the endotracheal tube suctioning/manual hyperventilation procedure on patients with severe closed head injuries. *Heart & Lung, 13*(4), 372–380.

Parsons, L. C., & Wilson, M. M. (1984). Cerebrovascular status of severe closed head injured patients following passive position changes. *Nursing Research, 33*(2), 68–75.

Parsons, L. C., Peard, A. L., & Page, M. C. (1985). The effects of hygiene interventions on the cerebrovascular status of severe closed head injured persons. *Research in Nursing & Health, 8*(2), 173–181.

Patman, S., Jenkins, S., & Stiller, K. (2009). Physiotherapy does not prevent, or hasten recovery from, ventilator-associated pneumonia in patients with acquired brain injury. *Intensive Care Medicine, 35*(2), 258–265. http://dx.doi.org/10.1007/s00134-008-1278-2

Pedersen, C. M., Rosendahl-Nielsen, M., Hjermind, J., & Egerod, I. (2009). Endotracheal suctioning of the adult intubated patient--what is the evidence? *Intensive Critical Care Nursing, 25*(1), 21–30. http://dx.doi.org/10.1016/j.iccn.2008.05.004

Poca, M. A., Sahuquillo, J., Barba, M. A., Anez, J. D., & Arikan, F. (2004). Prospective study of methodological issues in intracranial pressure monitoring in patients with hydrocephalus. *Journal of Neurosurgery, 100*(2), 260–265. http://dx.doi.org/10.3171/jns.2004.100.2.0260

Prendergast, V., Hagell, P., & Hallberg, I. R. (2011). Electric versus manual tooth brushing among neuroscience ICU patients: Is it safe? *Neurocritical Care, 14*(2), 281–286. http://dx.doi.org/10.1007/s12028-011-9502-2

Prendergast, V., Hallberg, I. R., Jahnke, H., Kleiman, C., & Hagell, P. (2009). Oral health, ventilator-associated pneumonia, and intracranial pressure in intubated patients in a neuroscience intensive care unit. *American Journal of Critical Care, 18*(4), 368–376. http://dx.doi.org/10.4037/ajcc2009621

Prendergast, V., Jakobsson, U., Renvert, S., & Hallberg, I. R. (2012). Effects of a standard versus comprehensive oral care protocol among intubated neuroscience ICU patients: Results of a randomized controlled trial. *The Journal of Neuroscience Nursing, 44*(3), 134–146; quiz 147–138. http://dx.doi.org/10.1097/JNN.0b013e3182510688

Prendergast, V., Kleiman, C., & King, M. (2013). The bedside oral exam and the barrow oral care protocol: Translating evidence-based oral care into practice. *Intensive Critical Care Nursing, 29*(5), 282–290. http://dx.doi.org/10.1016/j.iccn.2013.04.001

Price, A. M., Collins, T. J., & Gallagher, A. (2003). Nursing care of the acute head injury: A review of the evidence. *Nursing in Critical Care, 8*(3), 126–133.

Price, T., Miller, L., & deScossa, M. (2000). The Glasgow Coma Scale in intensive care: A study. *Nursing in Critical Care, 5*(4), 170–173.

Prins, M. M. (1989). The effect of family visits on intracranial pressure. *Western Journal of Nursing Research, 11*(3), 281–292; discussion 292–287.

Rao, V., Klepstad, P., Losvik, O. K., & Solheim, O. (2013). Confusion with cerebral perfusion pressure in a literature review of current guidelines and survey of clinical practise. *Scandinavian Journal of Trauma Resuscitation Emergency Medicine, 21*(1), 78. http://dx.doi.org/10.1186/1757-7241-21-78

Rauch, M. E., Mitchell, P. H., & Tyler, M. L. (1990). Validation of risk factors for the nursing diagnosis decreased intracranial adaptive capacity. *The Journal of Neuroscience Nursing, 22*(3), 173–178.

Rising, C. J. (1993). The relationship of selected nursing activities to ICP. *The Journal of Neuroscience Nursing, 25*(5), 302–308.

Ropper, A. H., O'Rourke, D., & Kennedy, S. K. (1982). Head position, intracranial pressure, and compliance. *Neurology, 32*, 1288–1291.

Rudy, E. B., Turner, B. S., Baun, M., Stone, K. S., & Brucia, J. (1991). Endotracheal suctioning in adults with head injury. *Heart & Lung, 20*, 667–674.

Schinner, K. M., Chisholm, A. H., Grap, M. J., Siva, P., Hallinan, M., & LaVoice-Hawkins, A. M. (1995). Effects of auditory stimuli on intracranial pressure and cerebral perfusion pressure in traumatic brain injury. *The Journal of Neuroscience Nursing, 27*(6), 348–354.

Shalit, M. N., & Umansky, F. (1977). Effect of routine bedside procedures on intracranial pressure. *Israel Journal of Medical Sciences, 13*(9), 881–886.

Simmons, B. J. (1997). Management of intracranial hemodynamics in the adult: A reserch analysis of head positioning and recommendations for clincial practice and future research. *Journal of Neuroscience Nursing, 29*(1), 44–49.

Snyder, M. (1983). Relation of nursing activities to increases in intracranial pressure. *Journal of Advanced Nursing, 8*(4), 273–279.

Sullivan, J. (2000). Positioning of patients with severe traumatic brain injury: Research-based practice. *The Journal of Neuroscience Nursing, 32*(4), 204–209.

Szabo, C. M. (2011). The effect of oral care on intracranial pressure: A review of the literature. *The Journal of Neuroscience Nursing, 43*(5), E1–E9. http://dx.doi.org/10.1097/JNN.0b013e318227f1e5

Talving, P., Karamanos, E., Teixeira, P. G., Skiada, D., Lam, L., Belzberg, H., et al. (2013). Intracranial pressure monitoring in severe head injury: Compliance with Brain Trauma Foundation guidelines and effect on outcomes: A prospective study. *Journal of Neurosurgery, 119*(5), 1248–1254. http://dx.doi.org/10.3171/2013.7.jns122255

Tasker, R. C., Fleming, T. J., Young, A. E., Morris, K. P., & Parslow, R. C. (2011). Severe head injury in children: Intensive care unit activity and mortality in England and Wales. *British Journal of Neurosurgery, 25*(1), 68–77. http://dx.doi.org/10.3109/02688697.2010.538770

Thompson, H. J., Kirkness, C. J., & Mitchell, P. H. (2007). Intensive care unit management of fever following traumatic brain injury. *Intensive Critical Care Nursing, 23*(2), 91–96. http://dx.doi.org/10.1016/j.iccn.2006.11.005

Thompson, H. J., McCormick, W. C., & Kagan, S. H. (2006). Traumatic brain injury in older adults: Epidemiology, outcomes, and future implications. *Journal of the American Geriatrics Society, 54*(10), 1590–1595. http://dx.doi.org/10.1111/j.1532-5415.2006.00894.x

Thompson, H. J., Rivara, F. P., Jurkovich, G. J., Wang, J., Nathens, A. B., & MacKenzie, E. J. (2008). Evaluation of the effect of intensity of care on mortality after traumatic brain injury. *Critical Care Medicine, 36*(1), 282–290. http://dx.doi.org/10.1097/01.ccm.0000297884.86058.8a

Thurman, D. J. (2014). The epidemiology of traumatic brain injury in children and youths: A review of research since 1990. *Journal of Child Neurology*. http://dx.doi.org/10.1177/0883073814544363 (August 14, epub ahead of print).

Treggiari, M. M., Schutz, N., Yanez, N. D., & Romand, J. A. (2007). Role of intracranial pressure values and patterns in predicting outcome in traumatic brain injury: A systematic review. *Neurocritical Care, 6*(2), 104–112. http://dx.doi.org/10.1007/s12028-007-0012-1

Treolar, D., Nalli, B., Guin, P., & Gary, R. (1991). The effect of familiar and unfamiliar voice treatments on intracranial pressure in head-injured patients. *Journal of Neuroscience Nursing, 23*(5), 295–299.

Tsementzis, S. A., Harris, P., & Loizou, L. A. (1982). The effect of Routine nursing care procedures on the ICP in severe head injuries. *Acta Neurochirurgica, 65*(3–4), 153–166.

Tume, L. N., Baines, P. B., & Lisboa, P. J. (2011). The effect of nursing interventions on the intracranial pressure in paediatric traumatic brain injury. *Nursing in Critical Care, 16*(2), 77–84. http://dx.doi.org/10.1111/j.1478-5153.2010.00412.x

Tume, L., & Jinks, A. (2008). Endotracheal suctioning in children with severe traumatic brain injury: A literature review. *Nursing in Critical Care, 13*(5), 232–240. http://dx.doi.org/10.1111/j.1478-5153.2008.00285.x

Turner, H. B., Anderson, R. L., Ward, J. D., Young, H. F., & Marmarou, A. (1988). Comparison of nurse and computer recording of ICP in head injured patients. *The Journal of Neuroscience Nursing, 20*(4), 236–239.

Ugras, G. A., & Aksoy, G. (2012). The effects of open and closed endotracheal suctioning on intracranial pressure and cerebral perfusion pressure: A crossover, single-blind clinical trial. *The Journal of Neuroscience Nursing, 44*(6), E1–E8. http://dx.doi.org/10.1097/JNN.0b013e3182682f69

Van Cleve, W., Kernic, M. A., Ellenbogen, R. G., Wang, J., Zatzick, D. F., Bell, M. J., et al. (2013). National variability in intracranial pressure monitoring and craniotomy for children with moderate to severe traumatic brain injury. *Neurosurgery, 73*(5), 746–752; discussion 752, quiz 752. http://dx.doi.org/10.1227/neu.0000000000000097

Wainwright, S. P., & Gould, D. (1996). Endotracheal suctioning in adults with severe head injury: Literature review. *Intensive Critical Care Nursing, 12*(5), 303–308.

Walker, J. S., Eakes, G. G., & Siebelink, E. (1998). The effects of familial voice interventions on comatose head-injured patients. *Journal of Trauma Nursing, 5*(2), 41–45.

Wall, B. M., Philips, J. P., & Howard, J. C. (1994). Validation of increased intracranial pressure and high risk for increased intracranial pressure. *Nursing Diagnosis, 5*(2), 74–81.

Walleck, C. A. (1992). Preventing secondary brain injury. *AACN Clinical Issues in Critical Care Nursing, 3*(1), 19–30.

Weich, M. (1992). Communication with patients--the effect of verbal and nonverbal communication on the unconscious patient. *Curationis, 15*(3), 27–30.

Williams, A., & Coyne, S. M. (1993). Effects of neck position on intracranial pressure. *American Journal of Critical Care, 2*(1), 68–71.

Yordy, M., & Hanigan, W. C. (1985). Cerebral perfusion pressure in the high-risk premature infant. *Pediatric Neurosciences, 12*(4–5), 226–231.

Zweifel, C., Dias, C., Smielewski, P., & Czosnyka, M. (2014). Continuous time-domain monitoring of cerebral autoregulation in neurocritical care. *Medical Engineering & Physics, 36*(5), 638–645. http://dx.doi.org/10.1016/j.medengphy.2014.03.002

CHAPTER 6

State of the Science of Pediatric Traumatic Brain Injury

Biomarkers and Gene Association Studies

Karin Reuter-Rice, Julia K. Eads, Suzanna Boyce Berndt, and Ellen Bennett

ABSTRACT

Objectives: Our objective is to review the most widely used biomarkers and gene studies reported in pediatric traumatic brain injury (TBI) literature, to describe their findings, and to discuss the discoveries and gaps that advance the understanding of brain injury and its associated outcomes. Ultimately, we aim to inform the science for future research priorities. *Data sources:* We searched PubMed, MEDLINE, CINAHL, and the Cochrane Database of Systematic Reviews for published English language studies conducted in the last 10 years to identify reviews and completed studies of biomarkers and gene associations in pediatric TBI. Of the 131 biomarker articles, only 16 were specific to pediatric TBI patients, whereas of the gene association studies in children with TBI, only four were included in this review. *Conclusion:* Biomarker and gene attributes are grossly understudied in pediatric TBI in comparison to adults. Although recent advances recognize the importance of biomarkers in the study of brain injury, the limited number of studies and genomic associations in the injured brain has shown the need for common data elements, larger sample sizes, heterogeneity, and common collection methods that allow for greater understanding of the injured pediatric

http://dx.doi.org/10.1891/0739-6686.33.185

brain. By building on to the consortium of interprofessional scientists, continued research priorities would lead to improved outcome prediction and treatment strategies for children who experience a TBI. *Implications for nursing research:* Understanding recent advances in biomarker and genomic studies in pediatric TBI is important because these advances may guide future research, collaborations, and interventions. It is also important to ensure that nursing is a part of this evolving science to promote improved outcomes in children with TBIs.

INTRODUCTION

Traumatic brain injury (TBI) is a major health concern and affects persons of all ages, races, ethnicities, and incomes. It is responsible for approximately one-third of all injury-related deaths in the United States and is the leading cause of morbidity and mortality in children and adolescents, with 7,400 children under the age of 19 dying annually from a TBI (Coronado et al., 2011; Center for Disease Control and Prevention, n.d.). Death rates are highest among children 0–4 years of age, boys, and minority populations (Coronado et al., 2011). The incidence of TBI is 35% higher in African Americans than in Whites and other races, and African Americans also have the highest death rate (Bruns & Hauser, 2003; Jager, Weiss, Coben, & Pepe, 2000). Acute and rehabilitative costs associated with TBI because of accidents and child abuse are estimated at $60 billion annually, with average lifetime costs ranging from $600,000 to $1,875,000 (Corso, Finkelstein, Miller, Fiebelkorn, & Zaloshnja, 2006; Schneier, Shields, Hostetler, Xiang, & Smith, 2006). In 2012, the second edition of the *Guidelines for the Acute Medical Management of Severe Traumatic Brain Injury in Infants, Children and Adolescents* was published to reflect once again the lack of Class I evidence to support the therapeutic interventions recommended (Kochanek et al., 2012). The role of biomarkers and gene association studies are important in the diagnosis of injury and inform future treatment strategies in pediatric TBI. However, there remain limitations with their use in children who have sustained a TBI. Thus, the financial, personal, and societal costs of pediatric TBI are immense, and the limited therapeutic interventions make a comprehensive research agenda a compelling need.

Injury as a result of head trauma in children occurs in two distinct phases. The *primary injury* phase occurs on impact and results from mechanical forces that cause direct disruption of the brain parenchyma. This injury phase may be preventable, which is why there is a heavy emphasis on education for injury prevention, such as protective headgear and seat belt use. Once the first irreversible injury is sustained, a *secondary injury* follows. Here, endogenous factors, such as metabolic, cellular, cytotoxic, and vasogenic edema, and biochemical derangements as well as exogenous factors, such as hypoxia and hypotension, lead to neuronal cell degeneration and, ultimately, neuronal death (Kochanek et al., 2000). The goal in the acute injury phase is to improve cerebral perfusion and to stabilize the injured brain while promoting neuroprotection strategies to optimize functional outcomes (Anderson, Brown, & Newitt, 2010; Coronado, et al., 2011; Langlois, Rutland-Brown, & Thomas, 2004; Oh & Seo, 2009; Faul, Xu, Wald, & Coronado, 2010). This acute phase may occur for days to weeks in the injured brain, and it is within this time frame that the majority of the biomarker study research has occurred, because associating a biomarker with cascading protein activity may lead to identifying outcomes (Papa et al., 2013).

Biomarkers are defined as "a characteristic that is objectively measured and evaluated as an indicator of normal biological processes, pathogenic processes, or pharmacologic responses to a therapeutic intervention" (Biomarkers Definitions Working Group, 2001, p. 91). The identification of biomarkers in injury and diseases has led others to consider their genetic association. Gene association studies are designed either as candidate gene approaches or as genome-wide association studies. In the candidate gene approach, the identification is of a single nucleotide polymorphism (SNP). SNPs are the most common type of genetic variations in a single base pair of deoxyribonucleic acid (DNA), and if found in an important gene, it can change the protein or biomarker structure, which may ultimately change an illness or injury or response (Kurowski, Martin & Wade, 2012). To date, the only published gene studied in children with head injury has been a candidate gene association by evaluating for the presence of the apolipoprotein E (APOE) gene, specifically allele 4 (APOE4). APOE4 has been associated with poor neurocognitive outcomes in adult patients with TBI, but has demonstrated mixed findings in children with a TBI (Blackman, Worley, & Strittmatter, 2005; Brichtova, & Kozak, 2008; Moran et al., 2009).

LITERATURE REVIEW

A systematic review was conducted in May 2014 of English language–published literature on pediatric TBIs, which included biomarker and genetic studies using PubMed, MEDLINE, CINAHL, and Cochrane Database of Systematic Reviews. The articles were narrowed down using the following MeSH search terms: pediatrics, children, traumatic brain injury, head injury, biomarkers, gene, genomics, and polymorphism. Studies were limited to the last 10 years and to children aged 18 years or younger who were hospitalized. Those studies that did not have pediatric TBI and biomarkers or a specific gene identified as their primary focus were excluded. Of the 131 biomarker articles, only 16 were specific to pediatric TBI patients, whereas of the gene association studies in children with TBI, only four were included in this review (Tables 6.1 and 6.2). The bibliographies and

TABLE 6.1
TBI Biomarkers Studies That Focused on Children 18 Years and Younger

Year/Author	Biomarker	Population (n)	Severity	Sample Collection Method	Outcome
Babcock et al. (2013)	S100B	n = 76; age range 5–18 years	Mild (GCS > 13)	Serum; samples were collected upon ED admission	• 28 children presented with PCS; mean (*SD*) S100B level 0.092 (0.376) μg/L, median was 0.008 μg/L (range 0–2.00 μg/L) • For patients with no PCS (n = 48), the mean (*SD*) S100B level was 0.022 (0.3756) μg/L and median was 0.012 μg/L (range 0–0.141 μg/L) • No association was seen between initial S100B levels measured in the ED and development of PCS or severity of PCS symptoms
Piazza et al. (2007)	S100B	n = 15; age range 1–15 years	Mild to severe (GCS 3–15)	Serum; samples were collected upon ED admission and after 48 hours	• 9 patients with mild TBI, 2 with moderate TBI, and 4 with severe TBI • S100B levels were higher in severe than in mild TBI patients • Correlation was seen between brain damage severity and serum S100B increase • No correlation was seen between serum S100B levels and outcome (GOSe = 8) • All patients had good 6-month neurological outcomes

Berger and Kochanek (2006)	S100B	$n = 29$ (9 HBI and 6 iTBI) and 14 healthy controls; age >17 years	Mild to severe (GCS 3–15)	Serum and urine; for TBI, initial level taken as quickly as possible after injury and then every 12 h for 3 days; for control, one serum and urine sample was collected	• Urinary S100B concentrations were detectable in 80% of patients with increased serum S100B; in 0% of controls • Increased urinary S100B was found in majority of TBI patients with abnormal serum S100B • Peak urinary S100B occurred later than peak serum S100B • No relationship was found between GCS and GOS or between GCS and initial or peak urinary S100B • Patients with undetectable urinary S100B and a normal serum S100B, independently, are more likely to have good outcome
Spinella et al. (2003)	S100B	$n = 163$ (136 healthy and 27 TBI); age range <18 years	Mild to severe (GCS 3–15)	Serum; TBI samples were collected within 12 h after injury; control samples collected preoperatively from outpatient surgery	• S-100B levels in healthy children had a mean of 0.3 µg/L and inversely correlated with age • In TBI children, 6 months after injury, outcome inversely correlated with GOS score and S-100B levels; comparing good outcome vs. poor outcome, median admission GOS scores (range) were 8 (3–15) and 3 (3–7), and median S-100B levels (range) were 0.85 µg/L (0.08–4.8 µg/L) and 3.6 µg/L (1.4–20 µg/L) • A serum S-100B level of >2.0 µg/L was associated with poor outcome • After TBI in children, the acute assessment of serum S-100B levels associated with outcome

(Continued)

TABLE 6.1
TBI Biomarkers Studies That Focused on Children 18 Years and Younger (Continued)

Year/Author	Biomarker	Population (n)	Severity	Sample Collection Method	Outcome
Berger et al. (2002)	S100B NSE	$n = 15$ (10 TBI [5 nTBI and 5 iTBI] and 5 meningitis LPs for comparison group); age range 0.1–9 years	Severe (GCS < 8)	CSF; for TBI, samples were collected at the time the catheter was placed and intermittently until catheter removal	• CSF S100B concentration/CSF NSE concentration increased in TBI versus the median value of control • 8/10 patients' S100B concentrations had a single peak with rapid decline; could be a correlation between early increases in S100B concentrations and primary BI at or near impact time • iTBI patients had initial peak in NSE concentration on Day 1 after injury followed by a second, higher peak sustained for up to 8 days; second peak may reflect delayed neuronal death • The mean and peak S100B concentration and time of peak were not associated with mechanism of injury • Mean S100B was associated with GCS • S100B concentrations for TBI were higher in patients (GCS > 4); could be a Type I error

Chiaretti et al. (2009)	NSE	*n* = 64 (32 TBI and 32 lumbar puncture controls); age range 1.3–15.6 years	Severe (GCS ≤ 8)	CSF; samples were collected at 2 h and 48 h after admission to PICU	• CSF concentrations of NSE measured 2 h after admission dramatically increased in TBI patients versus controls • At 48 h after injury, there was a sustained and delayed peak in NSE concentrations • An early and late peak suggests that there may be two waves of neuronal death, the second wave potentially representing neuronal apoptosis • Significant association was seen between increased NSE expression and poor outcome; this suggests that the production of NSE may indicate the extent of neuronal damage in patients with severe TBI

(*Continued*)

TABLE 6.1

TBI Biomarkers Studies That Focused on Children 18 Years and Younger (Continued)

Year/Author	Biomarker	Population (*n*)	Severity	Sample Collection Method	Outcome
Bandyopadhyay et al. (2005)	NSE	*n* = 86; age range 11 months to 18 years	Mild to severe (GCS 3–15)	Serum; sample was collected at ED evaluation and within 24 h of injury (average time interval = 3.8 h).	• The mean (±*SD*) NSE level was significantly higher with poor outcome (GOS < 5), 46.4 ± 12.7 ng/mL, versus good outcome (GOS = 5), 19.5 ±1.4 ng/mL. • Mean NSE levels (ng/mL; mean ± SE) were significantly higher in abnormal CT scan patients (26.9 ± 3.0) versus normal CT (16.8 ±1.1). • Levels (mean ± SE) were notably elevated in those with abnormal GCS score (< 15), 31.1 ± 3.6, than normal GCS (= 15), 16.7 ± 1.2. • NSE levels had suitable ability to predict good versus poor outcome. • NSE levels were poor predictors of abnormal CT scans.

Lo et al. (2009)	S100B NSE IL-6 IL-8	*n* = 28; age range [illegible] 3–14 years	Mild to severe (GCS 3–13)	Serum; samples were collected exactly 24 h after injury.	• Patients with unfavorable outcomes had significantly higher S100b, NSE, IL-6, and IL-8 concentrations. • Combinations using brain-specific proteins, S100B or NSE, as "screening markers" had higher predictive values for unfavorable outcome. • It was demonstrated that Day 1 serum levels of inflammatory mediators had higher prognostic values than brain-specific proteins, but best outcome predictive value was achieved with combinations of two biomarkers from different mediator families.
Chiaretti et al. (2008)	IL-6	*n* = 60 (29 TBI and 3[illegible] lumbar puncture controls); age range 1–16 years	Severe (GCS < 8)	CSF; samples were collected at 2 h and at 48 h after injury.	• NGF and IL-6 concentrations were significantly higher in TBI than controls 2 h after injury (T_1). • From 2 to 48 h (T_2), IL-6 concentrations declined. • At T_1, no correlation was found between GCS score and IL-6 (- 0.31). • T_1 IL-6 levels were not significantly lower in patients with better outcomes; at T_2, IL-6 was significantly higher in those with good outcome. • Correlation between the early upregulation of IL-6 and better outcomes may reflect internal effort at neuroprotection in response to TBI.

(Continued)

TABLE 6.1

TBI Biomarkers Studies That Focused on Children 18 Years and Younger (Continued)

Year/Author	Biomarker	Population (n)	Severity	Sample Collection Method	Outcome
Chiaretti et al. (2008)	IL-6	n = 48 (27 TBI and 21 bacterial meningitis LP controls); age range 1.3–15.6 years	Severe (GCS < 8)	CSF; samples were collected at 2 h and 48 h after injury.	• 2 h after injury (T_1), CSF IL-6 concentration in TBI patients was 10-fold higher than the control group. • There was a decrease in IL-6 concentration from T_1 to 48 h after injury. • No significant correlation was found between GCS score and IL-6 concentration. • The stronger the IL-6 upregulation early after initial injury, the better the outcome was for the TBI patient, confirming the neuroprotective role of IL-6 following TBI.
Whalen et al. (2000)	IL-8	n = 58 (27 TBI, 7 bacterial meningitis LP controls, and 24 normal LP controls); age range 0.1–16 years	Severe (GCS ≤ 8)	CSF; samples were collected within 12 h of injury and every 12 h until catheter removed.	• CSF IL-8 concentration in TBI patients 0–12 h after injury was much greater than concentration found in control group. • The median IL-8 level for TBI was 4,452.5 pg/mL (range 0–20,000); the median for control group was 14.5 pg/mL (range 0–250). • Median TBI IL-8 was similar to IL-8 in meningitis patients (median 5,300 pg/mL; range 1,510–22,000). • Strong correlation was seen between CSF IL-8 concentration and mortality.

Fraser et al. (2011)	GFAP	n = 27; age range 2–17 years	Severe (GCS < 8)	CSF and serum; samples were taken daily until arterial catheter was removed in PICU.	• GFAP was markedly elevated in CSF and serum after pediatric TBI. • Serum GFAP measured on PICU Day 1 correlated with functional outcome at 6 months. • Hypothermia therapy did not alter serum GFAP levels compared with normothermia after severe pediatric TBI. • Serum GFAP concentration, together with other biomarkers, may have prognostic value after pediatric TBI.
Su et al. (2012)	MBP	n = 84 (27 TBI and 57 LP controls); age range 3 days to 16 years	Severe (GCS score ≤ 8)	CSF; samples were collected daily for first 5 days after injury or until the EVD stopped draining and/or was removed.	• Mean CSF MBP concentration in TBI patients (50.49 ± 6.97 ng/mL) from all 5 days after injury was significantly greater than mean in controls (0.11 ± 0.01 ng/mL). • Mean CSF MBP concentration increased versus controls on the first day after injury (43.02 ± 15.34 vs. 0.11 ± 0.01 ng/mL) and concentration sustained through the first 5 days. • Correlation was found between age and CSF MBP concentrations in TBI patients; TBI patients ≥ 1 year old had higher mean than those who were younger (60.22 ± 8.26 vs. 19.18 ± 1.67 ng/mL).

(*Continued*)

TABLE 6.1

TBI Biomarkers Studies That Focused on Children 18 Years and Younger (Continued)

Year/Author	Biomarker	Population (*n*)	Severity	Sample Collection Method	Outcome
Berger et al. (2010)	S100B NSE MBP	*n* = 100 (72 TBI and 28 HIE); age <17 years	Mild to severe (GCS 3–15)	Serum; samples were collected as soon as possible after injury and then every 12 h for 120 h.	• 43% of the subjects had poor outcome 3 months after injury; there was no difference with regard to outcome by sex, race, or injury mechanism (HIE vs. TBI); the mean age ± *SD* of poor outcome was lower than a good outcome (2.3 ± 3.4 vs. 4.7 ± 4.6 years). • For each biomarker, the study validated 2-, 3-, and 4-group models for outcome prediction, using sensitivity/specificity; for S100B, the 3-group model predicted poor outcome 59%/100%; NSE, the 3-group model predicted poor outcome 48%/98%; and for MBP, the 3-group model predicted poor outcome 73%/61%. • When the models predicted a poor outcome, there was a very high probability of a poor outcome; conversely, 17% of subjects with a poor outcome were predicted to have good outcome by all 3 biomarker trajectories. • Data suggests trajectory analysis of biomarker data may be a useful approach for predicting outcome after pediatric BI.

Berger et al. (2007)	S100B NSE MBP	$n = 152$, age range 0.1–12.5 years	Mild to severe (GCS 3–15)	Serum; for mild and moderate TBI, sample was collected as soon as possible after injury and again 12–24 h after injury; for severe TBI, additional samples were collected approximately every 12 h for up to 5 days; 1 sample was collected from control.	• In all biomarkers, at any time point, higher concentration was associated with worse outcome. • The number of hours that NSE concentration was in abnormal range had highest correlation with 0–3 months GOS score. • Initial/peak NSE concentrations and initial MBP concentrations were more strongly correlated to outcome in ≤ 4-year-old TBI patients than in > 4-year–old TBI patients. • NSE, S100B, and MBP concentrations obtained at the time of TBI may be useful in predicting outcome.

(Continued)

TABLE 6.1

TBI Biomarkers Studies That Focused on Children 18 Years and Younger (Continued)

Year/Author	Biomarker	Population (*n*)	Severity	Sample Collection Method	Outcome
Berger et al. (2005)	S100B NSE MBP	*n* = 164 (100 TBI [56 nTBI and 44 iTBI] and 64 controls); age range 0.01–13 years	Mild to severe (GCS 3–15)	Serum; for mild and moderate TBI, sample was collected as soon as possible after injury and again 12–24 h after injury; for severe TBI, additional samples were collected approximately every 12 h for up to 5 days; 1 sample was collected from control.	• The initial median serum NSE/serum S100B concentrations were higher in TBI than in controls (24.29 ng/mL compared with 10.15 ng/mL)/(0.026 ng/mL compared with 0.016 ng/mL); no difference was seen in initial median MBP concentration in TBI compared with controls. • No difference was found in initial or peak NSE, S100B, and MBP concentrations between nTBI and iTBI. • The differences in the time course of all three for nTBI compared with iTBI suggests differences in the pathophysiology of the injuries; this may provide insight into the observed differences in outcome between children with nTBI and children with iTBI. • No relationship was seen between initial or peak NSE, S100B, and MBP concentrations and GCS score.

Note. BI = brain injury; CSF = cerebrospinal fluid; ED = emergency department; EVD = extraventricular drain; GCS = Glasgow Coma Scale; GFAP = glial fibrillary acidic protein; GOS = Glasgow Outcome Scale; GOSe = Extended Glasgow Outcome Scale; h = hour; HBI = hypoxemic brain injury; HIE = hypoxic ischemic encephalopathy; IL = interleukin; iTBI = inflicted traumatic brain injury; LP = lumbar puncture; MBP = myelin basic protein; NGF = nerve growth factor; NSE = neuron specific enolase; nTBI = noninflicted traumatic brain injury; PCS = postconcussion symptoms; PICU = pediatric intensive care unit; TBI = traumatic brain injury; T_1 = time 1; T_2 = time 2.

TABLE 6.2

TBI Gene Association Studies That Focused on Children 18 Years and Younger

Year/ Author	Gene	Population	Severity	Sample Collection Method	Outcome
Lo et al. (2009)	APOE	*n* = 225 (65 TBI and 160 healthy controls); age range undeclared	2 groups: "regained consciousness" (GCS>8) and "delayed return of consciousness" (GCS 8 or less)	Buccal smears	• The CPP insult level among E4 carriers with poor outcome was significantly less than non-E4 carriers. • Homozygotic E3 with good outcome did so with 26× more CPP insult than non-E3 homozygous. • 46 TBI children "regained consciousness" and 9 were in coma at discharge; at 6 months after injury, 8 had "poor outcome" and only 1 "regained consciousness" at discharge. • 3/38 of E3 homozygous had "poor outcome" at 6 months after injury; 3/16 of E2 carriers and 3/14 of E4 had "poor outcome." • The trend was for the E2 allele carriers to stay in coma at discharge.

(*Continued*)

TABLE 6.2

TBI Gene Association Studies That Focused on Children 18 Years and Younger (Continued)

Year/ Author	Gene	Population	Severity	Sample Collection Method	Outcome
Moran et al. (2009)	APOE	*n* = 99; age range 8–15 years	Mild (GCS 13–14)	Buccal swabs at 2 weeks after injury and 12 months after injury	• 28 children had APOE4 gene and 71 did not. • Presence of APOE4 was associated with lower GCS and with more severe injury. • There was little evidence to support that APOE4 has a great impact on injury severity or functional outcome. • There was evidence to suggest that APOE4 may be associated with negative early response to injury.
Brichtová and Kozák (2008)	APOE	*n* = 70; age range 1 month to 17 years	Mild to severe (GCS 3–15)	Serum	• 4 groups based on APOE genotype: E2/E3 (7 patients); E3/E3 (52); E2/E4 (2); E3/E4 (9). • There was a significant difference between the trauma severity and outcome for E2/E3 and E3/E3 genotype; no statistical difference in groups with the APOE4 allele. • Significant difference was seen between GCS and GOS in E3/E3 genotype groups and E2/E3 genotype.

Teasdale et al. (2005)	APOE	n = 1,094; age range 0–93 years; subset (n = 2[illegible]5 children <18[illegible]	Mild to severe (GCS 3–15)	Buccal swab; sample was collected at acute stage of injury	• Of 984 viable patients, 324 carriers of APOE4 allele; 660 non-APOE4 carriers. • No association was seen between having APOE4 allele and GOS. • There was no association between having APOE4 and unfavorable outcome: 118/324 (36%) of APOE4 carriers had unfavorable outcome versus 215/660 (33%) of noncarriers. • Association between unfavorable outcome and APOE4 carriers was strongest in patients aged 0–15 years; the adverse effect of being a APOE4 carrier decreased gradually with age and defused by age 55–60 years.

Note. APOE = apolipoprotein E; APOE4 = apolipoprotein E4; CPP = cerebral perfusion pressure; GCS = Glasgow Coma Scale; GOS = Glasgow Outcome Scale; TBI = traumatic brain injury.

reference lists of all articles were also reviewed for potentially relevant articles, which were independently reviewed by the three authors for further biomarker and genetic studies in association with pediatric TBI. No additional studies were identified or included; however, published literature reviews on the science of biomarkers and gene studies in pediatric TBI were included because they informed the state of the science and offered an additional historical foundation. There were no published biomarker or gene association research studies in pediatric TBI found in journals with nursing titles.

Biomarker Studies

The presence of biomarkers in the blood, cerebral spinal fluid (CSF), and/or urine can indicate a mediated cellular response to an injury (Feala et al., 2013). Although the number of biomarker studies were relatively few in children, as opposed to studies of adult TBI, there were six published comprehensive review articles since 2006 that specifically addressed the use of biomarkers in pediatric TBI (Berger, 2006; Daoud et al., 2014; Kochanek et al., 2008; Kovesdi et al., 2010; Sandelr, Figaji, & Adelson, 2010; Papa et al., 2013). The reviews addressed biomarkers and their use, prognostic value, clinical implications and applications, research utility, and outcome prediction. They included comprehensive tables that illustrated the most widely studied biomarkers, their time frame for discovery, values of measure, and referenced studies.

Although the majority of the biomarker research has only been within the last 15 years in children with head injury, the work of one group from the University of Pittsburgh has largely driven the focus on TBI (Kochanek et al., 2013). Along with colleagues from a number of institutions, the collaborative research led to the identification of a number of candidate molecular biomarkers (Table 6.3). Pediatric TBI biomarker research has reported the detection of viable candidate markers and their association with outcome prediction (Berger, 2006; Berger, Beers, Papa, & Bell, 2012; Kochanek et al., 2000; Kochanek et al., 2008). Having said that, only a few studies have reported a significant correlation between the biomarkers and an outcome measure, whereas others have determined those biomarkers to have poor prognostication qualities (Babcock et al., 2013; Bandyopadhyay et al., 2005; Berger & Kochanek, 2006; Chiaretti et al., 2008; Daoud et al., 2014; Geyer, Ulrich, Grafe, Stach, & Till, 2009). However, several biomarkers, such as S100B, neuron-specific enolase, and myelin basic protein, have been reported in some studies to have a correlative relationship with outcomes in children with TBI, while in others, they have been called into question.

The heterogeneity of TBI may bear on this conflicting evidence. Pediatric TBI classification (mild, moderate, and severe) does not accurately represent the actual injury type (noninflicted vs. inflicted) or the structural damage and

TABLE 6.3

Pediatric Traumatic Brain Injury Biomarkers

Biomarker	Mechanism of Action	CNS Source	Serum CSF Levels		Preclinical Work	Clinical Development	Knowledge Gap
			Mild TBI	Severe TBI			
GFAP	This protein is released upon cellular injury into the extracellular space.[a]	Glia	>0.033 μg/L increased[a]	>15.04 μg/L unfavorable outcome (death)[a]	May be useful for identifying various types of brain damage and is explicitly linked to CNS injury/not located outside CNS.[b,c]	Useful measurement immediately following TBI of predicted mortality and severity of injury[b]	Research is limited, as it is tough to apply this measure to peds due to its developmental chemical expression.[d]

(*Continued*)

TABLE 6.3

Pediatric Traumatic Brain Injury Biomarkers (Continued)

Biomarker	Mechanism of Action	CNS Source	Serum CSF Levels		Preclinical Work	Clinical Development	Knowledge Gap
			Mild TBI	Severe TBI			
IL-6	Injury induces release of T-cells and microphages, stimulating immune response, leading to inflammation.[e]	Neuron, astrocytes, endothelial, glia	No data	No data	May help stimulate NGF, which can indicate severity of head trauma[e]	IL-6 and NGF increase can repair damaged tissue and may lead to more positive outcomes in recovery.[e]	Studies are limited, which give contradictory results—upregulation of NGF and IL-6 has led to poor outcomes after TBI, or no relationship whatsoever.[e]
IL-8	Cooperates with G-protein–coupled receptors on neutrophils to induce chemotaxis and inflammation[f]	Endothelium, epithelium, leukocytes, and glia	No data	No data	Very elevated in peds TBI for first 108 h, indicating an acute inflammatory element in TBI[f]	May be involved in secondary injury. Also, inflammation could be a target of anti-inflammatory treatment.[f]	Limited research provides contradictory results—helpful versus hurtful to recovery[f]

MBP	Damaged myelin sheath releases elements of the sheath (MBP)[g]	Myelin sheath	No data	No data	Increases in MBP in CSF follow TBI[g]	Significantly elevated increases of MBP immediately following TBI were associated with poor outcomes[g]	There is a lack of study of mild TBI cases and MBP as it is most visible in CSF; age affects concentration levels in the control population (not as elevated).[g]
NSE	Emerges after damage to neuronal brain cells[a]	Neuron	>7–10 µg/L increased[a]	Mean 12.8 µg/L (Serum), mean 7.8 µg/L[a] (CSF)	Indicator of intracranial injury, as the enzyme appears after cellular damage within 6 h of injury[h]	May be used as predictor of short-term, physical disability in peds[h]	Focus is needed on long-term outcomes as well.[h]
S-100 beta (S100B)	Stimulates neuronal growth and enhances the survival of neurons after injury[i]	Glia	>0.25 µg/L increased[a]	>2–2.5 µg/L unfavorable outcome[a]	Served as markers of neuronal damage after TBI[i]	Increases in S100B serum concentrations were associated with brain damage severity.[i]	Variety of results makes it hard to conclusively use data for prognostic purposes.[i]

(*Continued*)

TABLE 6.3

Pediatric Traumatic Brain Injury Biomarkers (Continued)

Biomarker	Mechanism of Action	CNS Source	Serum CSF Levels		Preclinical Work	Clinical Development	Knowledge Gap
			Mild TBI	Severe TBI			
APOE	Found on chromosome 19. Alleles E2, E3, E4; associated with increased biochemical surrogates of inflammation.[a]	Neuron, glia	No data[a]	Mean 3.7 mg/L[a]	Possession of E4 allele in adults is shown to be related to poorer outcomes following brain injury.[k]	Possession of E4 allele may lead to poorer recovery outcomes in children with TBI.[k]	Very few research studies, which have resulted in contradictory evidence, and even fewer pediatric studies[k]

Note. APOE = apolipoprotein E; CNS = central nervous system; CSF = cerebrospinal fluid; h = hour; GFAP = glial fibrillary acidic protein; IL = interleukin; MBP = myelin basic protein; NGF = nerve growth factor; NSE = neuron-specific enolase; peds = pediatrics; TBI = traumatic brain injury.

[a]Kövesdi and colleagues (2010). [b]Pelinka and colleagues (2004). [c]Mondello and colleagues (2011). [d]Fraser and colleagues (2011); [e]Chiaretti and colleagues (2008); [f]Whalen and colleagues (2000); [g]Su and colleagues (2012); [h]Bandyopadhyay and colleagues (2005); [i]Piazza and colleagues (2007); [j]Berger and colleagues (2002); [k]Moran and colleagues (2009).

biomechanical and biochemical responses. These biochemical responses differ significantly based on the evolution of the secondary injury phase and the treatment delivered. Although there are standardized TBI guidelines for the treatment of severe head injury, the guidelines' singular pathway for approach may not appropriately address the different injuries and may also explain the contradiction in the biomarker findings (Bell & Kochanek, 2013; Kochanek, Bell, & Bayir, 2010; Kochanek, et al., 2012). The lack of clinical validation of defined biomarkers may contribute in part to the fact that the Food and Drug Administration has yet to approve any specific biomarkers for clinical evaluation in children with TBI (Berger et al, 2011; Papa et al., 2013).

Inconsistencies within the published research findings exist with respect to the relationships among study outcome measures, age groups, inclusion criteria, injury severity, and type of injury (accidental vs. nonaccidental/inflicted TBI [iTBI]). Reports of cognitive and functional outcomes have been limited by the absence or paucity of measures for children. Researchers are challenged by limited outcome assessment instruments designed for pediatric TBI, small study participant numbers and heterogeneous patients, dormant injury sequelae presenting after the injury occurrence, and outcome evaluation (Kövesdi et al., 2010). For example, one of the largest pediatric TBI studies suggested that biomarkers were associated with outcomes, when the Glasgow Outcome Scale-Extended Pediatrics (GOS-E Peds) was used as the outcome measure instead of the Glasgow Outcome Scale (GOS; Beers et al., 2012). Most other studies show different results because their outcomes are based either on survival or on a GOS score. The difference between these two measures is that the GOS-E Peds is specific to children with TBI and is considered the "gold" standard of measure. It has demonstrated validity in the pediatric TBI population (Beers et al., 2012), and yet, most studies still report outcomes based on survival or the GOS (Berger et al., 2011).

Although the prevalence of biomarker research in pediatric TBI has increased over the last decade, variable study methods have limited the accuracy of prediction and generalization (Berger et al., 2012; Papa et al., 2013). Analytic limitations in the published studies included small sample sizes, leading to underpowered studies, which prevent obtaining a direct association between the biomarker and the outcome measure (Daoud et al., 2014). Sample collection variability, including both the type of sample and the time of sample collection, has confounded the interpretation of biomarker effects, thereby creating increased complexity in attributing a biomarker change with an injury or predictive outcome. Some biomarkers, such as S100B, are dependent on age and time of injury (Filippidis, Papadopoulos, Kapsalaki, & Fountas, 2010). Additionally, depending on the severity of the injury, repeated collection of a biomarker may be inconsistent, thereby preventing repeated statistical measures. Other studies that collected biomarkers over time reported results by initial, mean, and/or peak concentration. Consistent reporting of concentrations has provided opportunities for comparison across studies, lending support to the finding that worse patient outcomes were associated with increasing biomarker concentrations (Berger et al., 2010).

An emerging science in pediatric TBI studies has focused on degradation products, specifically spectrin breakdown products (SBDPs), cleaved tau (c-tau), and amyloid-β1–42 (Kövesdi et al., 2010). This growing field of interest has also been subject to the limitations of the biomarker research in pediatric TBI, that is, small samples sizes, collection variation, and mixed severity of the injury.

Another new area of biomarker research is "rehabilomics," where biomarkers are collected to study the patient's biological and functional treatment response to rehabilitation (Berger et al., 2011; Kobeissy et al., 2011). This evolving field of biomarker discovery is rich for children with a TBI and opens the doors to promoting long-term, outcome-based treatments and research. It also supports the argument for pediatric neurocritical care and neurorehabilitation units (Pineda et al., 2013). These care units can promote health services and create environments that promote brain injury management and recovery by a standardized approach to TBI or neurologic insult (Kochanek et al., 2010).

Gene Association Studies

Studies of the gene association, specifically candidate gene identification in TBI in children are extremely limited. Kurowski and colleagues (2012) published a comprehensive literature review of APOE in children with TBI. Five of the studies described in that review focused on hospitalized children with TBI (Tables 6.2 and 6.3). The current review excluded one of these (Quinn et al., 2004), which focused on the presence of APOE in postmortem tissue samples. Although APOE4 was associated with younger age and unfavorable outcomes, the fact that all participants had died appears to have favored the outcome (Quinn et al., 2004).

The apolipoprotein gene, mapped to chromosome 19, consists of four exons and three introns, totaling 3597 base pairs. Three major isoforms of APOE are APOE2 (cys112, cys158), APOE3 (cys112, arg158), and APOE4 (arg112, arg158; Ghebranious, Ivacic, Mallum, & Dokken, 2005). Because the isoforms differ from each other, they change the APOE structure and function. Secreted locally by macrophages after a peripheral nerve injury and by astrocytes and oligodendrocytes after central nervous system insults, APOE polymorphisms have been associated with changes in neurocognitive and functional outcomes (Jofre-Monseny, Minihane, & Rimbach, 2008). The presence of the APOE genotype is associated with increased biochemical surrogates of inflammation. Evidence shows that the multifunctional nature of the APOE genotype may be in large part due to an impact on its oxidative status or the immunomodulatory/anti-inflammatory properties (Jofre-Monseny et al., 2008).

Studies examining APOE found that the possession of APOE4 allele led to poorer recovery outcomes in children with TBI. There were significant differences between the trauma severity and outcome for E2/E3 and E3/E3 genotype allele carriers. The presence of APOE4 was found to be associated with lower Glasgow Coma Scale and with more severe injury. Studies also found that there was little evidence to support that APOE4 has a greater impact on injury severity or functional outcome, whereas there was evidence to suggest that APOE4 may be associated with negative early response to injury. The presence of APOE4 in a child who happens to sustain a TBI may set him/her up for an exaggerated inflammatory process that maybe in part responsible for worse outcomes after injury. APOE4 has been associated with poor GOS scores (Blackman et al., 2005; Brichtová, & Kozák, 2008; Lo et al., 2009; Moran et al., 2009).

RESEARCH PRIORITIES

Common Data Elements

In 2009, the National Institute on Disability and Rehabilitation Research and the National Institute of Neurological Disorders and Stroke (NINDS) called for a review of the original TBI common data element (CDE) recommendations to ensure they were relevant to pediatric populations. An interprofessional work group composed of pediatric TBI experts developed and then revised the recommendations in 2012 (Papa et al., 2013). The work group published three descriptive articles to inform future study development (Adelson et al., 2012; Berger et al., 2012; Miller, Odenkirchen, Duhaime, & Hicks, 2012). At the University of Pittsburgh, Drs. Bell and Wisniewski received a $16.5 million grant from the NIH to lead the international Approaches and Decisions for Acute Pediatric TBI (ADAPT) trial (www.adapttrial.org). Funded for 5 years (2013–2017) as a comparative effectiveness study, CDEs will be collected from 1,000 children with severe TBI. The study will estimate the impact of strategies to lower intracranial pressure and treat secondary injuries and strategies to determine the delivery of nutrient treatments on outcomes up to 1 year after the injury, thereby determining what approach to clinical management works best. There is an opportunity for this body of work to include biomarkers and gene association studies. It may also be the needed step to defining predictive markers and polymorphism with this injury.

Research Methodologies

There is growing consensus that research conducted in pediatric TBI should have comparable methodologies. Small sample sizes and heterogeneous populations prevent collected biomarkers from being optimally sensitive and specific. The day-to-day variability of the patient's injury can be captured better by time-course collection of biomarkers, which has a higher specificity than point estimates, and can influence clinical validity and inform future treatment and recovery (Berger et al., 2011). Therefore, research may be served better if biomarkers that have demonstrated a positive relationship with patient outcomes are optimized in larger sample sizes to demonstrate their usefulness in informing the course of treatment. Additionally, developing programs of research that incorporate and more clearly elucidate the roles of degradation products in pediatric TBI may guide future treatment strategies.

Improving workgroups and multisite research communication will advance the field and ensure study designs and methodologies that can statistically support the research hypotheses. An example of this is the Pediatric Neurocritical Care Research Group (PNCRG). This group is dedicated to performing clinical and preclinical studies aimed at optimizing functional outcomes for critically ill children with neurological conditions. Its membership is international and interprofessional, comprising those who share a common passion for research that will ultimately lead to improved neurocritical care for children. Current research includes biomarkers and quality of life in children with TBI; determining the prevalence of acute critical neurologic disease in children; and computer tomography classification to guide therapeutic intervention and outcome prediction in children with severe TBI (www.pncrg.org).

As with biomarkers, gene association studies in TBI would benefit by being included in all TBI studies to promote comparison and combined analysis across studies. Kurowski and colleagues (2012) support gene association studies that would provide an opportunity to evaluate comprehensive and tailored outcomes. They suggest that pediatric TBI genetic research should include demographic, environmental, and genotypic characteristics to better contrast and compare patients and their outcomes (Kurowski et al., 2012). Multisite studies would also promote large sample sizes, thereby affecting the magnitude of the genetic polymorphism identification. The limited focus on gene association and polymorphism studies in children with TBI may be influenced in the future by a recent increase in such studies among adult TBI patients, as researchers have begun to recognize the importance of the interrelationships of genetics, recovery, rehabilitation, and promotion of functional outcomes. Improving the understanding of how genes are associated with phases of injury and how polymorphism influences outcomes is increasingly recognized as an important next step in pediatric TBI research.

Although there is more uniformity in preclinical (experimental) research than clinical research, researchers have developed animal models that explain some effects of injury such as impact, rotational, and repeat injury (Kochanek et al., 2010). Replications of developed injury models used in preclinical models have demonstrated utility in defining responses of the injured brain. However, limitations exist in the developing human brain, human biomarker response and identification, as well as gene associations studies.

To minimize the difficulty with tissue and biologic sample collection, Feala and colleagues (2013) suggest an important role for systems biology in TBI biomarkers. In this emerging science, systems biology researchers examine the interwoven molecular pathways and networks by computational modeling of diverse datasets. Sophisticated methods that create and measure protein-binding interaction (PPI) networks lead researchers to move heterogonous information from high-throughput molecular data sets of complex molecular TBI responses into testable hypotheses (Feala et al., 2013). By using protein/proteomic data sets for TBI, researchers can make new discoveries of biomarkers, and scientists would gain understanding into the underlying molecular mechanism of TBI as a promising frontier for improving TBI outcomes.

Biorepository

In 2010, an interagency TBI CDE Biospecimens Workgroup developed *Common Data Elements for TBI Research: Pediatric Considerations*, which presented recommendations for the best practice of the collection, processing, and storing of biological specimens collected in a child with TBI. The report stressed the importance of adopting standard practices for sample collection, processing, and storage, and for recording biomarker-specific data in all future pediatric biomarker studies (Berger et al., 2012; Papa et al., 2013). Highlights from these guidelines included the following: biospecimen collection should maintain a consistent volume collected at each sample time point and from the sample origin, appreciating that samples may be collected over a period of hours to months; if the TBI prevents assessment of time of injury, such as may occur in an iTBI, a consistent approach to timing should occur with all subjects; and internal review board approval should be sought for collection and storage; risk for hemolysis of samples, especially in younger children and infants, in whom hemolysis has been demonstrated to affect some biomarkers results. Collection of CSF collection may occur from existing drains; however, specialized attention should be taken with indwelling catheters. Additionally, lumbar puncture is not indicated unless for use with control subjects; processing of samples should include aliquots to avoid refreezing of samples; storage should ensure the protection of samples and rights of donors; and consent for sample storage must be revisited when the donor turns 18. Overall, the technologic and biotechnologic advances occurring daily strongly support the storage and development of biologic specimens so that future markers and gene associations may be defined in children with TBI.

IMPLICATIONS FOR NURSING RESEARCH

Understanding recent advances in biomarker and genomic studies in pediatric TBI is important because these advances may guide future research, collaborations, and interventions. It is also important to ensure that nursing is a part of this evolving science to promote improved outcomes in children with TBIs. Nurse scientists have been active in biologic and genetic work in adult TBI research. Many are fellows of the Summer Genetics Institute, National Institute of Nursing Research and have been integral in the development of the International Society of Nurses in Genetics (ISONG), which supports dissemination of biomarkers and gene association studies by nurses (www.isong.org). Nursing colleagues who study adult TBI have contributed widely, from the identification of mitochondrial polymorphism in severe TBI to the discovery of novel targets in human TBI by gene expression profiling (Barr, Alexander, & Conley, 2011; Conley et al., 2014). Others have evaluated the role of APOE4 in functional outcomes after severe TBI (Alexander et al., 2007). The opportunities are plenty for nurse researchers who are trained and eager to participate in the important discoveries to be made in pediatric TBI research.

CONCLUSION

The future is bright for pediatric TBI biomarker and gene association research. In order to improve the clinical utility of research, specific gaps must be closed and, most importantly, consistent outcomes must be demonstrated. This critical analysis of study designs revealed that large, homogeneous patient populations and more consistent use of similar injury and outcome measures may enable future studies to improve upon suspected associations (Kövesdi et al., 2010). The increased attention to the area can provide the impetus for a strong community of researchers to collaborate toward legitimizing biomarkers in pediatric TBI. As this subspecialty of research grows, groups such as ISONG and PNCRG provide opportunities to promote education, coordination, and dissemination, while multisite studies such as the ADAPT trial can foster consistent sample collection methods and ultimately more biomarker and gene association data. Equally important to the success of biomarker and gene association research is the continuation of training of the nurse fellows of the Summer Genetics Institute and the ongoing support of research strategies by the National Institute of Nursing

Research, National Institutes of Health. Continued exploration and validation of biomarkers and gene association studies for pediatric TBI should include robust research methodologies, CDEs, and biologic repositories. Biomarkers and gene association studies can contribute to illuminating the complexities of the brain injury process in children.

ACKNOWLEDGMENTS

Karin Reuter-Rice has center project support by NIH-NINR 1P30 NR014139-01 Adaptive Leadership for Cognitive Affective Symptom Science (ADAPT), Institute of Nursing Research Center of Excellence (2012–2015), in addition to funding by the Robert Wood Johnson Foundation as a Nurse Faculty scholar project 71244 (2013–2016).

Julia K. Eads has no disclosures.

Suzanna Boyce Berndt has no disclosures.

Ellen Bennett, PhD she is a consultant for Dr. Reuter-Rice's Robert Wood Johnson Foundation Nurse Faculty scholar project 71244.

The authors would like to acknowledge Judith C. Hays, RN, PhD, FGSA, Associate Professor Emeritus, Duke University, and Editor Emeritus, *Public Health Nursing*, for her gracious feedback on the development of this manuscript. They would also like to thank Elizabeth Flint, PhD, Research Analyst, for her assistance with formatting manuscript tables.

REFERENCES

Adelson, P. D., Pineda, J., Bell, M. J., Abend, N. S., Berger, R. P., Giza, C. C., et al. (2012). Common data elements for pediatric traumatic brain injury: Recommendations from the working group on demographics and clinical assessment. *Journal of Neurotrauma, 29*(4), 639–653. http://dx.doi.org/10.1089/neu.2011.1952

Alexander, S., Kerr, M. E., Kim, Y., Kamboh, M. I., Beers, S. R., & Conley, Y. P. (2007). Apolipoprotein E4 allele presence and functional outcome after severe traumatic brain injury. *Journal of Neurotrauma, 24*(5), 790–797. http://dx.doi.org/10.1089/neu.2006.0133

Anderson, V., Brown, S., & Newitt, H. (2010). What contributes to quality of life in adult survivors of childhood traumatic brain injury? *Journal of Neurotrauma, 27*(5), 863–870. http://dx.doi.org/10.1089/neu.2009.1169

Babcock, L., Byczkowski, T., Wade, S. L., Ho, M., & Bazarian, J. J. (2013). Inability of S100B to predict postconcussion syndrome in children who present to the emergency department with mild traumatic brain injury a brief report. *Pediatric Emergency Care, 29*(4), 458–461. http://dx.doi.org/10.1097/PEC.0b013e31828a202d

Bandyopadhyay, S., Hennes, H., Gorelick, M. H., Wells, R. G., & Walsh-Kelly, C. M. (2005). Serum neuron-specific enolase as a predictor of short-term outcome in children with closed traumatic brain injury. *Academic Emergency Medicine, 12*(8), 732–738. http://dx.doi.org/10.1111/j.1553-2712.2005.tb00940.x

Barr, T. L., Alexander, S., & Conley, Y. (2011). Gene expression profiling for discovery of novel targets in human traumatic brain injury. *Biological Research for Nursing, 13*(2), 140–153. http://dx.doi.org/10.1177/1099800410385671

Beers,S., Wisniewski,S., Garcia-Filion, P., Tian, Y., Hahner, T., Berger, R., Bell, M., et al. (2012). Validity of a pediatric version of the Glasgow outcome scale–extended. *Journal of Neurotrauma, 29*, 1126–1139. http://dx.doi.org/10.1089/neu.2011.2272

Bell, M. J., & Kochanek, P. M. (2013). Pediatric traumatic brain injury in 2012: The year with new guidelines and common data elements. *Critical Care Clinic, 29*, 223–238. http://dx.doi.org/10.1016/j.cc.2012.11.004

Berger, R. P. (2006). The use of serum biomarkers to predict outcome after traumatic brain injury in adults and children. *Journal of Head Trauma Rehabilitation, 21*(4), 315–333. http://dx.doi.org/10.1097/00001199-200607000-00004

Berger, R. P., Adelson, P. D., Pierce, M. C., Dulani, T., Cassidy, L. D., & Kochanek, P. M. (2005). Serum neuron-specific enolase, S100B, and myelin basic protein concentrations after inflicted and noninflicted traumatic brain injury in children. *Journal of Neurosurgery: Pediatrics, 103*(1), 61–68. http://dx.doi.org/10.3171/ped.2005.103.1.0061

Berger, R. P., Bazaco, M. C., Wagner, A. K., Kochanek, P. M., & Fabio, A. (2010). Trajectory analysis of serum biomarker concentrations facilitates outcome prediction after pediatric traumatic and hypoxemic brain injury. *Developmental Neuroscience, 32*, 396–405. http://dx.doi.org/10.1159/000316803

Berger, R. P., Beers, S. R., Papa, L., & Bell, M. (2012). Common data elements for pediatric traumatic brain injury: Recommendations from the biospecimens and biomarkers workgroup. *Journal of Neurotrauma, 29*(4), 672–677. http://dx.doi.org/10.1089/neu.2011.1861

Berger, R. P., Beers, S. R., Richichi, R., Wiesman, D., & Adelson, P. D. (2007). Serum biomarker concentrations and outcome after pediatric traumatic brain injury. *Journal of Neurotrauma, 24*(12), 1793–1801. http://dx.doi.org/10.1089/neu.2007.0316

Berger, R. P., Houle, J., Hayes, R. L., Wang, K. K., Mondello, S., & Bell, M. J. (2011). Translating biomarkers research to clinical care: Applications and issues for rehabilomics. *PM&R, 3*(6), S31–S38. http://dx.doi.org/10.1016/j.pmrj.2011.03.016

Berger, R. P., & Kochanek, P. M. (2006). Urinary S100B concentrations are increased after brain injury in children: A preliminary study*. *Pediatric Critical Care Medicine, 7*(6), 557–561. http://dx.doi.org/10.1097/01.PCC.0000244426.37793.23

Berger, R. P., Pierce, M. C., Wisniewski, S. R., Adelson, P. D., Clark, R. S., Ruppel, R. A., et al. (2002). Neuron-specific enolase and S100B in cerebrospinal fluid after severe traumatic brain injury in infants and children. *Pediatrics, 109*(2), E31–E31. http://dx.doi.org/10.1542/peds.109.2.e31

Biomarkers Definitions Working Group. (2001). Biomarkers and Surrogate Endpoints: Preferred Definitions and Conceptual Framework. *Clinical Pharmacology and Therapeutics*, *69*(3), 89–95. http://dx.doi.org/10.1067/mcp.2001.113989

Blackman, J. A., Worley, G., & Strittmatter, W. J. (2005). Apolipoprotein E and brain injury: Implications for children. *Developmental Medicine & Child Neurology, 47*(01), 64–70. http://dx.doi.org/10.1017/S0012162205000113

Brichtová, E., & Kozák, L. (2008). Apolipoprotein E genotype and traumatic brain injury in children—association with neurological outcome. *Child's Nervous System, 24*(3), 349–356. http://dx.doi.org/10.1007/s00381-007-0459-6

Bruns, J., & Hauser, W. A. (2003). The epidemiology of traumatic brain injury: A review. *Epilepsia, 44*, 2–10. http://dx.doi.org/10.1046/j.1528-1157.44.s10.3.x

Center for Disease Control and Prevention. (n.d.) Retrieved from http://www.cdc.gov/TraumaticBrainInjury/data/index.html

Chiaretti, A., Antonelli, A., Mastrangelo, A., Pezzotti, P., Tortorolo, L., Tosi, F., et al. (2008). Interleukin-6 and nerve growth factor upregulation correlates with improved outcome in children with severe traumatic brain injury. *Journal of Neurotrauma, 25*(3), 225–234. http://dx.doi.org/10.1089/neu.2007.0405

Chiaretti, A., Antonelli, A., Riccardi, R., Genovese, O., Pezzotti, P., Rocco, C. D., et al. (2008). Nerve growth factor expression correlates with severity and outcome of traumatic brain injury in children. *European Journal of Paediatric Neurology, 12*(3), 195–204. http://dx.doi.org/10.1016/j.ejpn.2007.07.016

Chiaretti, A., Barone, G., Riccardi, R., Antonelli, A., Pezzotti, P., Genovese, O., et al. (2009). NGF, DCX, and NSE upregulation correlates with severity and outcome of head trauma in children. *Neurology, 72*(7), 609–616. http://dx.doi.org/10.1212/01.wnl.0000342462.51073.06

Conley, Y. P., Okonkwo, D., Deslouches, S., Alexander, S., Puccio, A. M., Beers, S. R., et al. (2014). Mitochondrial polymorphisms impact outcomes after severe traumatic brain injury. *Journal of Neurotrauma, 31*(1), 34–41. http://dx.doi.org/10.1089/neu.2013.2855

Coronado, V., Xu, L., Basavaraju, S., McGuire, L., Wald, M., Faul, M., et al. (2011). Surveillance for traumatic brain injury–related deaths- United States, 1997–2007. Centers for Disease Control and Prevention, National Center for Injury Prevention and Control. *Morbidity and Mortality Weekly Report, 60*(5), 1–36. Retrieved from http://www.cdc.gov/mmwr/preview/mmwrhtml/ss6005a1.htm

Corso, P., Finkelstein, E., Miller, T., Fiebelkorn, I., & Zaloshnja, E. (2006). Incidence and lifetime costs of injuries in the United States. *Injury Prevention, 12*, 212–218. http://dx.doi.org/10.1136/ip.2005.010983

Daoud, H., Alharfi, I., Alhelali, I., Stewart, T. C., Qasem, H., & Fraser, D. D. (2014). Brain injury biomarkers as outcome predictors in pediatric severe traumatic brain injury. *Neurocritical Care Society, 20*, 427–435. http://dx.doi.org/10.1007/s12028-013-9879-1

Faul, M., Xu, L., Wald, M. M., & Coronado, V. G. (2010). Traumatic brain injury in the United States: Emergency department visits, hospitalizations and deaths 2002-2006. *Centers for Disease Control and Prevention, National Center for Injury Prevention and Control*. Retrieved from http://www.cdc.gov/traumaticbraininjury/pdf/blue_book.pdf

Feala, J. D., Abdulhameed, M. D., Yu, C., Dutta, B., Yu, X., Schmid, K., et al. (2013). Systems biology approaches for discovering biomarkers for traumatic brain injury. *Journal of Neurotrauma, 30*(13), 1101–1116. http://dx.doi.org/10.1089/neu.2012.2631

Filippidis, A. S., Papadopoulos, D. C., Kapsalaki, E. Z., & Fountas, K. N. (2010). Role of the S100B serum biomarker in the treatment of children suffering from mild traumatic brain injury. *Neurosurgical Focus, 29*(5), E2. http://dx.doi.org/10.3171/2010.8.FOCUS10185

Fraser, D. D., Close, T. E., Rose, K. L., Ward, R., Mehl, M., Farrell, C., et al. (2011). Severe traumatic brain injury in children elevates glial fibrillary acidic protein in cerebrospinal fluid and serum. *Pediatric Critical Care Medicine, 12*(3), 319–324. http://dx.doi.org/10.1097/PCC.0b013e3181e8b32d

Geyer, C., Ulrich, A., Grafe, G., Stach, B., & Till, H. (2009). Diagnostic value of S100B and neuron-specific enolase in mild pediatric traumatic brain injury. *Journal of Neurosurgery: Pediatrics, 4*(4), 339–344. http://dx.doi.org/10.3171/2009.5.PEDS08481

Ghebranious, N., Ivacic, L., Mallum, J., & Dokken, C. (2005). Detection of ApoE E2, E3 and E4 alleles using MALDI-TOF mass spectrometry and the homogeneous mass-extend technology. *Nucleic Acids Research, 33*(17), E149–E149. http://dx.doi.org/10.1093/nar/gni155

Jager, T. E., Weiss, H. B., Coben, J. H., & Pepe, P. E. (2000). Traumatic brain injuries evaluated in U.S. Emergency Departments, 1992-1994. *Academic Emergency Medicine, 7*(2), 134–140. http://dx.doi.org/10.1111/j.1553-2712.2000.tb00515.x

Jofre-Monseny, L., Minihane, A., & Rimbach, G. (2008). Impact of apoE genotype on oxidative stress, inflammation and disease risk. *Molecular Nutrition & Food Research, 52*(1), 131–145. http://dx.doi.org/10.1002/mnfr.200700322

Kobeissy, F. H., Guingab-Cagmat, J. D., Razafsha, M., O'steen, L., Zhang, Z., Hayes, R. L., et al. (2011). Leveraging biomarker platforms and systems biology for rehabilomics and biologics effectiveness research. *PM&R, 3*(6), S139–S147. http://dx.doi.org/10.1016/j.pmrj.2011.02.012

Kochanek, P. M., Bell, M. J., & Bayır, H. (2010). Quo vadis 2010 – carpe diem: Challenges and opportunities in pediatric traumatic brain injury. *Developmental Neuroscience, 32*(5–6), 335–342. http://dx.doi.org/10.1159/000323016

Kochanek, P. M., Berger, R. P., Bayir, H., Wagner, A. K., Jenkins, L. W., & Clark, R. S. (2008). Biomarkers of primary and evolving damage in traumatic and ischemic brain injury: Diagnosis, prognosis, probing mechanisms, and therapeutic decision making. *Current Opinion in Critical Care, 14*(2), 135–141. http://dx.doi.org/10.1097/MCC.0b013e3282f57564

Kochanek, P. M., Berger, R. P., Fink, E. L., Au, A. K., Bayır, H., Bell, M. J., et al. (2013). The potential for bio-mediators and biomarkers in pediatric traumatic brain injury and neurocritical care. *Frontiers in Neurology, 4*. http://dx.doi.org/10.3389/fneur.2013.00040

Kochanek, P. M., Carney, N., Adelson, P. D., Ashwal, S., Bell, M. J., Bratton, S., et al. (2012). Guidelines for the acute medical management of severe traumatic brain injury in infants, children and adolescents: Second edition. *Pediatric Critical Care Medicine, 13*(Suppl 1), S1–S2. http://dx.doi.org/10.1097/PCC.0b013e31823f435c

Kochanek, P. M., Clark, R. S., Ruppel, R. A., Adelson, P. D., Bell, M. J., Whalen, M. J., et al. (2000). Biochemical, cellular, and molecular mechanisms in the evolution of secondary damage after severe traumatic brain injury in infants and children: Lessons learned from the bedside. *Pediatric Critical Care Medicine, 1*(1), 4–19.

Kövesdi, E., Lückl, J., Bukovics, P., Farkas, O., Pál, J., Czeiter, E., et al. (2010). Update on protein biomarkers in traumatic brain injury with emphasis on clinical use in adults and pediatrics. *Acta Neurochirurgica, 152*(1), 1–17. http://dx.doi.org/10.1007/s00701-009-0463-6

Kurowski, B., Martin, L. J., & Wade, S. L. (2012). Genetics and outcomes after traumatic brain injury (TBI): What do we know about pediatric TBI? *Journal of Pediatric Rehabilitation Medicine: An Interdisciplinary Approach, 5*, 217–231. http://dx.doi.org/10.3233/PRM-2012-0214

Langlois, J., Rutland-Brown, W., & Thomas, K. (2004). Traumatic brain injury in the United States: Emergency department visits, hospitalizations, and deaths. *Centers for Disease Control and Prevention, National Center for Injury Prevention and Control.* Retrieved from www.cdc.gov/ncipc/pub-res/TBI_in_US_04/TBI-USA_Book-Oct1.pdf

Lo, T. Y., Jones, P. A., Chambers, I. R., Beattie, T. F., Forsyth, R., Mendelow, A. D., et al. (2009). Modulating the effect of apolipoprotein E polymorphisms on secondary brain insult and outcome after childhood brain trauma. *Child's Nervous System, 25*(1), 47–54. http://dx.doi.org/10.1007/s00381-008-0723-4

Miller, A. C., Odenkirchen, J., Duhaime, A., & Hicks, R. (2012). Common data elements for research on traumatic brain injury: Pediatric considerations. *Journal of Neurotrauma, 29*(4), 634–638. http://dx.doi.org/10.1089/neu.2011.1932

Mondello, S., Jeromin, A., Buki, A., Bullock, R., Czeiter, E., Kovacs, N., et al. (2011). Glial neuronal ratio (GNR): A novel index for differentiating injury type in patients with severe traumatic brain injury. *Journal of Neurotrauma, 29*(6), 1096–1104. http://dx.doi.org/10.1089/neu.2011.2092

Moran, L. M., Taylor, H. G., Ganesalingam, K., Gastier-Foster, J. M., Frick, J., Bangert, B., et al. (2009). Apolipoprotein E4 as a predictor of outcomes in pediatric mild traumatic brain injury. *Journal of Neurotrauma, 26*(9), 1489–1495. http://dx.doi.org/10.1089/neu.2008.0767

Oh, H., & Seo, W. (2009). Functional and cognitive recovery of patients with traumatic brain injury: Prediction tree model versus general model. *Critical Care Nurse, 29*(4), 12–22. http://dx.doi.org/10.4037/ccn2009279

Papa, L., Ramia, M. M., Kelly, J. M., Burks, S. S., Pawlowicz, A., & Berger, R. P. (2013). Systematic review of clinical research on biomarkers for pediatric traumatic brain injury. *Journal of Neurotrauma, 30*(5), 324–338. http://dx.doi.org/10.1089/neu.2012.2545

Pelinka, L. E., Kroepfl, A., Leixnering, M., Buchinger, W., Raabe, A., & Redl, H. (2004). GFAP versus S100B in serum after traumatic brain injury: Relationship to brain damage and outcome. *Journal of Neurotrauma, 21*(11), 1553–1561. http://dx.doi.org/10.1089/neu.2004.21.1553

Piazza, O., Storti, M., Cotena, S., Stoppa, F., Perrotta, D., Esposito, G., et al. (2007). S100B is not a reliable prognostic index in paediatric TBI. *Pediatric Neurosurgery, 43*(4), 258–264. http://dx.doi.org/10.1159/000103304

Pineda, J. A., Leonard, J. R., Mazotas, I. G., Noetzel, M., Limbrick, D. D., Keller, M. S., et al. (2013). Effect of implementation of a paediatric neurocritical care programme on outcomes after severe traumatic brain injury: A retrospective cohort study. *The Lancet Neurology, 12*(1), 45–52. http://dx.doi.org/10.1016/S1474-4422(12)70269-7

Quinn, T., Smith, C., Murray, L., Stewart, J., Nicoll, J., & Graham, D. (2004). There is no evidence of an association in children and teenagers between the Apolipoprotein E epsilon4 allele and post traumatic brain swelling. *Neuropathology and Applied Neurobiology, 30*(6), 569–575. http://dx.doi.org/10.1111/j.1365-2990.2004.00581.x

Sandler, S. J., Figaji, A. A., & Adelson, P. D. (2010). Clinical applications of biomarkers in pediatric traumatic brain injury. *Child's Nervous System, 26*(2), 205–213. http://dx.doi.org/10.1007/s00381-009-1009-1

Schneier, A. J., Shields, B. J., Hostetler, S. G., Xiang, H., & Smith, G. A. (2006). Incidence of pediatric traumatic brain injury and associated hospital resource utilization in the United States. *Pediatrics, 118*(2), 483–492. http://dx.doi.org/10.1542/peds.2005-2588

Spinella, P. C., Dominguez, T., Drott, H. R., Huh, J., McCormick, L., Rajendra, A., et al. (2003). S100beta protein-serum levels in healthy children and its association with outcome in pediatric traumatic brain injury. *Critical Care Medicine, 31*(3), 939–945. http://dx.doi.org/10.1097/01.CCM.0000053644.16336.52

Su, E., Bell, M. J., Kochanek, P. M., Wisniewski, S. R., Bayir, H., Clark, R. S., et al. (2012). Increased CSF concentrations of myelin basic protein after TBI in infants and children: Absence of significant effect of therapeutic hypothermia. *Neurocritical Care, 17*(3), 401–407. http://dx.doi.org/10.1007/s12028-012-9767-0

Teasdale, G. M., Murray, G. D., & Nicoll, J. A. (2005). The association between APOE 4, age and outcome after head injury: A prospective cohort study. *Brain, 128*(11), 2556–2561. http://dx.doi.org/10.1093/brain/awh595

Whalen, M. J., Carlos, T. M., Kochanek, P. M., Wisniewski, S. R., Bell, M. J., Clark, R. S., et al. (2000). Interleukin-8 is increased in cerebrospinal fluid of children with severe head injury. *Critical Care Medicine, 28*(4), 929–934. http://dx.doi.org/10.1097/00003246-200004000-00003

CHAPTER 7

The Relationship Between Coping and Psychological Adjustment in Family Caregivers of Individuals With Traumatic Brain Injury

A Systematic Review

Malcolm I. Anderson, Grahame K. Simpson, Maysaa Daher, and Lucinda Matheson

ABSTRACT

A systematic review was conducted to evaluate the association between coping (as measured by the Ways of Coping Questionnaire [WOCQ]) and psychological adjustment in caregivers of individuals with traumatic brain injury (TBI). A search conducted using the CINAHL, Medline, and PsycINFO databases yielded 201 citations between 1974 and 2014. A total of seven articles met the inclusion criteria; namely, the respondents who completed the WOCQ were family caregivers of individuals with TBI (including 66-item, 42-item, or 21-item versions). Reviews were conducted in accordance with the American Academy of Neurology guidelines (2011) for classifying evidence. The results found no Class 1 or Class II studies but only four Class III and three Class IV studies. The major finding across the better-rated Class III studies was that the use of

http://dx.doi.org/10.1891/0739-6686.33.219

emotion-focused coping and problem-focused coping was possibly associated with psychological adjustment in caregivers. The Class IV studies were determined to be inadequate or conflicting in determining the association between coping and psychological adjustment. Future studies need to employ carefully crafted designs, adhere to statistical procedure, apply advanced analytic techniques, and employ explicit models of coping, which will increase the accuracy and generalizability of the findings.

INTRODUCTION

Traumatic brain injury (TBI) is a relatively common cause of hospitalization and long-term disability, with the World Health Organization estimating that approximately 10 million people are affected annually (Hyder, Wunder, Puvanachandra, Gururaj, & Kobusingye, 2007). It is widely reported that TBI creates significant stress, burden, and loss of quality of life for families and the caregiver (Chan, Parmenter, & Stancliffe, 2009). Family caregivers, in the form of spouses, parents, siblings, or other relatives, frequently provide long-term support for the relative with TBI. Further, it is increasingly recognized that family members play a central role in the successful rehabilitation of the individual with TBI, while often being ill prepared to face the long-term demands of the caregiving role (Man, 2002). Family caregivers of people with disability play an important role in contributing to the economy. A report by Access Economics (2010) calculates the value of unpaid or informal care in Australia to be $40 billion per annum. In the United States, the economic value of informal care is estimated to be $450 billion per annum (Feinberg, Rienhard, Houser, & Choula, 2011). Given the central role that family caregivers play in the rehabilitation of people with disability, it is important that research is done to better understand coping and psychological adjustment in this population.

TBI refers to damage caused to the structure and/or functioning of the brain due to an external force (e.g., acceleration/deceleration forces in a car crash). It can result in physical, cognitive, and behavioral impairments, which may be temporary or permanent and can cause partial or total disability (Department of Human Services and Health, 1994). While most survivors make a good physical recovery (Marsh, Kersel, Havill, & Sleigh, 2002; McKinlay, Brooks, Bond, Martinage, & Marshall, 1981), it is the permanent cognitive and behavioral impairments that comprise usually the most disabling aspects of TBI (Lezak, 1988; Marsh et al., 2002; Thomsen, 1984). Characteristic neurobehavioral impairments span domains of cognition (e.g., attention, concentration, memory, executive functions, receptive and expressive aphasia) and personality (e.g., increased impulsivity, mood swings, temper outbursts, self-centeredness, lack of insight, decreased motivation; Anderson, Parmenter, & Mok, 2002; Ownsworth & Clare, 2006; Ponsford, Sloan, & Snow, 2012; Sabaz et al., 2014).

Generally, people with TBI have a relatively preserved life expectancy (Baguley et al., 2012), and given the preponderance of youth who sustain such injuries, there are profound economic, social, and personal costs for decades to come (Access Economics, 2009). Although returning to paid work is a major goal for people following TBI (Hofgren, Esbjörnsson, & Sunnerhagen, 2010), employment rates after brain injury are low with only 18%–41% able to find meaningful work within 1–5 years after the injury (Hofgren et al., 2010; van Velzen, van Bennekom, van Dormolen, Sluiter, & Frings-Dresen, 2011), a figure considerably lower than preinjury rates (Sander et al., 1996).

Problems with interpersonal relationships are all too common following TBI. Relationship breakdown is high when a partner has sustained a brain injury, with some studies reporting separation rates as high as 55%–78% (Godwin, Kreutzer, Arango-Lasprilla, & Lehan, 2011; Gosling & Oddy, 1999; Tate, Lulham, Broe, Strettles, & Pfaff, 1989; Thomsen, 1984; Wood & Yurdakul, 1997). Up to half of the people with TBI report that they rapidly lose friends and become more socially isolated after the injury (Olver et al., 1996; Rowlands, 2000; Tate et al., 1989). People with TBI may also experience a range of differing psychiatric reactions to the injury and changes in their lives. Psychiatric symptoms may include depression, mood disorders, panic disorder, anxiety disorder, and a high risk for suicide, with major depression seen as the most-recorded psychiatric issue after TBI (Chan et al., 2009; Gould, Ponsford, Johnston, & Schönberger, 2011; Simpson & Tate, 2007).

Given this range of problems and needs, family members (mostly parents or spouses) often play a pivotal role as caregivers for people with TBI over the long term. In the light of this, a substantial body of research has been carried out to better understand the impact of TBI on family caregivers. The neurobehavioral impairments associated with TBI can have multiple impacts on individual family members as well as the family system. For example, caregivers report high levels of depression, anxiety, and hostility (Anderson, Simpson, & Morey, 2013; Anderson, Simpson, Mok, Gosling, & Gillett, 2009; Gervasio & Kreutzer, 1997), ineffective family functioning (Anderson et al., 2009; Anderson et al., 2013; Ponsford, Olver, Ponsford, & Nelms, 2003); burden; and increased health-seeking behavior (Ponsford et al., 2003). Family caregivers report excessive demands on their time and having too little leisure time and too many responsibilities, to the point where caring for the relative with TBI becomes overwhelming (Douglas & Spellacy, 2000). Further, caregiver burden and mental health problems can persist for many years after the injury (Thomsen, 1984). Despite the multiplicity of challenges, there is considerable heterogeneity in the outcomes for caregivers.

This has led to the investigation of possible factors, such as coping or social support, that might mediate the relationship between neurobehavioral impairments of the person with TBI and the psychological state of caregivers.

The stress and coping model of Lazarus and Folkman (1984) has considerable utility as a conceptual framework for understanding factors mediating negative outcomes that are associated with family caregiving of people with illness/disability (e.g., Pakenham, Chiu, Bursnall, & Cannon, 2007) and survivors of TBI (Chronister, Chan, Sasson-Gelman, & Yi-Chiu, 2010; Chwalisz, 1996). The stress and coping model emphasizes the role of appraisal and personal resources, such as coping in moderating or mediating stress-related outcomes. Appraisal is an evaluative process that reflects the person's interpretation of the event. According to Lazarus and Folkman (1984), the person conducts a primary appraisal to evaluate what is at stake in the situation and then engages in a secondary appraisal to assess his or her coping resources and alternatives to manage the situation. Coping is defined as "constantly changing cognitive and behavioral efforts to manage specific external and/or internal demands that are appraised as taxing or exceeding the resources of the person" (Lazarus & Folkman, 1984, p. 141). Typically, coping is either problem focused or emotion focused. While problem-focused coping is orientated toward solving challenging problems, emotion-focused coping serves to decrease stressful emotions. This theory posits that appraisal and coping continually influence each other, resulting in a constant reevaluation of what is happening, its significance to the individual, and what can be done to manage the situation (Lazarus & Folkman, 1987).

Since the conceptualization of the stress and coping model (Lazarus & Folkman, 1984) a wide range of scales for measuring coping in caregivers have been derived (Pakenham et al., 2007). In spite of this, the Ways of Coping Scale (WOCQ 66-item; Folkman & Lazarus, 1988a), the original tool derived from the theoretical formulations of Lazarus and Folkman, has become the most widely used measure of coping (Rexrode, Petersen, & O'Toole, 2008). The scale comprises eight subscales representing different dimensions of coping. The eight subscales can be further grouped into emotionally focused coping (positive reappraisal, escape avoidance, accepting responsibility, distancing, self-controlling) and problem-focused coping (confrontive coping, planful problem-solving, seeking social support). The psychometric properties of the WOCQ are equal to or better than most other measures of coping processes (Folkman & Lazarus, 1988; Rexrode et al., 2008). Over the past two decades, a number of variants of the WOCQ (including full and briefer versions of the measure) have been used in caregiver research. The 21-item short version (Bouchard, Sabourin, Lussier, Richer, & Wright, 1995) is designed to measure coping (seeking social support, positive reappraisal/problem solving, and distance avoidance) in couples. The 42-item WOCQ (Lester, Smart, & Baum, 1994) measures coping flexibility as a strategy when confronting a stressful situation.

Within the field of TBI, research into coping has frequently employed a wide range of definitions and disparate variables without an underlying theoretical framework. Although most studies find that coping is a significant mediating factor between neurobehavioral impairments and psychological distress, the diversity of approaches has created difficulties in developing an integrated theoretically based picture of the specific functions and types of coping mechanisms that assist family members in adjusting to the caregiving role after TBI. As a step toward developing a more coherent understanding of coping, and given the theoretical and psychometric strengths of the WOCQ, the aim of the current review was to synthesize the findings of research that employed the WOCQ in studying coping among caregivers supporting relatives with TBI. The specific objectives were to (a) identify the literature available regarding the association between coping, as measured by the WOCQ, and psychological adjustment in family caregivers of individuals with TBI and (b) undertake a qualitative synthesis of the findings across these studies. Based on the results, potential areas for future research will be identified.

METHOD

The current review employed a systematic search strategy with a qualitative synthesis of the results. The steps included specifying the inclusion/exclusion criteria; developing and implementing the search strategy; data charting; and data extraction, synthesis, and study quality evaluation. A flow diagram as specified in the Preferred Reporting Items for Systematic Reviews and Meta-Analyses (PRISMA) guidelines (Moher, Liberati, Tetzlaff, Altman, & The PRISMA Group, 2010) was employed to document each stage of the study selection process.

Initial Inclusion/Exclusion Criteria

The research question that this review was addressing was "What ways of coping do family caregivers of individuals with TBI employ?" Study selection was based on the following inclusion criteria: (a) peer-reviewed articles published between 1974 and 2014; (b) articles written in English; (c) respondents who were family caregivers of individuals with TBI; and (d) research that implemented the WOCQ, including the 66-item, 42-item, or 21-item versions (all studies that used alternative measurement tools of coping were excluded). Non-peer–reviewed articles, dissertations, conference abstracts, and book chapters were excluded.

Developing and Implementing the Search Strategy

Articles were identified through electronic searches using the CINAHL, Medline, and PsycINFO databases. MeSH terms, subject headings, and keywords were generated for the five elements required to execute the search using the PICOS framework for identifying research gaps (Population, Intervention, Comparators, Outcomes, Setting). Selecting the Population of interest involved two steps: first identifying studies regarding caregivers, employing the terms *caregiver, carer, caregiving, family carer/caregiver, spouse,* and *spouse caregiver/carer.* These terms were then qualified to limit to TBI, by using the terms *brain injury* and *head injury.* There were no Intervention studies and all observational studies could be included, so there were no specified Comparators. Outcomes comprised caregiver well-being as mediated by coping. Therefore, the terms *stress, emotional distress, caregiver burden*, and *caregiver adjustment* were crossed with *coping*. The search words employed to identify coping comprised *coping, coping strategies, coping style, coping flexibility, adaptation process, resilience, social support, ways of coping inventory, ways of coping checklist*, and *ways of coping questionnaire.* No limitations were placed on Setting. Some overlapping terms were required because of the different terminology employed across the databases.

Data Charting

Four fields were identified and standardized information collected: (a) The type of study comprising descriptive characteristics and including the country where the study was conducted, the study design (cross-sectional, longitudinal), sample size, relationship of caregivers to the relative with TBI, sex of the participants, severity of the TBI, and time since injury that the study was conducted; (b) the use of the Ways of Coping measure including the version of the scale, the variables generated from the scale, and whether the variables were employed as predictors or outcome measures; (c) identification of theories underpinning the analyses; and (d) utilization of study-specific data on the psychometric properties of the WOCQ and the administration of the measure.

Data Extraction, Synthesis, and Quality Evaluation

Data extraction and synthesis was conducted by a consensus process, conducted at a meeting of the investigators (MA, GS, MD). At the meeting, each selected study was reviewed and information relevant to the four data fields extracted and entered onto a template. Data synthesis involved aggregating the results from each study. Prior to the meeting, the investigators had undertaken a rating of the selected studies using the quality criteria explained in the following text. The final component of the meeting involved reviewing the individual ratings, and in cases of different classifications, undertaking further discussion to reach a consensus rating.

For the quality evaluation, each article was reviewed independently by both teams (MA and GS/MD) using criteria (see Table 7.1) based on a modified version of the American Academy of Neurology (AAN) Guidelines (2011) for classifying the evidence for prognostic studies, which was redeveloped as part of a systematic review on the predictors of emotional distress in caregivers of individuals with TBI (Sander, Maestas, Clark, & Havins, 2013). As such, the revised criteria for classifying the evidence takes into account the subjective nature of the constructs of interest such as coping and the associated adjustment outcomes in family caregivers of individuals with TBI, which was suitable for our literature review.

TABLE 7.1
Criteria for Rating the Level of Evidence

Evidence Class	Criteria
Class I	Cohort survey with prospective data collection
	Includes a broad spectrum of persons with injury and caregivers at risk of developing distress and burden
	Inclusion criteria defined
	Current functional status (e.g., DRS, SPRS) of person with brain injury rated by examiner/clinician and used as a predictive factor in the analysis
	At least 80% of enrolled subjects have both risk factors and outcome measures (only relevant for studies with a baseline and follow-up)
	Outcome measurement objective or determined without knowledge of risk factor status (only relevant for studies with subjective rating by examiner or an independent rating of distress by a clinician)
Class II	Cohort study with retrospective data collection or case control study that meets other criteria for Class I
Class III	Cohort study with retrospective data collection or case control study with narrow spectrum (e.g., single-site study) of persons with or without the disease or negative outcome
Class IV	Convenience sample; does not involve a defined cohort (e.g., brain injury association, community support groups)
	Undefined or unaccepted measures of risk factor outcomes
	No measures of association or statistical precision presented or calculated

Note. DRS = Disability Rating Scale; SPRS = Sydney Psychosocial Reintegration Scale.

In consensus with Sander and colleagues (2013), recommended objective medical outcomes (objective presence or absence of diseases) were not part of the assessment criteria, but rather, outcomes based on self-report measures of adjustment were included. While acknowledging the importance of objective risk factors, the revised criteria gives credible weighting to subjective risk factors such as coping, given the importance of these types of factors in the rehabilitation process.

In this field of research, self-report measures are often used as both predictors and outcomes and as such, the need for a "blinded" rater for assessing outcomes is negated (Sander et al., 2013). Therefore, this criterion was not rated unless the study employed an assessment tool that was rated by a clinician. In brain injury rehabilitation, clinicians can employ various self-report measures or clinician-rated tools to rate the functional status of the person with the brain injury and assess family caregiver psychological responses. In our review, studies were not negatively rated if masked outcome assessment was not possible, due to the self-report nature of the variables, provided all the other criteria were met for a particular class of study.

In agreement with the AAN criteria for determining the class of evidence, at least 80% of the participants in a study need to have both risk factors (baseline) and later outcomes (follow-up) measured. Nonetheless, this criterion does not always apply in the context of assessing factors, such as coping and psychological adjustment in brain injury populations, because many studies are cross sectional, and as such, all measures are collected simultaneously (e.g., caregiver self-report of coping and psychological distress; Sander et al., 2013). Consequently, cross-sectional studies in this review were not rated down on the condition that the other criteria for a particular class of evidence were met.

Similar to the approach of Sanders and colleagues (2013) to their review, the quality of statistical analyses was also used as a means for determining the class of evidence. In this field of research, various statistical techniques are used, ranging from descriptive correlations to regression and structural equation modeling (SEM). The studies that employed exploratory or data-driven methods to select predictors, such as selecting variables for inclusion based on bivariate/correlational analyses, were rated a level down.

Once rated, the evidence-based classification was applied for different prognostic variables: Level A: Ways of coping is a highly probable predictor for psychological adjustment, as supported by two or more Class 1 studies; Level B: Ways of coping is a probable predictor for psychological adjustment as supported by at least one Class I study or two or more Class II studies; Level C: Ways of coping is a possible predictor for psychological adjustment, as supported by one Class II study or two or more Class III studies; and Level U: comprises

Class IV studies that are inadequate or conflicting for determining an association between coping and psychological adjustment in caregivers.

RESULTS

The selection of studies is illustrated in the flowchart provided (Figure 7.1), which summarizes each stage of the literature review. The electronic search of the CINAHL, Medline, and PsycINFO databases yielded 201 references. Abstracts were first reviewed by two authors (MA/LM) and the eligibility for inclusion was determined based on identified criteria. After screening, full copies of the remaining articles were retrieved. A search of the bibliographies of these articles and the author's (MA's) own collection found additional articles not identified by the database searches that required checking. The articles were then independently reviewed (MA and LM) and the final selection of articles determined.

Type of Studies

Details of all reviewed articles are available in Table 7.2. Six of the studies were conducted in North America (five in the U.S., one in Canada) and the other in Israel (Katz, Kravetz, & Grynbaum, 2005). All seven studies were observational

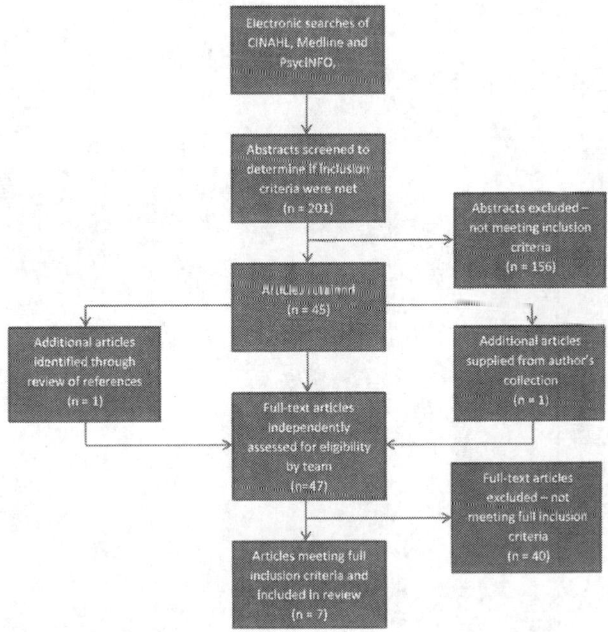

FIGURE 7.1 Literature review flowchart.

TABLE 7.2

Studies Examining Coping Using the Ways of Coping Questionnaire (WOCQ) in Caregivers Supporting Relatives With Traumatic Brain Injury (n = 7)

Study/Year/ Location	Design	Analysis	Sample	Time PI Injury Severity	WOCQ Version	Measures: Predictor (Independent)	Measures: Outcome (Dependent)	Research Findings	Level of Evidence
Davis et al. (2009) To investigate the relation of preinjury medical and psychiatric histories to perceived burden and emotional distress in caregivers of persons with TBI Location: U.S.A.	Prospective cohort	Multiple linear regression models to determine the contributions of medical and psychiatric history, social support, and coping strategies	114 parents/ spouses/ significant others (both English and Spanish speaking). TBI persons at one rehabilitation unit	Follow-up at 1 year Moderate-to-severe injury	WOCQ (66 items) Two subscales: • Escape-avoidance • Positive appraisal Stressor: injury-related situation	Coping as measured by WOCQ (escape-avoidance and positive appraisal subscales of the WOCQ) CGs were administered baseline interview (within 2 weeks of persons with TBI admitted) and within approximately 1 year after injury CG: gender, education, income, medical history, and psychiatric history Social support (MSPSS) Functional status of the individual with TBI, rated by examiner (DRS)	• BSI-GSI • MCAS	• Use of escape-avoidance coping strategy as a predictor of CG distress • Coping strategy escape-avoidance also a predictor of CG burden • Increased use of escape-avoidance associated with elevated CG burden • CGs' medical and psychiatric histories predicted global distress (after accounting for education, sex, income, and relationship) • DRS scores predictor of CG burden (poorer functional status of persons with injury associated with greater sense of burden) • Perceived social support also a predictor of CG burden • Increased perceived social support associated with decreased sense of burden	III

Chwalisz (1996) To develop and test a model of perceived stress and CG burden Location: U.S.A.	Prospective cohort	Structural equation modeling to test hypothesized model	135 spouses • At meetings sponsored by 2 Midwestern head injury associations • By mail, utilizing mailing lists of the same organizations. • In person by professionals working with brain-injured patients	<1 to 30years Severity of injury not identified	WOCQ (66 items) Problem-focused coping, emotion-focused coping, and seeking social support analyzed as indicators of overall coping capacity Stressor: general coping with spouse's injury	Coping (WOCQ) CG: age, gender, previous mental and physical health history Appraisal of patient (primary and secondary) Social support (SPS) Perceived stress (PSS)	• BSI/GSI • DUHP	• Coping and level of social support were associated with the degree of stress reported by the spouses, but did not find a significant association with the four CG characteristics of age, gender, prior mental health history, and appraisal of the degree of change in the partner with TBI • Chi-square and GFI were poor	IV

(*Continued*)

TABLE 7.2

Studies Examining Coping Using the Ways of Coping Questionnaire (WOCQ) in Caregivers Supporting Relatives With Traumatic Brain Injury (n = 7) (Continued)

Study/Year/ Location	Design	Analysis	Sample	Time PI Injury Severity	WOCQ Version	Measures: Predictor (Independent)	Measures: Outcome (Dependent)	Research Findings	Level of Evidence
Katz et al. (2005) To examine the moderating effect of wife's coping flexibility on the relation between time since husband's TBI and wife's perceived burden Location: Israel	Prospective cohort	Two-way ANOVA	40 wives Letters sent to various rehab facilities for persons with TBI inquiring whether attending rehabilitants would consider participating in study	2 groups: ≤7years and >7years Severity of injury not identified	WOCQ (42 items) Coping flexibility (high and low) Stressor: four hypothetical vignettes on stressful social situations	Time since husband's TBI (long and short)	• PBQ • WOCQ	• Significant interaction among time since injury, coping flexibility, and perceived burden of wife. • Wives with low levels of coping flexibility, whose husbands had more than 7-year duration TBI reported more burden than wives whose husbands had TBI since 7 or fewer years; wives with high coping flexibility had no significant difference in perceived burden • Significance between duration of marriage and wife's perceived burden; wives married longer experienced more burden • Significance between husband attending rehab and wife's burden (t test); husbands attending rehab had wives who experienced greater burden	IV

Sander et al. (2007) To compare emotional distress, appraisals of burden, and use of coping strategies between White and Black/Hispanic CGs of persons with TBI Location: U.S.A.	Prospective cohort	Multiple regression models to determine contribution of race/ethnicity/income to CG's distress, burden, and coping (age, education, and relationship adjusted) Chi-square determines demographic differences between racial groups t test determines if racial groups differ in age	195 CGs of persons with TBI. (parents, spouses/significant others) Recruited from patients admitted to one inpatient/outpatient rehabilitation unit	Follow-up at 1–2 years; mild, moderate, and severe injury	WOCQ (66 items) Four subscales: • Escape-avoidance • Accepting responsibility • Distancing • Self-controlling Stressor: injury-related situation	Coping strategies utilized by CG (WOCQ): • Escape-avoidance • Distancing • Accepting responsibility • Self-controlling CG: age, education, relationship to person with TBI, income, race/ethnicity (Black/Hispanic/White) Caregiver ideology subscale (traditional beliefs about the caregiving role; MCAS)	• BSI-Depression • BSI-Anxiety • GSI	• After adjusting for CG's relationship to injured person, age, education, and income, Black and Hispanic CGs made greater use of emotion-focused coping strategies, distancing, and accepting responsibility • Strategy of accepting responsibility was associated with greater emotional distress. no interactions noted • Black/Hispanic CGs reported more traditional CG ideology (interaction between race/ethnicity and traditional CG ideology); in Blacks/Hispanics, more traditional ideology was associated with greater distress, but the same did not apply to Whites	III

(*Continued*)

TABLE 7.2

Studies Examining Coping Using the Ways of Coping Questionnaire (WOCQ) in Caregivers Supporting Relatives With Traumatic Brain Injury (n = 7) (Continued)

Study/Year/ Location	Design	Analysis	Sample	Time PI Injury Severity	WOCQ Version	Measures: Predictor (Independent)	Measures: Outcome (Dependent)	Research Findings	Level of Evidence
Sander et al. (1997) To investigate the contribution of coping strategies, subjective burden, and social support to psychological health of CGs Location: U.S.A.	Prospective cohort	Multiple regression analyses to investigate relationship between CG's psychological health (GHQ) and predictor variables ANOVA (effect of time since injury to coping style, burden, social support, and psychological distress)	69 family members (parents, spouses/ significant others) Recruited from patients admitted to one inpatient/ outpatient rehab unit	Severe injury Acute: 0–6 months Intermediate: 6 months to 1.5 years Long term >1.5 years	WOCQ (66 items) CG scores from the 66 items were collapsed into mean scores for: • Problem-focused coping • Emotion-focused coping Stressor: injury-related situation	Coping strategies utilized by CG (emotion- focused and problem-focused scales of WOCQ) Time since injury Gender of CG Subjective burden measure, requesting family members to rate the amount of stress experienced Satisfaction with amount of social support (subscale of the SSQ) Patient's functional status (DRS)	• GHQ	• Confrontive coping strategies comprise approximately half of the problem-focused WOCQ items • No effect of time since injury on CG's coping style (trend noted for emotion-focused coping used more in acute period and relatively less in longer postinjury period) • CG's use of emotion-focused coping significantly predicted psychological health (the greater the use of emotion-focused coping, the greater was the psychological distress evident) • Problem-focused coping not significantly related to CG's psychological health • Burden and coping exert independent effects on psychological health	III

								• Best model to predict CG's emotional distress; included gender of CG, level of patient functioning, emotion-focused coping, subjective burden, satisfaction with social support, time since injury, coping × burden interaction (accounted for over half of the variance in psychological health) • Minimal relationship between patient's physical and cognitive deficit and CG adjustment	
Tarter (1990) Elucidating the factors associated with good and poor adjustment in the parents of adult head trauma victims Location: U.S.A.	Prospective cohort	Correlations computed between Hassles Scale of daily stress and three other measures Comparisons based on median split of sample according to Hassles Scale	48 parents of patients recruited from comprehensive rehab inpatient programs of three organizations, independent living programs, and the local chapter of a national head injury foundation	CHI at least 1 year prior to study Severity of injury not identified	WOCQ (66 items) Each item measured Stressor: standard administration (stressful event occurring over past week)	• WOCQ to determine whether coping style was associated with the severity of experienced stress • SIP to measure psychosocial and physical dysfunction of offspring	• SLC-90 • Hassles Scale	• Coping style involving avoidance/escape, self-control, and confrontation also related to magnitude of experienced stress • Coping strategy of accepting responsibility also related to high stress, indicating that high experienced stress related to ambivalence of situation • Behavioral impairment, not the physical disability of offspring, related to magnitude of parental stress	IV

(Continued)

TABLE 7.2

Studies Examining Coping Using the Ways of Coping Questionnaire (WOCQ) in Caregivers Supporting Relatives With Traumatic Brain Injury (n = 7) (Continued)

Study/Year/ Location	Design	Analysis	Sample	Time PI Injury Severity	WOCQ Version	Measures: Predictor (Independent)	Measures: Outcome (Dependent)	Research Findings	Level of Evidence
								• Impaired social interaction, reduced alertness, and emotional lability were correlated with parent stress, whereas ambulation, mobility, body care, eating, sleep, and communication disturbance were not associated • Psychiatric maladjustment in parents associated with increased experienced stress; virtually all major domains of psychiatric disorder correlated significantly with experienced stress • Underscores the complex dynamic and reciprocal relationship between parent and offspring with characteristics of one affecting reactions of the other	

Blais and Boisvert (2007) To verify the relationships between personal characteristics (coping and problem-solving strategies and perception of communication skills) of individuals with TBI and their spouses and their level of psychological and marital adjustment Location: Canada	Prospective cohort	Canonical correlations	70 couples where one partner had TBI; 70 control couples from general population where neither partner had TBI	Average = 3.11 years after injury Mild, moderate, and severe injury	WOCQ Short version (21 items) Stressor: stressful situations within couple's relationship over last 3 months	• Positive reappraisal/ problem-solving scale (WOCQ) • Social support seeking scale (WOCQ) • Distancing/ avoidance scale (WOCQ) • ICSI • SPSI-R • IRPS • SAC model	• MAT • KMMS • HADS- A • HADS-D • GWB	• CG spouses favored avoidance-coping strategies more than their matched group of wives • CG spouses who frequently used positive reappraisal/ problem-solving strategies adopted an effective attitude toward problems, had a positive perception of their communication skills and those of the injured partners, and when combined with infrequent use of avoidance strategies, were more likely to report lower levels of psychological distress and higher levels of well-being and marital satisfaction	III

Note. ANOVA = analysis of variance; BSI = Brief Symptom Inventory; CG = Caregiver; DAS = Dyadic Adjustment Scale; DRS = Disability Rating Scale; DUHP = Duke-UNC Health Profile; GFI = Goodness of Fit Index; GHQ = General Health Questionnaire; GSI = Global Severity Index; GWB = General Well-Being Scale; HADS = Hospital Anxiety and Depression Scale; HADS-A = Hospital Anxiety and Depression Scale-Anxiety; HADS-D = Hospital Anxiety and Depression Scale-Depression; ICSI = Interpersonal Communication Skills Inventory; IRPS = Inventory Revised Problem-Solving Scale; KMSS = Kansas Marital Satisfaction Scale; MAT = Marital Adjustment Test; MCAS = Modified Caregiver Appraisal Scale; MSPSS = Multidimensional Scale of Perceived Social Support; PBQ = Perceived Burden Questionnaire; PSS = Perceived Stress Scale; SCL-90 = Symptom Check List-90 questionnaire; SIP = Sickness Impact Profile; SPS = Social Provisions Scale; SPSI-R = Social Problem-Solving Inventory – Revised Scale; SSQ = Social Support Questionnaire; TBI = Traumatic Brain Injury; WOCQ = Ways of Coping Questionnaire.

and six employed a cross-sectional design, while the remaining study researchers (Davis et al., 2009) employed a longitudinal approach to their investigation. The sample sizes ranged from 40 to 195 family caregivers. Only three of the seven studies comprised mixed family samples (e.g., spouses, parents, and other relatives) of the individual with TBI, while the remaining focused on a single category of caregiver, namely, parents (Tarter, 1990), spouses (Blais & Boisvert, 2007; Chwalisz, 1996), and wives only (Katz et al., 2005). Participants were predominantly female. Relatives of the caregivers sustained mild, moderate, or severe TBI, albeit most of the injuries reported were in the severe category. Four studies did not report severity information (Blais & Boisvert, 2007; Chwalisz, 1996; Katz et al., 2005; Tarter, 1990). Time since injury ranged from a few months to over 30 years, with the majority of these families in the chronic phase of recovery.

Role of WOCQ

Six of the seven studies in this review employed coping as a predictor of psychological adjustment in family caregivers, with only one study employing coping as an outcome variable (Katz et al., 2005). Comparison of the studies was made more difficult due to the various versions of the WOCQ that were selected by the investigators. Furthermore, investigators then often made heterogeneous selections of specific subscales as variables in their research, rather than administer the whole scale.

Three studies employed subscales to measure both emotion-focused coping and problem-focused coping (Blais & Boisvert, 2007; Sander et al., 1997; Tarter, 1990). Sander and colleagues (1997) surveyed 69 primary caregivers with the 66-item WOCQ. They collapsed the participant's scores into a mean problem-focused score and a mean emotion-focused score. Tarter (1990) was the only researcher in this review who measured all eight dimensions of the 66-item WOCQ to assess coping as a predictor of adjustment in parents of adult children with TBI. In more recent research, Blais and Boisvert (2009) employed the 21-item version of the WOCQ, arguing that this is the most stable version for assessing couples. To this end, the three dimensions of this version of the scale were measured, namely, seeking social support, positive reappraisal/problem solving (problem-focused coping), and distance/avoidance (emotion-focused coping).

In contrast, two studies selected only subscales of emotion-focused coping from the 66-item WOCQ (escape-avoidance and positive appraisal in Davis et al., 2009; escape-avoidance, accepting responsibility, distancing, and self-controlling in Sander et al., 2007). These researchers argued that certain dimensions of emotion-focused coping had been found to predict emotional adjustment in caregivers and therefore warranted further investigation in the context of their studies.

Two studies measured coping as a single construct (Chwalisz, 1996; Katz et al., 2005). Chwalisz (1996) employed the 66-item WOCQ to measure coping as a major predictor (and mediating variable) within a theoretical model based on the integration of the stress appraisal–coping theory (Lazarus & Folkman, 1987) and previous empirical literature on caregiver burden. To this end, SEM was employed to test the model. Nonetheless, given the large number of variables relative to the sample size in the study, coping and other constructs in the model were measured as single composite variables rather than latent variables with multiple indicators. Katz and colleagues (2005) used a 42-item WOCQ to examine coping flexibility in wives of husbands with TBI.

The domains of adjustment that were measured across the six studies included anxiety, depression, general well-being, mental and physical health, marital satisfaction, perceived stress/burden, caregiver distress, and social support. In contrast, the remaining study (Katz et al., 2005) used coping as an outcome variable to examine coping flexibility in wives when confronting a stressful situation.

Theoretical Frameworks Underpinning the Analyses

To better understand the complex interaction that occurs between coping and psychological adjustment in caregivers, we investigated the predictive variables employed by the studies and whether they were derived from theoretical and/or empirical literature. Sander and colleagues (1997) and Chwalisz (1996) based their studies on clearly defined models of stress, coping, and adjustment. As mentioned previously, Chwalisz (1996) constructed her own model titled the "Perceived Stress Model of Caregiver Burden" to test the association between caregiver characteristics (stress appraisal, coping, social support) and psychological and physical health, which to our knowledge was the first study to employ a model of this kind in the brain injury literature. Shortly thereafter, Sander and colleagues (1997) also employed a theoretical model of coping (originally proposed by Graffi & Mines, 1989) to test the association among caregiver subjective burden, coping style, and social support and the outcome variable psychological health in caregivers.

The remaining five studies in this review did not engage explicit models of coping to operationalize their variables, but rather relied upon caregiver characteristics derived from the empirical literature and their contribution to psychological adjustment. Sander and colleagues (2007) studied the coping strategies, caregiver burden, and psychological distress among White versus Black/Hispanic caregivers of persons with TBI, given the paucity of research involving minority groups. In a follow-up study, Davis and colleagues (2009) employed the same data set to examine the contributions of pre-injury medical and psychiatric histories of caregivers to psychological distress. In the study by Davis and colleagues, the influence of these variables was determined after accounting for the functional status of the person with TBI, coping, and social support, which were factors known to be related to caregiver distress and burden.

Tarter (1990) investigated the association among coping, stress, and mental health in 48 parents of relatives with TBI, except that the relationship between coping and psychological distress was not assessed. Katz and colleagues (2005) examined the moderating effect of wives' coping flexibility on the relation between time since spouses' injury and wives' perceived burden. In contrast to the other studies in our review, Blais and Boisvert (2007) surveyed both partners (partner with TBI, noninjured spouse) rather than focusing solely on the caregiver of the person with TBI, something that had not been done before. Moreover, a control group was employed when examining the association between personal characteristics of the partners (coping, social problem solving, communication skills) and psychological distress and marital satisfaction.

Psychometrics and Administration of the WOCQ

Only three studies (Chwalisz, 1996; Davis et al., 2009; Katz et al., 2005) reported the internal consistencies for the scales based on data from their studies. The Cronbach alpha coefficients for the WOCQ were Escape-Avoidance Scale α = .71 and Positive Appraisal Scale α = .83 (Davis et al., 2009); Coping Flexibility α = 0.83 (Katz et al., 2005); and Coping α = .93 and primary and secondary appraisal in the context of measuring perceived stress and coping α = .50 in Chwalisz (1996). No other psychometric dimensions of the WOCQ were reported.

Standard administration of the WOCQ requires respondents to reflect on a stressful situation that occurred within the previous week and then complete the WOCQ items with reference to that situation. Only one study (Tarter, 1990) used this standard format, with the remaining studies varying the administration. Blais and Boisvert (2007) asked respondents to complete the questionnaire in relation to stressful situations within their couple relationships over the last 3 months. Katz and colleagues (2005) introduced four hypothetical vignettes (Lester, Smart, & Baum, 1994) to describe different stressful social events (ranging from arguing with a friend to something less stressful such as being caught in a traffic jam), which the caregivers were to consider when reporting their level of coping flexibility. The remaining studies (Chwalisz, 1996; Davis et al., 2009; Sander et al., 1997; Sander et al., 2007) focused on strategies used in stressful situations related directly to the injury. To confound matters further, among the studies that did adopt an injury-related approach, none included a time frame (e.g., past 7 days) as a parameter for measuring the caregiver's coping responses.

Quality Evaluation

Four of the studies selected for the review were rated as Class III (Blais & Boisvert 2007; Davis et al., 2009; Sander et al., 1997; Sander et al., 2007) and the remaining three as Class IV (Chwalisz, 1996; Katz et al., 2005; Tarter, 1990). The major finding across the studies rated better was that the use of emotion-focused coping strategies was found to be associated with psychological adjustment in three Class III studies. Problem-focused coping was also found to be associated with emotional adjustment in the remaining Class III investigation (Blais & Boisvert, 2007). The Class III studies were classified as Level C evidence, meaning that coping was a *possible* predictor of psychological adjustment in caregivers. The Class IV studies were classified as Level U evidence—data inadequate or conflicting for determining an association between coping and psychological adjustment in caregivers.

The contribution of coping to psychological distress in caregivers in the context of the four Class III studies is discussed in the following text. Sander and colleagues (1997) found that emotion-focused coping was significantly associated with psychological distress in caregivers as measured by the General Health Questionnaire (GHQ). In their study, the best model for predicting the caregiver's emotional distress included the gender of the caregiver, level of patient functioning, emotion-focused coping, subjective burden, satisfaction with social support, time since injury, and the interaction between coping and burden (multivariate regression). These factors accounted for 58% of the variance in the GHQ scores, but the individual weights for each of the predictor variables were not reported.

In the second Class III study, a more complete understanding of the contribution of coping strategies employed by caregivers and the subsequent psychological reactions was reported. At 1 year after injury, Davis and colleagues (2009) showed that higher levels of emotion-focused coping (escape-avoidance) were associated with increased caregiver burden and caregiver distress. Two multivariate regression models were employed to determine the association of medical and psychiatric history, social support, and coping strategies with psychological distress and perceived burden after controlling for the functional status (Disability Rating Scale) of the person with TBI, the caregiver's gender and education, and the relationship with the person with injury. In the model that examined the predictors of caregiver distress, escape-avoidance explained 16% of the variance in caregiver distress, a variation that was much higher than the remaining predictors (medical illness 7% and psychiatric illness 3.7%) of psychological distress in caregivers. Escape-avoidance and perceived social support explained 5% of the variance in caregiver burden. In contrast, functional status explained 15% of the variability in perceived burden in caregivers. Overall, the models accounted for 30% and 39% of the variance in caregiver distress and caregiver-perceived burden, respectively.

The relationship between positive emotion-focused coping and psychological adjustment in caregivers was supported by one Class III study (Blais & Boisvert, 2007). Employing the 21-item WOCQ (seeking social support, positive reappraisal–problem solving and distance/avoidance), the investigators interviewed both the caregiver and the partner with TBI as well as controls from the general population. Using canonical correlations, they found that spouse caregivers who frequently used positive reappraisal/problem-solving strategies adopted an effective attitude toward problems, had a positive perception of their communication skills and those of the injured partner, and when combined with the infrequent use of avoidance strategies, were more likely to report lower levels of psychological distress (anxiety and depression) and higher levels of well-being and marital satisfaction.

The final study rated as Class III (Sander et al., 2007) differed from the previous three in the use of the WOCQ emotional focus subscales as outcome variables. After taking into account the relationship with the person with brain injury, age, education, and income, race/ethnicity made an additional contribution, indicating that people from Black/Hispanic backgrounds were more likely to use the coping strategies of distancing (6% of the variance) and accepting responsibility (3% of the variance), in contrast to White people. The coping variable, accepting responsibility, was associated with emotional distress in caregivers, but the variance was not reported.

With reference to the three Class IV studies, each attempted to make unique contributions to understanding the relationship between coping and psychological adjustment in caregivers, but were found to have major methodological issues and hence received a Level U rating. In the first study, the conceptual model developed by Chwalisz (1996) was tested using SEM. This was an ambitious undertaking at the time of the study, but the procedure was not properly adhered to when testing the model. The model fit indices (chi-square and goodness of fit index [GFI]) were poor, which means the hypothesized model was not tenable and throws into doubt the validity of the findings. In order for a better understanding of the acceptability of the model, further exploration and the use of multiple measures of fit were warranted. In the second Class IV study, Tarter (1990) measured the 8 dimensions of the 66-item WOCQ, but the sample was small ($N = 48$), the inclusion criteria were not clearly defined, the internal consistency of the scales was not reported, the findings were based on simple correlations, and more important, the relationship between coping and psychological distress was not assessed. Similar methodological issues were noted in the study by Katz and colleagues (2005).

DISCUSSION

This chapter aimed to assess the literature on the association between coping as measured by WOCQ and psychological adjustment in family caregivers of individuals with TBI. There were no Class I or Class II studies identified in this review, which clearly indicates that the research into caregiver coping in the brain injury and disability field requires studies of higher quality. The studies in this review were rated as Class III or Class IV investigations because of the lack of conceptual and methodological rigor. Similar ratings were reported in a previous systematic review that examined the relationship between caregiver characteristics and psychological distress (Sander et al., 2013), which increases the validity of our findings.

A commonly identified limitation of the studies was the limited reporting of inclusion criteria to determine whether those involved in the study were representative of the population. For instance in this review, the term *spouse* was not clearly defined in one study (Chwalisz, 1996). There was a lack of clarity as to whether spouses were living together as a legally married couple, cohabiting as partners, or even living separately at the time of the interviews. Moreover, severity of injury and premorbid psychiatric or medical history were not consistently identified across the studies. Future studies using cross-sectional designs should be more precise in reporting on the demographic variables of the participants.

With respect to the theoretical aspects of coping, only two papers employed explicit theoretical models, which is a credit to the researchers, given the paucity of theoretically driven research in the rehabilitation field. The remaining studies relied upon a compilation of the empirical literature to develop research questions/hypotheses when examining the association between coping and psychological adjustment in caregivers, resulting in an assorted approach to measuring coping among caregivers, unfortunately making this area of research even more complex and difficult to interpret. For instance, one study focused specifically on emotion-focused coping, whereas others examined both emotion-focused coping and problem-focused strategies. Still others made heterogeneous selections of subscales rather than measuring the whole scale. To overcome this issue, future research must be driven by well-designed conceptual models of stress and coping.

The internal consistency of the WOCQ scales/subscales was generally robust in the three studies that reported this analysis (Chwalisz, 1996; Davies et al., 2009, Sander et al., 2007), with the coefficients (Cronbach's alpha) generally above .80, meeting an A rating for the reliability criterion in Andresen's 11 criteria for outcome measures in rehabilitation (Andresen, 2000). Studies in the review employed various statistical analyses to describe the contribution of coping and other predictive variables to psychological adjustment, which ranged from descriptive correlations and multiple regression to more sophisticated canonical analyses and SEM. One Class IV study relied upon simple correlations between variables, which is considered weak evidence and should be avoided in future research. The Class III studies utilized more sophisticated approaches, but the contribution of coping and other predictive variables was not always clearly delineated, and the internal consistency of the scales was not reported in three studies, which suggests that the interpretation of the findings should be done with caution. A further Class IV study (Chwalisz, 1996) employed SEM, but the hypothesized model was not a parsimonious representation of the sample, as indicated by the poor goodness of fit indices. Future research needs to place greater emphasis on statistical procedures when analyzing and reporting findings, which in turn will increase the accuracy and generalizability to other samples.

In relation to the clinical interpretation of the results, two Class III studies just echoed the terminology of the WOCQ without further extrapolation to the clinical context scale (Davis et al., 2009; Sander et al., 2007). In the studies that did provide further discussion, the main focus centered on the relative contributions of emotion-focused versus problem-focused coping on relative outcomes. Sander and colleagues (1997, Class III study) found that problem-focused strategies were not associated with psychological health. In trying to account for this, the authors observed that confrontive coping strategies comprised almost half of the items on the problem-focused coping and included items such as expressing anger at the person or trying to get the person to change his or her mind. They suggested that these strategies may not be particularly effective among people with impairment of executive functions who may lack the cognitive flexibility to easily change their mind or might react to anger from the caregiver by an escalation in their own anger due to an increased emotional lability.

Two studies took an alternative view about the role and value of problem-focused coping. Chwalisz and colleagues (1996, Class IV study) saw that the low association between problem-focused strategies and distress might indicate that such strategies played a constructive role, with the use of such strategies resulting in families having a greater sense of control in the caregiving situation. Further to this, Blais and Boisvert (2007, Class III study) found that the one strategy wives of partners with TBI used more frequently than the control group of wives was escape-avoidance. Escape-avoidance is classed as an emotionally focused coping strategy. Blais and Boisvert suggest that in the context of a partner with TBI who could display chronic unpredictable and impulsive reactions and behaviors (e.g., anger outbursts, mood swings), the traditional view would be to suggest that the wives gradually develop a learned helplessness in the caregiving situation, which then leads to coping by trying to avoid the problem (i.e., running away).

However, they propose an alternative view. The authors suggest that escape-avoidance could be reframed as a problem-focused positive coping strategy in the context of TBI. In clinical observation, escape-avoidance is associated with a range of caregiver behaviors (withdrawing until the storm has passed, rather than immediately responding or reacting in a conflict situation) that may in fact be a positive adaptation to the challenges of caregiving for a person with TBI. Finally, Katz and colleagues (2005, Class IV study) generated a single measure of coping flexibility from the WOCQ. They suggested that wives with high scores for flexibility may employ a gamut of strategies that could serve two different functions, namely, preventing the buildup of negative events arising from the brain injury (externally focused) or alternatively diffusing the stress associated with those negative events (internally focused).

FUTURE DIRECTIONS AND LIMITATIONS

In this review, the contribution of coping and other related factors showed the need for further research to better understand the nature of coping and associated psychological adjustment in caregivers of individuals with TBI. There are several reasons for this. First, from a clinical perspective, the results showed that problem-focused coping was not significantly associated with psychological distress in caregivers in the majority of the studies, either because problem-focused coping may have played a constructive role when caregivers were managing stressful brain injury–related situations or because emotion-focused strategies may actually work in the context of TBI populations, which is an outcome that needs further clarification. Second, the constructs being examined should be guided by conceptual models of coping, and third, SEM should be employed, which is an ideal approach for testing the direct and indirect effects of variables within an a priori model (Ho, 2006). Finally, and more important, the findings from this review suggested there are other factors yet to be explored that may be important when assessing the association between coping and psychological adjustment in caregivers.

To this end, researchers in brain injury may need to look further afield to determine the constructs that may be worthy of further exploration. Currently, there is a paradigm shift underway in the field of rehabilitation, with a new emphasis on investigating positive adaptation rather than psychological vulnerability among family caregivers. This includes a need to focus on caregiver resilience (Simpson & Jones, 2012) and other related constructs including personality, coping, self-efficacy, hope, and social support and their association with psychological adjustment among family members of people with TBI. Constructing a conceptual model to test the relationship among these variables may serve as a potential innovative framework for understanding caregiver outcomes following TBI.

Findings should be interpreted taking into consideration the limitations of the review. These include the search strategy adopted, which did not include gray literature such as theses or dissertations and textbooks; therefore, publication bias could be an issue. Only articles published in English were included, which may be culturally limiting. Further, we restricted this review to coping in caregivers based on the WOCQ; albeit the instrument has sound psychometric properties, the generalizability of our findings should be considered with caution. We also concur with Sander and colleagues (2013) that employing an adapted version of the AAN criteria for rating evidence has limitations in the context of evaluating studies that are mostly cross sectional, which are not as strong as a true prognostic study. Future research should be conducted by adopting prognostic models to predict caregiver coping and psychological adjustment.

CONCLUSION

This systematic review suggested that research into family caregiver coping in the brain injury and disability field requires studies of higher quality, given the lack of conceptual and methodological rigor. Emotion-focused coping and problem-focused coping were found to be possibly associated with emotional adjustment in caregivers. To strengthen the existing evidence base, studies need to employ carefully crafted designs, adhere to statistical procedure, apply advanced analytic techniques, and employ explicit models of coping, which will increase the accuracy and generalizability of the findings. Moreover, future work should consider the mediating effect of other variables such as resilience when assessing the relationship between coping and psychological adjustment in caregivers.

REFERENCES

Access Economics. (2009). *The economic cost of spinal cord injury and traumatic brain injury in Australia*. Report by Access Economics Pty Limited for the Victorian Neurotrauma Initiative.

Access Economics. (2010). *The economic value of informal care in 2010*. Report by Access Economics Pty Limited for Carers Australia.

American Academy of Neurology. (2011). *Clinical practice process manual*. St.Paul, MN: Author.

Anderson, M. I., Parmenter, T. R., & Mok, M. (2002). The relationship between neurobehavioural problems of severeve traumatic brain injury (TB), family functioning and psychological well-being of the spouse/caregiver: Path model analysis. *Brain Injury*, *16*(9), 743–757.

Anderson, M. I., Simpson, G. K., & Morey, P. J. (2013). The impact of neurobehavioural impairment of family functioning and the psychological well-being of male versus female caregivers of relatives with severe traumatic brain injury: Multigroup analysis. *Journal of Head Trauma Rehabilitation*, *28*(6), 453–463.

Anderson, M. I., Simpson, G. K., Morey, P. J., Mok, M. C., Gosling, T. J., & Gillett, L. E. (2009). Differential pathways of psychological distress in spouses vs. parents of people with severe traumatic brain injury (TBI): Multi-group analysis. *Brain Injury*, *23*(12), 931–943.

Andresen, E. M. (2000). Criteria for assessing tools of disability outcomes research. *Archives of Physical Medicine and Rehabilitation, 81*(Suppl 2), S15–S20.

Baguley, I., Nott, M. T., Howle, A. A., Simpson, G. K., Browne S., King, A. K., et al. (2012). Late mortality after severe traumatic brain injury in New South Wales: A multicentre study. *Medical Journal of Australia, 196*(1), 40–45.

Blais, M. C., & Boisvert, J.-M. (2007). Psychological adjustment and marital satisfaction following head injury. Which critical personal characteristics should both partners develop. *Brain Injury*, *21*(4), 357–372

Bouchard, G., Sabourin, S., Lussier, Y., Richer, C., & Wright, J. (1995). Nature des stratégies d'adatation au sein des relations conjugales: Prentation d'une version abrégée du Ways of Coping Questionnaire. *Revue Canadienne des Sciences du Comportement*, *27*, 371–377.

Chan, J., Parmenter, T. R., & Stancliffe, R. (2009). The impact of traumatic brain injury on the mental health outcomes of individuals and their family carers. *Australian e-Journal for the Advancement of Mental Health*, *8*(2), 1–10. Retrieved from www.auseinet.com/journal/vol8iss2/chan.pdf

Chronister, J., Chan, F., Sasson Gelman, F. J., & Chiu, C. Y. (2010). The association of stress-coping variables to quality of life among caregivers of individuals with traumatic brain injury. *Neurorehabilitation, 27*(1), 49–62.

Chwalisz, K. (1996). The perceived stress model of caregiver burden: Evidence from spouses of persons with brain injuries. *Rehabilitation Psychology, 41*(2), 91–111.

Davis, L. C., Sander, A. M., Struchen, M. A., Sherer, M., Nakase-Richardson, R., & Malec, J. F. (2009). Medical and psychosocial predictors of caregiver distress and perceived burden following traumatic brain injury. *Journal of Head Trauma Rehabilitation, 24*(3), 145–154. http://dx.doi.org/10.1097/HTR.0b013e3181a0b291

Department of Human Services and Health. (1994). *National policy on services for people with acquired brain injury*. Canberra: Department of Human services and Health.

Douglas, J. M., & Spellacy, F. J. (2000). Correlates of depression in adults w?ith severe traumatic brain injury and their carers. *Brain Injury, 14*(1), 71–88.

Feinberg, L., Rienhard, S. C., Houser, A., & Choula, R. (2011). *Valuing the invaluable: 2011 Update-The Growing Contributions and Costs of Family Caregiving, AARP Public Policy Institute*. Retrieved September 01, 2014 www.aarp.org/relationships/caregivers/info-07-2011/valuing-the-invaluable.html

Folkman, S., & Lazarus, R. S. (1988). The relationship between coping and emotion: Implications for theory and research. *Social Science Medicine, 26*(3), 309–317.

Folkman, S., & Lazarus, R. S. (1988a). Manual for the ways of coping questionnaire. Palo Alto, CA: Consulting Psychologists Press Inc.

Gervasio, A. H., & Kreutzer, J. S. (1997). Kinship and family members' psychological distress after traumatic brain injury: A large sample study. *Journal of Head Trauma Rehabilitation, 12*(3), 14–26.

Godwin, E. E., Kreutzer, J. S., Arango-Lasprilla, J. C., & Lehan, T. J. (2011). Marriage after brain injury: Review, analysis, and research recommendations. *The Journal of head trauma rehabilitation, 26*(1), 43–55.

Gosling, J., & Oddy, M. (1999). Rearranged marriages: Marital relationships after head injury. *Brain Injury, 13*(10), 785–796.

Gould, K. R., Ponsford, J. L., Johnston, L., & Schönberger, M. (2011). The nature, frequency and course of psychiatric disorders in the first year after traumatic brain injury: A prospective study. *Psychological medicine, 41*(10), 2099–2109.

Graffi, S., & Mines, P. (1989). Stress and coping in caregivers of persons with traumatic head injuries. *Journal ofd Applied Social Sciences, 13*, 293–316.

Ho, R. (2006). *Handbook of univariate and multivariate data analysis and interpretation with SPSS*. Boca Raton, FL: Chapman & Hall.

Hofgren, C., Esbjörnsson, E., & Sunnerhagen, K. S. (2010). Return to work after acquired brain injury: Facilitators and hindrances observed in a sub-acute rehabilitation setting. *Work, 36*, 431–439.

Hyder, A. A., Wunderlich, C. A., Puvanachandra, P., Gururaj, G., & Kobusingye, O. C. (2007). The impact of traumatic brain injuries: A global perspective. *Neurorehabilitation, 22*(5), 341–353.

Katz, S., Kravetz, S., & Grynbaum, F. (2005). Wives' coping flexibility, time since husbands' injury and the perceived burden of wives of men with traumatic brain injury. *Brain Inury, 19*(1), 59–66.

Lazarus, R. S., & Folkman, S. (1984). Stress, appraisal, and coping. New York, NY: Springer.

Lazarus, R. S., & Folkman, S. (1987). Transactional theory and research on emotions and coping. *European Journal of Personality, 1*(3), 141–169.

Lester, N., Smart, L., & Baum, A. (1994). Measuring coping flexibility. *Psychology and Health, 9*, 409–424.

Lezak, M. D. (1988). Brain damage is a family affair. *Journal of Clinical & Experimental Neuropsychology, 10*(1), 111–123.

Man, D. W. K. (2002). Family caregivers' reactions and coping for persons with brain injury. *Brain Injury, 16*(12), 1025–1037.

Marsh, N. V., Kersel, D. A., Havill, J. A., & Sleigh, J. W. (2002). Caregiver burden during the year following severe traumatic brain injury. *Journal of Clinical and Experimental Neuropsychology, 24*(4),434–447.

McKinlay, W. W., Brooks, D. N., Bond, M. R., Martinage, D. R., & Marshall, M. M. (1981). The short term outcone of severe blunt head injury as reported by relatives of injured persons. *Journal of Neurology, Neurosurgery and Psychiatry, 44*, 527–533.

Moher, D., Liberarty, A., Tetzlaff, J., Altman, D. G., & The PRISMA Group. (2010). Preferred repoting items for systematic and meta analyses: The PRISMA statement. *PLosMed* 6(6), e1000097. http://dx.doi.org/10.1371/journal.pmed1000097

Olver, J. H., Ponsford, J. L., & Curran, C. A. (1996). Outcome following traumatic brain injury: A comparision betweeen 2 and 5 years after injury. *Brain Injury, 10*(11), 842–848.

Ownsworth, T., & Clare, L. (2006). The association between awareness deficits and rehabilitation outcome following acquired brain injury. *Clinical Psychology Review, 26*(6), 783–795.

Pakenham, K. I., Chiu, J., Bursnall, S., & Cannon, T. (2007). Relations between social support appraisal and coping and both poisitive and negative outcomes in young carers. *Journal of Health Psychology, 12*(1), 89–102.

Ponsford, J., Olver, J., Ponsford, M., & Nelms, R. (2003). Long-term adjustment of families following traumatic brain injury where comprehensdive rehabilitation has been provided. *Brain Injury, 17*(6), 453–468.

Ponsford, J., Sloan, S., & Snow, P. (2012). *Traumatic Brain Injury: Rehabilitation for Everyday Adaptive Living* (2nd ed.). Hove, England: Psychology Press Ltd.

Rexrode, K. R., Peterson, S., & O'Toole, S. (2008). The ways of coping scale: A reliability generalisation study. *Educational and Psychological Measurement, 68*(2), 262–280.

Rowlands, A. (2000). Understanding social support and friendship: Implications for intervention after acquired brain injury. *Brain Impairment, 1*(02), 151–164.

Sabaz, M., Simpson, G. K., Walker, A. J., Rogers, J. M., Gillis, I., & Strettles, B. (2014). Prevalence, comorbidities, and correlates of challenging behavior among community-dwelling adults with severe traumatic brain injury: A multicenter study. *Journal of Head Trauma Rehabilitation, 29*(2), E19–E30.

Sander, A. M., Davis, L. C., Struchen, M. A., Atchison, T., Sherer, M., Malec, J. F., et al. (2007). Relationship of race/ethnicity to caregivers' coping, appraisals, and distress after traumatic brain injury. *Neurorehabilitation, 22*(1), 9–17.

Sander, A. M., High, W. M., Jr., Hannay, H. J., & Sherer, M. (1997). Predictors of psychological health in caregivers of patients with closed head injury. *Brain Injury, 11*(4), 235–249.

Sander, A. M., Kreutzer, J. S., Rosenthal, M., Delmonico, R., & Young, M. E. (1996). A multicenter longitudinal investigation of return to work and community integration following traumatic brain injury. *Journal of Head Trauma Rehabilitation, 11*, 70–84.

Sander, A. M., Maestas, K. L., Clark, A. N., & Havins, W. N. (2013). Predictors of emotional distress in family caregivers of persons with traumatic brain injury: A systemnatic review. *Brain Impairment, 14*(1), 113–129. http://dx.doi.org/10.1017/Brimp.2013.12

Simpson, G. K. & Jones, K. (2012). How important is resilience among family members supporting relatives with traumatic brain injury and spinalo cord injury? *Clinical Rehabilitation, 27*(4), 367–377.

Simpson, G., & Tate, R. (2007). Suicidality in people surviving a traumatic brain injury: Prevalence, risk factors and implications for clinical management. *Brain Injury, 21*(1–14), 1335–1351.

Tarter, S. B. (1990). Factors affecting adjustment of parents of head trauma victims. *Archives of Clinical Neuropsychology, 5*(1), 15–22.

Tate, R. L., Lulham, J. M., Broe, G. A., Strettles, B., & Pfaff, A. (1989). Psychosocial outcome for the survivors of severe blunt head injury: The results from a consecutive series of 100 patients. *Journal of Neurology, Neurosurgery and Psychiatry, 52*(10), 1128–1134.

Thomsen, I. V. (1984). Late outcome of very severe blunt head trauma: A 10-15 year follow-up. *Journal of Neurology, Neurosurgery, and Psychiatry, 4*(3), 260–268.

van Velzen, J. M., van Bennekom, C. A., van Dormolen, M., Sluiter, J. K., & Frings- Dresen, M. (2011). Factors influencing return to work experienced by people with acquired brain injury: A qualitative research study. *Disability and Rehabilitation: An International, Multidisciplinary Journal, 33*, 2237–2246.

Wood, R. L. & Yurdakul, L. K. (1997). Change in relationship status following traumatic brain injury. *Brain Injury, 11*(7), 491–502.

CHAPTER 8

Military Personnel With Traumatic Brain Injuries and Insomnia Have Reductions in PTSD and Improved Perceived Health Following Sleep Restoration

A Relationship Moderated by Inflammation

Taura Barr, Whitney Livingston, Pedro Guardado, Tristin Baxter, Vincent Mysliwiec, and Jessica Gill

ABSTRACT

Background: Up to one-third of deployed military personnel sustain a traumatic brain injury (TBI). TBIs and the stress of deployment contribute to the vulnerability for chronic sleep disturbance, resulting in high rates of insomnia diagnoses as well as symptoms of posttraumatic stress disorder (PTSD), depression, and declines in health-related quality of life (HRQOL). Inflammation is associated with insomnia; however, the impact of sleep changes on comorbid symptoms and inflammation in this population is unknown. *Methods:* In this study, we examined the relationship between reported sleep changes and the provision of the standard of care, which could include one or more of

http://dx.doi.org/10.1891/0739-6686.33.249

the following: cognitive behavioral therapy (CBT), medications, and continuous positive airway pressure (CPAP). We compared the following: (a) the group with a decrease in the Pittsburgh Sleep Quality Index (PSQI; restorative sleep) and (b) the group with no change or increase in PSQI (no change). Independent *t* tests and chi-square tests were used to compare the groups on demographic and clinical characteristics, and mixed between–within subjects analysis of variance tests were used to determine the effect of group differences on changes in comorbid symptoms. Linear regression models were used to examine the role of inflammation in changes in symptoms and HRQOL. *Results:* The sample included 70 recently deployed military personnel with TBI, seeking care for sleep disturbances. Thirty-seven participants reported restorative sleep and 33 reported no sleep changes or worse sleep. The two groups did not differ in demographic characteristics or clinical symptoms at baseline. The TBI + restored sleep group had significant reductions in PTSD and depression over the 3-month period, whereas the TBI + no change group had a slight increase in both PTSD and depression. The TBI + restored sleep group also had significant changes in HRQOL, including the following HRQOL subcomponents: physical functioning, role limitations in physical health, social functioning, emotional well-being, energy/fatigue, and general health perceptions. In a linear regression model using a forced entry method, the dependent variable of change in C-reactive protein (CRP) concentrations was significantly related to changes in PTSD symptoms and HRQOL in the TBI + restored sleep group, with $R^2 = 0.43$, $F_{33,3} = 8.31$, $p < .01$. *Conclusions:* Military personnel with TBIs who have a reduction in insomnia symptoms following a standard-of-care treatment report less severe symptoms of depression and PTSD and improved HRQOL, which relate to decreased plasma concentrations of CRP. These findings suggest that treatment for sleep disturbances in this TBI + military population is associated with improvements in health and decreases in inflammation. The contributions of inflammation-induced changes in PTSD and depression in sleep disturbances in TBI + military personnel require further study.

INTRODUCTION

Traumatic brain injuries (TBIs) are the hallmark injuries of Operation Enduring Freedom (OEF) and Operation Iraqi Freedom (OIF; Fisher 2010; Owens et al., 2008) and are linked to the onset of insomnia in one-third of the TBI + military personnel, as well as chronic neurological and psychological symptoms, including posttraumatic stress disorder (PTSD) and depression (Capaldi, Guerrero,

& Killgore, 2011; Insomnia, active component, U.S. Armed Forces, January 2000-December 2009., 2010; Seelig et al., 2010; Tsai, 2010). TBIs include injuries that result both from blunt forces and from blasts, which can result in neurological alterations/loss of consciousness or disruptions in memory (DePalma, Burris, Champion, & Hodgson, 2005; Warden et al., 2009). TBIs result in neuronal functional abnormalities that likely contribute to susceptibility to insomnia and comorbid disorders including PTSD and depression (Kou & Vandevord, 2014). However, few studies have examined the biological links that contribute to high rates of comorbidity as well as health declines in this population. In deployed military personnel, TBIs are linked to the onset of chronic disease and extensive use of medical services (Pugh et al., 2014), suggesting that chronic TBIs have long-lasting effects on health and well-being. Therefore, TBIs are common in military personnel, yet the mechanisms that underlie the risks for insomnia and comorbid symptoms and impairments are not well established.

Sleep disturbance is common during deployment due to alterations in sleep–wake schedules as well as the intensive psychological and physical conditions associated with deployment, all of which contribute to high rates of insomnia (Centers for Disease Control and Prevention, 2012; Ferrer, Bisson, & French, 1995; Joint Mental Health Advisory Team 7 [J-MHAT 7] Operation Enduring Freedom, 2010; Miller, Shattuck, & Matsangas, 2010; Peterson, Goodie, Satterfield, & Brim, 2008). We and other researchers have reported higher levels of inflammation, as assessed by the concentrations of interleukin-6 (IL-6) in participants with PTSD, depression, and insomnia, with the highest levels in those with the greatest severity of these comorbidites (Gill et al., 2014b). We also reported that recovery from PTSD and depression is associated with the resolution of inflammation in a community sample (Gill, Saligan, Lee, Rotolo, & Szanton, 2013). This has led us to question if sleep restoration in military personnel with a TBI might have a positive impact on the comorbid symptoms of PTSD and depression and if inflammation is related to sleep and comorbid symptom change.

In preclinical models, long-term consequences of TBI include inflammation, which contributes to neurological deficits and disruptions in sleep (Gola et al., 2013). This upregulated inflammatory response has also been shown to be present, albeit acutely in humans who have sustained a TBI (Das, Mohapatra, & Mohapatra, 2012). Through more investigative work, these two previous findings can be validated upon to establish that once an inflammatory response has been initiated, it will lead to a continued elevation of inflammation in those who have had a severe TBI or repeated exposure to TBIs; this is associated with a poor health-related quality of life (HRQOL). Previous studies report that declines in

HRQOL last even 10 years after the injury (Jacobsson, Westerberg, & Lexell, 2010) and that sleep problems contribute to observed health declines (Andelic et al., 2009). Furthermore, the severity of symptoms including sleep disturbance following a TBI predicts future HRQOL outcomes, including PTSD, depression, and HRQOL 24 months after discharge (Williamson et al., 2013).

The search for biomarkers in a brain injury is complicated. Many investigations have focused on the identification of biomarkers specific for brain tissue or the neurovascular unit. Although this approach is promising, it has proven to be the most difficult. At present, the clinical usefulness of these biomarkers has yet to be defined, and methodological challenges are immense (Jeter et al., 2013; Papa et al., 2014; Sharma & Laskowitz, 2012; Yokobori et al., 2013). Because of the nature of the blood–brain barrier and the tightly controlled cross talk between the brain and the periphery, only in severe injuries is it expected that brain-specific markers can be found in the peripheral blood. Cerebrospinal fluid is a preferred biological fluid, but not realistic for patients with mild-to-moderate injuries. In addition, the variety of symptoms that result from TBIs leads us and other researchers to question if there may be differences in biomarkers that relate to these differing symptom presentations following TBI. Thus a more beneficial approach to the identification of clinically useful biomarkers of brain injury may be the monitoring of the peripheral immune response to injury and determining how acute changes relate to differing symptom presentations over time. It is well established that peripheral immune cells migrate to the brain after ischemia and participate in localized inflammatory reactions (Chu et al., 2014; Sallusto et al., 2012). The signals that recruit these immune cells to the brain have been elusive, but may initiate from resident brain immune cells that signal in an intricate fashion to immune cells throughout the body (Chavarria & Cardenas, 2013). The immune system is classically divided into the innate (generalized, nonspecific, inflammatory) and the adaptive (learned, antibody response). However, sharp delineations between the two are disappearing. Factors once known to only participate in innate immune functions have been shown to play a role in the adaptive immune system and vice versa. Our current understanding of C-reactive protein (CRP) is primarily limited to its inflammatory properties; however, it can signal through toll-like receptors and complement to modulate adaptive immune processes, making it an interesting biomarker for the study of the immune response to brain injury (Du Clos & Mold, 2004).

It has been well established that sleep is created by a complex system of regulatory neuronal mechanisms influenced by inflammatory biomarkers in a bidirectional manner. In patients with cancer, the administration of interferon gamma (INF-g) results in sleep disturbance (Capuron et al., 2001). In preclinical models, stressors that mimic deployment result in increased inflammation, which contributes to a vulnerability to neurological alterations (e.g., reductions in the volume and function of stress-regulating centers including the hippocampus and amygdala), as well as the onset of anxiety and depression (Abazyan et al., 2010; Powell et al., 2009; Wohleb et al., 2011). The restriction of sleep for a short period in healthy individuals results in an increase in inflammatory cytokines (Axelsson et al., 2013; Chennaoui et al., 2011). Therefore, inflammation and sleep have complex interactions that affect the health and well-being of military personnel with TBIs, and the mechanisms underlying these risks have not been fully elucidated.

Previously, we and other researchers have shown that inflammation is associated with PTSD and depression (Gill et al., 2014a; Gill, Luckenbaugh, Charney, & Vythilingam, 2010; Maes, Mihaylova, Kubera, & Ringel, 2012; Rusiecki et al., 2013). Therefore, independent of the interactive mechanism of inflammation, sleep, and mental health, it is likely that chronic inflammation is common following deployment and may be a contributing factor to the increases in medical morbidity for the 2.4 million U. S. military personnel who have been deployed since 2010 (Edwards, 2010). This line of research is essential, because many military personnel might not have yet developed the morbidity and mortality risks linked to inflammation (Boscarino, 2008; Paulus, Argo, & Egge, 2013; Phillips et al., 2009; Scherrer et al., 2010; Zen, Whooley, Zhao, & Cohen, 2012), thus providing a window of opportunity to intervene to reduce the risk.

To address this critical issue, we examined military personnel who had a history of TBI and were established to have insomnia. We examined changes in sleep following standard of care interventions that include at least one of the following: cognitive behavioral therapy (CBT), pharmacological agents, and automatically adjusting positive airway pressure (APAP) over a 3-month period. We also examine changes in symptoms of PTSD and depression, and how they relate to sleep change and inflammation measured by concentrations of CRP.

METHODS

Study Design

This study is part of a larger, ongoing study of the U.S. military personnel who presented for evaluation of sleep disturbance at the Madigan Army Medical Center and were evaluated for PTSD, depression, and HRQOL using validated clinical instruments. Sixty-six participants who completed the study at baseline and 3-month follow-up and were determined to have insomnia in accordance with the second edition of the International Classification of Sleep Disorders, were included. Active duty military personnel who were deployed to OIF/OEF within the previous 18 months were eligible for participation, and participants were excluded from the study if they were undergoing active treatment or military administrative actions related to drug or alcohol abuse or unstable psychiatric conditions (i.e., schizophrenia or bipolar disorder). All participants underwent a clinical evaluation and polysomnogram as part of a sleep medicine evaluation; these findings were previously reported (Mysliwiec et al., 2013). These assessments resulted in the following diagnoses: insomnia and comorbid obstructive sleep apnea (OSA).

Assessment of Depression, PTSD, and HRQOL

The diagnosis of depression was determined using the Quick Inventory of Depressive Symptomatology (QIDS) questionnaire. A score of 11, which indicates a moderate severity of depression, was used as the cutoff for the diagnosis (Trivedi et al., 2004). The PTSD Checklist-Military Version (PCL-M) was used to assess for PTSD (Weathers, Keane, & Davidson, 2001). We used a score of 50 or higher to determine a PTSD diagnosis because this score provides the maximum specificity (0.98) and is consistent with the Structured Clinical Interview for the *Diagnostic and Statistical Manual of Mental Disorders* (3rd ed., *DSM-III-R*; Wilkins, Lang, & Norman, 2011).

The RAND 36-Item Health Survey (RAND-36), comprising 36 items that assess 8 health concepts, was used to determine HRQOL. The subcomponents of the instrument include the following: physical functioning, role limitations caused by physical health, role limitations caused by emotional problems, social functioning, emotional well-being, energy/fatigue, pain, and general health perceptions. A high score defines a more favorable health state. The RAND-36 is the most widely used measure of HRQOL and is both valid and reliable (test–retest correlation coefficient = 0.86) in traumatized participants (MacKenzie et al., 2002).

Blood Collection and Analysis

Blood was collected in a nonfasting state into ethylenediaminetetraacetic acid (EDTA) tubes that were immediately placed on ice, processed, and frozen at –80°C. Each sample was batch assayed at the same time by a technician who was blinded to the participant group. Plasma CRP levels (pg/mL) were measured using an antibody-coated tube radioimmunoassay (R&D Systems); the interassay and intra-assay coefficients of variation were 7.8% and 8.9%, respectively, with a lower limit detection of 0.78 pg/mL for CRP.

Statistical Analysis

The participants were first dichotomized, based on change in the Pittsburgh Sleep Quality Index (PSQI) scores between baseline and follow-up visits. Scores on the PSQI, a 19-item questionnaire about sleep quality (subsections: subjective sleep quality, sleep latency, sleep duration, habitual sleep efficiency, sleep disturbances, use of sleep medications, and daytime dysfunction), ranged from 0 to 21, with a difference of 4 points indicating significant improvement in sleep quality and scores less than an improvement of 4 indicating no significant change (Buysse, Reynolds, Monk, Berman, & Kupfer, 1989). Some participants demonstrated improved sleep quality (restorative sleep) and others demonstrated no change or decline in sleep quality (no change).

We used descriptive statistics to describe demographic characteristics (age, body mass index [BMI], gender, race, military rank) and clinical variables (sleep, TBI, depression, and PTSD diagnoses) using SPSS Statistics (IBM SPSS Inc., Chicago, IL). Comparisons were made between these two groups using independent *t* tests and chi-square tests for continuous and categorical variables, respectively. Mixed between–within subjects analysis of variance (ANOVA) tests were then used to determine the effect of group differences between the restorative and no change groups on changes in symptoms of depression and PTSD and all subcomponent scores of HRQOL; a priori p values < .05 were considered significant. Linear regression models were used to determine the relationship of CRP with HRQOL changes or changes in symptoms of PTSD and depression in the TBI + restored sleep group. In this model, the mean change in HRQOL was determined by combining all of the subcomponents of the Short Form 36 (SF-36). The change in CRP was determined by calculating the mean change from baseline to follow-up.

RESULTS

Demographics and Clinical Features

The demographic and clinical characteristics of the 70 participants are described in Table 8.1. The TBI + restorative sleep group (n = 37) and the TBI + no change group (n = 33) did not differ on demographic characteristics (age, BMI, gender, and race) and diagnoses of sleep disorders, and baseline symptoms of PTSD and depression (see Table 8.1). The sample was primarily male and White and demonstrated high rates of comorbid symptoms of sleep disorders, depression, and PTSD.

Symptom Change in HRQOL, Depression, and PTSD in TBI Participants Following Sleep Therapy

The TBI + restored sleep group (n = 37) had significant reductions in PTSD and depression over the 3-month period, whereas the TBI + no change (n = 33) had

TABLE 8.1

Demographics and Clinical Characteristics in TBI+ Military Personnel with Sleep Restoration (N = 37) and No Sleep Change (N = 33) Groups

	TBI + Restorative Sleep (*N* = 37)	TBI + No Sleep Change (*N* = 33)	Significance
Mean age in years (*SD*)	33.27 (7.52)	35.97 (9.84)	$F_{1,31} = 1.68$, $p = .20$
Mean BMI (*SD*)	29.47 (4.28)	30.26 (4.00)	$F_{1,31} = .625$, $p = .43$
Gender, % (no.)			N/A
Male	97.2% (37)	97.0% (32)	
Race, % (no.)			$\chi^2 = 2.47$, $p = .78$
White	62.2% (23)	57.6% (19)	
Mixed	16.2% (6)	18.1% (6)	
All Other	21.6% (8)	24.2% (8)	
Sleep diagnoses, % (no.)			$\chi^2 = 4.67$, $p = .20$
OSA	18.9% (7)	30.3% (10)	
Insomnia	18.9% (7)	33.3% (11)	
OSA + insomnia	51.3 % (19)	30.3% (10)	
None	10.8% (4)	6.1% (2)	

Note. BMI = body mass index; no. = number; OSA = obstructive sleep apnea; *SD* = standard deviation; TBI = traumatic brain injury.

a slight increase in both PTSD and depression (see Table 8.2). The TBI + restored sleep group also had significant changes in HRQOL, including the following HRQOL subcomponents: physical functioning, role limitations in physical health, social functioning, emotional well-being, energy/fatigue, and general health perceptions.

Relationship of Inflammation to HRQOL, Depression, and PTSD in TBI Participants Following Sleep Therapy

In a linear regression model using a forced entry method, the dependent variable of change in CRP concentrations was significantly related to changes in PTSD symptoms and HRQOL in the TBI + restored sleep group, with $R^2 = 0.43$, $F_{33,3} = 8.31$, and $p < .01$. PTSD symptom change was the strongest contributor with $\beta = 0.49$, $t = 3.44$, and $p < .01$, followed by HRQOL change, $\beta = 0.41$, $t = 2.92$, and $p < .01$. Depression symptom change was not related; $p = .55$.

TABLE 8.2

TBI + Military Personnel and Changes in PTSD and Depression Symptoms in Those with Restorative Sleep and No Change Between Baseline and Follow-up

	Restorative Sleep (N = 37)		No Change (N = 33)		Time and Group:	
	Baseline (mean ± *SD*)	Follow-Up (mean ± *SD*)	Baseline (mean ± *SD*)	Follow-Up (mean ± *SD*)	F^1	*p* value
RAND-36						
Physical functioning	73.11 ± 22.00	76.11 ± 23.85	73.33 ± 22.28	66.64 ± 26.33	8.57	.005
Role limitations: physical health	52.03 ± 43.45	52.78 ± 44.23	42.58 ± 44.71	44.70 ± 41.34	0.095	.76
Role limitations: emotional problems	54.92 ± 43.94	58.33 ± 44.66	60.61 ± 43.70	49.48 ± 45.76	1.89	.17
Social functioning	58.65 ± 27.48	63.99 ± 30.74	63.82 ± 28.24	55.77 ± 28.31	10.51	.002
Emotional well-being	53.51 ± 23.90	62.78 ± 21.25	60.00 ± 19.88	56.58 ± 24.18	11.84	.001
Energy/fatigue	28.51 ± 20.85	42.64 ± 23.98	33.79 ± 17.23	30.15 ± 16.51	17.0	.00
General health perceptions	56.08 ± 20.62	59.03 ± 19.52	54.09 ± 22.59	49.70 ± 24.01	5.32	.024
QIDS	12.03 ± 4.99	8.78 ± 5.41	10.67 ± 4.94	11.30 ± 5.37	12.93	.001
PCL-M	44.57 ± 16.73	38.46 ± 17.71	41.15 ± 15.90	44.88 ± 18.10	11.21	.001

Note. PCL-M = PTSD Checklist-Military Version; PTSD = posttraumatic stress disorder; QIDS = Quick Inventory of Depressive Symptomatology; *SD* = standard deviation; TBI = traumatic brain injury.

DISCUSSION

To our knowledge, this is the first study to report that sleep restoration in TBI + military personnel with insomnia is associated with decreased symptoms of depression and PTSD, improved HRQOL, and decreased concentrations of CRP. Large population-based studies have shown an association between high concentrations of CRP and symptoms of insomnia (Grandner et al., 2013; Laugsand, Vatten, Bjorngaard, Hveem, & Janszky, 2012). CRP elevations in young adults places these individuals at a high risk for increased morbidity and mortality (Shanahan, Freeman, & Bauldry, 2014), which suggests that therapeutic interventions to mitigate this risk are essential. Therefore, our data suggest that in in TBI + military personnel, 3 months of sleep restoration results in dramatic improvements in symptoms of PTSD and depression as well as reductions in inflammation. These findings suggest that sleep restoration in TBI + military personnel provides another avenue to promote the health and well-being of deployed military personnel.

Military personnel who sustain a TBI during deployment are at higher risk for developing chronic medical conditions. Previous reports link both blast and blunt force TBIs during deployment to higher rates of moderate-to-severe overall health disability, which relate to the severity of PTSD (Mac Donald et al., 2014). In this study, we found significant reductions in PTSD that related to HRQOL improvements and changes in inflammation in TBI + military personnel. In a recent Institute of Medicine report, increased intake of antioxidant food products has been advised as there is evidence that reduction of inflammation is therapeutic for the chronic symptoms of TBI (Institute of Medicine, 2013). While acute TBIs have been linked to higher concentrations of inflammation, less is known regarding chronic inflammation following TBI. We have consistently linked PTSD to inflammation, and HRQOL declines, providing the foundation to understand the links between chronic symptoms following trauma. Here, we extend these findings, by showing that decreased inflammation relates to improved HRQOL, in military personnel with TBI and insomnia, and to decreased symptoms of PTSD. Inflammation is likely a shared common mechanism related to symptoms associated with TBI, including insomnia, PTSD, and depression. It is interesting to consider whether the adaptive immune response to acute inflammation in these conditions has an effect on long-term symptoms. These relationships are essential to the understanding of TBI + military personnel who have high rates of comorbidities.

Although this is the first report of changes in inflammation following sleep restoration in TBI + military personnel, our findings are supported by previous studies that link sleep disturbance to inflammation. Specifically, measures of inflammation have been found to increase in healthy adults experiencing even brief periods of sleep deprivation (Axelsson et al., 2013; Chennaoui et al., 2011). Treating sleep disturbance may reduce CRP, which would, in turn, decrease morbidity and mortality in TBI + military personnel. Because of the stigma associated with PTSD, recent studies report that military personnel are more likely to seek treatment for sleep disturbance, one of the many symptoms of PTSD, rather than for PTSD (Fear, Seddon, Jones, Greenberg, & Wessely, 2012). With 2.5 million service members deployed since 2001, there are major ramifications for our findings about the reduction of CRP concentrations and sleep deprivation. Our key finding that sleep restoration can reduce inflammation and increase health and well-being suggests that there is a window of opportunity to provide interventions to mitigate the risks for morbidity and mortality by treating sleep disturbance and inflammation.

Increased concentrations of CRP have been consistently linked to morbidity and health mortality. Previous studies illustrate how inflammation plays a pivotal role in the development of morbidity and mortality in aging veterans with PTSD, placing them at twice the risk of developing cardiovascular disease, diabetes, hypertension, arthritis, and chronic pain, among others (Boscarino, Forsberg, & Goldberg, 2010; Boyko et al., 2010; Xue et al., 2012). It is estimated that the cost of medical care and diminished productivity in our military personnel as they age will be more than $4 trillion, with those with TBIs incurring the highest costs (Edwards, 2010). Therefore, efforts to reduce morbidity are crucial. Recently deployed military personnel with TBIs are still relatively young and do not yet display traditional morbidity or mortality risks. Thus, early intervention and treatment in TBI + military personnel with high combat exposure have already led to fewer reported symptoms of PTSD, depression, and sleep disturbance, providing further evidence that treating these personnel while they are relatively young is critical (Adler, Bliese, McGurk, Hoge, & Castro, 2009).

Second, we report that symptoms of depression are significantly reduced in the TBI + restorative sleep group, but that symptom change in depression is not related to CRP reductions. Increased CRP has been reported to be associated with depression in large studies (Chocano-Bedoya et al., 2014; Lopresti, Maker, Hood, & Drummond, 2014) and in older men with both sleep disturbance and depression (Smagula et al., 2014). In a large population-based study, patients with the highest CRP concentrations were at the highest risk for hospitalization for depression (Wium-Andersen, Orsted, Nielsen, & Nordestgaard, 2013). Previous studies that evaluated the impact of pharmacological agents used to treat depression report contradictory findings regarding CRP changes (Bot et al., 2011; Hamer, Batty, Marmot, Singh-Manoux, & Kivimaki, 2011; Pizzi et al., 2009), suggesting that changes in depression may not be strongly related to changes in CRP. No current study has examined the role of inflammation in depression following TBI, so it is not clear how CRP and other inflammatory markers relate to depression in TBI + military personnel. Therefore, our finding that treatment of sleep disturbance, with standard-of-care treatments of CBT, medication, or APAP, reduced depressive and also PTSD symptoms have substantial implications for improving the life and well-being of TBI + military personnel with insomnia who have high rates of comorbidity.

In this study, we also found that PTSD symptoms were significantly reduced in TBI+ military personnel with insomnia who reported restorative sleep. This finding supports recent data that combat-related PTSD in males is associated with higher levels of proinflammatory cytokines, even after accounting for depression and early-life trauma, suggesting that immune activation may be a core element of PTSD pathophysiology (Lindqvist et al., 2014). We expand on this finding by including an examination of the role of TBI and insomnia. We have reported that PTSD is associated with higher concentrations of IL-6 in those with comorbid depression in samples of civilians (Gill et al., 2010; Gill et al., 2013). This relationship is important to explore further because studies in veterans link health declines with increases in symptoms of PTSD (Aversa et al., 2012; Boscarino, 2008; Gill et al., 2013; Phillips et al., 2009) and a behavioral sleep intervention can improve sleep and reduce PTSD symptoms in military personnel (Germain et al., 2012). Thus, further studies are required in a larger sample of military personnel to investigate the potential impact of sleep treatment on these co-occurring disorders following deployment. In support of this, sleep disturbance following deployment has been shown to mediate one-third of the risk for PTSD or depression onset (Macera, Aralis, Rauh, & MacGregor, 2013).

There is a stigma attached to PTSD among military personnel, and therefore fewer active duty military personnel and veterans seek treatment for this disorder (Greene-Shortridge, Britt, & Castro, 2007). However, in military personnel with PTSD, pursuing treatment for sleep dysfunction is more likely as there is less stigma associated with insomnia (Fear et al., 2012). Findings suggest that PTSD symptoms are improved by first enlisting treatments focused on relieving sleep deprivation (Germain et al., 2012). By primarily treating insomnia, military personnel bypass the stigma while still reducing the symptoms of PTSD, depression, and other psychological symptoms. Finally, the high comorbidity of PTSD, depression, and insomnia in TBI + military personnel strongly suggests that comprehensive, multidisciplinary interventions are required to address this critical issue.

Limitations of this study include a small sample of participants from one military treatment facility who were only followed over a 3-month period. In addition, PTSD and depression were evaluated with validated questionnaires, which do not necessarily represent clinical diagnoses. We could not distinguish the potentially different impacts of CBT, medication, or APAP on comorbid symptoms and inflammation in our sample. Furthermore, we only included CRP as a marker of inflammation, which might not reflect the complete inflammatory milieu/spectrum in TBI + military personnel with mental health disorders. Nonetheless, our findings provide initial evidence that restorative sleep in TBI + military personnel is associated with reductions in CRP, a biological marker of inflammation and predictor of morbidity and mortality, decreases in symptoms of PTSD and depression, and improvements in health quality, warranting future studies to determine clinical interventions and functional mechanisms.

DISCLAIMER

The opinions and assertions in this chapter are those of the authors and do not necessarily represent those of the Department of the Army, Department of Defense, the U.S. Government, or the Center for Neuroscience and Regenerative Medicine.

ACKNOWLEDGMENTS

This study was funded, in part, by the Center for Neuroscience and Regenerative Medicine (Grant 60855). Taura Barr is a 2012 Robert Wood Johnson Foundation Nurse Faculty Scholar ID: 70319. Jessica Gill is an intramural researcher at the National Institute of Nursing Research, National Institutes of Health, and is supported by intramural funding.

No author has any conflicts of interest to disclose.

REFERENCES

Abazyan, B., Nomura, J., Kannan, G., Ishizuka, K., Tamashiro, K. L., Nucifora, F., et al. (2010). Prenatal interaction of mutant DISC1 and immune activation produces adult psychopathology. *Biological Psychiatry, 68*(12), 1172–1181. http://dx.doi.org/10.1016/j.biopsych.2010.09.022

Adler, A. B., Bliese, P. D., McGurk, D., Hoge, C. W., & Castro, C. A. (2009). Battlemind debriefing and battlemind training as early interventions with soldiers returning from iraq: Randomization by platoon. *Journal Consulting Clinical Psychology, 77*(5), 928–940. http://dx.doi.org/10.1037/a0016877

Andelic, N., Hammergren, N., Bautz-Holter, E., Sveen, U., Brunborg, C., & Roe, C. (2009). Functional outcome and health-related quality of life 10 years after moderate-to-severe traumatic brain injury. *Acta Neurologica Scandinavica, 120*(1), 16–23. http://dx.doi.org/10.1111/j.1600-0404.2008.01116.x

Aversa, L. H., Stoddard, J. A., Doran, N. M., Au, S., Chow, B., McFall, M., et al. (2012). Longitudinal analysis of the relationship between PTSD symptom clusters, cigarette use, and physical health-related quality of life. *Quality of Life Research, 22*(6), 1381–1389. http://dx.doi.org/10.1007/s11136-012-0280-x

Axelsson, J., Rehman, J. U., Akerstedt, T., Ekman, R., Miller, G. E., Hoglund, C. O., & Lekander, M. (2013). Effects of sustained sleep restriction on mitogen-stimulated cytokines, chemokines and T helper 1/ T helper 2 balance in humans. *PLoS One, 8*(12), e82291. http://dx.doi.org/10.1371/journal.pone.0082291

Boscarino, J. A. (2008). A prospective study of PTSD and early-age heart disease mortality among Vietnam veterans: Implications for surveillance and prevention. *Psychosomatic Medicine, 70*(6), 668–676. http://dx.doi.org/10.1097/PSY.0b013e31817bccaf

Boscarino, J. A., Forsberg, C. W., & Goldberg, J. (2010). A twin study of the association between PTSD symptoms and rheumatoid arthritis. *Psychosomatic Medicine, 72*(5), 481–486. http://dx.doi.org/10.1097/PSY.0b013e3181d9a80c

Bot, M., Carney, R. M., Freedland, K. E., Rubin, E. H., Rich, M. W., Steinmeyer, B. C., et al. (2011). Inflammation and treatment response to sertraline in patients with coronary heart disease and comorbid major depression. *Journal of Psychosomatic Research, 71*(1), 13–17. http://dx.doi.org/10.1016/j.jpsychores.2010.11.006

Boyko, E. J., Jacobson, I. G., Smith, B., Ryan, M. A., Hooper, T. I., Amoroso, P. J., et al. (2010). Risk of diabetes in U.S. military service members in relation to combat deployment and mental health. *Diabetes Care, 33*(8), 1771–1777. http://dx.doi.org/10.2337/dc10-0296

Buysse, D. J., Reynolds, C. F., III, Monk, T. H., Berman, S. R., & Kupfer, D. J. (1989). The Pittsburgh sleep quality index: A new instrument for psychiatric practice and research. *Psychiatry Research, 28*(2), 193–213.

Capaldi, V. F., II, Guerrero, M. L., & Killgore, W. D. (2011). Sleep disruptions among returning combat veterans from Iraq and Afghanistan. *Military Medicine, 176*(8), 879–888.

Capuron, L., Ravaud, A., Gualde, N., Bosmans, E., Dantzer, R., Maes, M., et al. (2001). Association between immune activation and early depressive symptoms in cancer patients treated with interleukin-2-based therapy. *Psychoneuroendocrinology, 26*(8), 797–808.

Centers for Disease Control and Prevention. (2012). *Morbidity and mortality monthly report: Great American smokeout, 61*(44), 889–908.

Chavarria, A., & Cardenas, G. (2013). Neuronal influence behind the central nervous system regulation of the immune cells. *Frontiers in Integrative Neuroscience, 7*, 64. http://dx.doi.org/10.3389/fnint.2013.00064

Chennaoui, M., Sauvet, F., Drogou, C., Van Beers, P., Langrume, C., Guillard, M., et al. (2011). Effect of one night of sleep loss on changes in tumor necrosis factor alpha (TNF-alpha) levels in healthy men. *Cytokine, 56*(2), 318–324. http://dx.doi.org/10.1016/j.cyto.2011.06.002

Chocano-Bedoya, P. O., Mirzaei, F., O'Reilly, E. J., Lucas, M., Okereke, O. I., Hu, F. B., et al. (2014). C-reactive protein, interleukin-6, soluble tumor necrosis factor alpha receptor 2 and incident clinical depression. *Journal of Affective Disorders, 163*, 25–32. http://dx.doi.org/10.1016/j.jad.2014.03.023

Chu, H. X., Kim, H. A., Lee, S., Moore, J. P., Chan, C. T., Vinh, A., et al. (2014). Immune cell infiltration in malignant middle cerebral artery infarction: Comparison with transient cerebral ischemia. *Journal of Cerebral Blood Flow & Metabolism, 34*(3), 450–459. http://dx.doi.org/10.1038/jcbfm.2013.217

Das, M., Mohapatra, S., & Mohapatra, S. S. (2012). New perspectives on central and peripheral immune responses to acute traumatic brain injury. *Journal of Neuroinflammation, 9*, 236. http://dx.doi.org/10.1186/1742-2094-9-236

DePalma, R. G., Burris, D. G., Champion, H. R., & Hodgson, M. J. (2005). Blast injuries. *The New England Journal of Medicine, 352*(13), 1335–1342. http://dx.doi.org/10.1056/NEJMra042083

Du Clos, T. W., & Mold, C. (2004). C-reactive protein: An activator of innate immunity and a modulator of adaptive immunity. *Immunologic Research, 30*(3), 261–277. http://dx.doi.org/10.1385/ir:30:3:261

Edwards, R. D. (2010). *A review of war costs in Iraq and Afghanistan* (Working Paper Series. 38). Cambridge, MA: National Bureau of Economic Research.

Fear, N. T., Seddon, R., Jones, N., Greenberg, N., & Wessely, S. (2012). Does anonymity increase the reporting of mental health symptoms? *BMC Public Health, 12*, 797. http://dx.doi.org/10.1186/1471-2458-12-797

Ferrer, C. F., Jr., Bisson, R. U., & French, J. (1995). Circadian rhythm desynchronosis in military deployments: A review of current strategies. *Aviation Space and Environmental Medicine, 66*(6), 571–578.

Fisher, H. (2010). *US military casualty statistics: Operation New Dawn, Operation Iraqi Freedom, and Operation Enduring Freedom. CRS report for Congress*. Washington, DC: Congressional Research Service.

Germain, A., Richardson, R., Moul, D. E., Mammen, O., Haas, G., Forman, S. D., et al. (2012). Placebo-controlled comparison of prazosin and cognitive-behavioral treatments for sleep disturbances in US Military Veterans. *Journal of Psychosomatic Research, 72*(2), 89–96. http://dx.doi.org/10.1016/j.jpsychores.2011.11.010

Gill, J., Lee, H., Barr, T., Baxter, T., Heinzelmann, M., Rak, H., et al. (2014a). Lower health related quality of life in U.S. military personnel is associated with service-related disorders and inflammation. *Psychiatry Research, 216*(1), 116–122. http://dx.doi.org/10.1016/j.psychres.2014.01.046

Gill, J., Lee, H., Barr, T., Baxter, T., Heinzelmann, M., Rak, H., et al. (2014b). Lower health related quality of life in U.S. military personnel is associated with service-related disorders and inflammation. *Psychiatry Research, 216*(1), 116–122. http://dx.doi.org/10.1016/j.psychres.2014.01.046

Gill, J., Luckenbaugh, D., Charney, D., & Vythilingam, M. (2010). Sustained elevation of serum interleukin-6 and relative insensitivity to hydrocortisone differentiates posttraumatic stress disorder with and without depression. *Biological Psychiatry, 68*(11), 999–1006. http://dx.doi.org/10.1016/j.biopsych.2010.07.033

Gill, J. M., Saligan, L., Lee, H., Rotolo, S., & Szanton, S. (2013). Women in recovery from PTSD have similar inflammation and quality of life as non-traumatized controls. *Journal of Psychosomatic Research, 74*(4), 301–306. http://dx.doi.org/10.1016/j.jpsychores.2012.10.013

Gola, H., Engler, H., Sommershof, A., Adenauer, H., Kolassa, S., Schedlowski, M., et al. (2013). Posttraumatic stress disorder is associated with an enhanced spontaneous production of pro-inflammatory cytokines by peripheral blood mononuclear cells. *BMC Psychiatry, 13*, 40. http://dx.doi.org/10.1186/1471-244x-13-40

Grandner, M. A., Buxton, O. M., Jackson, N., Sands-Lincoln, M., Pandey, A., & Jean-Louis, G. (2013). Extreme sleep durations and increased C-reactive protein: Effects of sex and ethnoracial group. *Sleep, 36*(5), 769–779E. http://dx.doi.org/10.5665/sleep.2646

Greene-Shortridge, T. M., Britt, T. W., & Castro, C. A. (2007). The stigma of mental health problems in the military. *Military Medicine, 172*(2), 157–161.

Hamer, M., Batty, G. D., Marmot, M. G., Singh-Manoux, A., & Kivimaki, M. (2011). Anti-depressant medication use and C-reactive protein: Results from two population-based studies. *Brain Behavior and Immunity, 25*(1), 168–173. http://dx.doi.org/10.1016/j.bbi.2010.09.013

Insomnia, active component, U.S. Armed Forces, January 2000-December 2009. (2010). *MSMR, 17*(5), 12–15.

Institute of Medicine. (2013). *Panel on Dietary Antioxidants and Related Compounds*. Retrieved from http://www.iom.edu/Activities/Nutrition/AntioxidantsPanel.aspx

Jacobsson, L. J., Westerberg, M., & Lexell, J. (2010). Health-related quality-of-life and life satisfaction 6-15 years after traumatic brain injuries in northern Sweden. *Brain Injury, 24*(9), 1075–1086. http://dx.doi.org/10.3109/02699052.2010.494590

Jeter, C. B., Hergenroeder, G. W., Hylin, M. J., Redell, J. B., Moore, A. N., & Dash, P. K. (2013). Biomarkers for the diagnosis and prognosis of mild traumatic brain injury/concussion. *Journal of Neurotrauma, 30*(8), 657–670. http://dx.doi.org/10.1089/neu.2012.2439

Joint Mental Health Advisory Team 7 (J-MHAT 7) Operation Enduring Freedom. (2010). *Office of the Surgeon General United States Army Medical Command, Office of the Command Surgeon HQ, USCENTCOM and Office of the Command Surgeon US Forces Afghanistan USFOR-A*. Retrieved from http://www.armymedicine.army.mil

Kou, Z., & Vandevord, P. J. (2014). Traumatic white matter injury and glial activation: From basic science to clinics. *Glia, 62*(11), 1831–1855. http://dx.doi.org/10.1002/glia.22690

Laugsand, L. E., Vatten, L. J., Bjorngaard, J. H., Hveem, K., & Janszky, I. (2012). Insomnia and high-sensitivity C-reactive protein: The HUNT study, Norway. *Psychosomatic Medicine, 74*(5), 543–553. http://dx.doi.org/10.1097/PSY.0b013e31825904eb

Lindqvist, D., Wolkowitz, O. M., Mellon, S., Yehuda, R., Flory, J. D., Henn-Haase, C., et al. (2014). Proinflammatory milieu in combat-related PTSD is independent of depression and early life stress. *Brain Behavior and Immunity, 42*, 81–88. http://dx.doi.org/10.1016/j.bbi.2014.06.003

Lopresti, A. L., Maker, G. L., Hood, S. D., & Drummond, P. D. (2014). A review of peripheral biomarkers in major depression: The potential of inflammatory and oxidative stress biomarkers. *Progress in Neuro-Psychopharmacology and Biological Psychiatry, 48*, 102–111. http://dx.doi.org/10.1016/j.pnpbp.2013.09.017

Mac Donald, C. L., Johnson, A. M., Wierzechowski, L., Kassner, E., Stewart, T., Nelson, E. C., et al. (2014). Prospectively assessed clinical outcomes in concussive blast vs nonblast traumatic brain injury among evacuated US military personnel. *JAMA Neurology, 71*(8), 994. http://dx.doi.org/10.1001/jamaneurol.2014.1114

Macera, C. A., Aralis, H. J., Rauh, M. J., & MacGregor, A. J. (2013). Do sleep problems mediate the relationship between traumatic brain injury and development of mental health symptoms after deployment? *Sleep, 36*(1), 83–90. http://dx.doi.org/10.5665/sleep.2306

MacKenzie, E. J., Sacco, W. J., Luchter, S., Ditunno, J. F., Staz, C. F., Gruen, G. S., et al. (2002). Validating the functional capacity index as a measure of outcome following blunt multiple trauma. *Quality of Life Research, 11*(8), 797–808.

Maes, M., Mihaylova, I., Kubera, M., & Ringel, K. (2012). Activation of cell-mediated immunity in depression: Association with inflammation, melancholia, clinical staging and the fatigue and somatic symptom cluster of depression. *Progress in Neuro-Psychopharmacology and Biological Psychiatry, 36*(1), 169–175. http://dx.doi.org/10.1016/j.pnpbp.2011.09.006

Miller, N. L., Shattuck, L. G., & Matsangas, P. (2010). Longitudinal study of sleep patterns of United States Military Academy cadets. *Sleep, 33*(12), 1623–1631.

Mysliwiec, V., Gill, J., Lee, H., Baxter, T., Pierce, R., Barr, T. L., et al. (2013). Sleep disorders in U.S. military personnel: A high rate of comorbid insomnia and obstructive sleep apnea. *Chest, 144*(2), 549–557. http://dx.doi.org/10.1378/chest.13-0088

Owens, B. D., Kragh, J. F., Jr., Wenke, J. C., Macaitis, J., Wade, C. E., & Holcomb, J. B. (2008). Combat wounds in operation Iraqi freedom and operation enduring freedom. *The Journal of Trauma Injury, Infection, and Critical Care, 64*(2), 295–299.

Papa, L., Robertson, C. S., Wang, K. K., Brophy, G. M., Hannay, H. J., Heaton, S., et al. (2014). Biomarkers improve clinical outcome predictors of mortality following non-penetrating severe traumatic brain injury. *Neurocritical Care*. http://dx.doi.org/10.1007/s12028-014-0028-2

Paulus, E. J., Argo, T. R., & Egge, J. A. (2013). The impact of posttraumatic stress disorder on blood pressure and heart rate in a veteran population. *Journal of Traumatic Stress, 26*(1), 169–172. http://dx.doi.org/10.1002/jts.21785

Peterson, A. L., Goodie, J. L., Satterfield, W. A., & Brim, W. L. (2008). Sleep disturbance during military deployment. *Military Medicine, 173*(3), 230–235.

Phillips, A. C., Batty, G. D., Gale, C. R., Deary, I. J., Osborn, D., MacIntyre, K., et al. (2009). Generalized anxiety disorder, major depressive disorder, and their comorbidity as predictors of all-cause and cardiovascular mortality: The Vietnam experience study. *Psychosomatic Medicine, 71*(4), 395–403. http://dx.doi.org/10.1097/PSY.0b013e31819e6706

Pizzi, C., Mancini, S., Angeloni, L., Fontana, F., Manzoli, L., & Costa, G. M. (2009). Effects of selective serotonin reuptake inhibitor therapy on endothelial function and inflammatory markers in patients with coronary heart disease. *Clinical Pharmacology & Therapeutics, 86*(5), 527–532. http://dx.doi.org/10.1038/clpt.2009.121

Powell, N. D., Bailey, M. T., Mays, J. W., Stiner-Jones, L. M., Hanke, M. L., Padgett, D. A., et al. (2009). Repeated social defeat activates dendritic cells and enhances Toll-like receptor dependent cytokine secretion. *Brain Behavior and Immunity, 23*(2), 225–231. http://dx.doi.org/10.1016/j.bbi.2008.09.010

Pugh, M. J., Finley, E. P., Copeland, L. A., Wang, C. P., Noel, P. H., Amuan, M. E., et al. (2014). Complex comorbidity clusters in OEF/OIF veterans: The polytrauma clinical triad and beyond. *Medical Care, 52*(2), 172–181. http://dx.doi.org/10.1097/mlr.0000000000000059

Rusiecki, J. A., Byrne, C., Galdzicki, Z., Srikantan, V., Chen, L., Poulin, M., et al. (2013). PTSD and DNA methylation in select immune function gene promoter regions: A repeated measures case-control study of U.S. military service members. *Frontiers in Psychiatry, 4*, 56. http://dx.doi.org/10.3389/fpsyt.2013.00056

Sallusto, F., Impellizzieri, D., Basso, C., Laroni, A., Uccelli, A., Lanzavecchia, A., & Engelhardt, B. (2012). T-cell trafficking in the central nervous system. *Immunological Reviews, 248*(1), 216–227. http://dx.doi.org/10.1111/j.1600-065X.2012.01140.x

Scherrer, J. F., Chrusciel, T., Zeringue, A., Garfield, L. D., Hauptman, P. J., Lustman, P. J., et al. (2010). Anxiety disorders increase risk for incident myocardial infarction in depressed and nondepressed Veterans Administration patients. *American Heart Journal, 159*(5), 772–779. http://dx.doi.org/10.1016/j.ahj.2010.02.033

Seelig, A. D., Jacobson, I. G., Smith, B., Hooper, T. I., Boyko, E. J., Gackstetter, G. D., et al. (2010). Sleep patterns before, during, and after deployment to Iraq and Afghanistan. *Sleep, 33*(12), 1615–1622.

Shanahan, L., Freeman, J., & Bauldry, S. (2014). Is very high C-reactive protein in young adults associated with indicators of chronic disease risk? *Psychoneuroendocrinology, 40*, 76–85. http://dx.doi.org/10.1016/j.psyneuen.2013.10.019

Sharma, R., & Laskowitz, D. T. (2012). Biomarkers in traumatic brain injury. *Current Neurology and Neuroscience Reports, 12*(5), 560–569. http://dx.doi.org/10.1007/s11910-012-0301-8

Smagula, S. F., Ancoli-Israel, S., Barrett-Connor, E., Lane, N. E., Redline, S., Stone, K. L., et al. (2014). Inflammation, sleep disturbances, and depressed mood among community dwelling older men. *Journal of Psychosomatic Research, 76*(5), 368–373. http://dx.doi.org/10.1016/j.jpsychores.2014.02.005

Trivedi, M. H., Rush, A. J., Ibrahim, H. M., Carmody, T. J., Biggs, M. M., Suppes, T., et al. (2004). The Inventory of Depressive Symptomatology, Clinician Rating (IDS-C) and Self-Report (IDS-SR), and the Quick Inventory of Depressive Symptomatology, Clinician Rating (QIDS-C) and Self-Report (QIDS-SR) in public sector patients with mood disorders: A psychometric evaluation. *Psychological Medicine, 34*(1), 73–82.

Tsai, J. C. (2010). Neurological and neurobehavioral sequelae of obstructive sleep apnea. *NeuroRehabilitation, 26*(1), 85–94. http://dx.doi.org/10.3233/nre-2010-0538

Warden, D. L., French, L. M., Shupenko, L., Fargus, J., Riedy, G., Erickson, M. E., et al. (2009). Case report of a soldier with primary blast brain injury. *Neuroimage, 47*(Suppl 2), T152–153. http://dx.doi.org/10.1016/j.neuroimage.2009.01.060

Weathers, F. W., Keane, T. M., & Davidson, J. R. (2001). Clinician-administered PTSD scale: A review of the first ten years of research. *Depress Anxiety, 13*(3), 132–156.

Wilkins, K. C., Lang, A. J., & Norman, S. B. (2011). Synthesis of the psychometric properties of the PTSD checklist (PCL) military, civilian, and specific versions. *Depress Anxiety, 28*(7), 596–606. http://dx.doi.org/10.1002/da.20837

Williamson, M. L., Elliott, T. R., Berry, J. W., Underhill, A. T., Stavrinos, D., & Fine, P. R. (2013). Predictors of health-related quality-of-life following traumatic brain injury. *Brain Injury, 27*(9), 992–999. http://dx.doi.org/10.3109/02699052.2013.801512

Wium-Andersen, M. K., Orsted, D. D., Nielsen, S. F., & Nordestgaard, B. G. (2013). Elevated C-reactive protein levels, psychological distress, and depression in 73, 131 individuals. *JAMA Psychiatry, 70*(2), 176–184. http://dx.doi.org/10.1001/2013.jamapsychiatry.102

Wohleb, E. S., Hanke, M. L., Corona, A. W., Powell, N. D., Stiner, L. M., Bailey, M. T., et al. (2011). beta-Adrenergic receptor antagonism prevents anxiety-like behavior and microglial reactivity induced by repeated social defeat. *The Journal of Neuroscience, 31*(17), 6277–6288. http://dx.doi.org/10.1523/JNEUROSCI.0450-11.2011

Xue, Y., Taub, P. R., Iqbal, N., Fard, A., Wentworth, B., Redwine, L., et al. (2012). Cardiac biomarkers, mortality, and post-traumatic stress disorder in military veterans. *The American Journal of Cardiology, 109*(8), 1215–1218. http://dx.doi.org/10.1016/j.amjcard.2011.11.063

Yokobori, S., Hosein, K., Burks, S., Sharma, I., Gajavelli, S., & Bullock, R. (2013). Biomarkers for the clinical differential diagnosis in traumatic brain injury--a systematic review. *CNS Neuroscience & Therapeutics, 19*(8), 556–565. http://dx.doi.org/10.1111/cns.12127

Zen, A. L., Whooley, M. A., Zhao, S., & Cohen, B. E. (2012). Post-traumatic stress disorder is associated with poor health behaviors: Findings from the heart and soul study. *Health Psychology, 31*(2), 194–201. http://dx.doi.org/10.1037/a0025989

Index

NOTE: Page references followed by *f* and *t* denote figures and tables, respectively.